Late effects of childhood cancer

Late effects of childhood cancer

Edited by

W Hamish B Wallace MD FRCPCH
Consultant Paediatric Oncologist, Department of
Child Life and Health, Developmental and
Reproductive Sciences, University of Edinburgh; and
Department of Haematology/Oncology, Royal Hospital for
Sick Children, Edinburgh

and

Daniel M Green MD
Pediatric Oncologist, Department of Pediatrics, Roswell
Park Cancer Institute, Buffalo, New York; and
Professor of Pediatrics, Department of Pediatrics,
School of Medicine and Biomedical Sciences,
State University of New York, Buffalo, New York

ARNOLD

A member of the Hodder Headline Group

LONDON

First published in Great Britain in 2004 by
Arnold, a member of the Hodder Headline Group,
338 Euston Road, London NW1 3BH

http://www.arnoldpublishers.com

Distributed in the United States of America by
Oxford University Press Inc.,
198 Madison Avenue, New York, NY10016
Oxford is a registered trademark of Oxford University Press

Whilst the advice and information in this book are believed to be
true and accurate at the date of going to press, neither the authors
nor the publisher can accept any legal responsibility or liability for any
errors or omissions that may be made. In particular (but without
limiting the generality of the preceding disclaimer) every effort has
been made to check drug dosages; however, it is still possible that
errors have been missed. Furthermore, dosage schedules are
constantly being revised and new side-effects recognized. For
these reasons the reader is strongly urged to consult the drug
companies' printed instructions before administering any of the
drugs recommended in this book.

British Library Cataloguing in Publication Data
A catalogue record for this book is available from the British Library

Library of Congress Cataloging-in-Publication Data
A catalog record for this book is available from the Library of Congress

ISBN 0 340 80803 9

1 2 3 4 5 6 7 8 9 10

Commissioning Editor: Joanna Koster
Development Editor: Sarah Burrows
Project Editor: Wendy Rooke
Production Controller: Deborah Smith
Cover Design: Lee-May Lim

Typeset in 10/12 pt Minion by Charon Tec Pvt. Ltd, Chennai, India
Printed in the UK by Butler & Tanner Ltd.

What do you think about this book? Or any other Arnold title?
Please send your comments to feedback.arnold@hodder.co.uk

Contents

Contributors

David Abramson MD
Director, Robert M Ellsworth Ophthalmic Oncology Center, Consultant, Memorial Sloan Kettering Cancer Institute, Weill Cornell Medical College, New York-Presbyterian Hospital, New York, NY, USA

Katherine Beaverson MS
Weill Cornell Medical College, New York-Presbyterian Hospital, Department of Ophthalmology, New York, NY, USA

E Claire Benton FRCP(Edin)
Consultant Dermatologist, Royal Infirmary of Edinburgh, Edinburgh, UK

Smita Bhatia MD MPH
Director, Epidemiology and Outcomes Research, Division of Pediatric Hematology, Oncology and Bone Marrow Transplantation, City of Hope National Medical Center, Duarte, CA, USA

Bernadette MD Brennan MD FRCPCH
Consultant Paediatric Oncologist, Royal Manchester Children's Hospital, Pendlebury, Manchester, UK

Ernest U Conrad III MD FACS
Director, Pediatric Bone Tumor Clinic, Children's Hospital and Regional Medical Center, University of Washington, Department of Orthopaedics and Sports Medicine, Seattle, Washington, USA

Hilary OD Critchley MD FRCOG
Professor of Reproductive Medicine, Reproductive and Developmental Sciences, Centre for Reproductive Biology, University of Edinburgh, Edinburgh, UK

Patricia M Crofton
Department of Paediatric Biochemistry, Royal Hospital for Sick Children, Edinburgh, UK

Ken H Darzy
Lecturer in Medicine, Department of Endocrinology, Diabetes and Metabolic Medicine, Queen Mary and Westfield College, University of London, London, UK

Sampada S Deshpande BS
Division of Pediatric Cardiology, Golisano Children's Hospital at Strong and University of Rochester Medical Center, Rochester, New York

Manuel Diezi MD
Division of Hematology and Oncology, Hospital for Sick Children, Toronto, Ontario, Canada

Patricia K Duffner MD
Professor of Neurology and Pediatrics, State University of New York at Buffalo, School of Medicine and Biomedical Sciences, Children's Hospital of Buffalo, Buffalo, New York, USA

Sarah A Duffy MS
Division of Pediatric Cardiology, Golisano Children's Hospital at Strong and University of Rochester Medical Center, Rochester, New York

Christine Eiser PhD
Professor of Psychology, University of Sheffield, Sheffield, UK

Carol A French MPH
Division of Pediatric Cardiology, Golisano Children's Hospital at Strong and University of Rochester Medical Center, Rochester, New York; and Department of Pediatrics, University of Rochester School of Medicine and Dentistry, Rochester, New York

Helena K Gleeson
Clinical Research Fellow, Department of Endocrinology, Christie Hospital, Withington, Manchester, UK

Daniel M Green MD
Department of Pediatrics, Roswell Park Cancer Institute, Buffalo, New York; and Professor, Department of Pediatrics, School of Medicine and Biomedical Sciences, University at Buffalo, State University of New York, Buffalo, New York, USA

John W Gregory MD FRCP FRCPCH DCH MB ChB
Reader in Pediatric Endocrinology, Department of Child Health, University of Wales College of Medicine, Cardiff, UK

Andrea S Hinkle MD
Division of Hematology/Oncology, Golisano Children's Hospital at Strong and University of Rochester Medical Center, Rochester, New York; and

Department of Pediatrics, University of
Rochester School of Medicine and Dentistry, Rochester,
New York

Melissa M Hudson MD
Director, After Completion of Therapy Clinic,
St Jude Children's Research Hospital, Pediatric
Hematology/Oncology, Memphis, Tennessee, USA

Christopher JH Kelnar MD FRCP FRCPCH
Section of Child Life and Health, Department of
Reproductive & Developmental Sciences,
University of Edinburgh, UK

Amy M Kozlowski BS
Division of Pediatric Cardiology, Golisano Children's
Hospital at Strong and University of Rochester Medical
Center, Rochester, New York

Alison D Leiper MB BS FRCP DCH
Associate Specialist in Paediatric Oncology,
Department of Haematology and Oncology,
Great Ormond Street Hospital for Children,
London, UK

Gill A Levitt BSc MBBS MRCP FRCPCH
Consultant in Oncology and Late Effects,
Great Ormond Street Hospital for Sick Children NHS
Trust, London, UK

Steven E Lipshultz MD
Division of Pediatric Cardiology, Golisano Children's
Hospital at Strong and University of Rochester Medical
Center, Rochester, New York; and
Department of Pediatrics, University of Rochester School
of Medicine and Dentistry, Rochester, New York

David Malkin MD FRCR
Research Scientist, National Cancer Institute/Canadian
Cancer Society; and Division of Hematology and
Oncology, Hospital for Sick Children, Toronto, Ontario,
Canada

Neyssa Marina MD
Professor of Pediatrics, Division of Hematology-Oncology,
Stanford University School of Medicine, Stanford,
CA, USA

Alexander McCall Smith LLB PhD FRSE
Professor of Medical Law, University of Edinburgh,
Edinburgh, UK

Nigel Meadows MD FRCP FRCPCH
Consultant Paediatric Gastroenetrologist, The Royal
London Hospital; and Honorary Senior Lecturer,
The Academic Department of Gastroenetrology,
Queen Mary College Westfield, University of London

Grace-Ann P Monaco JD
Director, Medical Care Ombudsman Program of the
Medical Care Management Corporation, Bethesda,
MD, USA

Hannah Morgan MD
Department of Orthopaedics and Sports Medicine,
University of Washington, Seattle, Washington, USA

Raymond K Mulhern PhD
Division of Behavioral Medicine, St Jude Children's
Research Hospital, Memphis, Tennessee, USA

Michael Ober MD
Weill Cornell Medical College, New York-Presbyterian
Hospital, Department of Ophthalmology, New York, NY, USA

Kevin C Oeffinger MD
Professor of Family Practice and Padiatrics,
The University of Texas Southwestern Medical Center at
Dallas, Department of Family Practice and Community
Medicine, Dallas, TX, USA

Sean Phipps PhD
Division of Behavioral Medicine, St Jude Children's
Research Hospital, Memphis, Tennessee, USA

Cindy B Proukou CPNP
Division of Hematology/Oncology, Golisano Children's
Hospital at Strong and University of Rochester Medical
Center, Rochester, New York; and
Department of Pediatrics, University of Rochester School
of Medicine and Dentistry,
Rochester, New York

R Beverly Raney MD
Professor of Pediatrics, MD Anderson Cancer Center,
Division of Pediatrics, University of Texas, Houston, Texas,
USA

John J Reilly BSc PhD
Reader in Pediatric Energy Balance, University of
Glasgow Department of Human Nutrition, Yorkhill
Hospitals, Glasgow, UK

Michael Ritchey MD
Professor of Surgery and Pediatrics, Director, Division of
Urology, University of Texas-Houston Health Sciences
Center, Houston, Texas, USA

Frank H Saran FRCR
Consultant in Clinical Oncology, Royal Marsden Hospital
NHS Trust, Sutton, Surrey, UK

Stephen M Shalet
Professor of Endocrinology, Department of Medicine &
Endocrinology, Christie Hospital NHS Trust, Withington,
Manchester, UK

Christine M Sharis MD
Instructor, Department of Radiation Oncology,
Massachusetts General Hospital, Boston, MA, USA

Patricia D Shearer MD MS
Division of Pediatric Hematology/Oncology, Ochsner for
Children, and Clinical Associate Professor of Pediatrics,
Tulane University School of Medicine,
New Orleans, LA, USA

Roderick Skinner MB ChB PhD FRCPCH MRCP DCH
Senior Lecturer and Honorary Consultant in Paediatric
Oncology, Sir James Spence Institute of Child Health,
University of Newcastle upon Tyne, Royal Victoria
Infirmary, Newcastle upon Tyne, UK

Charles Sklar MD
Department of Paediatrics,
Memorial Sloan Kettering Cancer Centre,
New York, NY, USA

Gilbert Smith JD
Associate Director, Business Development, MCMC,
Boston, MA, USA

Andrew L Sonis DMD
Senior Associate in Dentistry, Children's Hospital Boston;
and
Associate Clinical Professor in Growth and Development,
Harvard University School of Dental Medicine, Boston,
MA, USA

Helen A Spoudeas MBBS DRCOG FRCPCH FRCP MD
Consultant/Honorary Senior Lecturer in Paediatric
Neuro-Endocrinology, London Centre for Paediatric
Endocrinology, Neuroendocrine Division, University
College and Great Ormond Street Hospitals, London, UK

Nancy Tarbell MD
Professor of Radiation Oncology, Head, Pediatric
Radiation Oncology, Massachusetts General Hospital,
Boston, MA, USA

Angela B Thomson BSc MRCP(UK) MRCPCH
Section of Child Life and Health, Department of
Reproductive and Developmental Sciences,
University of Edinburgh; and
Department of Haematology/Oncology, Royal Hospital for
Sick Children, Edinburgh, UK

Michael J Tidman MD FRCP(Edin)
Consultant Dermatologist, Royal Infirmary of Edinburgh,
Edinburgh, UK

W Hamish B Wallace MD FRCPCH
Consultant Paediatric Oncologist, Child Life and Health,
Reproductive and Developmental Sciences, University of
Edinburgh; and
Department of Haematology/Oncology; Royal Hospital
for Sick Children; Edinburgh, UK

Holly White MS
Division of Behavioral Medicine, St Jude Children's
Research Hospital, Memphis, Tennessee, USA

Robin Zagone MD
Resident, Division of Urology, University of
Texas-Houston Health Sciences Center, Houston,
Texas, USA

Foreword

This timely book fills a void. It is a thorough and comprehensive review of those iatrogenic and societal consequences that can develop in children years after they have been cured of cancer. An outstanding roster of contributors provides detailed, up-to-the minute discussions of the many and varied adversities that can ensue. Less common complications such as the ocular sequelae of anticancer therapies can be found in these pages, but the more frequent questions asked by worried parents and patients themselves are addressed in detail.

They are chiefly concerned with possible untoward treatment-related effects on normal growth and development, competent neuropsychologic functioning especially cognition, and sexual maturation and reproductive capacity in both males and females. The sections of the book dealing with these issues provide the required, and very welcome, encompassing information. The data presented and the discussions of the issues can be read with profit by all those engaged in pediatric oncology.

Section 8, which deals with endocrine and fertility competence, is of particular interest and value. Much parental and patient disquiet revolves around these physiologic interplays, little remembered by busy practitioners from their fledgling days. Outstanding experts now give the reader a single source of precise information from which to restock their knowledge stores. Moreover, the editors have added a most compelling coda in Section 11. There, the ethical issues concerning fertility preservation are presented, outlining the valid and often impassioned debating points raised by various segments of society concerning these very topics.

*Ad astra per aspera** comes to mind, however, as one reads through the various chapters. It is well to remember that what are being described are *late* effects, that is, they reflect treatments given in the past. The difficulties described will be seen far less often if at all in the future. This is because pediatric oncologists and other specialists have traveled the rough road together, and have learned how to climb towards the stars through combined modality treatments. Less radical surgical procedures, lower doses of radiation therapy to smaller volumes, and less intensive courses of chemotherapy have led not only to

fewer long-term complications but also to better survival rates. These lessons have been learned through years of collaboration that give new meaning to 'less is more', the dictum of the late great architect Mies van der Rohe. Intensifying treatments in children with cancer, especially the antimitotic therapies, always carries a price because of their secondary effects. In the early days, as the cure rates in pediatric oncology began to climb, it was tempting to add a new agent or increase the field size and dose of radiation therapy. 'What we give now is doing something. Augmentation will surely be better. Let's add more and give the patient the benefit of the doubt' – of doubtful benefit most often when given only on that basis.

One of the glories of pediatric oncology is the fact that the clinical trial mechanism was adopted early and widely. More than 80 of 100 children with cancer in the United States are enrolled in a cooperative group study. This has brought science to the bedside. Modifications of management have been put to the test in carefully designed, completely ethical randomized studies to determine whether a new treatment is truly of benefit. Benefit in the short term as measured by better event-free survival rates has not been the only goal, however. The focus has also been on the potentially deleterious late consequences. The drive has therefore been to modulate therapeutic intensity according to well-defined risk estimates. Avoidance of routine cranial radiation therapy for 'prophylaxis' in children with ALL, and the use of doxorubicin only in those with Wilms tumor are just two of the many examples that could be cited.

Risk estimates are becoming increasingly precise. Molecular genetic markers have enabled accurate diagnoses than light or electron microscopy could ever achieve. The natural history and the response to available therapy for the specific tumor type or subtype within a particular entity has made it possible to tailor management much more exactly to the needs of the particular child.

Therefore, the information to be gained by those reading this book is of immense importance in understanding what to expect in a 20- or 30-year-old man or woman attending a long-term follow-up clinic today. But they represent past history – living history to be sure – but their severe complications will seldom if ever be seen

---

* Freely translated as 'To the stars though the road be rough.'

again 10, 20 or 30 years from now. The congestive heart failure secondary to doxorubicin or daunorubicin doses given 20 years ago will not be the heritage of therapy as it is given these days. Nor will the shortened legs, damaged lungs, or cirrhotic livers be encountered by the heirs of the pioneering pediatric radiation oncologists. They have smoothed the path and it is no longer so *aspera*. Indeed, the plot device in Dickens' 'Christmas Carol' needs to be borne in mind by those staffing follow-up clinics. They must think of treatments past, treatments present and treatments future – and prepare for these.

This is because the successes in pediatric oncology of yesteryear have created new – and happier – challenges today. The projections of a decade or two back have become a reality: one in a thousand young adults in the developed world is a childhood cancer survivor. This proportion will increase steadily as the years go by. The trickle of patients in long-term follow-up clinics has become a steady stream that presents new problems to those who must organize these clinics. Who on the team will become responsible for overseeing the continuing surveillance of the adolescent, shortly to become a young woman or man? This and collateral knotty issues will be solved differently from one center to the next, and from one country to its neighbor. More than socio-economic factors will be weighed. Cultural and even religious influences will play a part too. All lie atop simple, practical matters. These include proximity to competent specialists – gynecologists and cardiologists for instance – in accessible facilities where the adult age groups are seen.

The editors have wisely included Sections 14a and 14b that deal with these matters as they are viewed in North America and the United Kingdom. Helpful hints and insights are to be found in those pages that will prove useful to all those engaged in developing long-term follow-up facilities.

It is well to remember the broader psycho-socio-economic collateral adversities as well as the iatrogenic secondary effects. A family with a sick child is a sick family. The stresses on parents and their inter-personal relationships are impossible to quantify. More, there are the healthy siblings who may bear poorly healed emotional scars for a life-time. They have been aptly termed, 'the forgotten children.' Deprivation of parental attention during the acute phase of the patient's illness can lead to lasting resentment against both parents and the ill sibling. Pediatric oncologists must remember the forgotten children in their family conferences and counsel the parents accordingly. It is an essential part of 'total care'.

The rallying cry of pediatric oncology, 'cure is not enough' echoes within *all* the rooms of the home. Not only is the child with cancer to be cured, but his or her future as a functioning adult must also be safe-guarded along with the strength of the family unit. Nothing less will do.

Giulio J. D'Angio MD
Professor Emeritus
Department of Radiation Oncology
University of Pennsylvania
Philadelphia, PA 19104

Reference annotation

The reference lists are annotated, where appropriate, to guide readers to key primary papers and major review articles as follows:

Key primary papers are indicated by a ◆
Major review articles are indicated by a ●

We hope that this feature will render extensive lists of references more useful to the reader and will help to encourage self-directed learning among both trainees and practicing physicians.

Introduction

W HAMISH WALLACE AND DANIEL GREEN

Therapeutic advances for the management of childhood malignancies mean that the majority of affected children can realistically hope for long-term survival. It has been estimated that by the year 2010, 1 : 250 of the adult population will be a long-term survivor of childhood cancer. The successful treatment of childhood cancer using combinations of chemotherapy, surgery and radiotherapy may be associated with significant morbidity in later life. A major challenge faced by pediatric oncologists today is to sustain the excellent survival rates while striving to achieve optimal quality of life.

Improved survival has come about through pioneering national and international studies of rare childhood cancers. Multidisciplinary treatment has been the hallmark of success in pediatric oncology, with physicians and surgeons working together to improve the outcome and reduce the burden of treatment for these vulnerable patients. The last 40 years have shown us that many of the common childhood cancers are not only chemoresponsive, but also chemocurable. Centralization of treatment and high-quality supportive care have allowed our young patients to benefit from intensive chemotherapy and radiotherapy. While many challenges still remain, this book can rightly be considered a celebration of 40 years of effective cancer therapies for children.

Recent large epidemiological studies have analysed the subsequent mortality and its causes in children and adolescents, who survived 5 years from the diagnosis of cancer. Two landmark studies by Mertens *et al.*[1] and Möller *et al.*[2] in the *Journal of Clinical Oncology* found that 5-year survivors of childhood cancer have a standardized mortality ratio of 10.8. In other words, 5-year survivors of childhood and adolescent cancer have a 10.8-fold increased risk of death in the subsequent years when compared with age- and sex-specific expected rates for the general population. The American study described a cohort of 20 227, 5-year

survivors of cancer diagnosed between 1970 and 1986 before the age of 21, which included 208 947 person-years of follow-up. The risk of death in this cohort was statistically significantly higher in females (standardized mortality rate; SMR = 18.2), individuals diagnosed with cancer before the age of 5 years (SMR = 14.0) and those with an initial diagnosis of leukaemia (SMR = 15.5) or central nervous system (CNS) tumor (SMR = 15.7). The leading cause of death was recurrence of the original cancer with a statistically significant excess mortality rate seen due to subsequent malignancies (SMR = 19.4) as well as cardiac (SMR = 8.2), pulmonary (SMR = 9.2) and other causes (SMR = 3.3). Of the 20, 227 eligible for the American study, 90 per cent were alive at the time of the study, with death due to recurrent cancer accounting for 67 per cent of all deaths and more common between five and nine years after diagnosis, while treatment-related causes accounted for 21 per cent of all deaths, of which 12.7 per cent were due to a second cancer, 4.5 per cent due to cardiac toxicity and 1.8 per cent due to pulmonary complications. There was no excess mortality from external causes, for example, suicide or road traffic accidents. Unquestionably, these important studies will provide a rich resource for understanding how mortality may be reduced further, and how modifications of current therapy may reduce treatment-related mortality in the future.

In this book we have assembled a wide range of contributions from experts from all over the world to summarize the late effects of the treatment of childhood cancer. Each involved system is, in many respects, an innocent bystander that has received a non-selective cytotoxic hit as part of the necessary treatment that our patients have received. There remains a dearth of large multicenter interventional studies evaluating therapy to prevent, treat or modify late effects in our young survivors. If cure alone is not enough, then multidisciplinary, national and

international collaborative studies must be designed to improve the outcome for this large cohort of long-term survivors.

Perhaps the real challenge is to develop strategies for the long-term follow-up of survivors that addresses their needs, provide us with the opportunity to study and evaluate the long-term effects of treatment and give access to this population so that promising interventions can be assessed through collaborative multicenter studies.[3] It is our hope and belief that this book will catalyse these necessary collaborative ventures to improve the quality of the survival for the child treated for cancer.

REFERENCES

1. Mertens AC, Yasui Y, Neglia JP, *et al*. Late mortality experience in 5 year survivors of childhood and adolescent cancers – The Children's Cancer Survival Study. *J Clin Oncol* 2001; **19**:3163–3172.
2. Möller TR, Garwicz S, Barlow L, *et al*. Decreasing late mortality among 5 year survivors of cancer in childhood and adolescence: a population based study in the Nordic countries. *J Clin Oncol* 2001; **19**:3173–3181.
3. Wallace WHB, Blacklay A, Eiser C, *et al*. Developing strategies for long term follow up of survivors of childhood cancer. *Br Med J* 2001; **323**:271–274.

2

Neurological and special senses

2a

Long-term neurologic consequences of CNS therapy

PATRICIA K DUFFNER

PERIPHERAL NEUROPATHY

Certain chemotherapeutic agents, in particular vincristine, cisplatinum, paclitaxel and thalidomide are well known to cause peripheral neuropathies. The neurotoxicity associated with these agents is typically related to both the dose and duration of therapy, and hence limits their potential efficacy. Unfortunately, assessment of chemotherapy-induced peripheral neuropathies is exceedingly difficult in the young child. Most studies report a combination of subjective and objective criteria to assess peripheral neuropathies.[1] Subjective complaints include paresthesias and numbness, signs and symptoms, which are particularly difficult to elicit in young children. Although motor abnormalities, such as foot drop, may be identified on clinical examination, subtle weakness of dorsiflexion of the feet may be missed in a young child. This is particularly true in the infant or young child who is non-ambulatory. Furthermore, objective neurophysiologic evaluations of children with nerve conduction velocities and electromyography are obtained only when specifically indicated because the procedures are both painful and frightening. Therefore, much of the literature on chemotherapy-induced peripheral neuropathy in children is suboptimal. Extrapolating from adult studies is problematic because adults often have complicating neurotoxic factors, such as diabetes, alcohol use, remote effects of carcinoma, and other pre-existing diseases. Finally, most studies report neurotoxicity based on combination chemotherapy making firm conclusions regarding a single agent difficult. It is clear that, since the neurotoxicity of many agents is both dose- and time-dependent, the pediatric neurology community will need to develop a better system for assessing neurotoxicity in young children.

Vincristine neuropathy

Vincristine produces a distal symmetric sensory motor neuropathy, which is probably due to disruption of axoplasmic transport. Impaired ankle jerks are the first sign of vincristine neurotoxicity and may be recognized as early as 2 weeks following onset of therapy. Ultimately, the loss of ankle jerks is almost universal.[2] Paresthesias, first in the fingers and then in the feet, tend to occur 4–5 weeks following onset of treatment.[3] Sensory symptoms, most frequently impaired vibration sense, may occur in 75 per cent of treated patients.[3] Position sense, however, is never abnormal.[4] Motor weakness involves the extensor muscles of the fingers, wrists, toes and dorsiflexors of the feet.[1] The child may have difficulty running or walking, with associated foot drop.[5] If administration of high-dose vincristine is continued after the onset of mild distal weakness, a syndrome of rapidly progressive diffuse weakness may occur despite the fact that there is little increase in sensory disturbance. Muscle pain may also limit function. Cramps are present, particularly in the thighs and calves, while jaw pain may occur within 24–48 hours after the first dose.

Paralytic ileus, constipation and postural hypotension are the primary autonomic disturbances. Cranial neuropathies may occur in about 10 per cent of patients, typically after peripheral muscle weakness has first developed. Bilateral ptosis is the most common of these palsies.

Less common is paralytic strabismus. Some patients may develop changes in voice quality, dysarthria and dysphagia.[5] There is usually complete recovery of these deficits by 4 months following completion of treatment.[2] When the drug is stopped or the dose decreased, the weakness and paresthesias typically resolve, although ankle jerks may remain impaired.

A much more severe complication, that is, fulminant quadriparesis, has rarely been reported during vincristine therapy.[6] Profound motor weakness with arreflexia and moderate distal sensory disturbances have been identified along with elevation in cerebrospinal fluid (CSF) protein. In most cases, motor recovery eventually occurred. Some, if not all of these cases, may have had Guillain–Barré syndrome.[7]

The electromyogram (EMG) findings associated with typical vincristine neuropathy are denervation with fibrillation and decreased numbers of motor units in the distal muscles. The sensory nerve action potentials may remain abnormal even when clinical signs and symptoms have completely resolved.[4] Conduction studies reveal prolonged mean distal latencies with relatively preserved nerve conduction velocities.[3] On pathology, a distal axonopathy is recognized.

Infants, young children and adolescents are at greatest risk from vincristine neurotoxicity. Cachectic patients and those on bed rest are also typically more affected. The cachectic patient may have an underlying nutritional neuropathy, which is exacerbated by the vincristine, and the bedridden patient may be prone to traumatic compression injuries of the ulnar and peroneal nerves.[5] The concomitant use of itraconazole may also enhance vincristine neurotoxicity and should be avoided, if possible.[8]

An underlying peripheral neuropathy such as Charcot–Marie–Tooth (CMT) disease is another significant risk factor. The condition can be severely exacerbated following vincristine therapy. Although patients with other hereditary neuropathies may also be at risk, patients with CMT Type IA (17 p. 11.2–12 duplication) are at the highest risk. When patients have a family history of autosomal dominant neuropathy characterized by distal weakness and atrophy, arreflexia and pes cavus deformity with limited sensory involvement, CMT should be suspected and genetic testing performed. Vincristine is contraindicated in patients with this condition. It should be emphasized that, although the child may be presymptomatic and clinically normal, the gene will predispose them to a rapid course of vincristine-associated profound weakness, atrophy and arreflexia, which may be fatal.[9,10] High arched feet, hallucis recurvatum and tight heel cords with atrophy of the intrinsic muscles of the hands may be early signs of CMT. Prior to administering vincristine, a careful examination of the hands and feet should be performed and a detailed family history should be obtained.[11]

Thalidomide neuropathy

Thalidomide is associated with a predominantly sensory neuropathy characterized by paresthesias and numbness in a stocking glove distribution. The condition is symmetrical and not typically associated with weakness. When weakness is present, however, involved muscles are more proximal than distal in location. The incidence of neuropathy has ranged in various studies from 1 to 100 per cent.[12,13] Unfortunately, unlike vincristine neuropathy, symptoms and signs of peripheral neuropathy may resolve slowly or not at all. For example, in one study, 50 per cent of patients with peripheral neuropathy following thalidomide made no recovery as late as 4–6 years following completion of therapy. However, in the study by Molloy, clinical symptoms did improve upon discontinuation of the drug, perhaps because the drug was discontinued as soon as there were signs of peripheral neuropathy.[12] Unlike vincristine, where there is a clear-cut association with dose and duration of treatment, the data are less clear with thalidomide. In only one study has it been suggested that cumulative dose may be a risk factor.[12] Other risk factors are gender (female) and age (older).

The electrophysiologic abnormalities seen in thalidomide neuropathy are abnormalities of sensory nerve action potential amplitudes. It is recommended that sensory nerve action potentials be performed at baseline and then every 3 months. If there is a decline in amplitude by >40 per cent the drug should be discontinued immediately.[13] In addition, thalidomide should be stopped immediately at the first clinical sign of peripheral neuropathy. Even with clinical recovery, the sensory nerve action potentials only occasionally improve in amplitude.

Axonal degeneration of the peripheral nerves and degenerative changes in the dorsal root ganglion cells and posterior columns are identified on pathologic examination. The predominant changes are in the large diameter nerve fibers.

Cisplatinum neuropathy

Cisplatinum (CDDP) primarily produces a sensory peripheral neuropathy. The dorsal root ganglion is the primary target.[14] Paresthesias, dysesthesias, disturbance of position and vibration tend to occur with relative sparing of the motor units. Neuropathy has been reported to occur in as many as 76 per cent of patients, although some abnormalities are clinically silent, detected only by neurophysiologic testing or vibration thresholds. The severe acute neurotoxicity typically resolves but as many as 20–60 per cent of patients may have persistent paresthesias following completion of therapy.[14] Motor abnormalities are usually subtle but may increase in the presence of low serum levels of magnesium. The major identified

risk factor to date is cumulative dose. Amifostine was found to have a neuroprotective effect on subclinical neurotoxicity when given in conjunction with cisplatinum.[15]

Nerve conduction studies show a decrease or absence of sensory nerve action potentials, delayed sensory nerve conduction velocities, but normal motor nerve conduction and EMG.

Paclitaxel

The taxanes interfere with microtubule-based axonal transport. Paclitaxel (taxol) produces a reversible predominantly distal sensory neuropathy, which is dose dependent. It has primarily been studied in adults, usually when used in combination with agents such as doxorubicin, cyclophosphamide, carboplatin and/or cisplatinum. Markman reported 25 per cent of his patients developed peripheral neuropathy, with 40 per cent becoming symptomatic prior to the fourth treatment course.[16] Others have found a similar complication rate, e.g. 34 per cent of patients developed peripheral neuropathy, typically sensory in nature.[17] Motor involvement is rare. Because most reports include patients on combination therapy, particularly CDDP, it is hard to assign blame. It is clear that a severe peripheral neuropathy may occur in patients previously treated with neurotoxic chemotherapy.

Docetaxel (Taxotene) in combination with CDDP has also been reported to be associated with a predominantly sensory neuropathy.[18] At doses >200 mg/m^2, 74 per cent of patients in one study developed neuropathy, although most were considered mild. The neurotoxicity of docetaxel and CDDP in combination was worse than when either agent was given alone. In a study of docetaxel as monotherapy,[19] a reversible sensorimotor polyneuropathy occurred at a dose of 540 mg/m^2. Physiologic and pathologic studies have identified an axonal neuropathy with preferential loss of large myelinated fibers. Since the taxanes have such therapeutic promise, attempts have been made to reduce neurotoxicity. Glutamine, for example, was administered after high-dose paclitaxel (825 mg/m^2). Patients who had been given glutamine and paclitaxel had a significant decrease in the severity of neuropathy as measured by sensory symptoms, such as dysesthesias and numbness, motor weakness, gait disturbances, and activities of daily living compared to the control arm in which paclitaxel was given alone.[20] The study was not randomized or placebo controlled, but still of interest.

IFOSFAMIDE ENCEPHALOPATHY

Five to thirty per cent of patients treated with ifosfamide will develop central nervous system (CNS) toxicity, including seizures, visual disturbances, auditory and visual hallucinations, acute confusional state, mutism, extrapyramidal signs and, rarely, progressive irreversible coma. Symptoms will typically clear within 48–72 hours of cessation of drug, but fatalities have occurred. Hallucinations may occur in the face of a normal sensorium.[21] It is of interest that visual hallucinations tend to occur with the eyes closed and disappear with the eyes open. This toxicity is particularly important to recognize in children, as they may not be able to explain adequately what is frightening them. The encephalopathy may be related to both dose and regimen, as it appears to occur less frequently when continuous infusions are administered over several days.[22] The syndrome may be exacerbated when phenobarbital is used. Although the exact etiology for ifosfamide encephalopathy has not been identified, a previous event predicts recurrence and patients should never be retreated with the agent.[23] The related compound cyclophosphamide is not associated with this type of encephalopathy.

LEUKOENCEPHALOPATHY

Treatment-induced leukoencephalopathy develops most commonly as a consequence of cranial irradiation and/or methotrexate either when given alone or in combination. The pathology of leukoencephalopathy is demyelination with loss of oligodendroglia, focal or diffuse areas of white matter necrosis, mineralizing microangiopathy, dystrophic calcification and glial damage. Leukoencephalopathy spares the cortical gray matter and subcortical u fibers. The deep cerebral hemispheric and periventricular areas are most affected. On computed tomography (CT) scan, calcification (particularly in the basal ganglia), hypodense areas and widened subarachnoid spaces are characteristic (Figure 2a.1). The magnetic resonance imaging (MRI) pattern of leukoencephalopathy has been described and graded by Zimmerman et al.[24] Grade 4 is a diffuse irregular white matter abnormality on T2 extending from the ventricles to the cortical medullary junction. Grade 3 is a periventricular halo or band of hyperintensity of variable thickness forming smooth lateral margins around the ventricles. Grade 2 is a pencil-thin continuous line of hyperintensity around the ventricles. Grade 1 is a discontinuous area of periventricular hyperintensity and Grade 0 is normal.

Regardless of etiology, leukoencephalopathy may be associated with dementia, focal motor signs, seizures, ataxia and death. Although leukoencephalopathy by definition implies white matter damage, often the most striking clinical correlates suggest damage to gray matter, that is, memory loss and dementia. The cognitive abnormalities likely reflect the fact that white matter damage impacts on neurotransmission through neurobehavioral

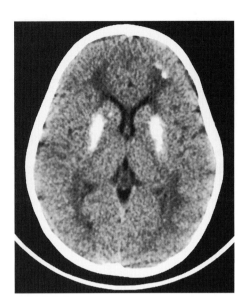

Figure 2a.1 *Axial CT scan of a 2-year-old boy who presented with seizures and dementia following treatment for ALL on POG 9001. He was never irradiated and had no history of CNS leukemia. CT reveals calcification in the basal ganglia and hypodense areas.*

pathways.[25] Even when leukoencephalopathy is considered mild, attention and memory retrieval are often abnormal. In moderate cases, a marked deficit in attention, memory, visuospatial skills and executive functions are found. Of interest, unlike dementing diseases such as Alzheimer's, language is typically preserved.[25]

Radiation-induced leukoencephalopathy has been correlated with dose, patient age, volume of radiation, fractionation schedule and time following radiation.[26] Patients who receive higher doses of radiation (i.e. >7000 cGy) are more likely to develop leukoencephalopathy than those who receive <6000 cGy. Whole-brain radiation is also more likely to be associated with Grade 3–4 leukoencephalopathy than is local radiation (50 per cent vs. 14 per cent).[26] Larger doses per fraction are also more toxic. Leukoencephalopathy does not typically develop earlier than 1 year following radiation.

Methotrexate-associated leukoencephalopathy has been receiving increased attention over the past few years. In 1978, Peylan Ramu reported a series of children with acute lymphoblastic leukemia (ALL) without CNS leukemia who had been treated with a methotrexate-containing protocol that included cranial irradiation.[27] Fifty-three per cent of her patients had abnormal CT scans characterized by hypodense areas, calcification (especially in the basal ganglia) and widened subarachnoid spaces. She attributed these changes to 'methotrexate leukoencephalopathy'. Subsequently, Ochs *et al.* studied a group of children with ALL treated at Roswell Park Cancer Institute (RPCI) with a chemotherapy regimen

that included both intravenous (IV) plus intrathecal (IT) methotrexate but no cranial irradiation.[28] CT scans were generally unremarkable with no cases of severe leukoencephalopathy (i.e. calcification or hypodensity). This suggested that methotrexate, in the absence of cranial irradiation, did not produce leukoencephalopathy and that it was the combination that was leukotoxic. In a subsequent analysis of the RPCI experience, >80 per cent of children treated for CNS leukemia, even in the absence of cranial irradiation, developed leukoencephalopathy, a proportion that reached 100 per cent if cranial irradiation had also been administered.[29] Ettinger, in an attempt to determine why this population was at such high risk, studied methotrexate clearance in children with and without CNS leukemia.[30] Methotrexate was injected into Ommaya reservoirs and sequential levels were obtained. Children with CNS relapse had significantly higher methotrexate levels at 24 and 48 hours compared to children without meningeal disease. Since the toxicity of methotrexate is related both to level and duration of exposure, the delay in clearance of methotrexate from the ventricles presumably permitted transependymal flow across the ventricles causing periventricular damage. The degree of CT leukoencephalopathy correlated in another study with delayed clearance.[29] Thus, until the mid-1990s the general belief was that risk factors for leukoencephalopathy included CNS leukemia and cranial irradiation and, in the absence of these risk factors, methotrexate could be given with impunity.

Even when studies surfaced in which transient white matter abnormalities on MRI were identified during ALL therapy, some queried the significance of these findings.[31] In one study, three of 33 children developed white matter changes during therapy that resolved by the end of treatment. These changes tended to occur in younger children. Correlations with the abnormal MRIs included limited attention span and changes on tests of executive function.[32] Others also identified transient white matter abnormalities on MRI. In one study, at mid-consolidation (15 weeks), 60 per cent of children (15 out of 25) had white-matter changes over baseline with 44 per cent moderate to severe. At 26 weeks (i.e. start of maintenance treatment), 60 per cent still had a change from baseline but 32 per cent were now moderate to severe. By 1 year, 52 per cent were abnormal compared to baseline but only one was moderate to severe. By 3 years, 40 per cent still had mild changes from baseline. The abnormalities did not predict neuropsychologic function except in children less than 5 years, in whom 10 of 11 had neuropsychological deficits and 8 of 11 had white-matter changes.[33]

In the mid-1990s, cases of children with standard risk leukemia without CNS disease and without prior cranial radiation therapy (CRT) were reported in whom both clinical and radiologic findings of leukoencephalopathy were present. Twenty-three patients treated at RPCI for

Figure 2a.2 *Axial MRI of same child as in Figure 2a.1. Note increased T2-weighted signals extending to the gray matter– white matter junction.*

ALL on Pediatric Oncology Group (POG) 9005 were evaluated. None of these children either had either CNS leukemia or cranial irradiation. The study consisted of three arms: arm A consisted of 1000 mg/m^2 IV methotrexate + 6-mercaptopurine; arm B received low-dose oral (PO) methotrexate + 6-mercaptopurine; and arm C received 1000 mg/m^2 IV methotrexate. Overall, 39 per cent of RPCI patients treated on 9005 had abnormal CT and MRI scans consistent with methotrexate leuko-encephalopathy, while 50 per cent of children treated on arms A and C were so affected (Figure 2a.2). Clinical correlates included frank mental retardation, learning disabilities, seizures and chorea. This led to a group-wide review of POG 9005.[34] CT or MRI scans were obtained only on the 7.8 per cent of patients who had had acute neurotoxicity, that is, seizures, paresis or paraplegia, dysarthria, ataxia, aphasia, altered state of consciousness, and/or severe postintrathecal headaches. As in the RPCI study, significantly more cases of leukoencephalopathy were identified in arms A and C in which 1000 mg/m^2 IV methotrexate was given (75 per cent of patients on A and 77 per cent on C vs. 15 per cent on arm B). The acute neurotoxicity rate of 7.8 per cent may have underestimated the true incidence of leukoencephalopathy, since in the RPCI experience some children with no history of acute neurotoxicity had both abnormal imaging and abnormalities on tests of neuropsychologic function.

Because of the experience with POG 9005, there is now a heightened level of awareness regarding the potential for neurotoxicity in children treated for standard risk leukemia. A study has been proposed to evaluate children on two other POG protocols, POG 9605 and POG 9201, which differ from each other in several ways. In POG 9605, the administration of IV methotrexate was separated by 1 week from IT methotrexate and hence leukovorin was not given following IT methotrexate, whereas on POG 9201, IT and IV methotrexate were given within 24 hours of each other and were accompanied by leukovorin. In addition, triple intrathecal therapy was given in POG 9605 while IT methotrexate alone was given in POG 9201. It is hoped that a comparison of these two studies will allow us to determine whether the differences in treatment have had an influence on the incidence of radiologic and clinical neurotoxicity.

The etiology of methotrexate leukoencephalopathy is likely multifactorial and includes the cumulative amount of methotrexate, the frequency of administration, the absence of leukovorin in patients receiving IT methotrexate alone and possibly the use of triple intrathecal therapy. The mechanism for methotrexate leukoencephalopathy is not fully known, but presumably relates to depletion of brain stores of folate with increased concentrations of homocysteine and excitotoxic neurotransmitters. The elevation of CSF and plasma homocysteine may, as in the model of homocystinuria, lead to vascular endothelial damage.[34]

SEIZURES AND BRAIN TUMORS

Seizures are a relatively frequent presenting symptom of children with hemispheric brain tumors. The Childhood Brain Tumor Consortium Database identified 3291 children with brain tumors.[35] Fourteen per cent had seizures prior to hospitalization. In that study, 22 per cent of children less than 14 years had seizures in association with supratentorial tumors, while in older children the prevalence increased to 68 per cent. The most epileptogenic areas are the temporal lobes and sensory motor regions. Seizures tend to occur more frequently with low-grade tumors, such as dysembryoplastic neuroepithelial tumors (DNET), oligodendrogliomas, gangliogliomas and pleomorphic xanthoastrocytomas (PXA), than with more malignant tumors, and are consequently considered to be a good prognostic sign.

Gangliogliomas are strongly associated with seizures, which were the presenting symptom in 49 per cent of 123 pediatric patients in one series.[36] Twenty-two per cent of patients undergoing epilepsy surgery in another study were found to have gangliogliomas.[37] Some patients with epilepsy have harbored gangliogliomas and other low-grade tumors for many years, which were either undetectable on CT or considered to represent encephalomalacia. With the advent of MRI, more of these lesions are being identified at an earlier stage.

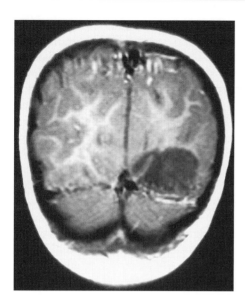

Figure 2a.3 *A 3-year-old girl who presented with partial seizures. MRI revealed low signal lesion in left occipital lobe. The mass does not enhance with gadolinium. Diagnosis: dysembryoplastic neuroepithelial tumor.*

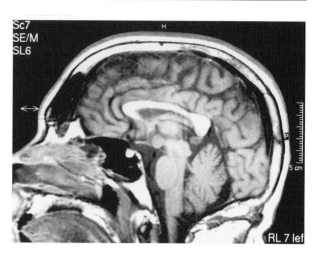

Figure 2a.4 *A 27-year-old followed for gelastic seizures since adolescence. Sagittal MRI reveals an elliptical mass posterior to the infundibulum and anterior to the mamillary body. Diagnosis: hypothalamic hamartoma.*

DNETs were first described by Daumas-Duport in 1988.[37] They are well-demarcated superficial tumors typically located in the temporal lobe. Cortical dysplasias are common. These tumors are strongly associated with intractable epilepsy (Figure 2a.3).

Pleomorphic xanthoastrocytomas are also superficial tumors involving the temporal lobe and overlying meninges. They have a malignant microscopic appearance with hypercellularity, multilobed and multiple nuclei, and rare mitoses, but are clinically benign. Up to 80 per cent of patients will present with seizures as their initial symptom.[38]

Partial seizures, either simple or complex, with or without secondary generalization, are the most common seizures associated with brain tumors. Infantile spasms have also been infrequently reported with brain tumors in babies. Of interest, in at least one study, a good response to adenocorticotrophic hormone (ACTH) was reported, comparable to those with cryptogenic infantile spasms. The tumors associated with infantile spasms are varied and include choroid plexus papillomas, gangliogliomas, gliomas, ependymomas, hamartomas and mixed oligoastrocytomas. They are also multifocal in location and include hemispheric, temporal lobe, parietal lobe, thalamic and hypothalamic locations.[39,40] An unusual seizure, the gelastic or laughing seizure, is typically associated with hypothalamic hamartomas. Generalized seizures may follow a gelastic event. This benign tumor has been underdiagnosed over the years because of the insensitivity of CT scan to tumors in this location (Figure 2a.4). Treatment of hypothalamic hamartomas can be quite difficult, and it is controversial as to whether surgery or even gamma knife radiation is appropriate versus a conservative watchful waiting approach.

Seizures and leukemia

The incidence of seizures in a population of children with ALL ranges from 4 to 13 per cent. Most seizures are partial with and without secondary generalization or primarily generalized. Etiologies are diverse. In one study, 10 per cent of 1289 children with ALL developed seizures. Defined etiologies included hemorrhage due to thrombocytopenia, thrombosis (associated with L-asparaginase), rapid cell lysis, infection and fever. Other patients developed seizures within a week following IT methotrexate and 50 per cent had prior meningeal leukemia.[41] Thirteen per cent of 127 children with ALL developed seizures in another study.[42] Sixteen of 17 children's seizures were attributed to either IT methotrexate or L-asparaginase. Seizures may also occur acutely due to administration of IT methotrexate (<2 per cent). Seizures may be isolated events or may occur in the presence of methotrexate-induced chemical meningitis, a syndrome characterized by fever, headache, dizziness, back pain, and nausea and vomiting. Neuroimaging reveals increased T2-weighted signals on MRI that may be transient. If concurrent CT reveals calcification, however, it is likely the patient has leukoencephalopathy and seizures will be chronic.

Seizures also may occur during administration of CDDP, typically due to inappropriate antidiuretic hormone (ADH) secretion and resulting hyponatremia. These seizures are transient, and resolve when fluid and electrolyte balance is achieved. In some cases, metabolic

derangements have not been present and the cause of the CDDP-induced seizures has not been identified.[43]

Vincristine is similarly associated with a syndrome of inappropriate ADH secretion that may induce seizures. There have, however, been reports of seizures developing 5–6 days following IV vincristine therapy, where metabolic factors and meningeal disease have been excluded.[44]

L-Asparaginase increases the risk of seizures in children with ALL.[41,42] This agent may be associated with the risk of cerebral hemorrhage (1–2 per cent), owing to reduced fibrinogen or thrombotic stroke due to depletion of antithrombin 3, protein C and plasminogen.[45] The presenting symptoms of both intracranial hemorrhage and thrombotic stroke are headache, seizures, vomiting, altered mental state and focal motor signs. A change in mental status is present in >60 per cent of patients. Not surprisingly, seizures are more common in children who suffer hemorrhagic rather than thrombotic stroke. In the thrombotic group, most cerebral infarcts are cortical. Thrombosis of cerebral veins or dural sinuses are also found. Recovery, partial or even complete, occurs in >60 per cent of patients. Risk of recurrence is low, but has been reported. Pretreatment with fresh frozen plasma is recommended by some authors.[46]

Metabolic causes of acute seizures in children being treated for cancer include hypoglycemia, hyponatremia, hypocalcemia and hypomagnesemia. Narcotics and antiemetics can lower the seizure threshold, also producing seizures. These disturbances are self-limited, if appropriate corrective treatment is administered. The prognosis of seizures in children with leukemia varies, depending on etiology. The best prognosis is in children with seizures that are acute and secondary to metabolic derangements, while the worst are associated with structural CNS disease, such as leukoencephalopathy and cerebrovascular accidents. As such, evaluation should include measurement of serum electrolytes (Na, Ca, Mg) and glucose, lumbar puncture with determination of CSF protein, glucose, cell count and differential, and culture, coagulation studies, and MRI, magnetic resonance venogram (MRV) and arteriogram (MRA).

Treatment

The choice of anticonvulsants is problematic when children are being treated with chemotherapy because of drug–drug interactions and the induction of hepatic microsomal enzyme systems. Platinum-based chemotherapy, for example, decreases levels of carbamazepine and phenytoin, while procarbazine will increase phenobarbital and phenytoin levels. More important, antiepileptic drugs (AEDs) can lower the serum levels of chemotherapeutic agents, making them less effective. Phenobarbital may alter the metabolism of cyclophosphamide, either

increasing or decreasing plasma levels. Also problematic is that both phenobarbital and phenytoin displace methotrexate from plasma proteins, and hence increase the risk of methotrexate toxicity. Both phenytoin and phenobarbital decrease the activity of steroids by increasing hepatic enzyme metabolism.[47] To further complicate matters, while patients receive AEDs on a daily basis, chemotherapy is administered in cycles, making it difficult to adjust the dose to ensure therapeutic levels of the agents.

Other concerns about the use of AEDs are their effects on blood and liver. For example, carbamazepine typically causes leukopenia, while valproic acid is associated with thrombocytopenia (usually in the presence of viral infections), abnormal bleeding times and hepatotoxicity. Hepatotoxicity is also a known idiosyncratic reaction of phenytoin and carbamazepine, albeit to a lesser extent. Children who already have hepatic or hematologic disorders may be difficult to assess when the physician is not certain whether the abnormalities are due to the primary disease, effects of chemotherapy or the antiepileptic drugs. Radiation may also pose problems. A syndrome of erythema multiforme and Stevens Johnson syndrome has been reported in patients receiving cranial irradiation and phenytoin. This combination should be avoided.[48] Children, especially those in younger age groups, who receive neuraxis radiation may also become leukopenic, making the use of agents with bone marrow toxicity (e.g. carbamazepine and felbamate) a poor choice.

The ideal anticonvulsant in this setting is one that is not metabolized by the liver and one with limited hematologic toxicity. Gabapentin, therefore, although typically not a first-line agent, should be considered for use in children with seizures who are simultaneously on chemotherapy.

EFFECTS OF RADIATION

Moyamoya disease

Radiation vasculopathy has been divided into two types: an early form occurring 1–20 weeks following radiation, which is associated with arterial disruption and hemorrhage and/or late onset type (7–24 years following CRT), which consists of vascular occlusive or stenotic disease. Moyamoya disease is an example of the late onset form of radiation vasculopathy, consisting of basilar occlusive disease. Patients present with a progressive syndrome of transient ischemic attacks, frank strokes, seizures, motor weakness and dementia.

Basilar stenotic and occlusive disease occurs in the large arteries of the Circle of Willis, the terminal parts of the internal carotid artery, the proximal portions of the middle cerebral artery and the anterior cerebral artery.

The stenosis is gradual, thus allowing the development of an extensive collateral circulation. The term for the angiographic appearance of the telangiectatic vessels is 'puff of smoke' or 'misty' ('moyamoya' in Japanese). The diagnosis may be made on cerebral angiograms as well as on MRAs.[49] In a 1995 review of the world's literature by Bitzer,[49] 40 cases of radiation-induced occlusive cerebral vasculopathy were identified. The most frequent location of the irradiated tumor was near the sella, with 34 per cent of cases occurring in children treated for optic gliomas. The majority of cases were in children, with 77 per cent occurring in those <18 years of age, 49 per cent in those <4 years and 18 per cent in those <1 year at the time of irradiation. In 85 per cent of cases, the symptoms appeared within 8 years following therapy. Adults with radiation-induced occlusive cerebral vasculopathy are less likely than children (33 per cent vs. 62 per cent) to develop a pattern of basal cerebral rete mirabile at the base of the brain and distal to the Circle of Willis. Transient ischemic attacks are more common as the presenting symptom in children, whereas intracranial hemorrhage is more common in adults. The patient at greatest risk for moyamoya disease is the young child (<5 years) with neurofibromatosis type 1 (NF1), who has been irradiated to the hypothalamic/chiasmatic regions with doses of >50 Gy. Although moyamoya disease may occur in irradiated children without NF1, higher radiation doses are required (5164 vs. 3927).[51] The propensity for this condition to occur in children with neurofibromatosis is a major problem because of the strong association of optic pathway tumors and NF1. Recognition of this potential complication has led to a reassessment of the appropriate therapeutic approach to these children. In particular, more aggressive chemotherapy, rather than radiation, has become the primary treatment modality.

The treatment for moyamoya disease is encephaloduroarteriosynangiosis (EDAS). This procedure involves the transposition of a segment of the scalp artery on to the surface of the brain to improve collateral flow. If successful, no further neurologic deterioration will occur.[52] It has been suggested that performing MRA screening for vasculopathy might be of use in the early identification of affected children. Failure to identify abnormalities on MRA, however, does not preclude the presence of disease.[49]

Radiation-induced intracranial aneurysms

Less common is the development of radiation-induced aneurysms. Although infrequent, these are now potentially treatable, if diagnosed in a timely fashion. As of 1997, there were 13 cases of radiation-induced intracranial aneurysms reported.[53] The aneurysms were either saccular, fusiform or giant, and occurred in both children and adults. The time to diagnosis (typically subarachnoid hemorrhage) ranged from 10 months to 21 years following radiation. In six patients, baseline angiography prior to radiation had been normal. There does not appear to be a direct relationship between dose and development of aneurysms.

The aneurysms can be differentiated from their non-radiation-induced counterparts. The fusiform aneurysms resemble aneurysms due to atherosclerosis, but differ in that they occur in a young age group, are located in the radiation field and contain large cells resembling histiocytes filled with foamy cytoplasm. The saccular aneurysms can be differentiated from the congenital type by location. They arise directly from a segment of the artery and rupture occurs at more than one site, usually near the aneurysm's origin or at points in which the arterial branches take off. Diagnosis can be made on arteriography and MRA, in most cases. Since subarachnoid hemorrhage is typically fatal in this setting, surgical intervention with clipping coils or wrapping is indicated.[53–55]

Radiation necrosis

Radiation necrosis is estimated to occur in 5 per cent of patients between 6 months and 2 years following cranial irradiation.[56] The risk increases with dose, occurring in 0 of 337 patients who received <54 Gy, but increasing rapidly for doses >60 Gy.[57] The risk also rises when larger fractions (>200 cGy/day) are given over a shorter period of time.[55,56,58] Symptoms range from memory loss, dementia, confusion, depression, agitation and personality change to symptoms that mimic recurrent tumor and increased intracranial pressure, such as headache, vomiting, diplopia, papilledema and focal motor signs.[59] The pathology of radiation necrosis is primarily vascular, affecting the endothelium of small arteries and arterioles. White matter is also selectively affected due to the sensitivity of oligodendroglia to radiation.[60] Pathologic findings include endothelial hyperplasia, telangiectasia, fibrinoid degeneration of the vascular walls, astrocytosis, perivascular lymphocytic infiltration and coagulation necrosis.[61] The exact pathophysiology of radiation necrosis is unknown, although increased vascular permeability, alterations in the blood–brain barrier, and resulting vasogenic edema are prominent. Over time, vessels thicken leading to thrombosis and resulting ischemia. Other factors in the development of radiation necrosis include selective damage to the oligodendroglia with resultant loss of myelin. Still others have identified changes in the fibrinolytic enzyme system, with an absence of tissue plasminogen activator and increased urokinase plasminogen activator. These enzymatic alterations may contribute to the vasogenic and cytotoxic edema. Finally, some have suggested an autoimmune

component in the development of radiation necrosis, with resulting vasculitis.[62]

Differentiating radiation necrosis from recurrent tumor may be difficult clinically and neuroradiologically. From a clinical point of view, both present with symptoms and signs of an expanding mass lesion including focal motor deficits, headache, diplopia, papilledema and mental status changes. Imaging may be indistinguishable as both lesions exert mass effect, enhance with intravenous contrast, are associated with edema and increase in size over time. Radiation necrosis often, but does not always, occurs at the site of the original tumor.[62] CSF protein may be elevated in both conditions and focal slowing is identified on the electroencephalogram (EEG) in both conditions. CT scans reveal a hypodense mass with irregular contrast enhancement.[63] MRI patterns include a single lesion at or near the site of the original tumor, multiple lesions, lesions in the contralateral hemisphere, subependymal lesions or lesions remote from the original site (e.g. in the cerebellum or brainstem) with the original tumor in the cerebral hemispheres. Kumar describes a 'Swiss cheese' pattern associated with diffuse necrosis of white matter and surrounding cortex. Enhancement of the margins is intermixed with areas of necrosis. Another pattern, the 'soap bubble' type is characterized by central areas of necrosis.[62]

Positron emission tomography (PET) scanning has been touted to distinguish radiation necrosis reliably from recurrent high-grade tumor, as the former is hypometabolic and the latter hypermetabolic. Some have found, however, that the sensitivity of PET in distinguishing the two entities is only approximately 43 per cent, which is insufficient to dispense with biopsy.[64]

Magnetic resonance spectroscopy may have a role in both differentiating radionecrosis from recurrent brain tumor and in providing insight into metabolic changes in the process. Lower N-acetyl aspartate (NAA)/choline (CHO) and NAA/creatine (Cr) ratios have been found in areas of even mild radionecrosis compared to brain prior to radiation. Furthermore, there is a trend of decreasing NAA with increasing severity of the process, suggesting continuous neuronal loss. Increased CHO/Cr ratios were found by Chan et al. in the most severe cases of radiation necrosis but others have shown the reverse.[65] Thus, the CHO/Cr ratio is not reliable at this time in differentiating necrosis from tumor. The most severe radiation necrosis is associated with elevation of lactate, which suggests ischemia as an etiology.[65]

The incidence of radionecrosis is rising with the use of interstitial brachytherapy, stereotactic radiosurgery and the gamma knife with abnormal pathology identified in 30–50 per cent of patients, although the incidence of clinical symptoms is much lower. For example, in one study, 5 per cent of patients treated with gamma knife developed radionecrosis but the risk varied with the lesion: glioma 17 per cent; brain metastases 5 per cent; and benign tumors 17.5 per cent. The greatest risk is in patients treated with 10 Gy total volume >10 cm^3 and those who have been retreated with radiosurgery. Of interest, prior whole-brain radiation is not considered a risk factor.[66]

Some cases of radiation necrosis spontaneously resolve, others stabilize while still others progress. Medical management has been attempted. Steroids in particular may reduce acute clinical symptoms due to swelling. Others have suggested anticoagulation, especially heparin and possibly hyperbaric oxygen. Additional agents, such as pentobarbital, desferrioxamine and pentoxifylline, are being studied. In case of significant mass effect, surgery is indicated.[58]

Radiation myelopathy

Early or (transient) radiation myelopathy occurs 6 weeks to 6 months following onset of radiation. Symptoms are mild and include L'Hermitte's sign, that is, sensation of an electric shock upon neck flexion. Complete recovery is anticipated in 2–9 months. The pathology is transient demyelination of the posterior columns and lateral spinothalamic tracts, presumably due to radiation damage to the oligodendroglia.

In contrast to the excellent prognosis associated with early radiation myelopathy, delayed radiation myelopathy has more serious consequences. This syndrome occurs in <1 to 12.5 per cent of patients and may occur months to years following radiation therapy. The condition is characterized by acute or progressive paraplegia or quadriplegia, a sensory level, and loss of bowel and bladder function.[67] Demyelination with loss of axons and spinal cord necrosis are identified at autopsy. Vascular changes include endothelial thickening, vasculitis, telangiectasia, fibrinoid necrosis and perivascular fibrosis.[68] The development of radiation myelopathy correlates with the total dose (>6000 cGy) and fraction size (>200 cGy).[67]

MRI has been helpful in the diagnosis of radiation myelopathy. Typical findings are spinal cord edema with ring enhancement on T1 and increased intramedullary signal on T2. Over time, spinal cord atrophy develops with normal signal intensity.[68] Cerebrospinal fluid typically shows an increased protein with lymphocytosis.[69] Somatosensory-evoked potentials can also be helpful, as they tend to correlate with the extent of the lesion, as does slowing of spinal conduction velocity.[68]

To make the diagnosis of radiation myelopathy, the neurologic symptoms should reflect the anatomical site of pathology, which must lie within the radiation port. In addition, other diagnoses such as tumor, hemorrhage and infection must be excluded. Finally, time elapsed after radiation, total radiation dose and fraction size should be consistent with the diagnosis.

The treatment of radiation myelopathy is rarely successful. Steroids are typically given during the acute phase to reduce edema. Recently, anticoagulation has been proposed for radiation necrosis of the brain as well as for radiation myelopathy. In at least one study, improvement was noted in the majority of patients. The theoretical reason to use anticoagulation is that it may prevent further damage and perhaps even reverse damage to the endothelium of small blood vessels.[67]

CHEMOTHERAPY-ASSOCIATED MYELOPATHY

Myelopathy has been reported following IT methotrexate with and without IT cytosine arabinoside. Initially, reports of chemotherapy-induced paraplegia were attributed to the benzyl alcohol preservative, which was a diluent for IT methotrexate. Unfortunately, by 1980, even when the preservative was changed, reports of methotrexate-associated paraplegia persisted.[70] The risk of developing myelopathy is highest in children with meningeal disease as the clearance of methotrexate is altered leading to not only elevated methotrexate levels, but prolonged duration of exposure. Myelopathy has also been reported, however, in the absence of CNS leukemia.

Cytosine arabinoside is another agent implicated in producing myelopathy.[71] Twenty-three patients were culled from the literature, including ten with no evidence of CNS disease. Only two of the 23 had complete recovery, while eight died, three were ventilator-dependent and ten remained paraplegic. Spinal cord necrosis was identified at autopsy. In this study, three patients had received cytosine arabinoside alone either intrathecally or in combination with high-dose IV cytosine arabinoside, suggesting that, even in the absence of methotrexate, it can also cause this phenomenon. Other risk factors include prior spinal cord irradiation as well as the total dose and frequency of drug administration.[72]

Clinically, myelopathy is characterized by weakness or paralysis, a sensory level usually in the lumbar thoracic region, and loss of bowel and bladder function. During the phase of spinal shock, the patient may be flaccid and arreflexic, but over time spasticity, hyperreflexia, clonus and Babinski responses will appear. Although paraparesis typically occurs rapidly either immediately or within a short time following therapy, there are cases of an ascending myelopathy and death, which may occur as late as 5 weeks following therapy, and even cases of progressive paraplegia occurring months following cessation of intrathecal therapy.[71]

Included in the differential diagnosis of chemotherapy-induced myelopathy is spinal cord compression due to space-occupying lesions, such as blood, tumor or infection. Epidural hematomas may develop secondary to trauma or from hemorrhage when a lumbar puncture is performed in the face of thrombocytopenia. Chloromas, although rare, can cause spinal cord compression in the leukemic population.[73] Finally, immune-suppressed patients are at risk for epidural abscesses. In addition to spinal cord compression, transverse myelitis – either viral (herpetic), postviral or idiopathic – are in the differential diagnosis. Patients will present in an identical fashion as with drug- or radiation-induced myelopathy. During the phase of spinal shock, when tone may be flaccid instead of spastic, and reflexes may be absent rather than increased, Guillain–Barré syndrome and poliomyelitis must also be considered. Neither of these will have a sensory level, however.

On pathologic examination, the brunt of the insult is usually in the thoracic cord, primarily affecting myelin with sparing of the axons.[74] A typical pattern of microvacuolization and degeneration in the absence of inflammation is identified.[75] Necrosis may be present in both the gray and white matter of the cord, although spongiotic degeneration of the white matter with preservation of gray matter has been reported. Price reported subacute necrotizing leukomyelopathy in children with leukemia, which was associated with the use of >200 mg of IT methotrexate.[76] In this description, myelin necrosis was present in the lateral and posterior columns similar in appearance to subacute combined degeneration of the cord secondary to vitamin B_{12} deficiency. More recent pathologic descriptions of cytosine arabinoside-induced myelopathy report microvacuolization without inflammation rather than necrosis of white matter. In contrast, methotrexate-associated myelopathy has, at least in some cases, been associated with white matter necrosis and sparing of the gray matter.[72] Acute damage to spinal nerve roots within the subarachnoid space likely reflects a direct toxic effect of either the diluent or the chemotherapeutic agent itself.[77] If the chemotherapeutic agent is able to penetrate the central gray matter of the spinal cord, necrosis may develop. A vascular etiology has been invoked in these cases.[78] Rarer still is a syndrome of anterior horn cell destruction associated with a rapidly ascending paralysis that resembles poliomyelitis.[79]

Examination of cerebrospinal fluid may reveal elevation in CSF protein in approximately half the patients. There have been studies suggesting that myelin basic protein is not only elevated at the time of myelopathy but may be predictive of the future development of myelopathy. In general, it appears that, if myelin basic protein is elevated, concern should be raised. The absence of an elevation of myelin basic protein, however, does not exclude the development of myelopathy in the near future.[75,80]

Somatosensory-evoked potentials have revealed spinal cord dysfunction in children with ALL after having

received IT methotrexate. Despite electrophysiologic abnormalities, the children are clinically normal. The association between these abnormalities of somatosensory-evoked responses and frank myelopathy has not yet been determined.[81]

The specific etiology for chemotherapy-induced myelopathy is unknown, but includes a direct toxic effect of the agents (methotrexate, cytosine arabinoside or thiotepa), reduced spinal cord folate levels (in the case of IT methotrexate) and high levels of drug, owing to either abnormal clearance or too frequent administration.

The prognosis of chemotherapy-induced myelopathy is generally very poor, with most children dying or permanently paraplegic, although rare cases of recovery have been reported. Although steroids have been used, there is no effective therapy.

KEY POINTS

- Vincristine, cisplatinum, paclitaxel and thalidomide may cause peripheral neuropathies, which relate to dose and duration of therapy.
- Risk factors for severe vincristine-induced neuropathy include young age, cachexia, bed rest and an underlying peripheral neuropathy, such as Charcot–Marie–Tooth disease.
- Radiation-induced leukoencephalopathy correlates with dose, patient age, volume of radiation, fractionation schedule and time following radiation.
- Methotrexate-induced leukoencephalopathy may develop in the absence of either cranial irradiation or leptomeningeal disease.
- The ideal anticonvulsant for patients with seizures who are on chemotherapy should be an agent not metabolized by the liver, and one with limited hematologic and hepatic toxicity.
- Patients at highest risk for radiation-induced moyamoya disease are children with neurofibromatosis Type I who are less than 5 years of age and have been irradiated to the hypothalamic/chiasmatic regions with doses of >50 Gy.
- Radiation necrosis occurs in 5 per cent of patients 6 months to 2 years following cranial irradiation. Risk factors include dose >60 Gy and larger fractions (>200 cGy) given over a shorter period of time.
- Intrathecal methotrexate and cytosine arabinoside (ARA-C) have been associated with myelopathy characterized by weakness, sensory level, and loss of bowel and bladder function. The prognosis for recovery is poor.

REFERENCES

1. Postma TJ, Heimans JJ. Grading of chemotherapy-induced peripheral neuropathy. *Ann Oncol* 2000; **11**:509–513.
2. Sandler SG, Tobin W, Henderson ES. Vincristine-induced neuropathy. *Neurology* 1969; **19**:367–374.
◆3. Pal PK. Clinical and electrophysiological studies in vincristine induced neuropathy. *Electromyog Clin Neurophysiol* 1999; **39**:323–330.
4. Casey EB, Jellife AM, LeQuesne PM, *et al.* Vincristine neuropathy. Clinical and electrophysiological observations. *Brain* 1973; **96**:69–86.
●5. Allen J. Medical progress: The effects of cancer therapy on the nervous system. *J Pediatr* 1978; **93**:903–909.
6. Moudgil SS, Riggs JE. Fulminant peripheral neuropathy with severe quadriparesis associated with Vincristine therapy. *Ann Pharmacother* 2000; **34**:1136–1138.
7. Norman M, Elinder G, Finkel Y. Vincristine neuropathy and a Guillain–Barré Syndrome: a case with acute lymphatic leukemia and quadriparesis. *Eur J Haematol* 1987; **39**:75–76.
8. Jeng MR, Feusner J. Itraconazole-enhanced vincristine neurotoxicity in a child with acute lymphoblastic leukemia. *Pediatr Hematol Oncol* 2001; **18**:137–142.
◆9. Graf WD, Chance PF, Lensch MW, *et al.* Severe vincristine neuropathy in Charcot–Marie–Tooth Disease Type 1A. *Cancer* 1996; **77**:1356–1362.
10. Neumann Y, Toren A, Rechavi G, *et al.* Vincristine treatment triggering the expression of asymptomatic Charcot–Marie–Tooth Disease. *Med Pediatr Oncol* 1996; **26**:280–283.
11. Igarashi M, Thompson EI, Rivera GK. Vincristine neuropathy in Type I and Type II Charcot–Marie–Tooth Disease (hereditary motor sensory neuropathy). *Med Pediatr Oncol* 1995; **25**:113–116.
12. Molloy FM, Floeter MK, Syed NA, *et al.* Thalidomide neuropathy in patients treated for metastatic prostate cancer. *Muscle Nerve* 2001; **24**:1050–1057.
13. Calabrese L, Fleischer AB. Thalidomide: current and potential clinical applications. *Am J Med* 2000; **108**:487–495.
14. Hartmann JT, Kollmannsberger C, Kanz L, *et al.* Platinum organ toxicity and possible prevention in patients with testicular cancer. *Int J Cancer* 1999; **83**:866–869.
15. Planting AST, Catimel G, deMulder PHM, *et al.* Randomized study of a short course of weekly cisplatin with or without amifostine in advanced head and neck cancer. *Ann Oncol* 1999; **10**:693–700.
16. Markman M, Kennedy A, Webster K, *et al.* Neurotoxicity associated with a regimen of carboplatin (AUC 5-6) and paclitaxel (175 mg/m^2 over 3 h) employed in the treatment of gynecologic malignancies. *J Cancer Res Clin Oncol* 2001; **127**:55–58.
17. Mayerhofer K, Bodner-Adler B, Bodner K, *et al.* Paclitaxel/carboplatin as first-line chemotherapy in advanced ovarian cancer: Efficacy and adverse effects with special consideration of peripheral neurotoxicity. *Anticancer Res* 2000; **20**:4047–4050.
18. Hilkens PHE, Pronk LC, Verweij J, *et al.* Peripheral neuropathy induced by combination chemotherapy of docetaxel and cisplatin. *Br J Cancer* 1997; **75**:417–422.
19. Fazio R, Quattrini A, Bolognesi A. Docetaxel neuropathy: a distal axonopathy. *Acta Neuropathol* 1999; **98**:651–653.
20. Vahdat L, Papadopoulos K, Lange D, *et al.* Reduction of paclitaxel-induced peripheral neuropathy with glutamine. *Clin Cancer Res* 2001; **7**:1192–1197.
21. DiMaggio JR, Brown R, Baile WF, *et al.* Hallucinations and ifosfamide-induced neurotoxicity. *Cancer* 1994; **73**:1509–1514.
22. Cerny T, Küpfer A. The enigma of ifosfamide encephalopathy. *Ann Oncol* (editorial) 1992; **3**:679–681.

◆23. Comandone A, Liboni W, Picci P, *et al.* Two episodes of ifosfamide-related neurotoxicity in the same patient following different schedules and doses of the drug. A case report. *Tumori* 2000; **86**:483–486.

24. Zimmerman RD, Fleming CA, Lee BCP, *et al.* Periventricular hyperintensity as seen by magnetic resonance: prevalence and significance. *Am J Neuroradiol* 1986; **7**:13–20.

25. Filley C, Kleinschmidt-DeMasters BK. Toxic leukoencephalopathy. *N Engl J Med* 2001; **345**:425–431.

◆26. Constine LS, Konski A, Ekholm S, *et al.* Adverse effects of brain irradiation correlated with MR and CT imaging. *Int J Radiat Oncol Biol Phys* 1988; **15**:319–330.

◆27. Peylan-Ramu N, Poplack DG, Pizzo PA, *et al.* Abnormal CT scans of the brain in asymptomatic children with acute lymphocytic leukemia after prophylactic treatment of the central nervous system with radiation and intrathecal chemotherapy. *N Engl J Med* 1978; **298**:815–818.

28. Ochs JJ, Berger P, Brecher ML, *et al.* Computed tomography brain scans in children with acute lymphocytic leukemia receiving methotrexate alone as central nervous system prophylaxis. *Cancer* 1980; **45**:2274–2278.

◆29. Duffner PK, Cohen ME, Berger P, *et al.* Abnormalities of CT scans and altered methotrexate clearance in children with central nervous system leukemia. *Ann Neurol* 1981; **10**:286–287.

30. Ettinger LJ, Chervinsky DS, Freeman AI, Creaven PJ. Pharmacokinetics of methotrexate following intravenous and intraventricular administration in acute lymphocytic leukemia and non-Hodgkin's lymphoma. *Cancer* 1982; **50**:1676–1682.

31. Bleyer WA. Leukoencephalopathy detectable by magnetic resonance imaging: Much ado about nothing? Regarding Matsumoto *et al.*, IJROBP **32**:913–918; 1995. *Int J Radiat Oncol Biol Phys* 1995; **32**:1251–1252.

32. Pääkkö E, Harila-Saari A, Vanionpää L, *et al.* White matter changes on MRI during treatment in children with acute lymphoblastic leukemia: Correlation with neuropsychological findings. *Med Pediatr Oncol* 2000; **35**:456–461.

33. Wilson DA, Nitschke R, Bowman ME, *et al.* Transient white matter changes on MR images in children undergoing chemotherapy for acute lymphocytic leukemia: correlation with neuropsychologic deficiencies. *Radiology* 1991; **180**:205–209.

◆34. Mahoney D, Shuster J, Nitschke R. Acute neurotoxicity in children with B-precursor acute lymphoid leukemia: an association with intermediate-dose intravenous methotrexate and intrathecal triple therapy – A Pediatric Oncology Group Study. *J Clin Oncol* 1998; **16**:1712–1722.

◆35. Gilles FH, Sobel E, Leviton A, *et al.* Epidemiology of seizures in children with brain tumors. *Neurooncology* 1992; **12**:53–68.

36. Johnson JH, Hariharan S, Berman J, *et al.* Clinical outcome of pediatric gangliogliomas: Ninety-nine cases over 20 years. *Pediatr Neurosurg* 1997; **27**:203–207.

37. Daumas-Dupont C, Scheithauek BW, Chodkiewitz JP, *et al.* Dysembryoplastic neuroepithelial tumor: a surgically curable tumor of young patients with intractable epilepsy. *Neurosurgery* 1988; **23**:545–556.

38. Pahapill PA, Ramsay DA, DelMaestro RF. Pleomorphic xanthoastrocytoma: case report and analysis of the literature concerning the efficacy of resection and the significance of necrosis. *Neurosurgery* 1996; **38**:822–829.

39. Ruggieri V, Caraballo R, Fejerman N. Intracranial tumors and West syndrome. *Pediatr Neurol* 1989; **5**:327–329.

◆40. Ochs JJ, Bowman P, Pui CH, *et al.* Seizures in childhood lymphoblastic leukemia patients. *The Lancet* 1984; **2**:1422–1424.

41. Maytal J, Grossman R, Yusuf FH, *et al.* Prognosis and treatment of seizures in children with acute lymphoblastic leukemia. *Epilepsia* 1995; **36**:831–836.

42. Mead GM, Arnold AM, Green JA, *et al.* Epileptic seizures associated with Cisplatin administration. *Cancer Treat Rep* 1982; **66**:1719–1722.

43. Johnson FL, Bernstein ID, Hartmann Jr, *et al.* Seizures associated with vincristine sulfate therapy. *J Pediatr* 1973; **82**:699–702.

44. Foreman NK, Mahmoud HH, Rivera GK. Recurrent cerebrovascular accident with L-asparaginase rechallenge. *Med Pediatr Oncol* 1992; **20**:532–534.

◆45. Feinberg WM, Swenson MR. Cerebrovascular complications of L-asparaginase therapy. *Neurol* 1988; **38**:127–133.

46. Warren RD, Bender RA. (Commentary) Drug interactions with antineoplastic agents. *Cancer Treat Rep* 1977. **61**:1231–1239.

47. Delattre JY, Safai B, Posner JB. Erythema multiforme and Stevens–Johnson syndrome in patients receiving cranial irradiation and phenytoin. *Neurology* 1988; **38**:194–198.

◆48. Omura M, Aida N, Sekido K. Large intracranial vessel occlusive vasculopathy after radiation therapy in children: Clinical features and usefulness of magnetic resonance imaging. *Int J Radiat Oncol Biol Phys* 1997; **38**:241–249.

49. Bitzer M, Topka H. Progressive cerebral occlusive disease after radiation therapy. *Stroke* 1995; **26**:131–136.

◆50. Kestle JRW, Hoffman HJ, Mock AR. Moyamoya phenomenon after radiation for optic glioma. *J Neurosurg* 1993; **79**:32–35.

51. Ross, IB, Shevell MI, Montes JL, *et al.* Encephaloduro-arteriosynangiosis (EDAS) for the treatment of childhood Moyamoya disease. *Pediatr Neurol* 1994; **10**:199–204.

52. Jensen FK, Wagner A. Intracranial aneurysm following radiation therapy for medulloblastoma. *Acta Radiol* 1997; **38**:37–42.

◆53. Scodary DJ, Tew JM, Thomas GM. Radiation-induced cerebral aneurysms. *Acta Neurochir (Wien)* 1990; **102**:141–144.

54. Azzarelli B, Moore J, Gilmor R, *et al.* Multiple fusiform intracranial aneurysms following curative radiation therapy for suprasellar germinoma. *J Neurosurg* 1984; **61**:1141–1145.

◆55. Marks JE, Baglan RJ, Prassad SC, *et al.* Cerebral radionecrosis: incidence and risk in relation to dose, time, fractionation, and volume. *Int J Radiat Oncol Biol Phys* 1980; **7**:243–252.

◆56. Marks JE, Wong J. The risk of cerebral radionecrosis in relation to dose, time and fractionation. *Prog Exp Tumor Res* 1985; **29**:210–218.

57. Tandon N, Vollmer DG, New PZ, *et al.* Fulminant radiation-induced necrosis after stereotactic radiation therapy to the posterior fossa. *J Neurosurg* 2001; **95**:507–512.

58. Glass JP, Hwang T-L, Leavens ME, *et al.* Cerebral radiation necrosis following treatment of extracranial malignancies. *Cancer* 1984; **54**:1966–1972.

59. al Mefty O, Kersh JE, Routh A, Smith RR. The long-term side effects of radiation therapy for benign brain tumors in adults. *J Neurosurg* 1990; **73**:502–512.

◆60. Martins AN, Johnston JS, Henry JM, *et al.* Delayed radiation necrosis of the brain. *J Neurosurg* 1977; **47**:336–345.

61. Takeuchi J, Hanakita J, Abe M, *et al.* Brain necrosis after repeated radiotherapy. *Surg Neurol* 1976; **5**:89–93.

62. Kumar AJ, Leeds NE, Fuller GN. Malignant gliomas: MR imaging spectrum of radiation therapy– and chemotherapy-induced necrosis of the brain after treatment. *Radiology* 2000; **217**:377–384.

63. Brismar J, Roberson GH, Davis KR. Radiation necrosis of the brain. Neuroradiological considerations with computed tomography. *Neuroradiology* 1976; **12**:109–113.

64. Thompson TP, Lunsford LD, Kondziolka D. Distinguishing recurrent tumor and radiation necrosis with positron emission tomography versus stereotactic biopsy. *Stereotact Funct Neurosurg* 1999; **73**:9–14.

65. Chan Y, Yeung DKW, Leung S. Proton magnetic resonance spectroscopy of late delayed radiation-induced injury of the brain. *J Magnetic Resonance Imaging* 1999; **10**:130–137.

66. Chin LS, DiBiase S. Radiation following gamma knife surgery: a case-controlled comparison of treatment parameters and long-term clinical follow up. *J Neurosurg* 2001; **94**:899–904.

67. Liu CY, Yim BT, Wozniak AJ. Anticoagulation therapy for radiation-induced myelopathy. *Ann Pharmacother* 2001; **35**:188–191.

68. Rampling R, Symonds P. Radiation myelopathy. *Curr Opin Neurol* 1998; **11**:627–632.

69. Chao MWT, Wirth A, Ryan G, *et al.* Radiation myelopathy following transplantation and radiotherapy for non-Hodgkin's lymphoma. *Int J Radiat Oncol Biol Phys* 1998; **41**:1057–1061.

◆70. Hahn AF, Feasby TE, Gilbert JJ. Paraparesis following intrathecal chemotherapy. *Neurology* 1983; **33**:1032–1038.

71. Dunton SF, Nitschke R, Spruce WE, *et al.* Progressive ascending paralysis following administration of intrathecal and intravenous cytosine arabinoside. A Pediatric Oncology Group Study. *Cancer* 1986; **57**:1083–1088.

◆72. Watterson J, Toogood I, Nieder M, *et al.* Excessive spinal cord toxicity from intensive central nervous system-directed therapies. *Cancer* 1994; **74**:3034–3041.

73. Keidan SE. Paraplegia in childhood malignant disease. *Acta Paediat Scand* 1967; Suppl. **172**:110–118.

74. McLean DR, Clink HM, Ernst P, *et al.* Myelopathy after intrathecal chemotherapy. *Cancer* 1994; **73**:3037–3040.

75. Bates SE, Raphaelson MI, Price RA, *et al.* Ascending myelopathy after chemotherapy for central nervous system acute lymphoblastic leukemia: correlation with cerebrospinal fluid myelin basic protein. *Med Pediatr Oncol* 1985; **13**:4–8.

◆76. Price RA, Jamieson PA. The central nervous system in childhood leukemia. *Cancer* 1975; **35**:306–318.

77. Saiki JH, Thompson S, Smith F, *et al.* Paraplegia following intrathecal chemotherapy. *Cancer* 1972; **29**:370–374.

78. Von der Weid NX, de Crousaz H, Beck D, *et al.* Acute fatal myeloencephalopathy after combined intrathecal chemotherapy in a child with acute lymphoblastic leukemia. *Med Pediatr Oncol* 1991; **19**:192–198.

79. Reznik, M. Acute ascending poliomyelomalacia after treatment of acute lymphocytic leukemia. *Acta Neuropathol (Berl)* 1979; **45**:153–157.

80. Werner RA. Paraplegia and quadriplegia after intrathecal chemotherapy. *Arch Phys Med Rehabil* 1988; **69**:1054–1056.

81. Vainionpaa L, Kovala T, Tolonen U, *et al.* Chemotherapy for acute lymphoblastic leukemia may cause subtle changes of the spinal cord detectable by somatosensory evoked potentials. *Med Pediatr Oncol* 1997; **28**:41–47.

2b

Neuropsychological outcomes

RAYMOND K MULHERN, SEAN PHIPPS AND HOLLY WHITE

INTRODUCTION

The present subchapter will focus on the neuropsychological aspects of the medical treatment of childhood cancer by discussing current knowledge of brain damage among patients and how it is reflected in their cognitive abilities. We will direct these efforts towards the two most common forms of childhood cancer, acute lymphoblastic leukemia (ALL) and brain tumors. In addition, we will discuss neuropsychological implications for bone marrow (stem cell) transplantation because of its increasing prevalence in the treatment of childhood cancers. For each of these three topics, we will first provide the reader with a brief medical background followed by a review of the current literature. The literature review will provide an in-depth analysis of the types of cognitive impairments observed, and known or suspected risk factors for impairments. Finally, we will close the subchapter with a section that discusses interventions with the potential to prevent or minimize cognitive deficits acquired in the course of cancer treatment and their impact on the quality of life of pediatric cancer survivors.

Our review will discuss primarily neuropsychological 'late effects' that are associated with childhood cancer and its treatment. The study of late effects presupposes that patients are long-term survivors, if not permanently cured, of their disease. Late effects are temporally defined as occurring after the successful completion of medical therapy, usually 2 or more years from the time of diagnosis, and it is generally assumed that late effects are chronic, if not progressive in their course. This definition serves to separate late effects from those effects of disease and treatment that are acute or subacute and time-limited, such as chemotherapy-induced nausea and vomiting or temporary cognitive changes induced by cranial irradiation.

Research interest in neuropsychological outcomes, as well as neurologic and other functional late effects, has shown an increase commensurate with improvements in effective therapy. For example, 30 years ago when few children were cured of ALL, questions relating to the ultimate academic or vocational performance of long-term survivors were trivial compared to the need for improved therapy. In contrast, today, more than 80 per cent of children diagnosed with ALL can be cured, and issues relating to their quality of life as long-term survivors have now received increased emphasis. There is at least comparable attention to the neuropsychologic status of children with primary brain tumors and growing interest in that of children receiving stem cell transplants.

ACUTE LYMPHOBLASTIC LEUKEMIA

Medical background

Approximately 20 000 children and adolescents under the age of 20 were diagnosed with cancer in 1999.[1] The most commonly diagnosed cancer in this age group is acute lymphoblastic leukemia, a malignant disorder of lymphoid cells found in the bone marrow that migrates to virtually every organ system, including the central nervous system (CNS), via the circulatory system. ALL accounts for one-fourth of all childhood cancers and 75 per cent of all cases of childhood leukemia.[2] In the USA, approximately 3000 children are diagnosed with ALL each year with an incidence of 3–4 cases per 100 000

white children. ALL is more common among white than black children, and is also more common among boys than girls with a peak incidence at 4 years of age. Although genetic, environmental, viral and immunodeficiency factors have been implicated in the pathogenesis of ALL, the precise causes of most cases of ALL remain largely unknown.

Presenting symptoms include fever, fatigue, pallor, anorexia, bone pain and bruising. Because the symptoms of ALL can mimic a number of non-malignant conditions, definitive diagnosis, usually made by bone marrow aspiration, is sometimes delayed. The duration of treatment varies from 30 to 36 months, and, in the modern era, is usually restricted to intervention with combination chemotherapy, reserving cranial irradiation for patients who experience a CNS relapse. A better prognosis is associated with female gender, age at diagnosis between 2 and 10 years, a lower white blood cell count and an earlier positive response to treatment. Treatment can be divided into four phases: remission induction, CNS preventative therapy, consolidation, and maintenance. The purpose of the remission induction phase is to eradicate leukemia cells from the bone marrow and circulatory system rapidly. CNS preventative therapy is necessary because the CNS is a sanctuary for occult leukemia. Traditionally, CNS therapy has included cranial radiation therapy (CRT) and intrathecal chemotherapy, usually with methotrexate (MTX) or methotrexate combined with other drugs. However, because of the risks for CNS toxicity to be discussed later in this subchapter, treatment is now usually restricted to intrathecal and systemic chemotherapy with equivalent success in the prevention of CNS relapses. Consolidation may be used to intensify therapy following remission induction. Maintenance therapy is required for a prolonged period because of the presence of undetectable levels of leukemia that, nevertheless, have the capacity to be fatal. After the completion of treatment, approximately 20 per cent of those children who will eventually relapse will do so in the first year off therapy with a subsequent risk of relapse in the remaining patients of 2–3 per cent per year for the next 3–4 years.

Neuropsychological outcomes: intellectual decline

Recent reviews indicate that an overwhelming majority of studies that have investigated the neurocognitive morbidity of CRT in leukemia patients have found significant adverse effects.[3,4] The primary literature also confirms that children treated for ALL demonstrate significant intellectual declines in response to a myriad of approaches to CNS therapy.[5–9] In general, recent reviews of this literature have concluded that children with intellectual decline

understandably have increasing difficulty with academic achievement, that intellectual declines are usually more severe among children who are younger at the time of treatment and those who receive more aggressive therapy (i.e. more intensive chemotherapy or irradiation), and that these adverse effects of treatment are delayed but progressive.[10] The strongest evidence comes from longitudinally designed studies with internal control or comparison groups.

For example, the group at Children's Hospital of Los Angeles reported on 24 patients treated for ALL who had received CNS prophylactic therapy with 18 Gy CRT, intrathecal MTX and intravenous MTX.[11] Patients were assessed with IQ testing prior to beginning CNS therapy and at 1 and 4 years later. Although IQ scores remained stable at the 1-year interval, significant declines in full-scale, verbal and performance IQ scores were noted at the 4-year follow-up testing, with a mean loss of 6–7 IQ points. Furthermore, 12 of the 24 children had received special educational services at the final assessment, with three of the 12 having repeated a grade prior to receiving special services. These results were disappointing because of the expectation that a reduction of the traditional CRT dose from 24 Gy to 18 Gy would minimize neurocognitive toxicity.

In a unique analysis across two institutional protocols at St Jude Children's Research Hospital, patients who had received 24 Gy CRT and those who had been randomized to receive 18 Gy CRT or no CRT were compared over time with regard to their neurocognitive development.[12] All patients also received intrathecal MTX and intravenous MTX therapy. With a median follow-up of 6.8–8.4 years for the groups, only small and non-significant changes in IQ values were noted with no significant differences between groups. However, 22–30 per cent of all patients showed a clinically significant decline of full-scale IQ over the study interval and scores on tests of arithmetic declined over time compared to normal expectations of same-age peers. Interestingly, one explanation for the lack of differences between CNS therapy groups were differences in parenteral MTX; the 18-Gy group had the lowest total dose, those in the 24-Gy group had approximately 1.5 times more, and those not receiving CRT received 10.7 times more MTX.

More recently, serial neurocognitive evaluations were performed on 30 children surviving ALL to 4-years post-diagnosis.[13] Patients had received CNS treatment with chemotherapy only. Although IQ scores remained stable, arithmetic achievement declined significantly as well as patients' verbal fluency and visual–motor skills. These results recapitulated earlier reports that intrathecal and/or intravenous MTX were not benign to the CNS. For example, one cross-sectional study of 47 long-term survivors of ALL treated with chemotherapy only found statistically significant deficits in performance IQ, as well

as perceptual organization, and freedom from distractibility scores, but no significant problems with academic achievement.[14]

It is worth noting that at least one prospective study failed to find IQ losses among patients treated without CRT at a 3-year follow-up.[15] Other types of chemotherapy, such as the use of dexamethasone instead of prednisone, in the treatment of children with ALL may also confer increased risk for neurocognitive impairment.[9]

Neuropsychological outcomes: mental processing

Unfortunately, it is often difficult to separate the late neurocognitive effects of treatment (e.g. IQ loss, academic failure) from the effects of other, non-biological factors associated with childhood illness such as loss of social and environmental stimulation and missed school days.[16] It would also be preferable to identify early cognitive changes that predict later IQ loss. For these reasons, several studies have attempted to measure cognitive functioning using mental processing paradigms rather than relying on IQ and achievement testing that depend heavily on previously learned skills and information.[17,18] The results have been mixed, presumably due to methodological variation and extreme within-sample variation. Despite these difficulties, recent findings are beginning to converge on specific cognitive processes that may underlie general cognitive impairments, typically summarized by the IQ score, observed in childhood ALL survivors. The majority of these cognitive processes fall under the umbrella of 'executive' or goal-directed cognitive processes. Executive functions are thought to be primarily mediated by control mechanisms in the frontal cortex, and include the ability to integrate multiple sources of information, keep track of multiple goals, ignore distracting information and focus on new information or activities.[19,20] The focus of this section will be to discuss several relevant empirical studies of cognitive processes involving two aspects of executive functioning, attention and working memory, with the aim of constructing a coherent picture describing the intellectual impairments associated with chemotherapy/CRT in pediatric ALL survivors.

'Attention' is a broad term that refers to a group of interrelated cognitive processes, including the ability to alert or orient to stimuli, selectively attend to stimuli while ignoring distracting information, sustain focused attention and disengage and reengage focus on new stimuli.[21] 'Working memory' is another broad concept that can be loosely defined as the ability to hold task-relevant information in mind (or 'online') while simultaneously performing operations on that information.[20] Working memory functions support higher cognitive functions (e.g. strategic, goal-directed activities), involving

active maintenance (i.e. sustained attention), regulation, and control (i.e. selective attention) of information. Clearly, attention and working memory are not independent constructs. The inhibitory processes associated with selective attention are also required to keep irrelevant information from disrupting the task-relevant contents of working memory.[22]

Contemporary models of attention deficit hyperactivity disorder (ADHD) theorize that poor inhibitory control underlies working memory deficits, which in turn impair attention.[23] This theory of ADHD is consistent with popular models of executive functioning that suggest a high degree of overlap between attention, working memory, and other executive processes.[21,24] In practice, clinicians and researchers often make a distinction between executive cognitive processes, either for simplicity or because many of the available tests to measure these constructs lend themselves to such a distinction. For consistency and clarity, we divided our review of late neurocognitive effects into sections on attention deficits and working memory deficits.

ATTENTIONAL DEFICITS

Studies of attention deficits in ALL survivors have used paradigms that range in complexity from simple detection tasks to more challenging tasks involving selective attention and task-switching. Brouwers et al.[25] examined attentional functioning in long-term survivors of ALL who had been treated with intrathecal chemotherapy and CNS-directed radiation therapy. Using a simple alerted reaction time (SRT) task, Brouwers et al. compared the performance of 13 ALL patients with computed tomography (CT) scan abnormalities of the brain against 10 ALL patients with normal CT scans. The abnormal CT scan group was further subdivided into a cerebral atrophy group ($n = 8$) and an intracerebral calcifications group ($n = 5$). The SRT task required subjects to perform a simple reaction, such as a key press, in response to a stimulus, such as a light or a tone. In this task, the stimulus onset is preceded by an alerting/warning signal. This study revealed reaction-time impairments for patients with abnormal scans relative to patients with normal scans. Specifically, patients with abnormal scans reacted more slowly, and with more variability (especially at longer inter-stimulus intervals), than those with normal scans. The authors noted that response variability across interstimulus intervals was indicative of an attentional, rather than motor, impairment. In addition, task performance was most impaired for patients with intracerebral calcifications. These lesions tended to occur in basal ganglia and parietal regions, consistent with observed deficits in processing speed and sustained attention.

Attention deficits may affect cognitive functioning in others areas, as well. A study conducted by Brouwers and

Poplack[26] examined verbal and non-verbal memory in long-term survivors of ALL treated with combination CRT/intrathecal chemotherapy. As in Brouwers et al.,[25] children were divided into three groups, according to level of CT scan abnormality, and presented with two stories from the Wechsler Memory Scale (WMS) to assess verbal memory. The results indicated that those patients with normal CT scans outperformed patients with abnormal CT scans. As in the earlier study, patients with intracerebral calcifications showed greater impairment than patients with atrophy and patients with normal scans. When the authors correlated these and other memory and learning scores with the attentional impairments reported in Brouwers et al.,[25] they found that median reaction time correlated significantly with accuracy scores on all the verbal and non-verbal learning and memory tests. When attentional impairment was controlled statistically, group differences were greatly attenuated, especially in the verbal–linguistic domain. The authors concluded that attentional deficits are a major factor in the learning impairments and intellectual decline demonstrated by ALL patients.

Rodgers et al.[27] used a clinical model of attention to examine attentional abilities in ALL survivors, divided into three primary processes: 'focus' (encode, execute), 'sustain' and 'shift'.[28] The investigators studied a group of 19 long-term survivors of childhood ALL who were treated with combined CRT/chemotherapy, and a group of 19 sibling controls. 'Focus encode' was measured using the arithmetic and digit span subtests of the Wechsler intelligence scale for children, and 'focus execute' was examined using the speed of information processing subtest of the British ability scales and the coding subtest of the Wechsler Intelligence Scale for Children – Revised (WISC-R). The Vigil Continuous Performance Test (VIGIL) test battery was used to measure 'sustain' and the Wisconsin card-sorting test (WCST) was used to measure 'shift'. Rodgers et al.[27] found that ALL survivors were impaired, relative to sibling controls, on the focus elements (encode and execute). However, no significant group differences were found for the sustain and shift elements of attention. Although the measure of shift was not impaired, the children in the ALL group had more difficulty in maintaining an appropriate task set during the WCST relative to sibling controls. Specifically, children in the ALL group were more likely than controls to process each trial independently and were less able to execute strategy across trials. The investigators interpreted these findings as indicating that perhaps the ALL survivors, because of their slower processing speed, were unable to modify behavior in response to experimenter feedback.

Lockwood et al.[18] conducted a study of the long-term effects of CRT on attention functioning in survivors of childhood leukemia, using a different theoretical model of attention than that used in the Rodgers et al. study.[27]

Lockwood et al.[18] separated attention into four components: 'sensory selection', 'response selection', 'attentional capacity' and 'sustained attention' using Cohen's model.[29] In this model, 'sensory selection' refers to stimulus filtering, simple focusing and automatic shifting of attention. 'Response selection' involves the inhibition and control of attention during goal-directed activity; this includes intentional, active switching. 'Attentional capacity' involves processing speed, temporal and spatial constraints, global resources, arousal and motivation. Finally, 'sustained attention' in Cohen's model of attention refers to the maintenance of attention and responses over time.

Lockwood et al.[18] tested 56 survivors of childhood leukemia whose treatment had been randomly assigned to chemotherapy only or combined chemotherapy/CRT treatment. The investigators observed better performance for the chemotherapy alone group, relative to the chemotherapy/CRT group, on measures indicative of sensory selection and attentional capacity. Taken together, the results of Lockwood et al.[18] and Rodgers et al.[27] indicate that children treated with CRT tend to show greater impairments in speed of information processing and selective (focused) attention compared to children not treated with CRT. However, the results are less straightforward with regard to the presence of deficits in attentional shifting. Irradiated children in the Lockwood et al.[18] study performed poorly on the TRAILS B, a measure of response selection (shift) that requires the participant to alternate between number searching and letter searching. These authors concluded that the CRT-treated children showed disrupted active mental shifting. In contrast, Rodgers et al.[27] did not find support for deficits in shift when using the WCST, despite the fact that this test has been found to correlate strongly with shifting ability as measured by tasks designed specifically to tap attention shifting.[30] Indeed, Rodgers et al.[27] found that ALL survivors had difficulty keeping task-relevant information in mind while performing the WCST. However, Rodgers et al.[27] used a different aspect of WCST performance (perseverations score) as the basis for their conclusions. Hence, the apparent contradiction between the Rodgers et al.[27] and Lockwood et al.[18] studies is probably an artifact of using different tests.

Working memory deficits

In addition to uncovering attentional deficits in survivors of ALL, empirical research has provided compelling evidence for working memory impairments in this population as well (e.g. Brouwers,[26] Cousens et al.[17]). In fact, some researchers argue that working memory impairment is primarily responsible for the intellectual decline in ALL survivors.[31]

Rodgers et al.[27] speculated that the attentional task-set disruption observed in their study occurred because ALL

survivors were unable to modify their responding, perhaps because of relatively slow processing speed. While this argument does not directly implicate working memory, it does suggest that processing speed deficits underlie the failure to maintain task set. This is consistent with the recent model of cognitive deficits in ALL survivors proposed by Schatz et al.[31] These researchers used statistical modeling to illustrate that IQ differences between ALL children treated with CRT versus non-irradiated controls were mediated by variations in working memory function, which in turn were partially accounted for by differences in processing speed. By this logic, the processing speed deficits observed in Rodgers et al.[27] may have indirectly contributed to the failure to maintain a task set by disrupting working memory, an interpretation that is consistent with the Schatz et al.[31] theoretical framework of cognitive dysfunction in ALL survivors.

Schatz et al. published a study examining delayed neurocognitive deficits in long-term survivors of acute lymphoblastic leukemia (ALL).[31] The results of this study revealed that survivors of ALL treated with CRT were impaired on tasks of processing speed, IQ and working memory, relative to matched healthy controls. The ALL survivors treated with chemotherapy alone did not differ from healthy controls on these measures. IQ differences between the CRT group and control group were mediated by differences in working memory. However, processing speed only partially accounted for the working memory deficits observed in the CRT group. Based upon these findings, Schatz et al. proposed a developmental model in which CRT affects processing speed and working memory, processing speed moderates working memory declines, and working memory mediates intellectual impairment (IQ).

Neuropathology of neuropsychological deficits

Unfortunately, the treatment of ALL is associated with adverse effects on healthy tissue in the CNS that place survivors at significant risk for serious cognitive impairments.[3,4] Combined chemotherapy/CRT is generally associated with greater declines in intellectual and academic functioning than chemotherapy alone.[16,32] Late effects of treatment-related CNS injury in ALL survivors may include diffuse and multifocal white matter abnormalities, demyelination, breakdown of the blood – brain barrier, microvascular occlusion, and calcifications in cortical gray matter and basal ganglia.[33,34] However, white matter injury is perhaps the principal factor in radiation- and chemotherapy-related CNS damage.

White matter is especially prone to radiation necrosis and demyelination is frequently observed in the CNS

following treatment.[35] Chemotherapy, especially methotrexate, is also associated with white matter injury and subsequent leukoencephalopathy.[36] Leukoencephalopathy generally emerges as a late effect of treatment. The clinical course of this pathology is gradual, characterized by decreased alertness and, eventually, intellectual decline.[37] Neuropathologically, multiple necrotic lesions in the periventricular white matter characterize leukoencephalopathy. As demyelination occurs, axons near the lesions become swollen without an inflammatory response. Patterns of white-matter loss in animal models of treatment-related CNS injury suggest the involvement of vascular impairment in the demyelination process.[38]

The course of white matter injury during cancer treatment and its impact on neurocognitive function is further complicated by significant variance in white-matter volume and distribution as a function of age and development. The development of myelin normally continues after birth into the third decade of life[39] and, while the cerebral hemispheres are about 50 per cent myelin, patterns of myelination differ across brain regions. The brainstem and cerebellar areas myelinate first, followed by the cerebral hemispheres and, finally, the anterior portions of the frontal lobes. Myelination of brain regions appears to parallel their functional maturation.[39] The interrelatedness of cognitive functions and the brain regions that support these functions is reflected in the rich connections between myelin in different brain areas; for example, frontal lobe white matter is linked extensively to posterior cortical and subcortical areas of the brain. White matter volumes vary from region to region. For example, the right frontal lobe is especially rich in myelin. For this reason, diffuse injury to white matter might disproportionately affect the cognitive processes of this region (e.g. attention, visuospatial ability). Hence, a global pathology of white matter can result in specific as well as non-specific impairments in cognitive function.[40]

For example, the loss of myelin in ALL survivors might be associated with relatively specific cognitive impairments (e.g. selective attention deficits), as well as widely distributed functions in the brain, such as information processing speed. In a related study, de Groot et al.[41] demonstrated that deficits in the speed of information processing correlated with the volume of white matter loss among older adults. New research findings are developing a link between white matter loss and neurocognitive outcome in survivors of pediatric cancer, as well.[42]

Risk factors for neurocognitive impairments

The well-documented findings of intellectual impairment in ALL survivors has prompted researchers to further investigate the risk factors that are associated with the development of cognitive dysfunction in long-term

survivors of childhood leukemia. Variables include age, gender, socioeconomic status (SES), baseline intelligence, age of diagnosis, therapeutic approach used to treat the cancer, and duration of therapy. When associated with a negative outcome, these variables are termed 'risk factors' and when linked to a positive outcome, they are termed 'protective factors'. The identification of these factors will potentially aid clinicians in making important decisions regarding treatment planning and intervention.

Waber et al.[43] examined the effects of age, gender, SES and treatment modality on cognitive impairment in a group of children treated for ALL. This study utilized a control group with solid tumors to assess the risks associated with CNS prophylaxis. The preventative therapy for the ALL group included CNS-directed radiation therapy and intrathecal methotrexate. The solid tumor control group had radiation at the site of the tumor and systemic chemotherapy. These investigators measured intellectual and academic functioning in both groups of children by administering the WISC-R, the Wide Range Academic Achievement Test – Revised (WRAT-R) and the Test of Reading Comprehension (TORC). The ALL group performed below average norms on all measures, while the solid tumor group performed above average on all measures. Group differences indicated that the ALL group was more cognitively impaired than the tumor group and females in both groups were more impaired than males. In addition, the correlation between age, SES and cognitive impairment within the ALL group differed as a function of gender. Specifically, early age of diagnosis and low SES were associated with more severe cognitive impairment in females, while these factors did not reliably correlate for males. The authors concluded that the major risk factor for CNS toxicity among children treated for ALL was gender; specifically, females were more impaired than males. Additionally, for females only, low SES and early age of diagnosis were predictive of greater impairment.

More recently, Waber et al.[44] investigated the relationship of treatment modality and gender to neurocognitive outcome in ALL. This newer study failed to replicate the age of diagnosis effect on cognitive outcome demonstrated in the 1990 study. However, consistent with earlier findings, the investigators showed dose-related, gender-dependent effects of treatment on cognitive functioning in ALL survivors. Specifically, higher doses of chemotherapy (intravenous methotrexate) were associated with IQ decline, but only for females. Performance on measures of language-based academic skill and memory for digit strings did not differ as a function of gender. However, only the females demonstrated an overall decline in cognitive function, as measured by IQ. Systemic chemotherapy was also associated with lower IQ, but only for females. Hence, this study suggested that systemic, as well as CNS, chemotherapy should be evaluated as a risk factor for cognitive impairment, especially for females.

Brown et al.[5] investigated the effects of prophylactic chemotherapy and time on cognitive functioning in survivors of childhood ALL. These investigators compared four groups of children: ALL patients recently diagnosed, ALL patients 1 year postdiagnosis, ALL patients off-therapy and healthy sibling controls. This design enabled the observation of the short-term and cumulative effects of systemic and intrathecal chemotherapy on cognitive functioning. The results were consistent with late effects of chemotherapy. Specifically, longer intervals between treatment and neurocognitive testing were associated with a more severe cognitive outcome. Indeed, children in the 1 year postdiagnosis group were not significantly impaired relative to healthy sibling controls. In addition, the effects associated with chemotherapy alone were less severe than those associated with the combined CRT/chemotherapy therapeutic approach. However, chemotherapy alone was associated with simultaneous and spatial processing deficits, impairments presumably linked with impaired right-hemispheric dysfunction. This study underscores the importance of continuing neurocognitive evaluation for all survivors of ALL, including those treated with chemotherapy alone.

The type of cancer therapy (e.g. radiation therapy versus chemotherapy) is not the only aspect of treatment strategy that affects the neurocognitive outcome of ALL survivors. Intellectual functioning among ALL survivors is also influenced by the dose of CRT and the drug combination and route of administration (i.e. systemic vs. intrathecal) of chemotherapy. A recent study by Waber et al.[9] found that two chemotherapeutic agents, dexamethasone and prednisone, were associated with different severities of neurocognitive outcome. While both of these drugs are glucocorticoid steroids, dexamethasone is more cytotoxic and CNS penetrating than prednisone. Because these characteristics enhance the clinical effectiveness of dexamethasone, this drug has recently been used in place of, or in addition to, prednisone in the treatment of ALL. Both dexamethasone and prednisone are toxic to neurons in the hippocampus and have the potential to cause damage to the memory system. Consistent with the regions of neurotoxicity associated with these drugs, the adverse effects of these agents are associated with tasks that involve a high demand on memory and learning processes.[9] However, children treated with dexamethasone showed greater cognitive deficits relative to children treated with prednisone. Hence, the lower incidence of relapse achieved with dexamethasone might be associated with more severe long-term cognitive dysfunction, a trade-off that should be considered when planning a therapeutic approach.

Age at diagnosis is another risk factor that has been studied extensively, in part because young children are generally at the greatest risk for traumatic events during development. This very young patient subgroup is at

high risk for CNS disease and, therefore, often requires aggressive prophylactic therapy to prevent relapse. Mulhern and colleagues conducted a cross-sectional study of 26 survivors of ALL treated in infancy and compared them to children surviving Wilm's tumor.[45] Overall, the patients treated for ALL performed significantly worse on testing of IQ, academic achievement, and memory than those treated for Wilm's tumor and had a higher incidence of special educational placement. There were trends noted for the severity of the neuropsychological deficits to be related to the dose of CRT used. A more recent study by Kaleita et al.[46] investigated cognitive functioning among ALL survivors who had been treated with very high-dose chemotherapy during infancy. Fortunately, the investigators reported favorable neurological outcomes for these children at follow-up (mean age = 5.2 years). Kaleita et al.[46] suggested that the neurocognitive outcome for ALL survivors treated during infancy is more favorable now than in the past. However, the authors acknowledge the possibility that late effects might emerge later in development. In summary, additional empirical research is necessary to clarify the role of risk factors in the neurocognitive outcome of ALL survivors.

Summary

The incidence and severity of neuropsychological impairments among children previously treated for ALL is variable, and depends upon the aggressiveness of CNS therapy, host factors, such as age of the patient at the time of treatment and possibly gender, time elapsed from completion of treatment, and methods of assessment. Clearly, the contemporary focus is on the assessment of executive functions, such as working memory, and other cognitive processes that affect learning for ALL survivors, but are not apparent until later captured by declining IQ and academic achievement test scores.

BRAIN TUMORS

Medical background

Pediatric brain tumors are considerably more heterogeneous than ALL in that they vary by histology as well as location. Next to ALL, brain tumors are the second most frequently diagnosed malignancy of childhood and the most common pediatric solid tumor with an annual incidence of 2.2–2.5 per 100 000.[47] The etiology of most pediatric brain tumors is unknown, although brain tumors can appear as a second malignancy following the treatment of ALL with cranial irradiation. Tumors are often characterized as being above (supratentorial) or below (infratentorial) the tentorium, a membrane that separates the cerebellum and brainstem from the rest of the brain. In approximate decreasing order of incidence, the most common tumors are supratentorial low-grade tumors, medulloblastoma, brainstem glioma, cerebellar astrocytomas, supratentorial high-grade tumors and craniopharyngioma.

Among the more common symptoms of a brain tumor are morning headaches, nausea and lethargy resulting from tumor obstruction of the ventricles and increased intracranial pressure. Problems with balance and cranial nerve findings are more common among patients with infratentorial tumors, whereas seizures are more common among patients with supratentorial tumors. Computed tomography and/or magnetic resonance imaging (MRI) are critical to the diagnosis of pediatric brain tumors, although surgical resection or biopsy of tissue is usually necessary for definitive histological diagnosis. In addition to maximal safe surgical resection of the tumor, chemotherapy with or without cranial or craniospinal irradiation is indicated for malignant tumors. Cranial irradiation is delivered once daily, 5 days each week for up to 6 weeks. The total dose delivered to the brain can be more than twice that given in the treatment of ALL.

Prognosis varies with the tumor type. For example, medulloblastoma, the most common malignant brain tumor in childhood, has a prognosis of approximately 65 per cent long-term survival, whereas children with intrinsic brainstem glioma have a prognosis of less than 10 per cent. Although this subchapter will focus on the neuropsychological toxicity of cranial irradiation, other potentially serious complications from irradiation (e.g. hormone deficiencies, growth retardation, second malignancies) are recognized in the literature as well as hearing loss from treatment with cisplatin chemotherapy.

Neuropsychological outcomes

The quality of life in survivors of pediatric brain tumors was reported by Mostow et al.[48] who studied 342 adults who had been treated for brain tumors before the age of 20 years and who had survived 5 years or more. When compared to their siblings, survivors were at significantly greater risk for unemployment, chronic health problems and inability to operate a motor vehicle. Specific risk factors included male gender, supratentorial tumors and treatment that included radiation therapy (RT). Treatment at a younger age was associated with a greater risk of poor school achievement, never being employed and never being married.

What, specifically, can account for the unacceptably high incidence of social and vocational problems among these survivors of pediatric brain tumors? An early review of intellectual outcomes among children treated for

brain tumors included 22 studies of the neuropsychological status in 544 children surviving treatment for brain tumors.[49] A quantitative reanalysis of IQ data from 403 children investigated the impact of age, tumor location and CRT. Although the mean IQ was 91.0, particular subgroups were clearly at greater risk. In particular, children who received CRT under the age of 4 years were very vulnerable to intellectual loss compared to older children (means 73.4 vs. 87.0).

A comprehensive assessment of risk factors in children was conducted in a longitudinal design by Ellenberg et al.[50] A total of 43 children with various brain tumors were followed with serial IQ testing. Univariate analyses found significantly lower IQs amongst those children who were younger at treatment, received a greater RT volume and had cerebral (vs. posterior fossa) tumors. IQ deficits were greater with more time elapsed post-treatment. Multivariate analysis revealed that IQ at 1 month following diagnosis, age at treatment and RT volume accounted for 80 per cent of the variance in IQ scores 1–4 years later.

Jannoun and Bloom[51] provided neuropsychological follow-up 3–20 years following irradiation in 62 children with a variety of brain tumors. Tumor location, RT volume (limited vs. full CRT), and patient gender had no discernible effect on IQ outcomes. The age of the patient at the time of treatment was the most powerful determinant of ultimate IQ with those under age 5 years at greatest risk (mean IQ = 72), those 6–11 years at intermediate risk (mean IQ = 93), and those older than 11 years functioning solidly in the normal range (mean IQ = 107). Although not statistically significant, children presenting with hydrocephalus had a 10-point decrement in IQ compared to those with normal pressure.

In the first randomized study comparing standard (36 Gy) and reduced (23.4 Gy) CRT in medulloblastoma, the Pediatric Oncology Group reported on the neuropsychological performance of 22 of 35 surviving eligible patients divided into four groups based upon CRT dose and age at CRT (younger or older than 9 years).[7] Although the number of patients in each of the four groups was small, there was a clear suggestion of both age and dose effects at the most recent testing: Younger children with standard dose CRT had a median IQ of 70, younger children with reduced dose CRT had a median IQ of 85, older children with standard dose CRT had a median IQ of 83 and older children with reduced dose CRT had a median IQ of 92. Similar, although not necessarily statistically significant, differences between groups were found with regard to measures of attention and academic achievement. Overall, the authors conclude that the 35 per cent dose reduction resulted in a measurable sparing of IQ for children diagnosed between the ages of 4 and 9 years of age.

A more recent study longitudinal study has been published by the Children's Cancer Group of 43 children who were survivors of average risk medulloblastoma treated with 23.4 Gy CRT and adjuvant chemotherapy at age 3 years or older.[52] Overall, full scale IQ declined a mean of 17.4 points or 4.3 points per year, verbal IQ declined a mean of 16.8 points or 4.2 points per year, and non-verbal IQ declined a mean of 16 points or 4.0 points per year. Although no significant age effects were found for full scale IQ changes, children under the age of 7 years at CRT lost a mean of 20.8 points over the interval of observation, placing in question the notion that younger children benefit from lower doses of CRT. However, without an internal comparison group, no definitive answer could be drawn.

Another recent longitudinal study of children surviving treatment for medulloblastoma elucidates the changes in learning that underly often noted declines in IQ in this group of children.[53] Forty-four children treated with CRT with or without chemotherapy received serial assessments of their full scale IQ up to 12 years post-treatment. The mean IQ score of the sample was 83.6 at the most recent testing with a rate of decline from diagnosis estimated at 2.2 points per year with children younger than 8 years at CRT having a more rapid decline than older children (means −3.2 vs. −1.2 points/year) and patients receiving CRT doses of 36 Gy or higher having a more rapid decline than those receiving lower CRT doses (−3.6 vs. −1.6 points/year). Importantly, the analysis of patient's performance using raw score values (uncorrected for age) demonstrated a positive learning slope, which was only 50–60 per cent of that necessary to maintain their original IQ scores. The above finding gives hope to the notion that the rate of learning could be accelerated in affected patients. In addition to IQ declines, specific problems with school achievement, dyslexia and memory functions were reported among children surviving temporal lobe gliomas.[54,55]

Risk factors for neurocognitive impairments

The analysis of risk factors for neurocognitive impairments is more complex among patients treated for brain tumors than among those treated for ALL because of the increased number and variety of putative sources of brain damage. In general, a young age at diagnosis, more aggressive CNS therapy, and tumor-associated factors, such as location, seizures and hydrocephalus are the most frequently cited risk factors.

Very young children treated for brain tumors, especially those below the age of 4 years, are exposed to potentially neurotoxic agents during a time of accelerated neuroanatomic as well as psychological development. Some of these neurotoxic events may be focal in nature, such as the tumor and associated mass effect as well as local RT; others may have a diffuse impact, such as

full CRT or chemotherapy. The prevailing opinion is that very young children are at greater risk as the CNS is still developing anatomically and functionally. Particularly in the young, diffuse insults may result in greater relative functional deficit, as those exposed to focal insults have greater adaptive capacity to shift developing functions to unimpaired areas of the brain. Recent independent reviews of the pediatric brain tumor literature and the radiotherapy literature are in agreement that young age plays a pre-eminent role with regard to risks for treatment-related neurocognitive impairments.[4,56]

Hydrocephalus, defined here as ventricular dilatation with increased intracranial pressure, is common as a presenting feature in newly diagnosed patients, especially those with obstruction of CSF flow through the 4th ventricle. This phenomenon is more common among children than adults with intracranial tumors, largely because of the greater prevalence of posterior fossa tumors in the younger age group.[57] Suprasellar tumors in both children and adults are often associated with hydrocephalus. If untreated, brain edema, periventricular white matter and vascular damage result. The association of chronic hydrocephalus with learning disability and mental retardation among children in settings other than that of brain tumors is well documented.[58] However, the effects of episodic and temporary increases in intracranial pressure are not well understood. Hydrocephalus has been variably reported as a risk factor for cognitive deficits in the setting of brain tumors. In Ellenberg's[50] mixed series of patients, 28 of 43 children presented with hydrocephalus at diagnosis. IQ deficits were documented at 1 and 4 months following tumor excision, whether or not a shunt was required. All children showed gains, but those receiving a shunt showed the greatest gains, suggesting that their initial IQ scores in part reflected the effects of excess intracranial pressure. Hydrocephalus at diagnosis had no significant effect on IQ measured 1–4 years later. In a later series of a heterogeneous group of children, 40 presenting with hydrocephalus at diagnosis were compared to 22 with normal ventricles and no differences were found between the two groups with regard to mean IQ at follow-up. However, children presenting with hydrocephalus were twice as likely to be functioning in the intellectually deficient range (IQ < 70).[51] In children with medulloblastoma, insertion of a ventriculo-peritoneal (VP) shunt was associated with less pronounced intellectual and academic deficits at follow-up.[59]

Infiltrative tumors invade and destroy normal brain structures, whereas non-invasive or encapsulated tumors displace and compress normal brain structures. Subsequent alterations of brain function related to the area of insult may be transient, durable or progressive. The manner in which tumor effects are manifested neuropsychologically may depend upon the developmental stage of the child. Two studies that investigated tumor location as

a risk factor had positive findings.[45,50] In each instance, patients surviving tumors of the cerebral hemispheres had lower IQ and/or quality of life than those with non-cerebral tumors. In two independent studies of children treated for temporal lobe tumors with surgery with or without RT, memory deficits and other cognitive changes have been associated with whether the tumor arose in the language dominant or non-dominant cerebral hemisphere.[55,60]

Investigators from France have reported a cohort of 42 consecutively diagnosed children with low-grade cerebral hemispheric gliomas.[61] Children were treated with surgery alone, comprising an important 'standard' for evaluating the late effects of other forms of treatment. Long-term follow-up revealed that 29 per cent of children had IQ levels below 80, often with major problems in school. Although the authors did not associate a 20 per cent incidence of poorly controlled postoperative seizures with low IQ or school problems, this additional influence cannot be ruled out. In contrast, Riva et al.[62] reported normal IQ among children with posterior fossa (largely cerebellar) astrocytoma similarly managed with surgery alone, implying that tumor location is important among non-irradiated children. In contrast, cognitive decline has been documented in children with low-grade tumors of the brainstem following often limited surgery with or without local CRT.[63]

The goal of CRT is the selective destruction of neoplastic cells. CT and MRI demonstrate white matter changes following irradiation that vary directly with the radiation dose.[34] Changes are often limited to the high-dose radiation volume, but may progress from focal to diffuse 'encephalopathy' including significant volumes of one or both cerebral hemispheres. The late deleterious effects of RT for brain tumors in children and adults have been demonstrated using a variety of designs, primarily comparing the effect of the presence versus absence of RT as a treatment component or comparing local RT to full CRT. Given the previous discussion of mechanisms of action, studies relating total dose and fraction size to cognitive function would be important.

Although one study failed to detect an effect of RT volume,[51] another has found that the IQ values of children given CRT were significantly lower than those given local RT or no RT; the latter groups did not differ from each other.[50] Mostow's[48] very long-term follow-up of adults who had been treated as children found the use of RT as part of the patient's treatment regimen was associated with an almost threefold increase in the risk of chronic unemployment. In general, the findings indicate that patients requiring whole-brain RT attain a lower level of cognitive function and quality of life than those treated with less than whole-brain RT or no brain RT . However, at least two qualifications to this statement must be made. Two studies from our group illustrate the potential for

unexpected cognitive changes among children treated with local RT for brainstem gliomas and gliomas of the temporal lobes apparently related to the impact on normal temporal lobe areas.[54,55]

Neurotoxicity has been related to several chemotherapeutic agents. Effects are generally acute and often self-limited for the CNS, typified by encephalopathies attributed to electrolyte disturbance (e.g. with cisplatinum) or direct drug effects (e.g. methotrexate or ifosfamide). Reduction of CRT-induced brain damage has been used to justify the use of primary chemotherapy, especially for very young children, with malignant or low-grade brain tumors. Neurotoxicities of chemotherapy in this clinical setting may relate to later functional change as in dose-related sensorineural hearing loss associated with cisplatin. Hearing loss extending into the speech frequencies can limit normal cognitive development and academic progress in children. In one study of infants and very young children treated for brain tumors with pre-irradiation chemotherapy, physical and psychological growth was abnormal in the majority of children and showed no 'catch up' effect during the time that CRT was delayed.[64] In the series of mixed intracranial tumors of children receiving neuraxis RT by Jannoun and Bloom,[51] 8 of the 13 patients also received chemotherapy. The chemotherapy was not specified, and patient function was not analyzed using chemotherapy exposure as a potential risk factor. Interpretation of the effects of whole-brain irradiation in this series is complicated by the high proportion of these patients who also received chemotherapy.

Other factors that may affect cognitive performance following treatment for brain tumors are mentioned only sporadically in the literature. These include family socioeconomic resources, premorbid levels of function, chronic sensory and motor deficits, and seizures. For example, in children without brain tumors, poorly controlled seizures are associated with abnormal intellectual and academic development.[65] Poorly controlled seizures among children surviving temporal lobe astrocytomas are associated with psychopathology and poor academic achievement.[54]

Surveys have found that a significant proportion of surviving patients have clinically significant visual (optic atrophy, hemianopsia), auditory and motor disabilities (hemiparesis, ataxia), or seizures that grossly affect performance of age-appropriate activities of daily living, such as self-care and socialization.[56] The precise etiology of these complications is many times unknown, but chronic increased intracranial pressure, operative complications and cisplatin-induced hearing loss are not uncommon. These deficits indirectly affect patient functional status because of the limitations placed on input and performance of tasks rather than on cognitive processing itself.

Neuropathology of neuropsychological deficits

Unlike patients treated for ALL, those treated for brain tumors are exposed to the mechanical trauma of an invasive, space-occupying lesion of the CNS as well as the trauma associated with surgical resection and secondary effects (e.g. visual field cuts, seizures, hemiplegia, etc.) of both of these processes. It has been demonstrated that secondary, perioperative deficits adversely affect neuropsychological performance after controlling for the effects of treatment.[56]

Similar to studies of patients with ALL, the shared neurobiological substrate for neuropsychological deficits attributed to CRT is thought to be loss of normal white matter or the failure to develop normal white matter at an age-appropriate rate.[42] For patients treated for malignant brain tumors, the adverse effects of ionizing irradiation on the cerebral microvasculature is thought to be the pathway leading to white matter loss as opposed to the direct effects of irradiation on glial cells or their precursors.[66] Although studies using qualitative methods of characterizing the type and frequency of brain abnormalities have sometimes resulted in ambiguous findings with respect to correlation with neuropsychological deficits, greater success has recently been achieved using quantitative methods of measuring brain morphology. For example, recent work from our institution has demonstrated that patients treated for medulloblastoma with craniospinal irradiation with or without chemotherapy following surgery exhibit smaller volumes of normal white matter than age-matched controls with low-grade posterior fossa tumors treated with surgery alone.[67] In addition, the patients had lower IQ scores as survivors than those treated for low-grade tumors, and increased volume of normal appearing white matter was significantly correlated with higher IQ scores among the patients treated for medulloblastoma but not those treated for low grade tumors,[42] implying that there is a threshold for normal white matter impacting on IQ.

One provocative hypothesis is that the development of normal white matter may explain the well-documented adverse effects of a young age at treatment for malignant brain tumors. A longitudinal study of patients treated for medulloblastoma with craniospinal irradiation and chemotherapy after surgical resection demonstrated a progressive loss of normal white matter in contradistinction to the normally expected increase of normal white matter in persons under the age of 20. Recently, this hypothesis was tested in a cross-sectional study of 42 survivors of medulloblastoma. IQ was positively correlated with white matter volume and inversely correlated with age at CRT, and white matter volume and age at CRT were inversely correlated. After statistically controlling for the impact of normal white matter on IQ, the effects

of age at CRT were no longer significant, implying that normal white matter mediated the relationship between age and IQ.[68]

Young age at treatment, perioperative complications, more aggressive treatment (e.g. greater doses and volumes of radiation therapy) and more adverse impact on future brain development are risk factors previously discussed in this subchapter that are probably not independent. Unlike research results with patients treated for ALL, patients treated for malignant brain tumors tend to have a greater number of potential sources of brain insult, more severe overall impairment as measured by IQ loss and a greater number of specific neuropsychological deficits identified.

Summary

The incidence of neurocognitive problems and resulting problems in attaining an adequate quality of life (e.g. employment, social relationships) is very high among persons treated for malignant brain tumors in childhood. Although neurocognitive problems are most often summarized by declining IQ values, one could use the ALL literature as a model for more in-depth studies of mental processing functions that may explain a lack of normal intellectual and academic development. Although demographic and clinical risk factors for neurocognitive deficits, such as young age at treatment and CRT, have been consistently identified, considerable work remains to be done regarding the biological substrates underlying these risks and methods of intervention.

STEM CELL TRANSPLANTATION

Medical background

Stem cell or bone marrow transplantation (SCT) has evolved over the past two decades from a heroic experimental therapy of last resort to a standard therapy for many high-risk leukemia patients, and the preferred first option after leukemic relapse.[69–72] Over 20 000 SCT procedures have been performed worldwide.[69] The indications for SCT have widened to include a number of other malignant disorders, including lymphomas, solid tumors and even brain tumors, as well as to a growing number of non-malignant disorders.[70,71,73] The growth of bone marrow registries that allow for wider use of unrelated donor transplants, and developments in stem-cell selection techniques that allow for haplotype transplants using parent donors, have greatly increased the availability of SCT as a viable treatment option for seriously ill children.[74] At the same time, advances in supportive care have led to improved survival outcomes and thus to rapidly growing number of long-term survivors of SCT.[70,71]

Patients receiving SCT will receive conditioning with aggressive chemotherapy with or without total body irradiation (TBI) to eradicate active and residual malignant cells.[69] Without SCT, conditioning would be fatal. The SCT procedure first involves harvesting bone marrow, the source of hematopioetic stem cells, from an identified suitable donor. This procedure, usually accomplished with the donor under general anesthesia, involves extracting marrow from the posterior ileac crests. The procedure is generally very safe and the donor usually leaves the hospital on the day of the harvest. The marrow may be processed prior to intravenous infusion into the patient. During the immediate post-transplant interval, the patient is at risk for a myriad of infections because of the immunosuppressive nature of the conditioning regimen and potential lack of engraftment. Graft-versus-host disease (GvHD) results when the donor cells reject the recipient's tissue(s). GvHD may occur at varying levels of seriousness, graded 1–4 depending upon the number of organ systems involved (e.g. skin, intestine, liver, etc.) and severity of symptoms.[69] The treatment of GvHD usually includes steroids and cytotoxic agents.

Neuropsychological outcomes and risk factors

Beyond specific neurological complications, research has focused on the risk for global cognitive and academic deficits in pediatric survivors of SCT. The concern regarding potential cognitive declines resulting from SCT has been based, in part, on extrapolation from studies of ALL survivors who received CNS therapy, because, until recently, empiric data from pediatric SCT survivors have been limited.[75] Survivors of SCT are thought to be at risk for cognitive deficits as a result of their exposure to numerous potentially neurotoxic agents. Among the agents used in pretransplant conditioning, TBI has been the primary focus of those assessing neurocognitive sequelae but other cytotoxic conditioning agents, such as busulfan and other high-dose ablative chemotherapies are potentially neurotoxic as well.[76–78] CNS toxicities are also associated with agents (e.g. cyclosporin) commonly used for the prophylaxis and/or treatment of GvHD.[79–82] More speculative is the possibility of direct adverse effects of GvHD on the CNS.[83,84]

The literature on neurocognitive outcomes in pediatric SCT's is only beginning to develop. The number of published studies is small, and they have frequently been limited by methodological difficulties, such as small sample size, or retrospective designs. The findings reported thus far have been somewhat contradictory, although a consensus is beginning to emerge. A few studies have indicated declines in cognitive or academic function following SCT,[85–87] but a somewhat larger number of

studies have reported normal neurodevelopment, with no evidence of declines in cognitive function.[88–92] Our interpretation is that many of the divergent findings in the literature may be related to age effects within and between cohorts, and that with due consideration of age effects, a relatively coherent picture of the neurocognitive late effects of SCT can be drawn. A summary of the published literature is provided in Table 2a.1. Studies are presented in chronological order of publication, and with a single entry per cohort; that is, multiple publications over time from ongoing longitudinal studies are included based on the most recent publication.

The earliest published reports indicated no evidence of cognitive deficits following SCT. Kalieta et al.[93] documented essentially normal development, 2–6 years post-SCT, in four children transplanted as infants: two with leukemia who were conditioned with single dose TBI (750 cGy), and two with aplastic anemia conditioned without TBI. Pot-Mees[91] reported on a group 43 children who were followed for a year post-SCT, and a subset of 23 for whom pre- and post-SCT cognitive evaluations were obtained. No significant changes were found in IQ scores post-SCT. The first study suggestive of possible post-SCT cognitive deficits was reported by Smedler et al.[94] They divided their initial cohort of 32 survivors into three groups based on their age at SCT: <3 years; 3–11 years; and 12–17. They reported normal neurodevelopment post-SCT in the 12–17-year-old group. The 3–11-year age group showed some suggestions of difficulties, particularly in the area of perceptual and fine motor skills. However, the youngest age group showed clear delays in sensorimotor development. Subsequent reports on a slightly larger cohort continued to confirm this picture and to point to TBI as the crucial determinant of adverse cognitive outcomes.[87,95] Of ten children transplanted at less than 3 years, all eight who received TBI showed some evidence of developmental delay, whereas the two children who did not receive TBI showed normal development.[95] Table 2a.1 provides a summary of studies of neuropsychological outcomes from pediatric SCT.

The age-related findings reported by Smedler et al. presaged the later results from larger cohorts and help to explain the apparent discrepant findings between the two largest prospective series of neurocognitive outcome in SCT survivors to date. Kramer and colleagues[86,96] in a well-designed, prospective longitudinal study reported on outcomes of 67 children assessed 1 year post-SCT, and a subset of 26 of these children who were reassessed at 3 years post-SCT. They reported a significant decline in IQ (a mean change of 6 points, or .4 standard deviation units) in their cohort at 1 year post-SCT. There were no further declines in the subset followed to 3 years post-SCT, but the deficits were maintained across time. In contrast, our group found no significant declines in global IQ or academic achievement in 102 survivors assessed at 1 year post-SCT, nor in a subset of 54 survivors followed 3 years post-SCT.[90,97] The discrepancies between these studies can be explained, in large part, by the differential age of the two cohorts. The Kramer et al.[86] cohort had a mean age of 45 months, compared with 10½ years in our cohort. Within our cohort, the subset of children under 6 years showed declines comparable to those reported by Kramer's group.[86,90,97] In fact, our youngest patients (<3 years) showed an even greater decline than that reported by Kramer et al.[86] and, moreover, their cognitive function continued to decline through 3 years.[97] In contrast to the report of Smedler et al.,[87] in neither the Kramer[86] nor the Phipps[97] studies was there any apparent effect of the use of TBI. In the Phipps et al.[97] cohort, the TBI and no TBI groups were large enough to detect relatively small effects, and none were apparent.

The findings from our cohort, in light of the previously published literature, led us to conclude that SCT, even with TBI, poses low to minimal risk for late cognitive and academic deficits in patients who are at least 6 years old at the time of transplant. For patients age 5 and under, and particularly for those younger than 3 years of age, the risk of cognitive impairment is increased, regardless of whether or not TBI is used in conditioning. The results of recently reported studies have continued to support this conclusion. Simms et al.[98,99] reported on a cohort of 25 patients followed prospectively through 2 years post-SCT, and found normal cognitive function and academic achievement, with no evidence of decline over this timeframe. However, three of the four children in their cohort who were <3 years at the time of SCT showed substantial declines in developmental indices post-SCT.[98] Likewise, Arvidson et al.[88] and Daniel Llach et al.[89] reported similar normal functioning and absence of declines over time in SCT survivors.

Neuropathology of neuropsychological deficits

Patients undergoing SCT are at risk for a number of adverse CNS events during the early post-SCT period, including cerebral hemorrhage, infectious complications, such as viral encephalitis, metabolic encephalopathy and other encephalopathies of unknown cause.[100–105] Although the mortality associated with these complications is quite high, the surviving children are likely to recover with significant neurological impairments. Estimates of the frequency of neurological complications in SCT patients have ranged from 11 per cent to as high as 70 per cent, depending on survey methods.[100,101,104] These surveys have generally involved only adult patients or mixed adult/pediatric populations, and no surveys have been reported focusing solely on children. One of the earliest reports of late effects of SCT on the CNS indicated an incidence of

Table 2b.1 *Studies of neurocognitive outcomes in survivors of pediatric stem cell transplantation (SCT)*

Study	Methods Subjects	Design/measures	Findings Results	Comments
1. Kaleita et al.[93]	Children <2 years old, n = 4	Prospective. Standardized measures of infant development administered pre- and 2–6 years post-SCT	Normal neurodevelopment in all cases; no change over time	First cases reported; 2 infants received TBI, 2 did not
2. Pot-Mees[91]	Children 5–18, n = 23 (from cohort of 75)	Prospective. Standardized measures of IQ, academic achievement given pre-SCT, and 6 months and 1 year post-SCT; 2 comparison groups	No changes in IQ or academic achievement at 1 year post-SCT. SCT group functioned lower than control group *before* SCT	Included some patients with genetic storage disorders, which makes results more difficult to interpret
3. Smedler et al.[87,94,95]	n = 36 in 3 groups; <3 years at SCT, n = 10; 3–11 years, n = 15; 12–17 years, n = 11	No pre-SCT assessment, but longitudinal survey of survivors 1–6 years post-SCT; donors as controls; standardized measures of development, IQ and neuropsychologic function	No deficits found in oldest group. Group age 3–11 showed trends towards declines in perceptual and fine-motor skill, and verbal skill. In group <3 years, all treated with TBI showed moderate developmental delay	Two children <3 years transplanted for SAA without TBI showed normal development
4. McGuire et al.[108]	Children through age 18 at SCT, n = 178	Retrospective, cross-section survey; compared 110 patients assessed pre-SCT to 68 patients assessed 1–12 years post-SCT on standardized measures of IQ achievement	No differences between pre- and post-SCT groups on any measures; across all patients, performance related to total amount of RT, age at first RT and time elapsed since RT	Published only as abstract
5. Kramer et al.[86,96]	Children <18 years, but with predominantly young (<6 years) population. n = 67 assessed at 1 year post-SCT and n = 26 at 3 years post-SCT (from cohort of 137 assessed pre-SCT)	Prospective, longitudinal design. Standardized measures of infant development and IQ obtained pre-SCT and at 1 year and 3 years post-SCT	Significant decline in IQ at 1 year post-SCT. No relationship of post-SCT function with diagnosis, type of SCT, TBI, age or gender. Deficits maintained at 3 years post-SCT but no further declines	Very young sample, with mean age of 45 months at SCT. Restricted age range limits ability to detect age effects
6. Phipps et al.[90,97]	Children through 18 years, n = 102 assessed at 1 year post-SCT, and n = 54 assessed at 3 years post-SCT (from cohort of 260 assessed pre-SCT)	Prospective, longitudinal design. Standardized measures of IQ, achievement and neuropsychological function obtained pre-SCT, and 1, 3 and 5 years post-SCT	In cohort as a whole, no significant declines in IQ or achievement at 1 or 3 years post-SCT. Age a significant predictor of outcome, with patients <3 years showing evidence of decline over time. TBI not related to outcome	Largest prospective study published to date. Adequate power to detect small (3 IQ points) effects. Concludes that SCT ± TBI entails minimal risk of neurocognitive sequelae in patients ≥6 years but younger children may be at some risk

(Continued)

Study	Sample	Design	Results	Conclusion
7. Cool[85]	Children through 18 years; $n = ?$; maximum $n = 45$ (of cohort of 76 assessed pre-SCT)	Prospective longitudinal study with pre-SCT assessment, and yearly follow-up through 4-years post-SCT. Standardized measures of IQ, achievement, neuropsychological function; brain CT scans obtained on some survivors	At pre-SCT evaluation, children already showing some deficits in IQ and achievement, related to prior CNS therapy. Overall, global IQ stable at 1 year post-SCT, some trends toward decline in academic achievement	Author concludes that by 4 years post-SCT, there is evidence of declines in IQ, achievement, attention, memory and fine-motor skills. However evidence from data is not persuasive. Presented as a series of studies, which makes interpretation difficult
8. Simms et al.[92,98]	$n = 25$ children assessed at pre-SCT, and 1 year and 2 years post-SCT (from cohort of 238 assessed pre-SCT)	Prospective, longitudinal study with pre-SCT, and 1-, 2- and 5 years post-SCT assessments. Standardized measures of IQ, achievement and neuropsychological function	No significant changes in any cognitive or academic achievement measures at either 1 year or 2 years post-SCT. No difference between TBI and non-TBI regimens; 3 of 4 children <3 years showed decline post-SCT of ≥ 10 points	No evidence of any decline in function, but possible risks for youngest children. Despite absence of declines, evidence that parents perceive difficulties in school functioning
9. Arvidson et al.[88]	Children <18 years; $n = 26$	Cross-sectional/longitudinal design. Children assessed at various intervals 2–11 years post-SCT, using measures of global IQ and neuropsychological function	Global IQ in normal range and generally unaffected over time. Slight increase in problems in 'executive function', attention and memory. No difference between TBI and non-TBI regimens. Age at diagnosis and time since SCT predictive of outcome	All patients underwent autologous transplant but the majority conditioned with TBI in a single 7.5 Gy dose
10. Daniel Llach et al.[89]	Children age 4–15; $n = 22$ (from cohort of 54)	Prospective. Children assessed pre- and 1 year post-SCT on global IQ	No significant changes in pre–post comparisons. Scores in the average range	Children scoring <100 pre-SCT showed gains, while those scoring >100 pre-SCT showed declines. Interpreted as reflective of anxiety effects

CNS, central nervous system; CT, computed tomography; RT, radiation therapy; SAA, severe aplastic anemia; TBI, total body irradiation.

leukoencephalopathy in 7 per cent of patients, but this occurred only in those patients who had both previous CNS therapy and TBI.[106] More recent studies that have included diagnostic imaging have indicated the presence of abnormalities on MRI in nearly two out of three of survivors.[79,81] The most common findings involve white matter lesions or mild cerebral atrophy. These abnormalities have not generally been associated with the use of TBI but relate to the occurrence of GvHD and, in particular, the use of corticosteroids and cyclosporine for the treatment of GvHD.[80,81,107] In one study, the incidence of abnormalities in MRI examinations (65 per cent) was higher than the incidence of cognitive deficits, and there was no significant relationship between MRI findings and cognitive function.[81] Again these studies have involved primarily adult patients.

Summary

Survivors of stem cell transplant in childhood represent a rapidly growing population who are at risk for adverse CNS outcomes and neurocognitive impairment. To date, studies of neurocognitive outcomes in specifically pediatric populations are few in number and suffer from a number of methodological limitations. Nevertheless, integration of the available literature leads to a reasonably coherent interpretation of the findings, with age at SCT a crucial determinant of outcome. For children age ≥ 6 years at the time of transplant, SCT, even with TBI, poses low to minimal risk for late cognitive and academic deficits. However, for children <6 years, and particularly for those ≤ 3 years, the risk of cognitive impairment is increased, regardless of whether or not TBI is used in conditioning.

INTERVENTIONS FOR NEUROPSYCHOLOGICAL DEFICITS

Although research on the patterns and risks for neuropsychological and educational deficits among survivors of childhood cancer has been progressing for the past three decades, the development of empirically validated interventions for these deficits has not been as rapid. Broadly speaking, interventions can be divided into two approaches: those intended to avoid or reduce the neuropsychological toxicity of therapy directed towards the CNS; and those intended to minimize or rehabilitate deficits that cannot be avoided.

A formal plan of prospective surveillance of neuropsychological status should be set forth for each patient based upon known or suspected risk for problems. This assumes that a qualified psychologist has been identified as a consultant to the institution. For example, a middle-aged adult with a supratentorial low-grade glioma treated with surgery alone may require formal assessment only once or twice during the 2-year period following diagnosis with the focus being whether there is evidence of loss of abilities. On the other hand, a young child with the same tumor and treatment should have a neuropsychological evaluation scheduled at the completion of therapy and 3–5 years later, whereas an infant with a brain tumor should probably be evaluated every 6 months until the age of 3 or 4 years and then yearly until 5 years post-therapy. Such plans should not depend upon the presentation of symptoms because presymptomatic assessments often allow for early educational interventions that may minimize deficits.

Contemporary treatment protocols for children treated for cancer generally show an enlightened concern for the potential neurotoxicity of therapy, especially among very young patients. The elimination of CRT, delay of CRT until the patient is older, or CRT dose/volume reduction to spare more normal brain are the most frequently considered approaches. Several studies have documented benefit of CRT dose reduction in terms of IQ and achievement functioning in survivors of ALL and brain tumors. The benefits of more recent technological improvements, such as the use of three-dimensional conformal CRT, are not yet known. However, with ever-increasing cure rates, this approach to toxicity reduction is likely to continue to be very active.

If neuropsychological impairments are unavoidable, one may attempt to minimize their impact by direct intervention with cognitive rehabilitation or pharmacotherapy, and/or through more indirect approaches involving manipulations of the patient's environment. Cognitive rehabilitation is a term used to describe interventions intended to restore lost cognitive functions or to teach the patient skills to compensate for cognitive losses that cannot be restored. Although some evidence for efficacy is available from the child closed head injury literature, we are aware of only one program in the USA that is attempting to validate a standardized, 20-session program of cognitive rehabilitation for survivors of ALL and brain tumors in a seven-institution consortium funded by the National Cancer Institute.[109]

Pharmacotherapy, especially the use of psychostimulants, such as methylphenidate (Ritalin), has recently received interest. Impressive gains in activity level and quality of life were shown in one study of adult glioma patients treated with methylphenidate at the University of Texas/M.D. Anderson Cancer Center.[110] A subsequent study at our institution investigated the acute effects of methylphenidate on the cognitive functioning of pediatric patients treated for cancer.[111] In this double-blind placebo-controlled study, patients given 0.6 mg/kg methylphenidate showed significant improvement on measures of attention when compared to those receiving placebo. Our current study, funded by the National Cancer Institute, expands

upon these findings by conducting a 3-week crossover trial of two doses of methylphenidate and placebo in the home and school environments to establish the potential for efficacy prior to 12 months of treatment. Parent and teacher ratings of behavior as well as objective testing of the patients will allow the evaluation of effects on academic achievement and social relations.

Finally, one should not minimize the potential positive impact of optimal communication and education on the patient's caregivers.[112] Routine communication between the cancer treatment center and the patient's school should be the standard of care, especially in cases in which neurological (e.g. hearing loss in the speech frequencies, visual field cuts) or neuropsychological deficits (e.g. problems with attention, memory or processing speed) can impair the patient's ability to function in a normal classroom environment. Because all of the deficits listed above are unobservable to teachers, there may be a tendency to misinterpret the patient's behavior in the absence of knowledge of the deficits. For example, we have experience with children labeled as having attitude problems, or as being daydreamers or unmotivated to learn when, in fact, the patient had neurological and neuropsychological disabilities that were unknown to the teacher. Although parents can have an important role in facilitating communication between the cancer center and the school, we have found that a telephone call or visit from a representative from the cancer center teacher or social worker can have a profound impact on the adaptation of the classroom environment to meet the patient's needs.

CONCLUSIONS

This subchapter has highlighted the most important issues relevant to neurocognitive late effects in childhood cancer; specifically, those associated with ALL, malignant brain tumors and stem cell transplantation. Although neurocognitive problems have been traditionally defined by late IQ and achievement deficits, more recent studies, particularly with survivors of ALL, are defining the particular mental processing factors that antedate these late changes. However, clinical research in the area of late neuropsychological effects could be facilitated by several factors. These include improving methods of identifying the basis for declines in IQ and academic achievement, developing a better understanding of which children are at greatest risk for these changes, increasing our understanding of the biological substrates underlying neurocognitive deficits and, most importantly, developing interventions at several levels to avoid or remediate deficits. Reaching these goals will be expedited by removing barriers to third-party payment for protocol-driven clinical neuropsychological evaluations of patients. The discovery

of effective interventions will facilitate the achievement of our ultimate goal for survivors of childhood cancer; that is, returning them to the quality of life that they would have had if they had never had cancer.

KEY POINTS

- The severity of neurocognitive deficits in childhood cancer survivors, particularly acute lymphoblastic leukemia and malignant brain tumors, are directly related to the aggressiveness of central nervous system therapy.
- Many factors, including the age of the child at the time of treatment, time elapsed from treatment, socioeconomic status and neurological problems can modify the impact of central nervous system treatment for leukemia and brain tumors.
- For children receiving bone marrow transplantation with or without total body irradiation, only those 3 years of age or less appear vulnerable to neurocognitive deficits.
- The most common neurocognitive phenotype is characterized by problems with attention, working memory and executive functions, which eventually are manifested by decreased rates of academic achievement and intellectual development.
- Efforts to eliminate neurocognitive deficits have traditionally been focused on decreasing the intensity of central nervous system therapy, although contemporary studies are testing the efficacy of treatment of learning problems using cognitive/behavioral therapy and stimulant medications.
- Pediatric cancer centers should provide school liaison services for patients at risk for neurocognitive deficits to maximize the patient's learning potential.

ACKNOWLEDGEMENT

Preparation of this subchapter was supported in part by the American Lebanese Syrian Associated Charities and grants CA 21765 and CA 20180 from the National Cancer Institute.

REFERENCES

1. Steen G, Mirro J. *Childhood cancer: a handbook from St. Jude Children's Research Hospital.* Cambridge, MA: Perseus Publishing, 2000.

2. Margolin JF, Poplack DG. Acute lymphoblastic leukemia. In: Pizzo PA, Poplack DG (eds) *Principles and practice of pediatric oncology*, 3rd edn. Philadelphia, PA: Lippincott-Raven, 1997:409–462.

3. Moleski M. Neuropsychological, neuroanatomical, and neurophysiological consequences of CNS chemotherapy for acute lymphoblastic leukemia. *Arch Clin Neuropsychol* 2000; **15**:603–630.

●4. Roman DD, Sperduto PW. Neuropsychological effects of cranial irradiation: current knowledge and future directions. *Int J Radiat Oncol Biol Phys* 1995; **31**:983–998.

5. Brown RT, Madan-Swain A, Pais R. Cognitive status of children treated with central nervous system prophylactic chemotherapy for acute lymphocytic leukemia. *Arch Clin Neuropsychol* 1992; **7**:481–497.

◆6. Cetingul N, Aydmok Y, Kantar M, *et al.* Neuropsychologic sequelae in the long-term survivors of childhood acute lymphoblastic leukemia. *Pediatr Hematol Oncol* 1999; **16**:213–220.

◆7. Mulhern RK, Kepner JL, Thomas, PR, *et al.* Neuropsychologic functioning of survivors of childhood medulloblastoma randomized to receive conventional or reduced-dose craniospinal irradiation: A pediatric oncology group study. *J Clin Oncol* 1998; **16**:1723–1728.

8. Raymond-Speden E, Tripp G, Lawrence B, Holdaway D. Intellectual, neuropsychological and academic functioning in long-term survivors of leukemia. *J Pediatr Psychol* 2000; **25**:59–68.

9. Waber DP, Carpentieri SC, Klar N, *et al.* Cognitive sequelae in children treated for acute lymphoblastic leukemia with dexamethasone or prednisone. *J Pediatr Hematol Oncol* 2000; **22**:206–213.

10. Mulhern RK, Phipps S, Tyc VL. Psychosocial Issues. In: Pui CH (ed.) *Childhood leukemias*. Cambridge: Cambridge University Press, 1999: 520–541.

11. Rubenstein CL, Varni JW, Katz ER. Cognitive functioning in long-term survivors of childhood leukemia: a prospective analysis. *Dev Behav Pediatr* 1990; **11**:301–305.

12. Mulhern RK, Fairclough D, Ochs J. A prospective comparison of neuropsychologic performance of children surviving leukemia who received 18-Gy, 24-Gy, or no cranial irradiation. *J Clin Oncol* 1991; **9**:1348–1356.

13. Espy KA, Moore IM, Kaufmann PM, *et al.* Chemotherapeutic CNS prophylaxis and neuropsychologic change in children with acute lymphoblastic leukemia: a prospective study. *J Pediatr Psychol* 2001; **26**:1–9.

14. Brown RT, Madan-Swain A, Walco GA, *et al.* Cognitive and academic late effects among children previously treated for acute lymphocytic leukemia receiving chemotherapy as CNS prophylaxis. *J Pediatr Psychol* 1998; **23**:333–340.

15. Copeland DR, Moore BD, Francis DJ, *et al.* Neuropsychologic effects of chemotherapy on children with cancer: a longitudinal study. *J Clin Oncol* 1996; **14**:2826–2835.

16. Brown RT, Madan-Swain A. Cognitive, neuropsychological, and academic sequelae in children with leukemia. *J Learn Disabil* 1993; **26**:74–90.

17. Cousens P, Ungerer JA, Crawford JA, Stevens MM. Cognitive effects of childhood leukemia therapy: a case for four specific deficits. *J Pediatr Psychol* 1991; **16**: 475–488.

◆18. Lockwood KA, Bell TS, Colegrove RW. Long-term effects of cranial radiation therapy on attention functioning in survivors of childhood leukemia. *J Pediatr Psychol* 1999; **24**:55–66.

19. Baddeley AD. Exploring the central executive. *Q J Exp Psychol* 1996; **49**:5–28.

20. Shah P, Miyake A. Models of working memory: an introduction. In: Miyake A, Shah P (eds) *Models of working memory: mechanisms of active maintenance and executive control*. New York: Cambridge University Press, 1999:1–27.

21. Posner MI, Peterson SE. The attention system of the human brain. *Annu Rev Neurosci* 1990; **13**:25–42.

22. Engle RW, Kane MJ, Tulholski SW. Individual differences in working memory capacity and what they tell us about controlled attention, general fluid intelligence, and functions of the prefrontal cortex. In: Miyake A and Shah P (eds) *Models of working memory: mechanisms of active maintenance and executive control*. New York: Cambridge University Press, 1999:102–134.

23. Barkley RA. Attention-deficit/hyperactivity disorder, self-regulation, and time: toward a more comprehensive theory. *Dev Behav Pediatr* 1997; **18**:271–279.

24. Baddeley AD, Logie RH. Working memory: the multiple-component model. In: Miyake A and Shah P (eds) *Models of working memory: mechanisms of active maintenance and executive control*. New York: Cambridge University Press, 1999.

25. Brouwers P, Riccardi R, Poplack D, Fedio P. Attentional deficits in long-term survivors of childhood acute lymphoblastic leukemia. *J Clin Neuropsychol* 1984; **6**:325–336.

◆26. Brouwers P, Poplack D. Memory and learning sequelae in long-term survivors of acute lymphoblastic leukemia: Association with attention deficits. *Am J Pediatr Hematol Oncol* 1990; **12**:174–181.

◆27. Rodgers J, Horrocks J, Britton PG, Kernahan J. Attentional ability among survivors of leukaemia. *Arch Dis Child* 1999; **80**: 318–323.

28. Mirsky AF, Anthony BJ, Duncan CC, *et al.* Analysis of the element of attention: A neuropsychological approach. *Neuropsychol Rev* 1991; **2**:109–145.

29. Cohen RA. *The neuropsychology of attention*. New York: Plenum Press, 1993.

30. Miyake A, Shah P. Toward unified theories of working memory: emerging general consensus, unresolved theoretical issues, and future research directions. In: Miyake A and Shah P (eds) *Models of working memory: mechanisms of active maintenance and executive control*. New York: Cambridge University Press, 1999:444–481.

◆31. Schatz J, Kramer JH, Ablin A, Matthay KK. Processing speed, working memory, and IQ: a developmental model of cognitive deficits following cranial radiation therapy. *Neuropsychology* 2000; **14**:189–200.

32. Cousens P, Waters B, Said J, Stevens M. Cognitive effects of cranial irradiation in leukaemia: a survey and meta-analysis. *J Child Clin Psychiatr* 1988; **29**:839–852.

33. Tsuruda JS, Kortman KE, Bradley WG, *et al.* Radiation effects on white matter: MR evaluation. *Am J Roentgenol* 1987; **149**:165–171.

34. Corn BW, Yousem DM, Scott CB, *et al.* White matter changes are correlated significantly with radiation dose. *Cancer* 1994; **74**:2828–2835.

35. Burger PC, Boyko OB. The pathology of central nervous system radiation injury. In: Gutin PH, Leibel SA and Sheline GE (eds) *Radiation injury to the nervous system*. New York: Raven Press, 1991:3–15.

36. Hudson M. Late complications after leukemia therapy. In Pui CH (ed.) *Childhood leukemias*. Cambridge: Cambridge University Press, 1999:463–481.

37. Lee YY, Nauert C, Glass P. Treatment-related white matter changes in cancer patients. *Cancer* 1986; **57**:1473–1482.

38. Mildenberger M, Beach TG, McGeer EG, Ludgate CM. An animal model of prophylactic cranial irradiation: histological effects at acute, early, and delayed stages. *Int J Oncol Biol Phys* 1990; **18**:1051–1060.

39. Sowell ER, Thompson PM, Holmes CJ, *et al.* In vivo evidence for post-adolescent brain maturation in frontal and striatal regions. *Nature Neurosci* 1999; **2**:859–861.

◆40. Filley CM. The behavioral neurology of cerebral white matter. *Neurology* 1998; **50**:1535–1540.

41. de Groot, JC, de Leeuw FE, Oudkerk M, *et al.* Cerebral white matter lesions and cognitive function: The Rotterdam scan study. *Ann Neurol* 2000; **47**:145–151.

42. Mulhern RK, Reddick WE, Palmer SL, *et al.* Neurocognitive deficits in medulloblastoma survivors and white matter loss. *Ann Neurol* 1999; **46**:834–841.

43. Waber DP, Urion DK, Tarbell NJ, *et al.* Late effects of central nervous system treatment of acute lymphoblastic leukemia in childhood are sex-dependent. *Dev Med Child Neurol* 1990; **32**:238–248.

◆44. Waber DP, Tarbell NJ, Kahn CM, *et al.* The relationship of sex and treatment modality to neuropsychologic outcome in childhood acute lymphoblastic leukemia. *J Clin Oncol* 1992; **10**:810–817.

45. Mulhern RK, Kovnar E, Langston J, *et al.* Long-term survivors of leukemia treated in infancy: factors associated with neuropsychological status. *J Clin Oncol* 1992; **10**:1095–1102.

46. Kaleita TA, Reaman GH, MacLean WE, *et al.* Neurodevelopmental outcome of infants with acute lymphoblastic leukemia: a Children's Cancer Group report. *Cancer* 1999; **85**:1859–1865.

47. Heideman RL, Packer RJ, Albright LA, *et al.* Tumors of the central nervous system. In: Pizzo PA, Poplack DG (eds) *Principles and practice of pediatric oncology*, 3rd edn. Philadelphia: Lippincott-Raven, 1997:633–681.

48. Mostow EN, Byrne J, Connelly RR, Mulvihill JJ. Quality of life in long-term survivors of CNS tumors of childhood and adolescence. *J Clin Oncol* 1991; **9**:592–599.

49. Mulhern RK, Hancock J, Fairclough D, Kun LE. Neuropsychological status of children treated for brain tumors: a critical review and integrative analysis. *Med Pediatr Oncol* 1992; **20**:181–191.

50. Ellenberg L, McComb JG, Siegel SE, Stowe S. Factors affecting intellectual outcome in pediatric brain tumor patients. *Neurosurgery* 1987; **21**:638–644.

51. Jannoun L, Bloom HJG. Long-term psychological effects in children treated for intracranial tumors. *Int J Radiat Oncol Biol Phys* 1990; **18**:747–753.

52. Ris MD, Packer R, Goldwein J, *et al.* Intellectual outcome after reduced-dose radiation therapy plus adjuvant chemotherapy for medulloblastoma: a Children's Cancer Group study. *J Clin Oncol* 2001; **19**:3470–3476.

53. Palmer SL, Goloubeva O, Reddick WE, *et al.* Patterns of intellectual development among survivors of pediatric medulloblastoma: a longitudinal analysis. *J Clin Oncol* 2001; **19**:2302–2308.

54. Mulhern RK, Kovnar EK, Kun LE, *et al.* Psychologic and neurologic function following treatment for childhood temporal lobe astrocytoma. *J Child Neurol* 1988; **3**:47–52.

55. Carpentieri S, Mulhern RK. Patterns of memory dysfunction among children surviving temporal lobe tumors. *Arch Clin Neuropsychol* 1993; **8**:345–357.

●56. Ris MD, Noll RB. Long-term neurobehavioral outcome in pediatric brain-tumor patients: review and methodological critique. *J Clin Exp Neuropsychol* 1994; **16**:21–42.

57. Klein DM. Principles of neurosurgery. In: Cohen M, Duffner P (eds) *Brain tumors in children*. New York: Raven Press, 1984:92–102.

58. Willis KE. Neuropsychological functioning in children with spina bifida and/or hydrocephalus. *J Clin Child Psychol* 1993; **22**:247–265.

59. Johnson DL, McCabe MA, Nicholson HS, *et al.* Quality of long-term survival in young children with medulloblastoma. *J Neurosurg* 1994; **80**:1004–1010.

60. Cavazzuti V, Winston K, Baket R, Welch K. Psychological changes following surgery for tumors in the temporal lobe. *J Neurosurg* 1980; **53**:618–626.

61. Hirsch JF, Rose CS, Pierre-Kahn A, *et al.* Benign astrocytic and oligodendrocytic tumors of the cerebral hemispheres in children. *J Neurosurg* 1989; **70**:568–572.

62. Riva D, Pantaleone C, Milani N, Belani FF. Impairment of neuropsychological functions in children with medulloblastomas and astrocytomas in the posterior fossa. *Childs Nerv Syst* 1989; **5**:107–110.

63. Mulhern RK, Heideman RL, Khatib ZA, *et al.* Quality of survival among children treated for brain stem glioma. *Pediatr Neurosurg* 1994; **20**:226–232.

64. Horowitz ME, Mulhern RK, Kun LE, *et al.* Brain tumor in the very young child: postoperative chemotherapy in combined-modality treatment. *Cancer* 1988; **61**:428–434.

65. Rankin EJ, Adams RL, Jones HE. Epilepsy and nonepileptic attack disorder. In: Adams RL, Parsons OA, Culbertson JL, Nixon SJ (eds) *Neuropsychology for clinical practice: etiology, assessment, and treatment of common neurological disorders*. Washington, DC: American Psychological Association, 1996:131–173.

◆66. Hopewell JW, van der Kogel AJ. Pathophysiological mechanisms leading to the development of late radiation-induced damage to the central nervous system. In: Wiegel T, Hinkelbein W, Brock M, Hoell T (eds) *Controversies in neuro-oncology: frontiers of radiation therapy and oncology*. Basel: Karger, 1999:265–275.

67. Reddick WE, Mulhern RK, Elkin TD, *et al.* A hybrid neural network analysis of subtle brain volume differences in children surviving brain tumors. *Magn Reson Imaging* 1998; **16**:413–421.

◆68. Mulhern RK, Palmer SL, Reddick WE, *et al.* Risks of young age for selected neurocognitive deficits in medulloblastoma are associated with white matter loss. *J Clin Oncol* 2001; **19**:472–479.

69. Sanders, JE. Bone Marrow transplantation in pediatric oncology. In: Pizzo PA, Poplack DG (eds) *Principles and practices of pediatric oncology*, 3rd edn. New York: Lippincott-Raven, 1997: 357–373.

70. Santos GW. Historical background to hematopoetic stem cell transplantation. In: Atkinson K (ed.) *Clinical bone marrow and blood stem cell transplantation*, 2nd edn. New York: Cambridge University Press, 2000:1–12.

71. Treleaven J, Barrett J. Introduction. In: Barrett J, Trealeaven J (eds) *The clinical practice of stem-cell transplantation*, Volume 1. Oxford: ISIS, 1998:2–16.

72. Wingard JR. Bone marrow to blood stem cells: past, present, future. In: Whedon MB, Wujcik D (eds) *Blood and marrow stem cell transplantation: principles, practice, and nursing insights*, 2nd edn. Boston: Jones and Bartlett Publishers, 1997:3–24.

73. Meller S, Pinkerton, R. Solid tumors in children. In: Barrett J, Trealeaven J (eds) *The clinical practice of stem-cell transplantation*, Volume 1. Oxford: ISIS, 1998: 173–190.

74. Mehta J, Powles R. The future of blood and marrow transplantation. In: Atkinson K (ed.) *Clinical bone marrow and blood stem cell transplantation*, 2nd edn. New York: Cambridge University Press, 2000:1457–1465.

●75. Phipps S, Barclay D. Psychosocial consequences of pediatric bone marrow transplantation. *Int J Pediatr Hematol Oncol* 1996; **3**:171–182.

76. Chou RH, Wong GB, Kramer JH, *et al.* Toxicities of total-body irradiation for pediatric bone marrow transplantation. *Int J Radiol Onc Biol Phys* 1996; **34**:843–851.

77. Miale TD, Sirithorn S, Ahmed S. Efficacy and toxicity of radiation in preparative regimens for pediatric stem cell transplantation. In: Clinical applications and therapeutic effects. *Med Oncol* 1995; **12**:231–249.

78. Peper M, Schraube P, Kimming C, *et al.* Long-term cerebral side-effects of total body irradiation and quality of life. *Recent Results Cancer Res* 1993; **130**:219–230.

79. Coley SC, Jager HR, Szydlo RM, Goldman JM. CT and MRI manifestations of central nervous system infection following allogeneic bone marrow transplantation. *Clin Radiol* 1999; **54**:390–397.

80. Pace MT, Slovis TL, Kelly JK, Abella SD. Cyclosporin A toxicity: MRI appearance of the brain. *Pediatr Radiol* 1995; **25**:180–183.

81. Padovan CS, Gerbitz A, Sostak P, *et al*. Cerebral involvement in graft-versus-host disease after murine bone marrow transplantation. *Neurology* 2001; **56**:1106–1108.

82. Reece DE, Frei-Lahr DA, Shepherd JD, *et al*. Neurologic complications in allogeneic bone marrow transplant patients receiving cyclosporin. *Bone Marrow Transplant* 1991; **8**:393–401.

83. Garrick R. Neurologic Complications. In: Atkinson K (ed.) *Clinical bone marrow and blood stem cell transplantation*, 2nd edn. New York: Cambridge University Press, 2000:958–979.

84. Rouah E, Gruber R, Shearer W, *et al*. Graft-versus-host disease in the central nervous system. A real entity? *Am J Clin Pathol* 1988; **89**:543–546.

85. Cool VA. Long-term neuropsychological risks in pediatric bone marrow transplant: what do we know? *Bone Marrow Transplant* 1996; **18**(Suppl. 3):S45–S49.

◆86. Kramer JH, Crittenden MR, DeSantes K, Cowan MJ. Cognitive and adaptive behavior 1 and 3 years following bone marrow transplantation. *Bone Marrow Transplant* 1997; **19**:607–613.

87. Smedler AC, Bolme P. Neuropsychological deficits in very young bone marrow transplant recipients. *Acta Pediatr* 1995b; **84**:429–433.

88. Arvidson J, Kihlgren M, Hall C, Lonnerholm G. Neuropsychological functioning after treatment for hematological malignancies in childhood, including autologous bone marrow transplantation. *Pediatr Hematol Oncol* 1999; **16**:9–21.

89. Daniel Llach M, Perez Campdepadros M, Baza Ceballos N, *et al*. Secuelas neuropsicologicas a medio y largo plazo del trasplante de medula osea en pacientes con enfermedades heamtologicas. *Anales Pediatria* 2001; **54**:463–467.

◆90. Phipps S, Brenner M, Heslop H, *et al*. Psychological effects of bone marrow transplant on children: preliminary report of a longitudinal study. *Bone Marrow Transplant* 1995; **16**:829–835.

●91. Pot-Mees CC. *The psychological aspects of bone marrow transplantation in children*. Delft: Eburon, 1989.

92. Simms S, Kazak AE, Golumb VA, *et al*. Cognitive and psychological outcome in 2 year survivors of childhood bone marrow transplantation, paper presented at the *University of Pennsylvania Cancer Center Annual Symposium*, March, 1999.

93. Kaleita TA, Shields WD, Tesler A, Feig S. Normal neurodevelopment in four young children treated for acute leukemia or aplastic anemia. *Pediatrics* 1989; **83**:753–757.

94. Smedler AC, Ringden K, Bergman H, Bolme P. Sensory-motor and cognitive functioning in children who have undergone bone marrow transplantation. *Acta Paediatr Scand* 1990; **79**:613–621.

95. Smedler AC, Nilsson C, Bolme P. Total body irradiation: a neuropsychological risk factor in pediatric bone marrow transplant recipients. *Acta Pediatr* 1995; **84**:325–330.

96. Kramer JH, Crittenden MR, Halberg FE, *et al*. A prospective study of cognitive function following low-dose cranial radiation for bone marrow transplantation. *Pediatrics* 1992; **90**:447–450.

◆97. Phipps S, Dunavant M, Srivasatava DK, *et al*. Cognitive and academic functioning in survivors of pediatric bone marrow transplantation. *J Clin Oncol* 2000; **18**:1004–1011.

98. Simms S, Kazak AE, Gannon T, *et al*. Neuropsychological outcome of children undergoing bone marrow transplantation. *Bone Marrow Transplant* 1998; **22**:181–184.

99. Simms S, Kazak AE, Golumb VA, *et al*. Cognitive and psychological outcome in 2 year survivors of childhood bone marrow transplantation, paper presented at the *University of Pennsylvania Cancer Center Annual Symposium*, March, 1999.

100. Graus F, Saiz A, Sierra J, *et al*. Neurologic complications of autologous and allogeneic bone marrow transplantation in patients with leukemia: a comparative study. *Neurology* 1996; **46**:1004–1009.

101. Meyers CA, Weitzer M, Byrne K, *et al*. Evaluation of the neurobehavioral functioning of patients before, during and after bone marrow transplantation. *J Clin Oncol* 1994; **12**:820–826.

102. Marks PV. Neurological aspects of stem cell transplantation. In: Barrett J, Trealeaven J (eds) *The clinical practice of stem-cell transplantation*, Volume 1. Oxford: ISIS, 1998:787–794.

103. Padovan CS, Tarek YA, Schleuning M, *et al*. Neurological and neuroradiological findings in long-term survivors of allogeneic bone marrow transplantation. *Ann Neurol* 1998; **43**:627–633.

104. Patchell RA, White CL, Clark AW, *et al*. Neurologic complications of bone marrow transplantation. *Neurology* 1985; **35**:300–306.

105. Wiznitzer M, Packer R, August C, *et al*. Neurological complications of bone marrow transplantation. *Ann Neurol* 1984; **16**:569–576.

106. Thompson CB, Sanders JE, Flournoy N, *et al*. The risks of central nervous system relapse and leukoencephalopathy in patients receiving marrow transplants for acute leukemia. *Blood* 1986; **67**:195–199.

107. Coley SC, Porter DA, Calamante F, *et al*. Quantitative MR diffusion mapping and cyclosporin-induced neurotoxicity. *Am J Neuroradiol* 1999; **20**:1507–1510.

108. McGuire T, Sanders JE, Hill JD, *et al*. Neuropsychological function in children given total body irradiation for marrow transplantation. *Exp Hematol* 1991; **19**:578 (abstract).

◆109. Butler R, Copeland DR. Attentional processes and their remediation in children treated for cancer: a literature review and the development of a therapeutic approach. *J Int Neuropsychol Soc* 2002; **8**:115–124.

110. Meyers CA, Weitzner MA, Valentine AD. Methylphenidate therapy improves cognition, mood, and function of brain tumor patients. *J Clin Oncol* 1998; **16**:2522–2527.

◆111. Thompson SJ, Leigh L, Christensen R, *et al*. Immediate neurocognitive effects of methylphenidate on learning-impaired survivors of childhood cancer. *J Clin Oncol* 2001; **19**:1802–1808.

●112. Armstrong FD, Blumberg MJ, Toledano SR. Neurobehavioral issues in childhood cancer. *School Psychol Rev* 1999; **28**:194–203.

Ocular complications

MICHAEL OBER, KATHERINE BEAVERSON AND DAVID ABRAMSON

ANATOMY AND PHYSIOLOGY OF THE EYE

The purpose of this section is to provide the reader with sufficient ocular anatomy and physiology to interpret the remainder of the subchapter properly (see also Figures 2c.1 and 2c.2). It is intended only as a basic review detailing those aspects pertinent to cancer treatment.

Eyelids

The skin on the outer surface of the eyelids is the thinnest in the body. In addition, it is devoid of subcutaneous fat, allowing fluid accumulation to cause rapid swelling. The eyelids are separated anatomically into anterior and posterior segments. The anterior segment contains skin and the orbicularis oculi muscle, which acts as the main protractor of the eyelids. The posterior segment consists of the tarsal plates and conjunctiva. The tarsal plates are found in both the upper and lower eyelids, and consist of dense connective tissue, which functions as the support structure of the eyelids.

Conjunctiva

The conjunctiva contains many structures vital to maintain proper function of the eye. It covers both the posterior aspect of the eyelids (palpebral conjunctiva) and the anterior surface of the eye (bulbar conjunctiva) extending from the mucocutaneous junction of the lids to the corneal limbus. The areas between the palpebral and

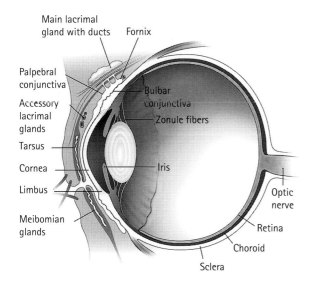

Figure 2c.1 *Sagittal anatomy of the eye.*

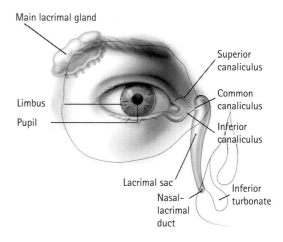

Figure 2c.2 *Frontal view of the eye.*

bulbar conjunctiva are known as the superior and inferior fornices. In these areas, conjunctival tissue is folded and redundant to allow for adequate movement of the globe without impedance. The main lacrimal gland ducts empty into the superior fornix along with many of the accessory lacrimal glands.

The conjunctiva contains a stratified non-keratinized epithelium overlying a multilayered stroma, known as the substancia propria. Intermixed with epithelial cells are mucin-producing goblet cells, which supply one portion of the tear film. The conjunctiva also plays a role in host defenses. Besides acting as a physical barrier, the conjunctiva contains many immune cells, including lymphocytes, mast cells, plasma cells and neutrophils, all of which reside within the substancia propria.

Cornea

The cornea is an optically transparent, avascular tissue, which refracts and transmits light to the inner structures of the eye. It provides approximately 60 per cent of the refractive power of the eye. The conjunctiva borders the cornea in a region known as the limbus. This zone is believed to contain corneal stem cells; therefore, compromise of this area will lead directly to the loss of corneal transparency and often corneal integrity. Because it is avascular, the cornea is dependent on the limbal vessels and aqueous fluid of the anterior chamber for nutrients and waste removal.

The cornea contains five layers, including (from the anterior) epithelium, Bowman's membrane, stroma, Descemet's membrane and, finally, endothelium. The epithelium consists of stratified non-keratinized cells, which turn over approximately every 5–7 days. The stroma provides roughly 90 per cent of the overall corneal thickness including a small superficial specialized region known as Bowman's layer. The regular orderly arrangement of type 1 collagen lamellae within the stroma is partially responsible for the corneal transparency. Descemet's membrane is a thickened periodic acid Schiff (PAS)-positive basement membrane secreted by the endothelium. The endothelium cells form a non-regenerating monolayer containing the ionic pumps that control stromal deturgence. These pumps are essential to maintain transparency, as small changes in stromal thickness drastically change its optical properties. Inflammation of the cornea, known as keratitis, also causes changes in corneal thickness.

Lens

The lens contains 35 per cent protein and 65 per cent water; it is devoid of both blood vessels and nerves. The biconvex shape and colorless transparent nature of the lens provides the second major refractive surface of the eye after the cornea. It is suspended circumferentially by a ligament known as the zonule and is immersed anteriorly in aqueous humor and posteriorly in vitreous humor. The lens capsule is a semipermeable membrane surrounding the lens, which admits water and nutrients. Throughout life, the lens epithelial cell progeny migrate inward from the anterior subcapsular epithelium, known as the germinal center, forming the dense nucleus. The younger outer fibers constitute the cortex. Unlike other epithelial structures, the cells of the lens are never shed. Rather they are incorporated into the nucleus and thus injured cells leave permanent visible defects within the structure of the lens.

The crystalline lens is particularly susceptible to cancer treatment, such as radiation and pharmacological therapy, evident in the form of cataract. A cataract simply refers to loss of the optical clarity of the lens. It is usually caused by disruption of the regular structure of the lamellar fibers or by swollen abnormal cells themselves. They are classified by location, with names such as nuclear, cortical and subcapsular, and can vary widely in severity.

Tear film production and drainage

The tear film covers the anterior surface of the cornea and the conjunctiva. It supplies moisture and nutrients to the cornea in addition to carrying protein signals and immunoglobulins as part of the host defense mechanism. It allows the cornea and conjunctiva to maintain their epithelium as non-keratinized. Furthermore, it comprises the smooth refractive coating vital to vision by covering corneal epithelial irregularities.

The tear film consists of three basic layers. The aqueous layer comprises the bulk of the tear volume. The accessory lacrimal glands of Krause and Wolfring, found in the substancia propria of the conjunctiva, provide the basal secretion, while the main lacrimal glands are located in the superior temporal orbits and produce reflex tearing. The aqueous layer consists of proteins, electrolytes and water. The proteins include immunoglobulins, lactoferrin, lysozyme and many others, which function as part of the host defense mechanism among other proposed actions. The electrolytes provide lubrication and nourishment to the anterior cornea and conjunctiva. Meibomian glands located within the tarsal plate of the upper and lower lids produce the second layer, a thin oily film that coats the aqueous layer. This oily layer is believed to have several vital functions including prevention of tear spillover and reducing evaporation in open eyes. The mucous layer secreted by the goblet cells of the conjunctiva represents the third distinct layer of the tear film. It lays on the outer surface of the cornea and conjunctiva, and functions to stabilize the aqueous layer

along with preventing desiccation. The overall function of the tear film is intimately dependent on each individual layer such that a deficiency in any stratum will adversely affect the entire ocular surface.

Tears are drained from the ocular surface via two puncta located in the medial canthus on the upper and lower lids. These puncta lead to the canaliculi, which merge as the common canaliculus and empty into the lacrimal sac. The lacrimal sac in turn drains into the nose via the nasolacrimal duct.

Optic nerve and retina

The retina is a thin transparent structure made up of many highly specialized cells. The macula, located temporal to the optic disc, is responsible for central vision and contains a central avascular zone known as the fovea. It consists mainly of cone photoreceptors responsible for color perception, while the peripheral retina contains mostly rod cells, which function in low light situations.

The optic nerve contains 1 100 000 axons of the superficial layer of the retina. These axons comprise the pathway through which visual stimuli reach the brain. It enters the orbit via the optic canal and the eye through an area known as the optic disc, where fibers are dispersed throughout the posterior pole of the globe to form the retina.

Amblyopia

The brain has only a finite period of time during which the visual pathways develop. When the central nervous system is presented with altered visual stimuli during this critical period, such as through a cataracterous lens, the potential visual acuity is diminished. This phenomenon is termed amblyopia. The vital time begins before or at birth, and is believed to end somewhere between age 7 and 13. In young patients, visual deprivation as short as a week or two is believed to cause some degree of amblyopia. Once development is complete, alterations in stimuli no longer change the potential vision. When identified early in its course, amblyopia is potentially reversible through various treatment modalities. It is for this reason that visually impairing complications in children must be recognized early.

CHEMOTHERAPY

The eye has a potentially high degree of sensitivity to cancer chemotherapy. In children, the long-term ramifications may be visually devastating. Several sources in the literature provide thorough reviews of both acute and chronic

ocular side effects of antineoplastic medications.[1–4] The following summarizes the long-term ocular complications of chemotherapeutic agents with an emphasis on pediatric treatments (see also Figure 2c.3, Plate 1).

Alkyl sulfonates

BUSULFAN

Posterior subcapsular cataracts (PSC) are a well-documented complication of busulfan therapy (Figures 2c.4 and 2c.5). These lens changes appear pathologically comparable to those found in corticosteroid-induced cataracts. Podos and Canellos found two cases of definite PSC cataracts following a mean of 113.5 months of continuous treatment and six cases with early lens changes after a mean 27.2 months. Both incidence and severity of lens changes increased with the total dose and duration of treatment.[5]

In addition, the development of keratoconjunctivitis sicca has been correlated with busulfan therapy. One patient developed total loss of vision secondary to dry eyes following 9 years of treatment.[6]

NITROSOUREA

Long-term ocular complications are rarely seen in patients treated with intravenous nitrosourea therapy at recommended doses; however, severe visual complications may develop following high-dose or combination therapy in association with bone marrow transplantation. Several cases of bilateral blindness have been reported following high-dose 1,3-bis(2-chloroethyl)-1-nitrosourea (BCNU) and cisplatin therapy secondary to retinal arterial occlusion and optic nerve necrosis.[7] In addition, optic neuroretinitis developed in patients treated with high-dose BCNU alone.[8]

The majority of cases demonstrating ocular toxicity to nitrosourea compounds involve ipsilateral intracarotid infusion, where incidence and severity increase with higher doses and injection rates. Reported complications include optic neuropathy, pupil abnormalities, internal ophthalmoplegia, and blindness with optic atrophy.[9] Several authors have attempted to circumvent these complications by using supraophthalmic infusions of BCNU; however, optic nerve degeneration, pupil abnormalities and visual loss were still reported, although with lesser frequency.[10]

Antibiotics

DOXORUBICIN

No long-term side effects of this medication have been reported in the literature.

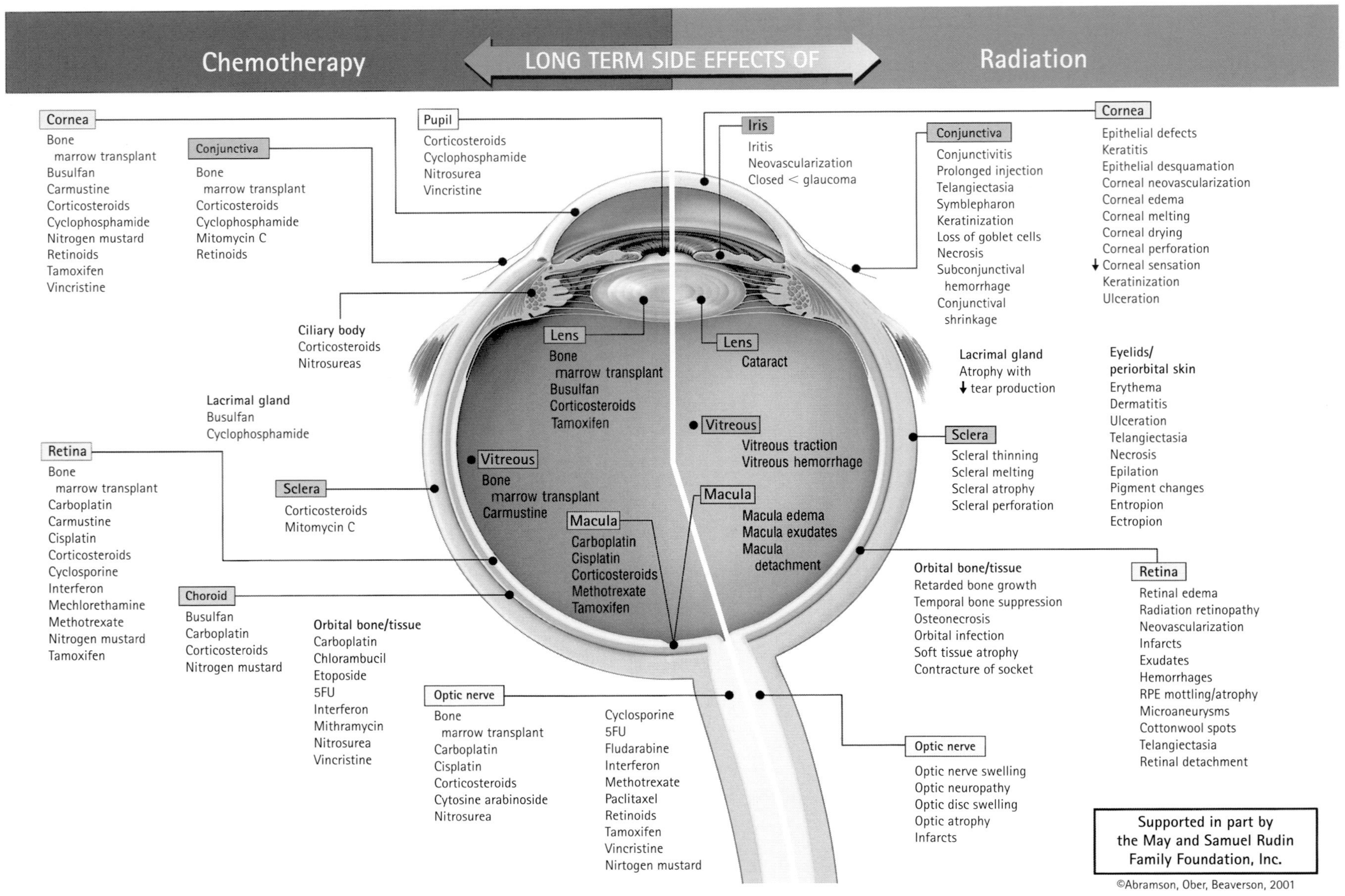
Chemotherapy
LONG TERM SIDE EFFECTS OF
Radiation
Cornea
Bone
marrow transplant
Busulfan
Carmustine
Corticosteroids
Cyclophosphamide
Nitrogen mustard
Retinoids
Tamoxifen
Vincristine
Conjunctiva
Bone
marrow transplant
Corticosteroids
Cyclophosphamide
Mitomycin C
Retinoids
Pupil
Corticosteroids
Cyclophosphamide
Nitrosurea
Vincristine
Ciliary body
Corticosteroids
Nitrosureas
Lacrimal gland
Busulfan
Cyclophosphamide
Lens
Bone
marrow transplant
Busulfan
Corticosteroids
Tamoxifen
Vitreous
Bone
marrow transplant
Carmustine
Macula
Carboplatin
Cisplatin
Corticosteroids
Methotrexate
Tamoxifen
Retina
Bone
marrow transplant
Carboplatin
Carmustine
Cisplatin
Corticosteroids
Cyclosporine
Interferon
Mechlorethamine
Methotrexate
Nitrogen mustard
Tamoxifen
Sclera
Corticosteroids
Mitomycin C
Choroid
Busulfan
Carboplatin
Corticosteroids
Nitrogen mustard
Orbital bone/tissue
Carboplatin
Chlorambucil
Etoposide
5FU
Interferon
Mithramycin
Nitrosurea
Vincristine
Optic nerve
Bone
marrow transplant
Carboplatin
Cisplatin
Corticosteroids
Cytosine arabinoside
Nitrosurea
Cyclosporine
5FU
Fludarabine
Interferon
Methotrexate
Paclitaxel
Retinoids
Tamoxifen
Vincristine
Nirtogen mustard
Iris
Iritis
Neovascularization
Closed < glaucoma
Conjunctiva
Conjunctivitis
Prolonged injection
Telangiectasia
Symblepharon
Keratinization
Loss of goblet cells
Necrosis
Subconjunctival
hemorrhage
Conjunctival
shrinkage
Cornea
Epithelial defects
Keratitis
Epithelial desquamation
Corneal neovascularization
Corneal edema
Corneal melting
Corneal drying
Corneal perforation
↓ Corneal sensation
Keratinization
Ulceration
Lens
Cataract
Lacrimal gland
Atrophy with
↓ tear production
Eyelids/
periorbital skin
Erythema
Dermatitis
Ulceration
Telangiectasia
Necrosis
Epilation
Pigment changes
Entropion
Ectropion
Vitreous
Vitreous traction
Vitreous hemorrhage
Sclera
Scleral thinning
Scleral melting
Scleral atrophy
Scleral perforation
Macula
Macula edema
Macula exudates
Macula
detachment
Orbital bone/tissue
Retarded bone growth
Temporal bone suppression
Osteonecrosis
Orbital infection
Soft tissue atrophy
Contracture of socket
Retina
Retinal edema
Radiation retinopathy
Neovascularization
Infarcts
Exudates
Hemorrhages
RPE mottling/atrophy
Microaneurysms
Cottonwool spots
Telangiectasia
Retinal detachment
Optic nerve
Optic nerve swelling
Optic neuropathy
Optic disc swelling
Optic atrophy
Infarcts
Supported in part by
the May and Samuel Rudin
Family Foundation, Inc.
©Abramson, Ober, Beaverson, 2001

Figure 2c.3 *Long-term side effects of chemotherapy and radiation. 5FU, 5-fluorouuracil; RPE, refinal pigment epithelium.*

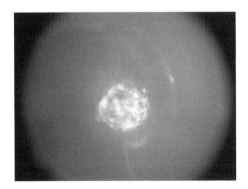

Figure 2c.4 *Photograph of a posterior subcapsular cataract.*

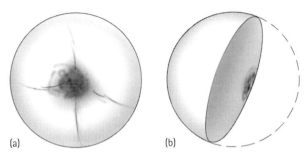

(a)   (b)

Figure 2c.5 *(a) Schematic drawing of posterior subcapsular cataract (frontal view). (b) Schematic drawing of posterior subcapsular cataract (cut-away view).*

Mitomycin C

Systemic use of mitomycin C has produced few reports of ocular toxicity, none with long-term ramifications. While many authors have observed severe ocular complications of topical treatment with mitomycin, it is not currently employed for antineoplasic therapy in the pediatric population.

MITHRAMYCIN

The national registry of drug-induced ocular side effects mentions periorbital pallor as an adverse reaction to mithramycin, although no details are given as to dose or duration of effect.[2]

Antimetabolites

CYTOSINE ARABINOSIDE

As with other antimetabolites, the majority of reports of ocular toxicity associated with intravenous cytosine arabinoside involve reversible corneal and conjunctival irritation. To decrease the incidence and severity of this reaction, concurrent administration of glucocorticoid containing drops has been adopted as standard practice at some institutions, although some reports show artificial

tears to be equally effective.[11] Intrathecal injections in association with radiation therapy, however, have been shown to induce severe visual loss from optic neuropathy.[12] It is unclear whether this represents a toxic effect of cytosine arabinoside or rather an example of the radiopotentiation of chemotherapy.

5-FLUOROURACIL

Excess tearing secondary to cicatricial ectropion and canalicular fibrosis has been reported as a complication of 5-fluorouracil therapy developing either acutely or up to 6–14 months after treatment.[13] This may occur because of excretion of 5-fluorouracil into tears. Silastic intubation of the nasal lacrimal system has resulted in improvement for patients with similar complications.[14] Two patients have also reportedly developed extraocular muscle dysfunction owing to cranial nerve palsy.[15] Chan *et al.* reported 5-fluorouracil may also potentiate the effects of radiation on the eye.[16]

METHOTREXATE

Ocular toxicity associated with methotrexate involves short-term corneal and conjunctival irritation resolving in weeks to months following cessation of therapy. When combined with carotid arterial infusion of mannitol and intravenous cyclophosphamide, however, methotrexate was reported to cause retinal pigment epithelial changes and macular edema.[17] As with other antimetabolites, methotrexate is excreted in measurable amounts within tears. Methotrexate has also been observed to potentiate the radiosensitivity of the eye.

FLUDARABINE

Visual loss has been attributed to fludarabine therapy believed to be secondary to optic neuritis or cortical blindness.[18] Bowyer reported a case of fungal endophthalmitis in a patient treated with fludarabine. The infection was believed to result from immunosuppression secondary to fludarabine treatment and underlying chronic lymphocytic leukemia.[19]

CORTICOSTEROIDS

The ocular complications related to corticosteroids are well established. Black *et al.* first described the most frequently reported side effect, the posterior subcapsular cataract in 1960.[20] The overall incidence of steroid induced cataracts ranges from 15 to 52 per cent with dose and duration of therapy influencing the figures. It has been suggested that children treated with corticosteroids are more susceptible to the development of cataracts;[21] however, this may simply reflect a relative dose increase as the opposite has also been reported.[22] One large study followed 693 patients of various ages and found that dose

and length of treatment were the major risk factors for development of cataracts. Other studies have found no relation between steroid dose and PSC development in children, suggesting a possible genetic susceptibility.[23] Although subject to wide variability, the approximate threshold dose for PSC formation is 10 mg prednisone daily for 1 year.[24] Rare reports document that some corticosteroid-induced cataracts in children are reversible.[25] The majority of secondary PSCs are not visually significant; however, some will require cataract extraction in order to maintain satisfactory vision and prevent amblyopia. It should also be mentioned that steroid-induced PSC has been seen with systemic, inhaled, topical and skin formulations.

An elevation in intraocular pressure (IOP) with the associated development or exacerbation of open-angle glaucoma is another well-described side effect of corticosteroid therapy. The susceptibility to develop an IOP increase following steroid treatment is genetically predetermined.[26] While pressure rises may be found in the normal population, patients with pre-existing glaucoma show greater increases in IOP from equivalent therapy.[27] Older patients also display a higher relative IOP than children and young adults.[28] A time–response relationship has also been established for steroid-induced ocular hypertension, where a clinically significant rise in IOP usually requires greater than 2 weeks of therapy. Although an increase in aqueous production has been proposed as a possible mechanism of steroid-induced IOP elevation, a greater body of evidence advocates an effect on the outflow mechanism. The increase in IOP by steroids is generally felt to be reversible; however, irreversible glaucoma has also been demonstrated.[29]

The immunosuppressive effects of corticosteroids are believed to have caused or enhanced many opportunistic infections, including *Herpes simplex* keratouveitis, *Varicella zoster* keratoconjuctivitis or retinitis, *Candida* endophthalmitis, cytomegalovirus retinitis, toxoplasmosis chorioretinitis, pseudomonal corneal ulcers and fungal keratitis. Patients subject to initiation of treatment with or rapid tapering of corticosteroids may also develop pseudotumor cerebri. In addition, ptosis has been reported following long-term corticosteroid use.[30] Furthermore, chronic corticosteroid therapy has been implicated in causing exophthalmos.[31]

NITROGEN MUSTARDS

Few ocular side effects have been reported after treatment with nitrogen mustard when given topically, intravenously or intracavitary; however, a single case of bilateral papilledema with retinal hemorrhages and diplopia was attributed to treatment with chlorambucil. In addition, patients treated with chlorambucil have developed keratitis after several years of oral therapy.[2] Anderson

et al. found 25 per cent of patients ($n = 12$) developed an ipsilateral necrotizing uveitis following intracarotid infusion of mechlorethamine. Pathology revealed a necrotizing vasculitis of the choroid.[32]

OXAZOPHOSPHORINES

Dry eye syndrome and blepharoconjunctivitis comprise the long-term complications associated with cylophosphamide therapy.[33] While transient blurring of vision and conjunctivitis have been associated with ifosfamide therapy, a search of the literature produced no cases demonstrating ocular toxicity beyond 1 year after treatment.

Plant alkaloids

VINCRISTINE AND VINBLASTINE

Vincristine and vinblastine have been associated with many acute, reversible ophthalmic changes including ptosis, cranial nerve palsy, lagophthalmos, corneal hypoesthesia and transient cortical blindness. Albert *et al.* reported one case with persistent extraocular muscle weakness and esotropia 34 months after onset.[34] Optic neuropathy has also been attributed to therapy with vincristine. The symptoms resolve in a majority of patients after discontinuation of treatment; however, one patient who received a combination of vincristine (2 mg/dose for six courses over 4 weeks), cyclophosphamide and prednisone remained completely blind despite cessation of therapy.[35] Partially reversible optic atrophy with optic disc pallor has also been seen following vincristine therapy. The authors suggest that increased central nervous system penetration secondary to concomitant radiation and surgery potentiate vincristine toxicity.[36]

Platinum complexes

CISPLATIN

Intravenous cisplatin therapy has been associated with papilledema, retrobulbar neuritis, optic disc edema and optic neuritis at doses as low as $120 \, mg/m^2$.[37–39] While some of these complications appeared to reverse with cessation of therapy, electrophysiological testing revealed permanent ocular toxicity correlating with decreased vision.[2] Wilding *et al.* also reported retinal toxicity, manifest as altered color perception and blurred vision, with associated macular pigmentation changes resulting from intravenous cisplatin. Visual dysfunction was localized to the retina by characteristic changes on electroretinogram (ERG). Following completion of therapy, patients reported full resolution of symptoms within 16 months.[40]

Intracarotid infusion of cisplatin in doses of 90–200 mg/treatment has resulted in ipsilateral visual loss from optic

nerve and/or retinal ischemia, cavernous sinus syndrome and one case of uveal effusion with exudative retinal detachment and periorbital edema.[28,41]

CARBOPLATIN

Carboplatin has caused significantly fewer reported cases of ocular toxicity than cisplatin at comparable doses. Several cases of visual loss, however, have been reported from chorioretinitis, maculopathy and optic neuropathy.[42] In addition, severe orbital inflammation has been described resulting in permanently decreased corrected visual acuity from ischemia of the optic nerve and glaucoma secondary to uveal effusion in a patient treated with intracarotid etoposide and carboplatin.[43]

Taxanes

PACLITAXEL

While reproducible photopsia and scintillating scotoma have been reported as short-term reversible consequences to paclitaxel therapy, one report suggested a more ominous long-term toxicity of optic nerve damage.[44] Peripapillary atrophy was seen on examination and electrophysiologic testing revealed abnormal visual evoked potential (VEP) despite a normal ERG consistent with results seen in ischemic optic neuropathy. This side effect was noted at doses of $225 \, mg/m^2$ by 3-hour infusion for a total of six courses.

DOCETAXEL

Although a relatively new medication, Esmaeli et al. has already reported three cases of punctual and canalicular stenosis secondary to treatment with docetaxel.[45] Patients were treated with weekly injections of $35 \, mg/m^2$ along with dexamethasone coverage for 14–20 weeks before presentation. The mechanism was thought to be either from direct contact with the drug in the tear film or through systemic fibrosis as seen elsewhere in the body. The authors recommended punctoplasty or intubation of the canalicular system early to prevent complete fibrosis.

Other agents

CYCLOSPORINE

Patients treated with cyclosporine have been reported to develop a variety of ocular toxicities including optic neuropathy, ophthalmoplegia, nystagmus, optic disc edema and cortical blindness.[46,47] Porges et al. reported a case of severe bilateral visual loss secondary to irreversible optic neuropathy in a patient with a toxic cyclosporine blood level of 1290 mg/ml. While some authors have implicated

cyclosporine in the development of a microvascular retinopathy,[48] it remains unclear whether this is an effect from cyclosporine alone or results from concurrent use with radiation therapy and bone marrow transplantation.

HYDROXYUREA

While several authors have reported skin toxicities of hydroxyurea therapy, such as icthyosis, a search of the literature revealed one case with manifestations limited to the eyelids with associated conjunctival injection. The patient received long-term doses 1–1.5 g of hydroxurea when he developed right eye discomfort and was found to have an erythematous eyelid with dry, flaking skin and adjacent conjunctival injection. Cessation of treatment was followed by full recovery within 4 months.[49]

RETINOIDS

Fraunfelder et al. reviewed 2379 reported adverse events by patients on isotretinoin.[50] He found several cases of permanent loss of dark adaptation occurring between 10 days and 4 months after treatment, and 16 cases of decreased color vision developing after 3–14 months of therapy. A similar color vision abnormality has also been reported with etretinate.[51] Other long-term toxicities Fraunfelder regards as 'certain' included blepharoconjunctivitis, keratoconjunctivitis sicca, meibomian gland dysfunction, corneal opacities and decreased vision.

INTERFERON α

Guyer et al. first reported retinopathy associated with interferon therapy manifest as cotton-wool spots with intraretinal hemorrhages.[52] This finding has been corroborated by many authors and is now believed to result from high-dose regimens, such as 20 million units/m^2 induction three times weekly for 4 weeks followed by maintenance doses of 10 million units/m^2 five times per week.[53] These findings usually present in patients complaining of blurry or decreased vision; however, Esmaeli et al. showed that retinopathy may develop in asymptomatic patients up to a year following initiation of treatment.[54] Visual loss and retinal findings are normally reversible upon prompt cessation of interferon; however, with progression of retinopathy, visual deficits may become irreversible. One case of exophthalmos attributed to interferon has been reported, which led to severe exposure necessitating eventual enucleation.[55]

TAMOXIFEN

High-dose tamoxifen use, $60 \, mg/m^2$ twice weekly, has been linked to corneal opacities, macular edema with corresponding funduscopic changes, and associated decreased visual acuity.[56] Pathologic specimens revealed intraretinal vesicles composed of glycosaminoglycans.[57,58]

Further experience with tamoxifen has led to reports of ocular toxicity associated with lower dosages. One study found evidence of decreased vision associated with corneal changes and macular edema in two patients taking 30 mg daily for 9–14 months.[59] Another study found similar changes in patients treated with 20 mg per day for an average of 35 months.[60] Although there has been some disagreement regarding regular ophthalmic screening examinations for patients taking tamoxifen, Heier *et al.* concluded that ocular toxicity was relatively uncommon and did not require special screening.[61] During his examination of 135 asymptomatic patients, he found two with characteristic retinal changes. There is also some evidence linking tamoxifen use with cataract development; however, the statistical and clinical significance of this association continues to be debated.[4,62]

RADIOTHERAPY

The long-term side effects of radiation are summarized in Figure 2c.3 and Plate 1.

Eyelids and periorbital skin

Late effects of radiation therapy include hyperpigmentation, depigmentation, telangiectasia, sun sensitivity, epilation, necrosis, ulceration and structural position changes, such as entropion and ectropion. Fibrosis and blockage of the lacrimal drainage system have also resulted from exposure to 30–60 Gy.[63] Loss of eyelashes occurs at 10–14 days following five doses of radiation and may persist as a chronic complication. Lid necrosis caused by excess sun exposure in areas previously treated with radiation may develop months to years after treatment.[64]

Conjunctiva

Vascular changes comprise the majority of long-term radiation side effects on the conjunctiva. Exposure to 30–50 Gy has resulted in prolonged injection developing 1–2 months after exposure with friable telangiectatic vessels following 3 months to 6 years later. Typical changes described as 'pearl string' involve irregular vascular dilations alternating with constrictions. These vessels tend to bleed spontaneously as subconjunctival hemorrhages with minor trauma. One relatively common side effect that may occur at minimal doses involves tear film instability from loss of goblet cells and accessory lacrimal glands. Conjunctival keratinization can occur with doses of 50 Gy. These keratin plaques may constantly irritate adjacent cornea leading to scarring and visual loss. Contracture of conjunctiva leading to symblepharon (adhesions between bulbar and palpebral conjunctiva),

shortening of the fornices, trichiasis (turning of the lashes on to the ocular surface) and lid malpositioning is seen following treatment with 60 Gy. Late conjunctival necrosis has also been documented after exposure to 90–300 Gy from radioactive plaque treatment.[63,64]

Cornea

The cornea is susceptible to visually significant changes from radiation toxicity. Acute keratitis is often self-limited following exposure to 30 Gy;[64] however, corneal abrasions may persist for months after 40 Gy.[63] Impaired corneal nerve function often accompanies a deep keratitis generally seen with greater than 50 Gy. The decreased sensation exacerbates corneal damage both by impairing reflex tearing with its accompanying nourishment, lubrication and host defenses, and by delaying complaints from the patient. The corneal edema associated with radiation exposure is thought to result from both lymphocyte infiltration into the stroma and loss of the endothelial cell pumping mechanism.[65] Additional complications include neovascularization, lipid infiltration, stromal keratitis and corneal melting.[63] Many of the corneal surface changes are exacerbated or caused solely by tear film insufficiency and/or hypoesthesia. Damage to conjunctival goblet cells, lacrimal glands and meibomian glands lead to inadequate tear stability and subsequent corneal erosion. In this setting, the cornea heals poorly and becomes colonized with bacteria, potentially leading to ulceration.

Lens

The posterior subcapsular cataract is a characteristic late complication of radiation exposure. The lens is especially susceptible to radiation exposure because of perpetual mitotic activity and inability to remove injured cells or disperse heat efficiently. Abnormal lens cells from the metabolically active germinative zone located immediately behind the anterior capsule migrate to the posterior pole of the lens form the distinctive opacity. Merriam and Focht's analysis in 1957 of lens changes in patients treated with radiation therapy yielded results which remain clinically relevant.[66] They found that a single exposure to 200 R, fractionated doses of 400 R over 3 weeks to 3 months, or a dose of 550 R divided over greater than 3 months provided the threshold to developing lenticular opacities. Furthermore, they reported that 100 per cent of those patients exposed to a single treatment of ⩾200 R, fractionated doses of >1000 R over 3 weeks to 3 months, or those receiving a total of >1100 R over greater than 3 months developed cataracts. The lens in children less than 1 year of age is more sensitive to radiation than adults, presumably from greater cell proliferation. Rates approach those for adults in children greater than 1 year old.[67]

Retina

Retinopathy is a well-documented consequence of radiation treatment characterized by specific fundoscopic findings including microaneurysms, hard exudates, cotton-wool spots, optic disc swelling, vascular occlusion, capillary non-perfusion, neovascularization, and retinal and vitreous hemorrhages. These changes are clinically indistinguishable from diabetic retinopathy. Radiation maculopathy is a term applied to non-proliferative radiation retinopathy that displays microvascular changes within 3 mm of the center of the fovea and carries significant visual consequences. The development of neovascularization, known as proliferative radiation retinopathy, is associated with a poor visual prognosis and leads to surgical removal of the eye in a significant percentage of patients secondary to glaucoma, pain and chronic retinal detachments. Other less typical complications of radiation retinopathy include choroidal neovascularization, and retinal artery and vein occlusion.

Radiation retinopathy develops as early as 3 weeks and as late as 15 years after treatment, although more typically it is seen between 1 and 3 years. As little as 15 Gy of external beam radiation has resulted in retinopathy, 30–60 Gy are more typically required.[63,68] In the author's experience, fewer than 5 per cent of children treated with external-beam radiation for retinoblastoma develop radiation retinopathy, making it a rather uncommon finding within this subgroup. A level of 50 Gy is regarded as the threshold for retinopathy development following radioactive plaque exposure.[68,69]

Several factors are believed to increase susceptibility to radiation retinopathy. Many reports have concluded that patients with diabetes mellitus will both develop retinal changes after exposure to a lesser dose of radiation and demonstrate more severe pathology.[69,70] The potentiation of radiation retinopathy by chemotherapy has also been well demonstrated with a suggestion that it may even predispose patients to blindness.[68–70] Chemotherapy not given concurrently may still potentiate the effects of radiation on the retina.[68]

Sclera

Scleral thinning, melting and atrophy may occur several years after exposure to 900 Gy.[69,71]

Orbital bones and soft tissue

Suppression of bony orbit growth can become a devastating lifelong complication of radiation treatment. Typical cases involve patients with bilateral retinoblastoma treated at a very young age with 40–70 Gy fractionated over 3–7 weeks. These patients develop a hollow temple,

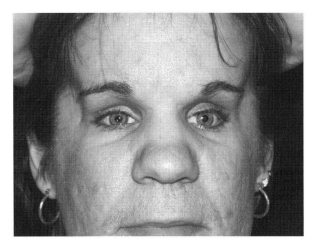

Figure 2c.6 *Patient treated with external beam radiation for bilateral retinoblastoma with characteristic bony orbital growth suppression. Printed by kind permission of the patient.*

prominent brows from a sunken orbit, shortening and narrowing of the midface, along with a saddle-nose (Figure 2c.6). Rarely, bony necrosis associated with chronic osteochondritis can occur.[63,64]

BONE MARROW TRANSPLANTATION

There are numerous reports of long-term ocular complications following bone marrow transplantation (BMT). Most develop secondary to intensive exposure to radiation or chemotherapy agents and thus are included in discussions elsewhere. The changes associated with graft-versus-host disease (GvHD), are distinct from medication and radiation toxicity and are considered unique to patients undergoing BMT.

Ocular complications occur in 60 per cent of patients with GvHD. Although the acute form of GvHD develops within 3 months of treatment, many of the side effects become long lasting or permanent. Keratoconjunctivitis sicca (KCS) from conjunctival and lacrimal gland involvement are the most commonly reported manifestations. A total of 59–75 per cent of patients with GvHD reportedly develop dry eye syndrome from either lacrimal stasis or inflammatory involvement within the gland itself.[72–76] While some relate this finding to chemotherapy toxicity, Jabs *et al.* link it to PAS-positive material deposited within the ductules secondary to GvHD.[75] In addition, the histopathology of GvHD reveals a lymphocyte infiltration of the main lacrimal gland resembling Sjogren's syndrome with inflammatory destruction followed by fibrosis.[77] Patients with either acute or chronic GvHD commonly develop a self-limited hemorrhagic pseudomembraneous conjunctivitis leading to cicatrical fibrotic scarring of the tarsus, and secondary destruction of accessory lacrimal

and meibomian glands. This severely affects tear film production and leads directly to dry eye symptoms.[75] Those under 20 years old tend to have less tear dysfunction and resulting corneal damage from dry eye syndrome.[74,78] KCS also causes corneal breakdown manifest as epithelial defects, keratinization, punctuate keratitis with chronic sterile and infectious ulceration with occasional perforation.[79] GvHD-related lid changes, such as entropion and ectropion, often exacerbate these corneal changes.

Several studies conclude cataracts are the most common ocular complication of BMT; however, the reported incidence varies greatly from 8.5 to 80 per cent.[78] Radiation, corticosteroids, busulfan and GvHD have all been reported as instigating factors in the development of BMT-related cataracts.[74,78,80,81] Dunn et al. wrote that the association with GvHD may be related to its treatment with corticosteroids rather than an immune reaction directed against lens particles,[81] while Bray et al. found a higher incidence of cataracts in patients with GvHD despite lower average levels of steroid use.[74] Despite the controversy over etiology, cataracts remain a significant cause of ocular pathology following BMT.

Uveitis in the form of iridocyclitis and/or choroiditis has been demonstrated in patients with GvHD, and is believed to be related to a direct immunologic reaction of donor lymphocytes against host histocompatability agents.[73] Uveitis itself has potentially devastating effects on the eye including cataracts, glaucoma and retinal changes.

Posterior segment complications occur in 13 per cent of patients undergoing BMT.[77,82] Most retinal and vitreous hemorrhages occur concurrent with episodes of pancytopenia and generally resolve without long-term sequelae. Cotton wool spots with ischemic retinopathy develop up to 1 year following BMT.[81,83] One study found chronic GvHD to be the only statistically significant risk factor for development of cotton wool spots.[81] These spots are often accompanied by focal intraretinal hemorrhages, telangiectatic vessels, capillary non-perfusion and, rarely, neovascularization to comprise a characteristic ischemic retinopathy termed bone marrow transplant retinopathy.[83] While radiation can account for all these findings, a similar clinical appearance may be seen in patients following BMT who have not received radiation.[48,84] Optic disc edema is also reported after BMT; however, this has been linked to cyclosporine treatment or concurrent development of meningitis.[81] In addition, rare cases of serious retinal detachments from central serous chorioretinopathy have been linked to BMT and GvHD.[85]

All BMT recipients develop a severe immune deficiency and thus become highly susceptible to ocular infections. GvHD causes inherent persistent abnormalities of the immune system further inhibited by its treatment with immunosuppressant medications. Pseudomonal corneal ulcers, *Herpes simplex* keratitis, *Herpes zoster* retinitis, cytomegalovirus chorioretinitis, *Toxoplasma* chorioretinitis,

fungal endophthalmitis and infectious subretinal abscesses have all been reported following BMT, often leading to permanent visual deficits.[72,73,77,78,81]

KEY POINTS

- Ocular complications of cancer therapy are *not* uncommon.
- Common manifestations include, but are not limited to, tear film deficiency, conjunctivitis, keratitis, cataracts, uveitis and chorioretinopathy.
- Knowledge of adverse reactions allows for prevention and reduced severity of symptoms in some cases.
- Certain complications will require lifelong treatment.
- Consultation with an ophthalmologist should be considered when symptoms arise, especially changes in vision.

REFERENCES

● 1. Al-Tweigeri T, Nabholtz JM, Mackey JR. Ocular toxicity and cancer chemotherapy. A review. *Cancer* 1996; **78**:1359–1373.
● 2. Grant WM. *Toxicology of the eye*, 3rd edn. Springfield, IL: Charles C Thomas, 1986.
● 3. Fraunfelder FT, Meyer SM (eds). *Drug induced ocular side effects and drug interactions*. Philadelphia: Lea & Febiger, 1989.
4. Burns LJ. Ocular side effects of chemotherapy. In: Perry MC (ed.) *The chemotherapy source book*. Baltimore: Lippincott Williams & Wilkins, 2001.
5. Podos SM, Canellos GP. Lens changes in chronic granulocytic leukemia. Possible relationship to chemotherapy. *Am J Ophthalmol* 1969; **68**:500–504.
6. Sidi Y, Douer D, Pinkhas J. Sicca syndrome in a patient with toxic reaction to busulfan. *JAMA* 1977; **238**:1951.
7. Wang MY, Arnold AC, Vinters HV, *et al.* Bilateral blindness and lumbosacral myelopathy associated with high dose carmustine and cisplatin therapy. *Am J Ophthalmol* 2000; **130**:367–368.
8. Shingleton BJ, Bienfang DC, Albert DM, *et al.* Ocular toxicity associated with high-dose carmustine. *Arch Ophthalmol* 1982; **100**:1766–1772.
9. Miller DF, Bay JW, Lederman RJ. Ocular and orbital toxicity following intra-carotid injection of BCNU and cisplatin for malignant gliomas. *Ophthalmology* 1985; **92**:402–406.
10. Shirmamura Y, Chikama M, Tanimoto Y, *et al.* Optic nerve degeneration caused by supraophthalmic carotid artery infusion with cisplatin and ACNU. *J Neurosurg* 1990; **72**:285–288.
11. Higa GM, Gockerman JP, Hunt AL. The use of prophylactic eye drops during high-dose cytosine arabinoside therapy. *Cancer* 1991; **68**:1691–1693.
12. Margileth DA, Poplack DG, Pizzo PA. Blindness during remission in two patients with acute lymphoblastic leukemia. A possible complication of multimodality therapy. *Cancer* 1977; **39**: 58–61.
13. Straus DJ, Mausolf FA, Ellerby RA. Cicatricial ectropian secondary to 5-fluorouracil therapy. *Med Pediatr Oncol* 1977; **3**:15–19.

14. Seiff SR, Shorr N, Adams T. Surgical treatment of punctual-canalicular fibrosis from 5-fluorouracil therapy. *Cancer* 1985; **56**:2148–2149.

15. Bixenman WW, Nicholls JV, Warwick OH. Oculomotor disturbances associated with 5-fluorouracil chemotherapy. *Am J Ophthalmol* 1968; **83**:604–608.

16. Chan RC, Shukorsky LJ. Effects of irradiation on the eye. *Radiology* 1976; **120**:673–675.

17. Millay RH, Klein ML, Shults WT. Maculopathy associated with combination chemotherapy and osmotic opening of the blood brain barrier. *Am J Ophthalmol* 1986; **102**:626–632.

18. Chun JH, Leyland-Jones BR, Caryk SM, et al. Central nervous sytem toxicity of fludarabine phosphate. *Cancer Treat Rep* 1986; **70**:1225–1228.

19. Bowyer JD, Johnson EM, Horn EH, et al. Ochroconis gallopava endophthalmitis in fludarabine treated chronic lymphocytic leukaemia. *Br J Ophthalmol* 2000; **84**:117.

◆20. Black RL, Oglesby RB, von Sallman L, et al. Posterior subcapsular cataracts induced by corticosteroids in patients with rheumatoid arthritis. *JAMA* 1960; **174**:166–171.

21. Braver DA, Richards RD, Good TA. Posterior subcapsular cataracts in steroid treated children. *Arch Ophthalmol* 1967; **77**:161.

◆22. Spaeth GL, von Sallman L. Corticosteroids and cataracts. *Int Ophthalmol Clin* 1966; **6**:915–929.

23. Limaye SR, Pillai S, Tina LU. Relationship of steroid dose to degree of posterior subcapsular cataracts in nephritic syndrome. *Ann Ophthalmol* 1988; **20**:225–227.

24. Loredo A, Rodriguez RS, Murillo L. Cataracts after short-term corticosteroid treatment. *N Engl J Med* 1972; **286**:160.

25. Forman AR, Loreto JA, Tina LU. Reversibility of corticosteroid-associated cataracts in children with the nephritic syndrome. *Am J Ophthalmol* 1977; **84**:75–78.

26. Armaly MF. The heritable nature of dexamethasone-induced ocular hypertension. *Arch Ophthalmol* 1966; **75**:32–35.

27. Armaly MF. Effect of corticosteroids on intraocular pressure and fluid dynamics II. The effect of dexamethasone in the glaucomatous eye. *Arch Ophthalmol* 1963; **70**:492–499.

28. Armaly MF. Effect of corticosteroids on intraocular pressure and fluid dynamics I: Effect of dexamethasone in the normal eye. *Arch Ophthalmol* 1963; **70**:482–490.

29. Spaeth GL, Rodriques MM, Weinreb S. Steroid induced glaucoma. A: Persistent elevation of intraocular pressure. B: Histopathological aspects. *Trans Am Ophthalmol Soc* 1977; **75**:353–381.

30. Miller D, Pecxon JD. Corticosteroid and functions in the anterior segment of the eye. *Am J Ophthalmol* 1965; **59**:31.

31. Katz G, Carmody R. Exophthalmos induced by exogenous steroids. *J Clin Neuro-Ophthalmol* 1986; **6**:250–253.

32. Anderson B, Anderson B Jr. Necrotizing uveitis incident to perfusion of intracranial malignancies with nitrogen mustard and related compounds. *Trans Am Ophthalmol Soc* 1960; **58**:95–104.

◆33. Fraunfelder FT, Meyer MS. Ocular toxicity of antieneoplastic agents. *Ophthalmology* 1983; **90**:1–3.

34. Albert DM, Wong VG, Henderson ES. Ocular complications of vincristine therapy. *Arch Ophthalmol* 1967; **78**:709–713.

35. Awidi AS. Blindness and vincristine. *Ann Intern Med* 1980; **93**:781.

36. Shurin SB, Rekate HL, Annable W. Optic atrophy induced by vincristine. *Pediatrics* 1982; **70**:288–291.

37. Ostrow S, Hohn D, Wiernik PH, et al. Ophthalmologic toxicity after cis-dichlorodiamine platinum II therapy. *Cancer Treat Rep* 1978; **62**:1591–1593.

38. Becher R, Schutt P, Osieka R, et al. Peripheral neuropathy and ophthalmologic toxicity after treatment with cis-dichlorodiamine platinum II. *J Cancer Res Clin Oncol* 1980; **96**:219–221.

39. Walsh TJ, Clark AW, Parhad IM, et al. Neurotoxic effects of cisplatin therapy. *Arch Neurol* 1982; **39**:719–720.

40. Wilding G, Caruso R, Lawrence TS, et al. Retinal toxicity after high-dose cisplatin therapy. *J Clin Oncol* 1985; **3**:1683–1689.

41. Margo CE, Murtagh FR. Ocular and orbital toxicity after intra-carotid cisplatin therapy. *Am J Ophthalmol* 1993; **116**:508–509.

42. Rankin EM, Pitts JE. Ophthalmic toxicity during carboplatin therapy. *Ann Oncol* 1993; **4**:337–338.

43. Lauer AK, Wobig JL, Shults WT, et al. Severe ocular and orbital toxicity after intracarotid etoposide phosphate and carboplatin therapy. *Am J Ophthalmol* 1999; **127**:230–233.

44. Capri G, Munzone E, Tarenzi E, et al. Optic nerve disturbances: a new form of paclitaxel neurotoxicity. *J Natl Cancer Inst* 1994; **86(14)**:1099–1101.

45. Esmaeli B, Valero V, Ahmadi A, et al. Canalicular stenosis secondary to docetaxel (taxotere). A newly recognized side effect. *Ophthalmology* 2001; **108**:994–995.

46. Porges Y, Blumen S, Fireman Z, et al. Cyclosporine-induced optic neuropathy, ophthalmoplegia, and nystagmus in a patient with Crohn's disease. *Am J Ophthalmol* 1998; **126(4)**:607–609.

47. Ghalie R, Fitzsimmons WE, Bennett D, et al. Cortical blindness: a rare complication of cyclosporine therapy. *Bone Marrow Transplant* 1990; **6**:147–149.

48. O'Riordam JM, FitzSimon S, O'Connor M, et al. Retinal microvascular changes following bone marrow transplantation: the role of cyclosporine. *Bone Marrow Transplant* 1994; **13**:101–104.

49. Puri P, Woodcock BE, O'Donnell NP. Localised chronic eyelid disease resulting from long term hydroxurea therapy. *Br J Ophthalmol* 2001; **85**:371.

50. Fraunfelder FT, Fraunfelder FW, Edwards R. Ocular side effects possibly associated with isotretinoin usage. *Am J Ophthalmol* 2001; **132**:299–305.

51. Brown RD, Grattan CH. Visual toxicit of synthetic retinoids. *Br J Ophthalmol* 1989; **73**:286–288.

52. Guyer D, Tiedeman J, Yannuzzi J, et al. Interferon-associated retinopathy. Arch Ophthalmol 1993; **111**:50–56.

53. Hejny C, Sternberg P, Lawson DH, et al. Retinopathy associated with high-dose interferon alfa-2b therapy. *Am J Ophthalmol* 2001; **131**:782–787.

54. Esmaeli B, Koller C, Papadopoulos N, et al. Interferon-induced retinopathy in asymptomatic cancer patients. *Ophthalmology* 2001; **108**:858–860.

55. Yamada H, Mizobuchi K, Isogal Y. Acute onset of ocular complication with interferon. *Lancet* 1994; **343**:914.

56. Kaiser-Kupfer MI, Lippman ME. Tamoxifen retinopathy. *Cancer Treat Rep* 1978; **62**:315–320.

57. Kaiser-Kupfer MI, Kupfer C, Rodrigues MM. Tamoxifen retinopathy: a clinicopathologic report. *Ophthalmology* 1981; **88**:89–93.

58. McKeown CA, Swartz M, Blom J, et al. Tamoxifen retinopathy. *Br J Ophthalmol* 1981; **65**:177–179.

59. Vinding T, Nielsen NV. Retinopathy caused by treatment with tamoxifen in low dosage. *Acta Ophthalmol* 1983; **61**:45–50.

60. Pavlidis NA, Petris C, Briassoulis E, et al. Clear evidence that long-term, low-dose tamoxifen treatment can induce ocular toxicity. *Cancer* 1992; **69**:2961–2964.

61. Heier JS, Dragoo RA, Enzenauer RW, et al. Screening for ocular toxicity in asymptomatic patients treated with tamoxifen. *Am J Ophthalmol* 1994; **117**:772–775.

62. Gorin MB, Day R, Costantino JP. Long-term tamoxifen citrate use and potential ocular toxicity. *Am J Ophthalmol* 1998; **125**:493–501.

63. Servodidio CA, Abramson DH. Acute and long-term effects of radiation therapy to the eye in children. *Cancer Nursing* 1993; **16**:371–381.

64. Haik BG, Jereb B, Abramson DH, *et al.* Ophthalmic radiotherapy. In: Iliff NT (ed.) *Complication in ophthalmic surgery.* New York: Churchill Livingstone 1983:449–485.

65. Blondi FC. The late effects of x-radiation on the cornea. *Trans Am Ophthalmol Soc* 1958; **56**:413–450.

◆66. Merriam GR, Focht EF. A clinical study of radiation cataracts and the relationship to dose. *Am J Roentgenol.* 1957; **77**:759–785.

◆67. Donnenfeld ED, Ingraham HJ, Abramson DH. Effects of ionizing radiation on the conjunctiva, cornea, and lens. In: Alberti WE, Sagerman RH (eds) *Medical radiology. Radiotherapy of intraocular and orbital tumors.* Berlin: Springer-Verlag, 1993:261–270.

68. Brown GC, Shields JA, Sanborn G, *et al.* Radiation retinopathy. *Ophthalmology* 1982; **89**:1494–1501.

69. Gunduz K, Shields CL, Shields JA, *et al.* Radiation retinopathy following plaque radiotherapy for posterior uveal melanoma. *Arch Ophthalmol* 1999; **117**:609–614.

70. Parsons JT, Bova FJ, Fitzgerald CR. Radiation retinopathy after external-beam irradiation: analysis of time-dose factors. *Int J Radiation Oncology Biol Phys* 1994; **30**:765–772.

71. Brady LW, Shields J, Augusburger JJ, *et al.* Complications from radiation therapy to the eye. *Front Radiat Ther Oncol* 1989; **23**:238–250.

72. Hirst LW, Jabs DA, Tutschka PJ, *et al.* The eye in bone marrow transplantation I. Clinical study. *Arch Ophthalmol* 1983; **101**:580–584.

73. Franklin RM, Kenyon KR, Tutschka PJ, *et al.* Ocular manifestations of graft-vs-host disease. *Ophthalmology* 1983; **90**:4–13.

74. Bray LC, Carey PJ, Proctor SJ, *et al.* Ocular complications of bone marrow transplantation. *Br J Ophthalmol* 1991; **75**:611–614.

75. Jabs DA, Hirst LW, Green R, *et al.* The eye in bone marrow transplantation II. Histopathology. *Arch Ophthalmol* 1983; **101**:585–590.

76. Jabs DA, Wingard J, Green R, *et al.* The eye in bone marrow transplantation III. Conjunctival graft-vs-host disease. *Arch Ophthalmol* 1989; **107**:1343–1348.

77. Jack MK, Jack GM, Sale GE, *et al.* Ocular manifestations of graft-vs-host disease. *Arch Ophthalmol* 1983; **101**:1080–1084.

78. Suh DW, Ruttum MS, Stuckenschneider BJ, *et al.* Ocular findings after bone marrow transplantation in a pediatric population. *Ophthalmology* 1999; **106**:1564–1570.

79. Jack MK, Hicks JD. Ocular complications in high-dose chemoradiotherapy and marrow transplantation. *Ann Ophthalmol* 1981; **13**:709–711.

80. Calissendorff BM, Bolme P. Cataract development and outcome of surgery in bone marrow transplanted children. *Br J Ophthalmol* 1993; **77**:36–38.

81. Dunn JP, Jabs DA, Wingard J, *et al.* Bone marrow transplantation and cataract development. *Arch Ophthalmol* 1993; **111**:1367–1373.

82. Coskuncan NM, Jabs DA, Dunn JP, *et al.* The eye in bone marrow transplantation IV. Retinal complications. *Arch Ophthalmol* 1994; **112**:372–379.

83. Lopez PF, Sternberg P, Dabbs CK, *et al.* Bone marrow transplant retinopathy. *Am J Ophthalmol* 1991; **112**:635–646.

84. Cunningham ET, Irvine AR, Rugo HS. Bone marrow transplantation retinopathy in the absence of radiation therapy. *Am J Ophthalmol* 1996; **122**:268–270.

85. Fawzi AA, Cunningham ET. Central serous chorioretinopathy after bone marrow transplantation. *Am J Ophthalmol* 2001; **131**:804–805.

2d

Hearing impairment

PATRICIA D SHEARER

INTRODUCTION

As more pediatric oncology patients survive, satisfactory academic achievement becomes an important long-range goal. Because both expressive and receptive language reflect auditory verbal input, treatment-related hearing loss may pose a significant obstacle to mastery of language skills and to overall academic performance. Patients at particular risk of hearing loss include those treated with cisplatin-, carboplatin- and/or ifosfamide-containing chemotherapy regimens, particularly when combined with cranial irradiation.

CISPLATIN

Cisplatin may directly cause a sensorineural high-frequency hearing loss, which is often associated with tinnitus. The mechanism of hearing loss is blockage of signal transduction of impulses from the outer hair cells (OHCs) in the organ of Corti, particularly those in the first row of the basal turn.[1,2] Hair cell injury tends to be sporadic and non-continuous,[2] and fused and disarrayed stereocilia are noted.[3] Other sites of injury may include the spiral ganglion cells, cochlear neurons[4] and stria vascularis.[2]

Because the stria vascularis provides the main blood supply to the cochlea, cisplatin may cause ototoxicity indirectly through metabolic derangements that affect this organ. Magnesium, which is required to maintain hair cell permeability[5,6] and blood flow to the cochlear arteries,[7] may be deficient after administration of cisplatin because of renal wasting or decreased intestinal absorption. Magnesium deficiency also affects the ionic concentration of both endolymph[8] and perilymph[9] in the stria vascularis, and also lowers the threshold for stimulating a cochlear action potential.[6] Hypoalbuminemia, which decreases the number of binding sites for cisplatin, may contribute to increased plasma concentration of free drug.[10] Decreased hemoglobin concentration,[10] dark skin pigmentation and brown iris color[11] have also been associated with susceptibility to cisplatin-related hearing loss.

Berg *et al.* summarize 11 studies that describe factors reported to be associated with cisplatin toxicity in pediatric patients.[12] These factors include bolus administration of drug,[13] prior cranial irradiation[14,15] and central nervous system neoplasia.[16] Although certain studies show a relationship between young age at time of treatment and cisplatin ototoxicity,[14,16] other reports do not confirm this association.[17] Similarly, most studies, but not all, associate cumulative cisplatin dose with ototoxicity.[12,14–16]

According to Schell *et al.*, cisplatin-related hearing loss appears to have a triphasic pattern.[16] Hearing remains normal until a certain amount of drug has been delivered. After this point, damage to OHCs in the basal turn progresses until maximal effect is reached. This damage usually affects hearing at approximately 75 dB.[19] Once the maximal threshold for stimulation of OHCs occurs, inner hair cells (IHCs) are then stimulated. However, because these structures are relatively resistant to the effects of cisplatin, a plateau occurs in the progression of damage (Figure 2d.1).

The net result of cisplatin ototoxicity is impaired understanding of high-frequency consonants that give speech its clarity and enhance discrimination between words (Figure 2d.2). Children who have this complication may

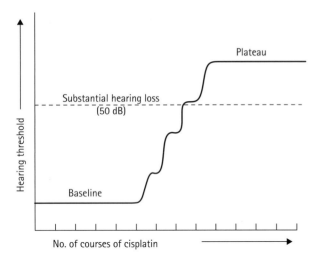

Figure 2d.1 *Schematized plot of hearing threshold as a function of the number of courses of cisplatin for a typical non-irradiated patient tested at 4000 kHz. (Source: Figure 2d.1 from MJ Schell, VA McHaney, AA Green, et al: Hearing loss in children and young adults receiving cisplatin with or without prior cranial irradiation.* J Clin Oncol *7;1989:754–760. (Reprinted with permission of the American Society of Clinical Oncology.)*

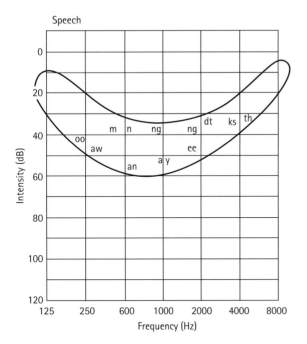

Figure 2d.2 *Speech frequencies superimposed on a standard audiogram. The letters correspond to phonemes. High-frequency hearing loss renders some speech sounds inaudible, particularly in a background of noise. (Reproduced with permission from Macdonald* et al. J Otolaryngol *1994; 23:151–160.)*

experience difficulties in educational, social and psychological adaptation. These include the need for amplification and/or preferential classroom seating, an increased sense of isolation, and an overall decrease in quality of life.[12,18]

Although cochlear function in guinea pigs[2,20] and rhesus monkeys[1] has been reported to improve after discontinuation of cisplatin,[20] most studies in humans do not demonstrate recovery of hearing after cessation of drug therapy.[12,14–16] Patients may be at risk of developing hearing loss as late as 50 months after the last dose of cisplatin.[12]

The extent of hearing loss after cisplatin therapy is usually considered to be dose-dependent. Pasic and Dobie[18] showed that, in 33 pediatric cancer patients, hearing thresholds at 6000 and 8000 kHz were 20–25 dB after cumulative doses of 201 and 300 mg/m² but progressed to 35–40 dB after cumulative doses of 301–400 mg/m². Auditory thresholds at 4000 kHz were not affected until patients had received as much as 401–500 mg/m². Similarly, Schell *et al.*[16] reported hearing thresholds in excess of 50 dB at 4000–8000 kHz in approximately 70 pediatric patients treated at St Jude Children's Research Hospital (SJCRH) with 167–575 mg/m² cisplatin (but not with cranial irradiation). In contrast, Berg *et al.* noted hearing loss in nine of 28 children who received only 60–120 mg/m² of cisplatin and did not receive irradiation.[12]

CRANIAL IRRADIATION

Cranial irradiation alone is generally thought to exert minimal ototoxic effects.[14–16] McHaney reported that none of 23 pediatric patients treated at SJCRH with 54–60 Gy cranial irradiation alone experienced hearing loss.[14] In a follow-up report from the same institution, Schell *et al.* noted that only two of 32 patients who received cranial irradiation but no cisplatin had hearing losses of 25–50 dB at frequencies lower than 6000 kHz.[16] However, among patients in that series who subsequently received cisplatin, cumulative doses as low as 270 mg/m² were associated with high probability of hearing loss across the frequency spectrum of 1000–8000 kHz. Preliminary data from SJCRH in 27.4 per cent of 157 pediatric patients treated exclusively with cranial irradiation, including the cochlea, indicate that hearing loss may appear as long as 5 years after treatment (J. Thompson, SJCRH, personal communication).

CARBOPLATIN

Carboplatin is considered to be less ototoxic than cisplatin, but may cause or exacerbate high-frequency hearing loss, particularly when given in high doses (Figure 2d.3). Studies in guinea pigs and chinchillas revealed that carboplatin may selectively damage IHCs[21] or OHCs[22] in the basal turn of the cochlea, or may have no effect on these structures.[23] There are no available reports of the effects of carboplatin on human temporal bones.

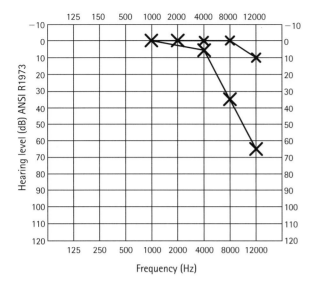

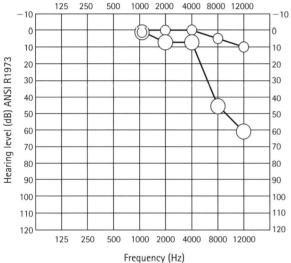

Figure 2d.3 *Representative audiograms (X = left ear, O = right ear) in a patient who received five doses of carboplatin for osteogenic sarcoma. A significant deterioration in hearing is noted in the high frequencies between the baseline audiogram (small x, o) and the audiogram after the fifth dose (large X, O). (Reproduced with permission from Macdonald et al. J Otolaryngol 1994; 23:151–160.)*

Freilich *et al.* reported high-frequency sensorineural loss in seven of 11 evaluable pediatric patients with brain tumors who had received multiagent induction chemotherapy that included cisplatin and had subsequently received carboplatin as a conditioning agent for autologous bone marrow transplantation (ABMT).[24] Five patients (one of whom had undergone cranial irradiation) experienced auditory threshold shifts of up to 65 dB between 2000 and 8000 kHz. Three patients required hearing aids.

Parsons *et al.* documented worsening of hearing in all 11 evaluable heavily pretreated patients with advanced stage neuroblastoma who received 2 g/m²carboplatin as part of a conditioning regimen for ABMT.[25] After ABMT, 9 of the 11 required amplification to compensate for loss in the speech frequency range (500–2000 kHz).

Macdonald *et al.* described a dose-dependent pattern of hearing loss in 11 of 22 pediatric patients at the Hospital for Sick Children in Toronto, who were treated for a variety of solid tumors with individual doses of 500 mg/m² of carboplatin.[21] Three of these patients had received cranial irradiation. All of the four patients who received eight or more doses of carboplatin developed a hearing loss of 15 dB or greater between 4000 and 12 000 kHz. Eleven patients demonstrated a loss at 2000 kHz. Twenty-two patients sustained loss between 8000 and 12 000 kHz after only two doses of carboplatin.

IFOSFAMIDE

Ifosfamide may exacerbate cisplatin-related hearing loss. Meyer *et al.* compared hearing loss in patients treated for osteosarcoma at SJCRH with multidrug regimens that contained either cisplatin, or both cisplatin and ifosfamide.[26] Functional impairment was sufficient to require amplification (a threshold of at least 30 dB at 2000 kHz) in 12 of 25 patients treated with cisplatin and ifosfamide, but in only 4 of 24 cases treated without ifosfamide. In contrast, Bajwa *et al.* reported no auditory toxicity in 48 children with a variety of solid tumors treated with ifosfamide given alone or in combination with other drugs.[27]

AUDITORY TESTING

Auditory toxicity may not be apparent to the patient, parent or treating physician.[12] Therefore, hearing must be assessed by behavioral audiometry (conventional pure tone audiometry with headphones, play audiometry using operant conditioning, visual evoked response audiometry or sound field testing) and/or by electrophysiology. Electrophysiological methods include measurement of auditory brainstem responses (ABRs), otoacoustic emissions (OAEs) and/or distortion product otoacoustic emissions (DPOAEs). Behavioral audiometry requires patient cooperation but provides meaningful responses to stimuli at various test frequencies. Behavioral techniques other than sound field testing may separately distinguish the responses of the two ears.

Electrophysiological methods, although they are not tests of hearing *per se*, may be used to evaluate auditory function in children too young or too ill to participate in behavioral assessment. ABR measures synchronous discharge of neural units in response to a click or tone pip centered around a particular frequency.[28] Abnormal

ABRs have been reported in association with IHC loss in premature infants at autopsy.[29] OAEs and DPOAEs are cochlear responses generated in response to two simultaneous stimuli of known frequency relationship. They reflect the function of OHCs and are, therefore, well suited to provide reliable information about changes in these structures after cisplatin administration.[30,31] Combined ABR and OAE testing may distinguish neural from cochlear (hair cell) pathology.[30]

In patients treated with cisplatin, OAEs and behavioral audiometry have shown good correlation.[32] Littman et al. reported that in pediatric patients with medulloblastoma, DPOAEs detected hearing loss before it was identified by behavioral methods.[31] Because OHCs contribute both to amplification of low-level acoustic inputs (e.g. high-frequency consonants) and compression of high-level inputs (e.g. vowels), patients with absent OAEs may be ideal candidates for dynamic compression hearing aids that optimize consonant–vowel relationships.[19]

CYTOPROTECTIVE AGENTS

Cytoprotective agents, including sodium thiosulfate,[33,34] D-methionine,[35;36] 4-methylthiobenzoic acid[37] and amifostine[38–41] may reduce the auditory toxicity of chemotherapy, particularly that of platinum-containing compounds and alkylating agents. Calcium supplementation has been used without benefit to prevent hearing loss in patients receiving cisplatin.[42]

Amifostine

Amifostine, first synthesized in the 1950s as a radioprotectant by the US Walter Reed Army Institute of Research, is an analog of cysteamine.[39] It is dephosphorylated by membrane-bound alkaline phosphatase to its active metabolite, WR-1065. This is a free thiol, which protects normal cells from damage caused by platinum-containing compounds, alkylating agents, anthracyclines, taxanes or radiation by scavenging free radicals and by binding to reactive nucleophiles that would ordinarily cross-link and damage DNA. Normal organs are selectively protected because their vasculature contains a greater concentration of alkaline phosphatase than does tumor vasculature and amifostine is thus converted to its active metabolite more effectively in the organs. Steady-state concentrations of the metabolite may be as much as 100 times greater in normal tissues than in neoplastic cells.[38,39]

Clinical studies in adults report that amifostine offers protection against myelosuppression,[41] nephrotoxicity,[41] mucositis,[43] and xerostomia[44] caused by chemotherapy and radiotherapy. Studies of human and murine xenografts demonstrated no reduction in antitumor effect.[45,46] In fact,

in Phase II trials in patients with melanoma and small-cell lung cancer antitumor responses were greater than expected.[47,48]

Data regarding the ability of amifostine to protect patients from auditory toxicity are limited. A single Phase III randomized trial in 242 adult patients with ovarian cancer treated with cyclophosphamide and cisplatin, with or without amifostine, showed a 43 per cent lower incidence of auditory toxicity in patients who received amifostine.[41] One Phase I/II trial in 12 pediatric patients with solid tumors treated with ifosfamide, carboplatin and etoposide established that amifostine was well tolerated at a dose of 600 mg/m^2 when administered before and again half way through cisplatin infusion.[49] Additional studies are under way in pediatric patients with brain tumors to evaluate the pharmacokinetics of amifostine and its role in protection from auditory toxicity (M. Fouladi, SJCRH, personal communication).

The toxic effects of amifostine are dose-related. They include nausea, emesis, sneezing, hiccups, warmth, somnolence, metallic taste, occasional allergic reaction, hypocalcemia and hypotension.[50] Of these, the last two are most significant. Hypocalcemia is caused by inhibition of parathyroid hormone secretion and resultant inhibition of bone resorption.[51] The mechanism for hypotension is unknown. However, this complication may be reduced by prehydration, maintenance of the patient in a supine position during drug administration and careful monitoring during the infusion.

ACKNOWLEDGEMENTS

The author wishes to acknowledge Dr Charles Berlin, Director of the Kresge Hearing Research Laboratory, Louisiana State University School of Medicine, New Orleans, Louisiana, and Sharon Naron of the Scientific Editing Department of St Jude Children's Research Hospital, University of Tennessee, Memphis, Tennessee, for their helpful contributions to preparation of this manuscript.

KEY POINTS

- Hearing loss from cancer treatment impacts on speech, language and psychosocial function.
- Hearing loss may occur after administration of cisplatin, carboplatin, ifosfamide and/or cranial irradiation.
- Hearing loss may not be apparent to the patient, family or physician.
- Hearing loss may be preventable with amifostine and/or other cytoprotective agents.

REFERENCES

◆1. Stadnicki SW, Fleischman RW, Schaeppi U, Merriam P. Cis-dichlorodiammine platinum (II) (NSC-119875): hearing loss and other toxic effects in rhesus monkeys. *Cancer Chemother Rep* 1975; **59**:467–480.

◆2. Nakai Y, Konishi K, Chang KC, *et al.* Ototoxicity of the anticancer drug cisplatin: an experimental study. *Acta Otolaryngol (Stockholm)* 1982; **93**:227–232.

3. Comis SD, Rhys-Evans PH, Osborne MP, *et al.* Early morphological and chemical changes induced by cisplatin in the guinea pig organ of Corti. *J Laryngol Otol* 1986; **100**:1375–1383.

4. Boheim K, Bichler E. Cisplatin-induced ototoxicity: audiometric findings and experimental cochlear pathology. *Arch Otorhinolaryngol* 1985; **242**:1–6.

5. Trump BF, Berezesky IK, Sato T, *et al.* Cell calcium, cell injury, and cell death. *Environ Health Perspect* 1984; **57**:281–287.

6. Brusilow SW, Gordes E. The mutual independence of the endolymphatic potential and the concentrations of sodium and potassium in endolymph. *J Clin Invest* 1973; **52**:2517–2521.

7. Altura BM, Altura BT, Gebrewold A, *et al.* Magnesium deficiency and hypertension: correlation between magnesium-deficient diets and microcirculatory changes *in situ*. *Science* 1984; **223**:1315–1317.

8. Brown RD. Ethacrynic acid and furosemide: possible cochlear sites and mechanisms of ototoxic action. *Medikon* 1975; **4**:33–40.

9. Joachims Z, Babisch W, Ising H, *et al.* Dependence of noise-induced hearing loss upon perilymph magnesium concentration. *J Acoust Soc Am* 1983; **74**:104–108.

10. Blakley B, Gupta A, Myers S, Schwan MA. Risk factors for ototoxicity due to cisplatin. *Arch Otolaryngol Head Neck Surg* 1994; **120**:541–546.

11. Todd W, Alvarado C, Brewer D. Cisplatin in children: hearing loss correlates with iris and skin pigmentation. *J Laryngol Otol* 1995; **109**:926–929.

12. Berg A, Spitzer J, Garvin J. Ototoxic impact of cisplatin in pediatric oncology patients. *Laryngoscope* 1999; **109**:1806–1814.

13. Reddell R, Kefford R, Grant J, *et al.* Ototoxicity in patients receiving cisplatin: importance of dose and method of drug administration. *Cancer Treat Rep* 1982; **66**:19–23.

14. McHaney V, Thibadoux M, Hayes A, Green A. Hearing loss in children receiving cisplatin chemotherapy. *J Pediatr* 1983; **102**:314–317.

15. McHaney V, Kovnar E, Meyer W, *et al.* Effects of radiation therapy and chemotherapy on hearing. In: Green DM, D'Angio GJ (eds) *Late effects of treatment for childhood cancer.* New York: Wiley–Liss, Inc., 1991:7–10.

●16. Schell M, McHaney V, Green A, *et al.* Hearing loss in children and young adults receiving cisplatin with or without prior cranial irradiation. *J Clin Oncol* 1989; **7**:754–760.

●17. Kretschmar C, Warren M, Lavally B, *et al.* Ototoxicity of preradiation cisplatin for children with central nervous system tumors. *J Clin Oncol* 1990; **8**:1191–1198.

●18. Pasic T, Dobie R. Cis-platinum ototoxicity in children. *Laryngoscope* 1991; **101**:985–991.

19. Berlin C, Hood L, Hurley A, Wen H. Hearing aids: only for hearing impaired patients with abnormal otoacoustic emissions. In: Berlin CI (ed.) *Hair cells and hearing aids.* San Diego: Singular Publishing Group, 1996.

20. Stengs C, Klis S, Huizing E, Smoorenburg G. Cisplatin-induced ototoxicity; electrophysiological evidence of spontaneous recovery in the albino guinea pig. *Hear Res* 1997; **111**:103–113.

21. Macdonald M, Harrison R, Wake M, *et al.* Ototoxicity of carboplatin: comparing animal and clinical models at the Hospital for Sick Children. *J Otolaryngol* 1994; **23**:151–159.

22. Saito T, Saito H, Saito K, *et al.* Ototoxicity of carboplatin in guinea pigs. *Auris Nasus Larynx* 1989; **16**:13–21.

23. Taudy M, Syka J, Popelar J, Ulehlova L. Carboplatin and cisplatin ototoxicity in guinea pigs. *Audiology* 1992; **31**:293–299.

◆24. Freilich R, Kraus D, Budnick A, *et al.* Hearing loss in children with brain tumors treated with cisplatin and carboplatin-based high-dose chemotherapy with autologous bone marrow rescue. *Med Pediatr Oncol* 1996; **26**:95–100.

◆25. Parsons S, Neault M, Lehmann L, *et al.* Severe ototoxicity following carboplatin-containing conditioning regimen for autologous marrow transplantation for neuroblastoma. *Bone Marrow Transplant* 1998; **22**:669–674.

26. Meyer W, Ayers D, McHaney V, *et al.* Ifosfamide and exacerbation of cisplatin-induced hearing loss. *Lancet* 1993; **341**:754–755.

27. Bajwa R, Price L, Roberts A, *et al.* Auditory function is unaffected by treatment with ifosfamide in children and adolescents. *Med Pediatr Oncol* 2000; **35**:156.

28. Hood L. Auditory neuropathy: what is it and what can we do about it? *Hearing J* 1998; **51**:10–18.

29. Amatuzzi M, Northrup C, Liberman M, *et al.* Selective inner hair cell loss in premature infants and cochlea pathological patterns from neonatal intensive care unit autopsies. *Arch Otolaryngol Head Neck Surg* 2001; **127**:629–636.

30. Sie K, Norton S. Changes in otoacoustic emissions and auditory brain stem response after cis-platinum exposure in gerbils. *Otolaryngol Head Neck Surg* 1997; **116**:585–592.

◆31. Littman T, Magruder A, Strother D. Monitoring and predicting ototoxic damage using distortion-product otoacoustic emissions: pediatric case study. *J Am Acad Audiol* 1998; **9**:257–262.

◆32. Allen G, Tiu C, Koike K, *et al.* Transient-evoked otoacoustic emissions in children after cisplatin chemotherapy. *Otolaryngol Head Neck Surg* 1998; **118**:584–588.

33. Saito T, Zhang Z, Manabe Y, *et al.* The effect of sodium thiosulfate on ototoxicity and pharmacokinetics after cisplatin treatment in guinea pigs. *Eur Arch Otorhinolaryngol* 1997; **254**:281–286.

34. Maduso R, Ruckenstein M, Leake F, *et al.* Ototoxic effects of supradose cisplatin with sodium thiosulfate neutralization in patients with head and neck cancer. *Arch Otolaryngol Head Neck Surg* 1997; **123**:978–981.

35. Gabaizadeh R, Staecker H, Lui W, *et al.* Protection of both auditory hair cells and auditory neurons from cisplatin induced damage. *Acta Otolaryngol (Stockholm)* 1997; **117**:232–238.

36. Campbell K, Rybak L, Meech R, Hughes L. D-Methionine provides excellent protection from cisplatin ototoxicity in the rat. *Hear Res* 1996; **102**:90–98.

37. Rybak L, Husain K, Evenson L, *et al.* Protection by 4-methylthio-benzoic acid against cisplatin-induced ototoxicity: antioxidant system. *Pharmacol Toxicol* 1997; **81**:173–179.

38. Hensley M, Schuchter L, Lindley C, *et al.* American Society of Clinical Oncology clinical practice guidelines for the use of chemotherapy and radiotherapy protectants. *J Clin Oncol* 1999; **17**:3333–3355.

●39. Capizzi R, Oster W. Chemoprotective and radioprotective effects of amifostine: an update of clinical trials. *Int J Hematol* 2000; **72**:425–435.

40. Santini V. Amifostine: chemotherapeutic and radiotherapeutic protective effects. *Expert Opin Pharmacother* 2001; **2**:479–489.

41. Kemp G, Rose P, Lurain J, *et al.* Amifostine pretreatment for protection against cyclophosphamide-induced and cisplatin-induced toxicities: results of a randomized control trial in patients with advanced ovarian cancer. *J Clin Oncol* 1996; **14**:2101–2112.

42. Grau J, Estape J, Cuchi M, *et al.* Calcium supplementation and ototoxicity in patients receiving cisplatin. *Br J Clin Pharmacol* 1996; **42**:233–235.
43. Taylor C, Briggs A, Epner E, List A. Amifostine cytoprotection in an outpatient high-dose chemotherapy regimen for breast cancer [abstract]. *Proc Am Soc Clin Oncol* 1999; **18**:137a.
44. Brizel D, Wasserman T, Henke M, *et al.* Phase III randomized trial of amifostine as a radioprotector in head and neck cancer. *J Clin Oncol* 2000; **18**:3339–3345.
45. Yuhas J, Spellman J, Jordan S, *et al.* Treatment of tumors with the combination of WR-2721 and cisdichlorodiammineplatinum (II) or cyclophosphamide. *Br J Cancer* 1980; **42**:574–585.
46. Grdina D, Hunter N, Kataoka Y, *et al.* Chemoprotective doses of amifostine confer no cytoprotection to tumor nodules growing in the lungs of mice treated with cyclophosphamide. *Semin Oncol* 1999; **26**(2 Suppl 7):22–27.
47. Glover D, Glick J, Weiler C, *et al.* WR-2721 and high-dose cisplatin: an active combination in the treatment of metastatic melanoma. *J Clin Oncol* 1987; **5**:574–578.
48. Schiller J. High-dose cisplatin and vinblastine plus amifostine for metastatic non-small cell lung cancer. *Semin Oncol* 1996; **23**:78–82.
◆49. Fouladi M, Koren G, Greenberg M, *et al.* Safety and monitoring guidelines of amifostine in the pediatric population: results of a phase I/II trial of ICE with amifostine. *Clin Invest Med* (Suppl) 1998; S8.
50. Schuchter L, Glick J. The current status of WR-2721 (Amifostine): a chemotherapy and radiation therapy protector. *Biol Ther Cancer* 1993; **3**:1–10.
51. Glover D, Riley L, Carmichael K, *et al.* Hypocalcemia and inhibition of parathyroid hormone secretion after administration of WR-2721 (a radioprotective and chemoprotective agent). *N Engl J Med* 1983; **309**:1137–1141.

3

Secondary primary cancers

3a

Epidemiology

SMITA BHATIA

Approximately one in every 350 individuals living in the USA develops cancer before the age of 20 years. With current risk-based multimodality therapeutic approaches, more than 70 per cent of these children can be expected to be long-term survivors, with the 5-year survival rates ranging from more than 90 per cent to less than 50 per cent, depending on the specific diagnosis.[1] As a result of this improvement in survival over the last three decades, increasing attention is now being focused on the growing population of individuals who have survived several years from their primary treatment. Sixty to seventy per cent of young adult survivors of childhood cancer are reported to develop at least one health-related complication as a result of their cancer or therapy. These complications include endocrine dysfunction, cardiopulmonary compromise, neurocognitive dysfunction and second primary cancers.[2] A second primary cancer is defined as a histologically distinct second neoplasm that develops after the first neoplasm.

SECOND PRIMARY CANCERS AFTER FIRST PRIMARY CANCERS IN ADULTS

Several large epidemiological studies have demonstrated that the risk of second cancers after primary cancers diagnosed and treated in adulthood is modest at best. A cohort of 470 000 cancer patients diagnosed between 1953 and 1991 in Finland was not at an increased risk of developing a second cancer, when compared with the risk of cancer in an age- and gender-matched healthy population.[3] Similarly, evaluation of a cohort of 633 964 cancer patients diagnosed between 1958 and 1996 in Sweden revealed a less than twofold increased risk when compared with the general population.[4] A third cohort of 250 000 patients from the USA had a 1.3-fold increased risk of developing a second cancer, when compared with the general population.[5]

SECOND PRIMARY CANCERS AFTER FIRST PRIMARY CANCER IN CHILDHOOD

There are several reports describing the risk of second primary cancers after a primary cancer in childhood, with the estimated cumulative probability of approximately 3 per cent, representing a 3–10-fold increased risk when compared to the general population.[6,7] A Nordic cohort of 30 880 patients diagnosed with their primary cancer at 21 years of age or less between 1947 and 1987 was followed for the development of a second cancer.[6] The estimated cumulative incidence of second cancers in this cohort was 3.5 per cent at 25 years, and the cohort was at a 3.6-fold increased risk of developing a second cancer when compared with an age- and gender-matched healthy population. A recent report of a cohort of 13 581 children diagnosed between 1970 and 1986 with common cancers in the USA before the age of 21 years, and surviving at least 5 years, constituting the Childhood Cancer Survivor Study Cohort, demonstrated that the cohort was at a 6.4-fold increased risk of developing a second cancer.[7] The estimated cumulative probability of developing a

second cancer was 3.2 per cent at 20 years, an estimate similar to the previous reports.

Burden of second cancers following childhood cancer

Data from the Surveillance, Epidemiology and End Results program were used to calculate the influence of subsequent neoplasms on incidence trends in childhood cancer.[8] Increasing annual incidence rates were found for all childhood cancers combined, acute lymphoblastic leukemia and brain tumors, but not for other cancer types. However, excluding subsequent neoplasms from the analysis had a negligible effect on the observed trends.

The Childhood Cancer Survivor Study Cohort reported the absolute excess risk of second primary cancers following a first primary cancer diagnosed and treated during childhood to be 1.9 per 1000 patient-years of follow-up.[7] This study, as well as the previous study, demonstrate that, although the relative risk of second cancers following a primary cancer in childhood may be high, the absolute risk is not high. However, the morbidity and mortality associated with second primary cancers is very high and, therefore, the need to characterize this complication and identify associated risk factors.

RISK FACTORS FOR SECOND CANCERS

Subsets of patients exposed to radiation therapy or to specific chemotherapeutic agents and patients with known genetic predisposition to malignancy have been shown to be at an increased risk of second primary cancers.[7,9–13] The types of second cancers vary with the primary diagnosis, the type of therapy received, presence of genetic predisposition and the time from initial treatment.

Primary diagnosis

Hereditary retinoblastoma, Hodgkin's disease and soft tissue sarcomas are the most common first cancers associated with the development of second cancers, and are over-represented among patients with second cancers relative to their incidence in the general population.[7,13] For subjects with hereditary retinoblastoma and soft tissue sarcoma, this is due to an interaction between a genetic predisposition to develop cancer and specific cancer therapies, such as radiation.[13,14] For individuals with Hodgkin's disease, it is not clear whether the primary diagnosis is an independent risk factor for the development of second cancers or whether the specific therapy required to treat the primary cancer is a major contributor to the development of second cancer. The associations between first and second cancers are summarized in Table 3a.1.

Host-related risk factors

AGE AT DIAGNOSIS AND TREATMENT OF PRIMARY CANCER

Younger age at diagnosis of the primary cancer has been reported to be associated with an increased risk of second cancers,[7,10,15] with the exception of secondary myelodysplasia and acute myeloid leukemia, where the risk increases with older age at diagnosis and treatment of primary cancer.[16,17] The association of younger age at diagnosis of the primary cancer with an increased risk of a second cancer is seen primarily among radiation-associated second cancers.[7,10,15]

Table 3a.1 *Second cancers and their relationship with primary cancers*

Second cancers	Primary cancers	Latency (median)	Risk factors
Brain tumors	ALL; brain tumors; HD	9–10 years	Radiation; younger age
MDS/AML	ALL; HD; bone tumors	3–5 years	Topoisomerase II inhibitors; alkylating agents
Breast cancer	HD; bone tumors; soft tissue sarcomas; ALL; brain tumors; Wilms tumors; NHL	15–20 years	Radiation; female gender
Thyroid cancer	ALL; HD; neuroblastoma; soft tissue sarcoma; bone tumors; NHL	13–15 years	Radiation; younger age; female gender
Bone tumors	Retinoblastoma (heritable); other bone tumors; Ewing's sarcoma; soft tissue sarcomas; ALL	9–10 years	Radiation; alkylating agents; splenectomy
Soft tissue sarcomas	Retinoblastoma (heritable); soft tissue sarcoma; HD; Wilms tumor; bone tumors; ALL	10–11 years	Radiation; younger age; anthracyclines

ALL, acute lymphocytic leukaemia; AML, acute myeloid leukaemia; HD, Hodgkin's disease; MDS, myelodysplasia; NHL, non-Hodgkin's lymphoma.

GENDER

Female sex is associated with an increased risk of second primary cancers, contributed primarily by the excess of secondary breast and thyroid cancers among the female cancer survivors.[18,19] Moreover, some studies indicate an increased susceptibility of women to known carcinogens, such as cigarette smoke.[20] Possible mechanisms that underlie this increased susceptibility include greater activity of cytochrome P450 enzymes, enhanced formation of DNA adducts, and the effects of hormones, such as estrogen on tumor promotion.[20]

Therapy-related risk factors

RADIATION

Although ionizing radiation is capable of causing most types of cancer, different organs vary in their susceptibility. The risk is highest when exposure occurs at a younger age, and increases with increasing doses of radiation and with increasing follow-up from radiation.[21] Radiation-associated second cancers have a long latency period, and typically develop within or at the edge of the radiation field. Some of the well-established radiation-associated second cancers include breast cancer (after Hodgkin's disease), thyroid cancer (following Hodgkin's disease and acute lymphoblastic leukemia), lung cancer (after Hodgkin's disease), brain tumors (following other brain tumors, and acute lymphoblastic leukemia), osteosarcoma (retinoblastoma, Ewing's sarcoma and other soft tissue sarcomas) and non-melanoma skin cancers (Table 3a.1).

Radiation-associated bone tumors and sarcomas exhibit a clear relationship with radiation dose. The secondary bone tumors develop within the radiation field typically after a latency period of 10 years. The radiation-associated bone tumors and sarcomas may be aggressive and respond poorly to therapy.[12,22,23]

Breast cancer has been increasingly reported among patients receiving radiation for Hodgkin's disease. The latency is typically between 15 and 20 years from primary diagnosis, and the risk is highest among patients diagnosed at a younger age, with the risk decreasing to that of the general population for patients receiving radiation for their primary cancer after the age of 30 years. Again, the risk appears to increase with radiation dose and the tumors typically develop within or at the edge of the radiation field.[7,10,24-28]

Patients receiving radiation to the neck region are at an increased risk of developing thyroid cancers. Radiation therapy at a young age has been identified as a risk factor for the development of secondary thyroid cancers. Thyroid cancer has also been reported among patients receiving radiation to the craniospinal axis for acute lymphoblastic leukemia.[23,29-31]

Brain tumors have been reported following cranial radiation for histologically distinct brain tumors or for prophylaxis or treatment of central nervous system disease among patients with acute lymphoblastic leukemia. Patients identified to be at greatest risk were those receiving radiation at age less than 6 years.[7,15,32-36]

CHEMOTHERAPEUTIC AGENTS

Exposure to certain chemotherapeutic agents, such as alkylating agents and topoisomerase II inhibitors have been shown to increase the risk of secondary myelodysplasia and acute myeloid leukemia.[10,37,38] Alkylating agents have also been linked with bone tumors[22,23] and bladder cancer.[39] The incidence of therapy-related myelodysplasia and acute myeloid leukemia typically peaks between 4 and 6 years from diagnosis of the primary cancer and reaches a plateau after 15 years (Figure 3a.1). Blaney et al. first suggested that the risk of myeloid malignancy after treatment for Hodgkin's disease might be confined to a limited time period; consistent data across reported studies including more than 11 716 exposed patients, suggest that the observed plateau in incidence of myeloid malignancy which occurs after 15 years truly reflects a biological limitation on risk.[40] The clinical observation that the risk of therapy-related leukemia does not extend beyond 15 years, despite an increasing risk of second neoplasms at other sites, indicates that the 'at-risk' population of cells is no longer present. It may be that this period of time allows early pluripotential hematopoietic progenitors to undergo clonal extinction and be replaced from the compartment of resting stem cells by clonal succession. It would be

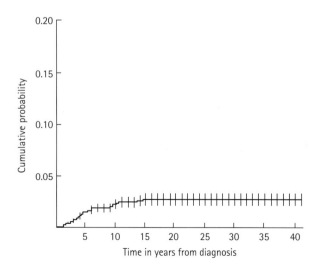

Figure 3a.1 *Cumulative probability of therapy-related myelodysplasia/acute myeloid leukemia in a cohort of 1380 patients with Hodgkin's disease in childhood and adolescence. The vertical bars indicate standard errors.*

expected that stem cells in the resting phase of the cell cycle would be protected from the genotoxic effects of chemotherapy and radiation and that the excess risk of therapy-related leukemia would cease as undamaged cells were recruited into active hematopoiesis. Therapy-related leukemia is associated with a very poor outcome, with an estimated 12-month survival of 10 per cent.[41]

Alkylating agent associated acute myeloid leukemia/myelodysplasia

Table 3a.2 summarizes the incidence, risk factors and outcomes among patients with therapy-related leukemia following alkylating agent exposure.[10,37,42–48] Increasing dose of alkylating agent and older age at exposure have been identified as risk factors. The incidence is typically

less than 5 per cent, and patients with therapy-related myelodysplasia and acute myeloid leukemia following alkylating agent exposure have characteristic clinical and morphologic features.[10,15–17,37,49,50] (Table 3a.3). Cytogenetic abnormalities in patients who develop myeloid malignancies after therapy with alkylating agents characteristically involve losses or deletions of chromosomes 5 and 7.[37] The 5q31–33 region of the long arm of chromosome 5 contains at least nine genes involved in hematopoiesis. Defects in any of these genes could disrupt the balance between cell growth and differentiation and play a role in initiation and progression of leukemia. Complete or partial deletions of the long arm of chromosome 7 (7q- and -7) are nonrandom abnormalities observed in therapy-related leukemia.

Table 3a.2 *Characteristics of cases of therapy-related myelodysplasia or acute myeloid leukemia after treatment with alkylating agents and topoisomerase II inhibitors*

Study	Primary cancer	Cohort size	Follow-up	Cases of MDS/AML	Latency period	Cumulative probability (%) (year)	Risk factors	Outcome (% alive)
Associated with alkylating agent exposure								
42	HD	694	13.1 years	8	51.6 (16–148)	1.5 (20)	Chemotherapy; relapse	0
43	HD	1 641	17 000 person-years	7	NA	0.8 (30)	NA	NA
44	HD	667	8.3 years	5	49 (31–125)	1.1 (15)	Alkylating agents	0
45	Childhood cancer	9 170	5.5 years	19	NA	0.8 (20)	Increasing age; HD, Ewing's; alkylating agents; doxorubicin	NA
10	HD	1 380	11.4 years	24	48 (10–168)	2.8 (14)	Alkylating agents; older age	0
Associated with topoisomerase II inhibitor exposure								
46	ALL	734	NA	21	39.5 (15–100)	3.8 (6)	Etoposide: weekly/ twice weekly	14
47	ALL	205	NA	10	32	5.9 (4)	Etoposide	50
48	NHL	38	15 years	5	21	18.4 (4)	Etoposide; twice weekly	60
38	Pediatric malignancies	16 422	7.7 years	10	NA	0.5 (5)	Etoposide; alkylating agents; radiation	NA

Table 3a.3 *Features of chemotherapy-induced haematopoietic malignancies*

Property	Alkylating agents	Epipodophyllotoxins	References
Median latency	4–6 years (range 1–20 years)	1–3 years (range 0.5–4.5 years)	10, 15, 17, 37, 49
Presentation	Myelodysplasia	Abrupt, no preleukemia	37, 49, 50
Cytogenetic abnormalities	Loss of genetic material, often from chromosomes 5 and 7	Balanced translocations (often include 11q23)	37, 50
Age	Typically older patients	Younger patients	37, 50

Topoisomerase II inhibitor–associated acute myeloid leukemia

There is a wide variation in the estimates of risk of therapy-related leukemia, reflecting small sample size, differences in susceptibility among different patient populations, varying schedules of drug administrations and different cumulative doses (Table 3a.2). Studies from St Jude Children's Research Hospital (SJCRH) have demonstrated that the risk of secondary leukemia associated with epipodophyllotoxins is related to the intensity of the dosing schedule.[46] The overall cumulative risk of secondary leukemia reported from SJCRH was 3.8 per cent, but within the subgroups of patients who received epipodophyllotoxins [etoposide (VP-16) or teniposide (VM-26)] twice weekly or weekly, the cumulative risks were 12.3 per cent and 12.4 per cent, respectively. Of the remaining subgroups that included patients who received epipodophyllotoxins every 2 weeks, did not receive epipodophyllotoxins or received them only during remission induction, the cumulative risk was 1.6 per cent. After adjustment for the frequency of treatment, there was no apparent independent effect of the total dose of epipodophyllotoxins in this study.[46] The Cancer Therapy Evaluation Program (CTEP) of the National Cancer Institute (NCI) developed a monitoring plan to obtain reliable estimates of the risk of secondary leukemia after epipodophyllotoxins.[51] Twelve NCI-supported cooperative group clinical trials were identified that used epipodophyllotoxins at low ($<1.5\,g/m^2$ etoposide), moderate (1.5–$2.99\,g/m^2$ etoposide), or higher ($>3.0\,g/m^2$ etoposide) cumulative doses. Cases of secondary leukemia were reported to CTEP and cumulative incidence calculated. The cumulative risks at 6 years for the development of secondary leukemia were 3.3 per cent, 0.7 per cent and 2.2 per cent at the low, moderate and high doses of etoposide, suggesting a lack of dose–response relationship. Acute myeloid leukemia associated with exposure to topoisomerase II inhibitors is characterized by short latency (median, 24–36 months), predominance of monocytic phenotypes (M4 and M5), and an acute onset, often with a high blast count, rather than an initial myelodysplastic presentation (Table 3a.3).

Topoisomerase II inhibitors induce chromosomal fragmentation, sister chromatid exchange, DNA deletions and DNA rearrangements. Most of the translocations characteristic of leukemia disrupt a breakpoint cluster region between exons 5 and 11 of the *MLL* gene at chromosome band 11q23 and fuse *MLL* with a partner gene.[52]

Genetic predisposition

Members of families with Li–Fraumeni syndrome have been reported to be at increased risk of multiple subsequent cancers compared with the general population.[11] The risk was highest among survivors of childhood cancer, and the excess risk was mainly for cancers characteristics of Li–Fraumeni syndrome. This study suggests that germline mutations in tumor suppressor genes might interact with therapeutic exposures to result in an increased risk of second primary cancers.

Patients with soft-tissue sarcomas who develop a second cancer are more likely to have a family history of cancer, when compared with those without a second cancer.[14] The tumor types occurring in excess in family members are similar to those observed as second cancers, such as cancers of the breast, bone, joint or soft tissue, thus indicating that the risk of second cancers is associated with a familial predisposition.

Genetic predisposition also plays a significant role in increasing the risk of second cancers among patients receiving radiation therapy for hereditary retinoblastoma, with the risk increasing with increasing doses of radiation.[13]

Another example of genetic characteristics interacting with treatment is the presence of polymorphism in a drug-metabolizing enzyme, such as thiopurine S-methyltransferase (*TPMT*). *TPMT* catalyzes the S-methylation of thiopurines, including 6-mercaptopurine and 6-thioguanine. *TPMT* activity exhibits genetic polymorphism, with about 1/300 individuals inheriting *TPMT* deficiency as an autosomal recessive trait. There is emerging evidence that *TPMT* genotype might influence the risk of second cancers, including brain tumors[53] and acute myeloid leukemia.[54]

Several other genetic polymorphisms of enzymes capable of metabolic activation or detoxification of anticancer drugs, such as NAD(P)H:quinone oxireductase (NQO1), glutathione S-transferase (GST)-M1, -T1 and -P1, and CYP3A4, have been examined for their role in the development of therapy-related leukemia and myelodysplasia.[55–58] There is evidence that an NQO1 polymorphism may be associated with an increased risk of therapy-related myelodysplasia.[55] Individuals with CYP3A4-W genotype may be at increased risk of treatment-related leukemia, by increasing the production of reactive intermediates that might damage DNA.[56] Recently, Allan *et al.* reported data suggesting that inheritance of at least one Val allele at GST-P1 codon 105 confers an increased risk of developing therapy-related leukemia.[57]

Environmental/lifestyle factors

Environmental exposures and lifestyle factors, such as tobacco, alcohol, diet and hormonal factors, and their association with second cancers have been most commonly studied in survivors of adult-onset cancers. Smoking has been linked with lung cancer occurring as a second primary cancer among survivors of Hodgkin's disease, with

the risk increasing with increasing doses of radiation received, suggesting a positive interaction on a multiplicative scale.[59] Moreover, the increase in risk of lung cancer with increasing radiation dose was much greater among the patients who smoked after the diagnosis of Hodgkin's disease than among those who refrained from smoking ($p = 0.04$).[60] Alcohol consumption has been shown to be a risk factor for oral, esophageal and liver cancers occurring as second cancers.[61–63] There are several anatomic sites such as colon, breast, ovary, uterus and prostate, where nutritional and hormonal factors play a role in carcinogenesis. Bidirectional associations across several hypothesized nutrition- and hormone-related cancers have been demonstrated across many registries. However, these studies are generally lacking in specific exposure information, and the support for a given etiologic hypothesis is usually indirect, because the correlations between cancers hypothesized to share a common risk factor are examined without directly measuring either the putative common risk factors or potential confounders. Moreover, since the environmental exposures and lifestyle factors seem to be associated with primarily adult-onset cancers, a sufficiently large cohort of childhood cancer survivors need to be followed long enough so as to reach the age at which they would be at risk for the development of such cancers.

The next section will focus on certain primary cancers that are associated with a significantly increased risk of second primary cancers (e.g. retinoblastoma and Hodgkin's disease). It will also focus on primary cancers; with large well-characterized cohorts of patients followed for sufficiently long periods of time for the development of second primary cancers (e.g. acute lymphoblastic leukemia and Wilms' tumor).

Retinoblastoma

Children with hereditary retinoblastoma are at exceptionally high risk of developing multiple primary cancers, especially osteosarcoma and soft tissue sarcomas.[13,64] On the other hand, patients with non-hereditary retinoblastoma appear not to be at increased risk for second cancers. The high risk of multiple primary cancers in hereditary retinoblastoma patients is attributable primarily to germline mutations in the retinoblastoma tumor suppressor gene, *RB1*. Wong *et al.* examined the long-term risk of second primary cancers in survivors of childhood retinoblastoma and attempted to quantify the role of radiotherapy in second primary sarcoma development. A total of 1604 patients with retinoblastoma diagnosed between 1914 and 1984, who survived at least 1 year were identified from hospital records in Massachusetts and New York. The incidence of second cancers was statistically significantly elevated among 961 patients with hereditary

retinoblastoma, in whom 190 second cancers were diagnosed [relative risk (RR) 30, 95 per cent confidence interval (95% CI), 26–47]. The cumulative incidence of a second cancer at 50 years after diagnosis was 51 per cent ($\pm$6.2 per cent) for hereditary retinoblastoma and 5 per cent ($\pm$3 per cent) for nonhereditary retinoblastoma. A radiation risk for all sarcomas was evident at doses above 5 Gy, rising to 10.7-fold at doses of 60 Gy or greater. For second primary soft tissue sarcomas, the relative risks showed stepwise increase for all dose categories of radiation therapy, and were statistically significant at 10–29.9 Gy and 30–59.9 Gy.

The development of third and additional nonocular tumors among patients with retinoblastoma who developed a second primary cancer was examined by Abramson *et al.*[65] The 5- and 10-year incidence rates were reported to be 11 per cent and 22 per cent, respectively, among the 211 patients with retinoblastoma who had developed a second tumor. The third and subsequent tumors were reported among patients who had received radiation for retinoblastoma, and included soft tissue sarcomas, bone tumors and skin cancers.

Eng *et al.* sought to quantify the mortality from second primary cancers among long-term survivors of retinoblastoma and to identify factors that predispose to these deaths.[66] The cumulative probability of death from a second primary cancer was 26 per cent at 40 years after bilateral retinoblastoma diagnosis and additional cancer deaths occurred thereafter. Radiotherapy for retinoblastoma further increased the risk of mortality from second cancers.

These studies indicate that genetic predisposition has a substantial impact on risk of subsequent cancers in retinoblastoma patients, which is further increased by radiation therapy. Moreover, patients with retinoblastoma are at an increased risk for the development of third and fourth tumors, although the location and other risk factors are similar to those described for second primary cancers.

Hodgkin's disease

There are several reports of large, well-characterized cohorts of patients diagnosed with Hodgkin's disease in childhood and adolescence that describe the incidence of and risk factors for second primary cancers among the survivors (Table 3a.4).[7,10,18,27,42,43,67–69]

Metayer *et al.* analyzed data from 5925 patients with Hodgkin's disease diagnosed before 21 years of age and reported to 16 population-based cancer registries in North America and Europe between 1935 and 1994.[26] A total of 157 solid (RR = 7.0, 95% CI, 5.9–8.2) and 26 acute leukemias (RR = 27.4, 95% CI, 17.9–40.2) were reported. The risk of solid tumors remained elevated among 20-year survivors (RR = 6.6) and persisted for 25 years

Table 3a.4 *Second cancers following childhood Hodgkin's disease*

Reference	Cohort size	Time–period studied	Number of second cancers	Cumulative probability (%) (years)	Standardized incidence ratio
26	5925	1935–1994	195	Solid tumors: 11.7% (25 years)	7.7
10	1380	1955–1986	135	31.2% (30 years)	17.9
42	694	1960–1995	59	Males 9.7% (20 years); females 16.8% (20 years)	Males 10.6; females 15.4
43	1641	1940s to 1991	62	18% (30 years)	7.7
19	191	1969–1988	15	12% (15 years)	Males 18.0; females 57.0
69	182	1960–1989	28	26.7% (30 years)	9.4
18	499	1962–1993	25	7.7% (15 years)	—[a]

[a]Information not available.

(RR = 4.6). Temporal trends for cancers of thyroid, female breast, bone and connective tissue, stomach and esophagus were consistent with the late effects of radiotherapy. Greater than 50-fold increased risks were observed for tumors of the thyroid and respiratory tract among children treated before age 10. At older ages (10–16 years), the largest number of second cancers occurred in the digestive tract (RR = 19.3) and breast (RR = 22.9).

Sankila et al. defined the risk of second cancers in a cohort 1641 patients diagnosed before the age of 20 years in the five Nordic countries.[43] A total of 62 second malignancies were diagnosed (RR = 7.7, 95% CI, 5.9–9.9). The overall cumulative risk of subsequent neoplasms was 1.9 per cent at 10 years, 6.9 per cent at 20 years and 18 per cent at 30 years. High risks were observed for breast cancer (RR = 17, 95% CI, 9.9–28), thyroid cancer (RR = 33, 95% CI 15–62), secondary leukemia (RR = 17, 95% CI, 6.9–35) and non-Hodgkin's lymphoma (RR = 15, 95% CI, 4.9–35).

A cohort of 694 children and adolescents, diagnosed and treated at Stanford University were monitored for a median of 13 years for the development of second primary cancers.[42] Fifty-six patients developed 59 second primary cancers: 48 solid tumors, eight leukemias and three non-Hodgkin's lymphomas. The relative risk of developing a second cancer was 15.4 (95% CI, 10.6–21.5) for females and 10.6 (95% CI, 6.6–16.0) for males. Breast cancer (n = 16) and soft tissue (n = 13) sarcomas were the most common solid tumors. The actuarial risk of second cancers at 20 years of follow-up was 9.7 per cent for males and 16.8 per cent for females, and 9.2 per cent for breast cancer.

The Late Effects Study Group (LESG) followed a cohort of 1380 children with Hodgkin's disease diagnosed within North America and Europe between 1955 and 1986 to determine the incidence of second malignant neoplasms and associated risk factors.[10] Median age at diagnosis was 11 years (range 0.3–16) and the median length of follow-up was 11.4 years. Eighty-eight second cancers occurred in this cohort, as compared with 4.4 expected based on rates in the general population

(RR = 18.1, 95% CI, 14.3–22.3). The estimated actuarial incidence of any second malignancy by 15 years was 7.0 per cent, of which 3.9 per cent was due to solid tumors. The cohort was recently updated to extend the median length of follow-up to 15.1 years.[70] The median age of the cohort at last follow-up was 26 (range 1–55). With the recent update, an additional 58 new second cancers were observed bringing the total to 146 second cancers. These included solid tumors (n = 112), leukemia (n = 28) and non-Hodgkin's lymphoma (n = 6). The solid tumors included breast cancer (n = 29), thyroid cancer (n = 19), basal cell carcinoma (n = 17), colorectal cancer (n = 7), lung cancer (n = 5), bone and brain tumors (n = 5, each), gastric cancer (n = 4), and others (n = 21). The median time to development of any second cancer was 14.6 years and the median age at diagnosis of a second cancer was 27.2 years. The cumulative probability of developing a second cancer approached 31.2 per cent at 30 years from diagnosis. This represented a 17.9-fold excess of second cancers when compared to the general population. The most common second cancer was breast cancer (females, n = 28; males, n = 1). Thyroid cancer was the second most common solid tumor, with the cumulative probability approaching 6.7 per cent at 30 years. This cohort was at a 37-fold increased risk of developing a thyroid cancer, when compared to the general population. Colorectal (n = 7, RR = 32.3, 95% CI, 12–63) and lung cancers (n = 5, RR = 37.2, 95% CI, 12–77) were also reported as second cancers in this cohort. The median age at diagnosis of patients who developed colorectal cancer was 32.4 years, while the median age at diagnosis of lung cancer was 31.8 years. The secondary leukemias occurred at a median of 4.3 years from diagnosis of Hodgkin's disease, with the cumulative probability approaching 2.9 per cent at 15 years, with no events reported thereafter.

Follow-up of these large cohorts of survivors of childhood Hodgkin's disease for extended periods of time documents the increasing occurrence of radiation-associated solid tumors, especially breast and thyroid cancers and

Table 3a.5 *Second cancers following childhood acute lymphoblastic leukemia*

Study	Cohort size	Time–period studied	Number of patients with second cancers	Cumulative incidence (%) (years)	Standardized incidence ratio
15	9 720	1972–1988	43	2.5% (15 years)	7.0
32	1 597	1972–1995	13	2.7% (18 years)	–[a]
33	981	1958–1985	8	2.9% (20 years)	5.9
34	1 815	1962–1988	20	5.0% (15 years)	–[a]
35	5 006	1979–1995	52	3.3% (15 years)	–[a]
36	8 831	1983–1995	70	1.3% (10 years)	7.0

[a]Information not available.

the emergence of other cancers common in the adult population, such as colon and lung at a younger age than expected in the general population.

Acute lymphoblastic leukemia

For survivors of childhood acute lymphoblastic leukemia, the estimated actuarial risk of developing a second neoplasm has been reported to be between 2.5 per cent and 5 per cent at 15 years from diagnosis (Table 3a.5).[7,15,32–36] Among the second neoplasms observed after treatment of acute lymphoblastic leukemia, central nervous system tumors in patients treated with cranial irradiation, acute myeloid leukemia and thyroid cancer are most commonly reported. Children under 6 years of age at the time of radiation to the central nervous system are at an increased risk of developing second primary brain tumors.[7,15]

Loning *et al.* evaluated the incidence and type of second primary cancers after Berlin–Frankfurt–Munster (BFM) treatment in 5006 children with acute lymphoblastic leukemia diagnosed between 1979 and 1995.[35] The median follow-up time from diagnosis was 5.7 years and 52 second primary cancers were observed. These included 16 patients with acute myeloid leukemia, 13 patients with central nervous system tumors and 23 other neoplasms. This cohort was at a 14-fold increased risk of developing a second cancer, when compared to the general population, and at a 19-fold increased risk of developing a brain tumor. The cumulative risk of second primary cancers was 3.3 per cent at 15 years. It was 3.5 per cent among patients treated with cranial irradiation and significantly lower in non-irradiated patients at 1.2 per cent.

A cohort of 8 831 children diagnosed with acute lymphoblastic leukemia and enrolled on Children's Cancer Group (CCG) therapeutic protocols between 1983 and 1995, were followed to determine the incidence of second primary cancers and associated risk factors.[36] The median age at diagnosis of acute lymphoblastic leukemia was 4.7 years. The cohort had accrued 54 883 person-years of follow-up. Seventy patients developed second cancers, including leukemia ($n = 16$), lymphoma ($n = 15$), brain tumors ($n = 19$) and other solid malignancies ($n = 20$).

The estimated cumulative probability ($\pm$SE) of any second neoplasm was 1.3 ± 0.2 per cent (at 10 years), representing a 7.9-fold increased risk, as compared with the general population. The risk was significantly increased for acute myeloid leukemia (RR = 52.3), non-Hodgkin's lymphoma (RR = 20.8), parotid gland tumors (RR = 33.4), thyroid cancer (RR = 13.3), brain tumorsz (RR = 10.1) and soft-tissue sarcoma (RR = 9.1). Multivariate analysis revealed relapse of primary disease (RR = 3.5, 95% CI, 2.1–5.8), female gender (RR = 1.8, 95% CI, 1.1–2.8) and radiation to craniospinal axis (RR = 1.6, 95% CI, 1.0–2.6) to be independently associated with increased risk of second neoplasms. Actuarial survival at 10 years from diagnosis of second neoplasms was 39 per cent.

Follow-up of these large cohorts of children treated with contemporary risk-based therapy documents that the incidence of second neoplasms remains low following diagnosis of childhood acute lymphoblastic leukemia.

Wilms' tumors

Between 1969 and 1991, 5278 patients were enrolled onto the National Wilms Tumor Study (NWTS) and, by the end of 1993, had contributed 39 461 person-years of follow-up. Forty-three second neoplasms were observed, whereas only 5.1 were expected (RR = 8.4, 95% CI, 6.1–11.4).[71] The cumulative incidence of a second primary cancer after Wilms' tumor was 1.6 per cent after 15 years from diagnosis of Wilms' tumor. Abdominal irradiation received as part of initial therapy was associated with an increased risk of a second cancer (RR = 1.4 per 10 Gy; 95% CI, 1.1–1.8). Doxorubicin potentiated the radiation effect. Among 234 patients who received doxorubicin and >35 Gy of abdominal radiation, eight second cancers were observed, whereas only 0.22 were expected (RR = 36, 95% CI, 16–72). Treatment for relapse further increased the risk for second cancers. Seven of the 43 patients with second cancers were identified to have acute myeloid leukemia at a median of 3 years from diagnosis of Wilms' tumor (range 1.2–4 years).[72] All seven patients had received chemotherapy

regimens that included doxorubicin or etoposide, and six of the seven patients had received infradiaphragmatic irradiation. One patient developed an 11q23 translocation. These results demonstrate the importance of current efforts to limit the use of intensive chemotherapy and radiation therapy to patients with aggressive disease.

COMMONLY REPORTED SECOND PRIMARY CANCERS

This section is devoted to the more commonly reported second primary cancers, such as breast, bone and thyroid cancers, with the focus being on the incidence and associated risk factors for these second cancers.

Bone tumors

The risk of subsequent bone tumors was estimated among 9170 patients who had survived 2 or more years after the initial diagnosis of a cancer in childhood.[23] As compared with the general population, the patients had a 133-fold increased risk of developing a bone tumor (95% CI, 98–176) and an estimated 20-year cumulative risk of 2.8 ± 0.7 per cent. Detailed data on treatment were obtained on 64 patients with subsequent bone tumor after childhood cancer. As compared with 209 matched controls who had survived cancer in childhood but not developed bone cancer later, patients who had received radiation therapy had a 2.7-fold risk (95% CI, 1–7.7) of developing a bone tumor, and a sharp dose–response gradient reaching a 40-fold risk after doses to the bone of more than 60 Gy. After adjustment for radiation therapy, treatment with alkylating agents was also linked to bone cancer (RR = 4.7, 95% CI, 1.0–22.3), with the risk increasing as cumulative drug exposure rose.

Hawkins et al. used the population-based National Registry of Childhood Tumours in Britain to investigate the incidence and etiology of second primary bone cancer after childhood cancer, using both a cohort and case-control study design.[22] The cohort study of 13 175 3-year survivors of childhood cancer diagnosed in Britain between 1940 and 1983 revealed 55 subsequent bone cancers. The cumulative probability of 3-year survivors developing bone cancer within 20 years did not exceed 0.9 per cent, except following hereditary retinoblastoma (7.2 per cent), Ewing's sarcoma (5.4 per cent) and other malignant bone tumors (2.4 per cent). The risk of bone cancer increased substantially with increased cumulative dose of radiation to the bone ($p < 0.001$, linear trend). At the highest level of exposure, the risk appeared to decline ($p = 0.065$, non-linearity). The risk of bone cancer increased linearly ($p = 0.04$, one-tailed test) with increased cumulative dose of alkylating agents.

A cohort study of 4400 3-year survivors of a first solid cancer during childhood diagnosed in France or UK between 1942 and 1986 revealed 32 subsequent osteosarcomas.[12] In a nested case-control study, the authors matched 32 cases and 160 controls for sex, type of first cancer, age at first cancer and the duration of follow-up. The risk of osteosarcoma was found to be a linear function of the local dose of radiation. Bilateral retinoblastoma, Ewing's sarcoma and soft tissue sarcoma were associated with an increased risk of subsequent osteosarcoma.

These three studies, therefore, demonstrate that the risk of second primary bone tumors among survivors of childhood cancer is not very high, except among certain specific tumor types, and that the risk is associated with the use of radiation therapy and alkylating agents. These studies, therefore, provide a rational basis for targeted surveillance and consideration regarding modification of therapeutic protocols in certain high-risk groups.

Breast cancer

Women with Hodgkin's disease who receive mantle irradiation are at an increased risk of breast cancer. Results from several registries show that 10 or more years after radiation, the overall breast cancer risk is increased approximately fourfold,[7,25–27,73–80] and can be as high as 33–75-fold, in girls exposed to radiation at puberty.[10] The risk of developing breast cancer remains elevated for a considerable length of time.[10] Table 3a.6 shows the risk of breast cancer as a second neoplasm following Hodgkin's disease, according to age at diagnosis of Hodgkin's disease, and latency from treatment for Hodgkin's disease.

Follow-up of a cohort of female Hodgkin's disease survivors diagnosed and treated for Hodgkin's disease before 16 years of age showed that the actuarial estimated cumulative probability of developing breast cancer approached 28 per cent at 30 years from diagnosis (Figure 3a.2).[70] The median age at diagnosis of Hodgkin's disease was 14 years, while the median age at diagnosis of breast cancer was 32 years. The median latency between the diagnosis of Hodgkin's disease and diagnosis of second primary breast cancer was 18 years (range 4–28 years). Twenty-seven of the 29 cancers developed within the radiation field. Ten of the 29 patients with breast cancer subsequently developed cancer in the contralateral breast. The estimated cumulative probability of developing breast cancer among women receiving irradiation approached 25 per cent by 40 years of age.

The Childhood Cancer Survivor Study Cohort has evaluated the risk of breast cancer among 13 581 5-year survivors of childhood cancer.[7] Breast cancer was the most frequent second primary cancer ($n = 60$). The majority of second primary breast cancers occurred among survivors of childhood Hodgkin's disease. The cohort was at

Table 3a.6 *Risk of breast cancer by age and latency*

Study	Size of cohort	Length of follow-up	Number of BC	Median age at Dx of HD/BC	Years to BC (median)	Relative risk	Risk factors	Outcome (% alive)
25	885	10 years	26	28/40 years	15 years	13 (<15years at Dx)	Age < 30 years; radiation therapy	73%
10	483	11 years	17	11/32 years	19 years	75	10–16 years; radiation therapy	82%
27	257	10 years	6	14/28 years	14 years	20	Radiation therapy	—[a]
28	3 869	—[a]	55	All ages/_years	>10 years	61	Age < 16 years at Dx of HD	—[a]
7	13 851	15.4 years	60	—[a]	—[a]	16	Radiation therapy	—[a]
26	5 925	10.5 years	52	—[a]	—[a]	14	Radiation therapy	—[a]

BC, breast cancer; Dx, diagnosis: HD, Hodgkin's disease; RR, relative risk.
[a]Information not available.

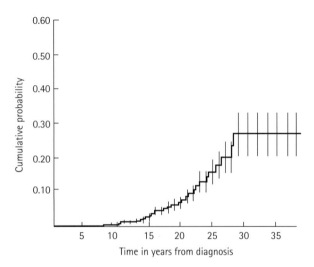

Figure 3a.2 *Cumulative probability of second primary breast cancer in a cohort of 1380 patients with Hodgkin's disease in childhood and adolescence. The vertical bars indicate standard errors.*

a 16.2-fold increased risk of developing a second primary breast cancer when compared with the general population. The median time to development of breast cancer was 15.7 years. The risk of developing a breast cancer appeared to remain elevated throughout the follow-up period (RR = 10.1 at 5–9 years of follow-up and 10.1 at 20–30 years of follow-up).

For women treated after the age of 30, however, no excess breast cancers have occurred.[25] The high risk of breast cancer in women exposed to radiation for the treatment of Hodgkin's disease at younger ages raises important issues about cooperative efforts among institutions to mount prospective screening programs including breast physical examination, sonography, mammography or quantitative magnetic resonance imaging for these patients.

Thyroid cancers

The thyroid gland is among the most radiosensitive organs. The risk of thyroid cancer has been described after radiation therapy for several primary cancers, including Hodgkin's disease, acute lymphoblastic leukemia, brain tumors and after total body irradiation for bone marrow transplantation. De Vathaire *et al.* have studied the long-term risk of developing a thyroid tumor in 4096 3-year survivors of childhood cancer treated between 1942 and 1985 in France and Britain.[30] After a mean follow-up of 15 years, 14 patients developed a thyroid carcinoma, all of whom had received radiation therapy. The risk increased with increasing dose of radiation: a dose of 0.5 Gy was associated with a 35-fold increased risk of developing a thyroid cancer, when compared with the general population, while the risk increased to 73-fold when the exposure increased to 3.6 Gy.

Radiation therapy at a young age has been identified as a risk factor for the development of secondary thyroid cancers. In a cohort of 9170 survivors of childhood cancer, Tucker *et al.* reported a 53-fold increased risk of thyroid cancer.[29] Sixty-eight per cent of the secondary thyroid cancers arose in previously irradiated fields, and the risk factors included increasing dose of radiation and young age at irradiation.

The risk of thyroid cancer was evaluated among 1 791 5-year survivors of Hodgkin's disease followed as part of the Childhood Cancer Survivor Study Cohort. Thyroid cancer was diagnosed in 20 survivors (RR = 18.1).[31] Thyroid cancer has also been reported among patients receiving radiation to the craniospinal axis for acute lymphoblastic leukemia.[8,15,36]

IMPLICATIONS AND FUTURE DIRECTIONS

The absolute risk of second cancers is small with less than two excess second cancers occurring per 1000

patient-years of follow-up.[7] The ongoing endeavors to strive constantly for improvement in survival following childhood cancer must not be overshadowed by the risk of second cancers. However, of all the possible late sequelae, second cancers can be the most devastating. It is, therefore, imperative that patients and health-care providers are aware of risk factors for second cancers as well as the populations at increased risk for the development of second cancers, so that surveillance is focused and early prevention strategies can be implemented.

Some of the primary prevention strategies that are currently being implemented include use of gender-specific therapy for patients with Hodgkin's disease. Adolescent females with Hodgkin's disease are offered primarily chemotherapy-based regimens, and radiation therapy to the chest area among females is reserved for patients considered at high risk of local relapse. This strategy is aimed to reduce the risk of radiation-associated breast cancer among female survivors of Hodgkin's disease. Another example of a primary prevention strategy would be identification of patients heterozygous for drug-metabolizing enzymes before initiation of therapy for the primary cancer. This could lead to modification of therapy resulting potentially in a decrease in the incidence of second cancers.

Secondary prevention measures currently under consideration include programs to educate clinicians and survivors about the risk of second cancers and about ways to decrease the risk of development of second cancers by adopting healthy lifestyles. For example, both the patients and health-care providers need to be educated regarding the increased risk of breast cancer among the female survivors of childhood cancer. The importance of properly conducted self-examination as the foundation of breast cancer screening needs to be impressed upon the patients. In addition, clinical and mammographic screening should be instituted at a younger age and performed more frequently than recommended for the general population.[27] Other measures include intervention programs for smoking cessation, screening for breast, lung and cervical cancers, chemoprevention for specific cancers, and avoidance of unnecessary exposure to sunlight.

Finally, second cancers provide us with a unique opportunity to understand the pathogenesis of the disease process. The exact timing and magnitude of the primary exposure (i.e. cancer therapy) is known, and following the patients closely can possibly lead to a better understanding of the progression of events and perhaps the identification of biomarkers that would identify patients who ultimately do develop second cancers.[37] Several such studies that involve prospective longitudinal follow-up of patients are currently being undertaken to better understand the sequence of events that ultimately lead to the development of second cancers.

KEY POINTS

- Survivors of childhood cancer are at a 3–6-fold increased risk of developing a second primary cancer when compared to the general population but the absolute excess risk of second cancers is not very high.
- Younger age at diagnosis, female gender and certain primary diagnoses, such as hereditary retinoblastoma, Hodgkin's disease and soft tissue sarcomas, are associated with an increased risk of second cancers.
- Exposure to radiation therapy, specific chemotherapeutic agents and certain genetic syndromes are associated with an increased risk of second primary cancers.
- Radiation-associated risk is highest when the exposure occurs at a young age, and increases with the dose of radiation and with increasing follow-up from radiation.
- Radiation-associated second primary cancers include bone tumors, breast cancer, thyroid cancer, brain tumors and basal cell carcinoma.
- Exposure to certain chemotherapeutic agents, such as alkylating agents and topoisomerase II inhibitors, have been shown to increase the risk of secondary myelodysplasia and acute myeloid leukemia. These second cancers are characterized by a short latency period and a finite period of increased risk.
- Polymorphisms in certain drug metabolizing enzymes, such as glutathione S-transferase, Cytochrome P 450 and NAD(P)H:quinone oxireductase are being explored to understand the role of gene–environment interactions in the risk of chemotherapy-associated secondary leukemia.
- Primary and secondary prevention measures are being explored to reduce the morbidity and mortality associated with second primary cancers.

REFERENCES

1. Reis LAG, Eisner MP, Kosary CL, et al. (eds). SEER cancer statistics review, 1973–1998. Bethesda, MD: National Cancer Institute, 2001.
2. Sklar CA. An overview of the effects of cancer therapies: the nature, scale, and breadth of the problem. Acta Paediatr Scand Suppl. 1999; 433:1–4.
3. Sankila R, Pukkala E, Teppo L. Risk of subsequent malignant neoplasms among 470,000 cancer patients in Finland, 1953–1991. Int J Cancer 1995; 60:464–470.
4. Dong C, Hemminki K. Second primary neoplasms in 633,964 cancer patients in Sweden, 1958–1996. Int J Cancer 2001; 93:155–161.

5. Curtis RE, Boice JD Jr, Kleinerman RA, Flannery JT, *et al.* Summary: Multiple primary cancers in Connecticut, 1935–82. *Natl Cancer Inst Monogr* 1985; **68**:219–242.

♦6. Olsen JH, Garwicz S, Hertz H, *et al.* Second malignant neoplasms after cancer in childhood or adolescence. Nordic Society of Paediatric Haematology and Oncology Association of the Nordic Cancer Registries. *Br Med J* 1993; **307**:1030–1036.

♦7. Neglia JP, Friedman DL, Yutaka Y, *et al.* Second malignant neoplasms in five-year survivors of childhood cancer: childhood cancer survivor study. *J Natl Cancer Inst* 2001; **93**:618–629.

8. Gurney JG, Davis S, Severson RK, Robison LL. The influence of subsequent neoplasms on incidence trends in childhood cancer. *Cancer Epidemiol Biomarkers Prev* 1994; **3**:349–351.

9. Robison LL. Second primary cancers after childhood cancer [editorial]. *Br Med J* 1996; **12**:861–862.

♦10. Bhatia S, Robison LL, Oberlin O, *et al.* Breast cancer and other second neoplasms after childhood Hodgkin's disease. *N Engl J Med* 1996; **334**:745–751.

11. Hisada M, Garber JE, Fung CY, *et al.* Multiple primary cancers in families with Li–Fraumeni syndrome. *J Natl Cancer Inst* 1998; **90**:606–611.

12. Le Vu B, de Vathaire F, Shamsaldin A, *et al.* Radiation dose, chemotherapy and risk of osteosarcoma after solid tumours during childhood. *Int J Cancer* 1998; **77**:370–377.

♦13. Wong FL, Boice JD Jr, Abramson DH, *et al.* Cancer incidence after retinoblastoma. Radiation dose and sarcoma risk. *JAMA* 1997; **278**:1262–1267.

♦14. Strong LC, Stine M, Norsted TL. Cancer in survivors of childhood soft tissue sarcoma and their relatives. *J Natl Cancer Inst* 1987; **79**:1213–1220.

♦15. Neglia JP, Meadows AT, Robison LL, *et al.* Second neoplasms after acute lymphoblastic leukemia in childhood. *N Engl J Med* 1991; **325**:1330–1336.

16. Bhatia S, Ramsay NKC, Steinbuch M, *et al.* Malignant neoplasms following bone marrow transplantation. *Blood* 1996; **87**:3633–3639.

17. Darrington DL, Vose JM, Anderson JR, *et al.* Incidence and characterization of secondary myelodysplastic syndrome and acute myelogenous leukemia following high-dose chemoradiotherapy and autologous stem cell transplantation for lymphoid malignancies. *J Clin Oncol* 1994; **12**:2527–2534.

18. Beaty O 3rd, Hudson MM, Greenwald C, *et al.* Subsequent malignancies in children and adolescents after treatment for Hodgkin's disease. *J Clin Oncol* 1995; **13**:603–609.

19. Tarbell NJ, Gelber RD, Weinstein HJ, Mauch P. Sex differences in risk of second malignant tumours after Hodgkin's disease in childhood. *Lancet* 1993; **341**:1428–1432.

20. Zang EA, Wynder EL. Differences in lung cancer risk between men and women: examination of the evidence. *J Natl Cancer Inst* 1996; **88**:183–192.

21. Garwicz S, Anderson H, Olsen JH, *et al.* Second malignant neoplasms after cancer in childhood and adolescence: a population-based case-control study in the 5 Nordic countries. The Nordic Society for Pediatric Hematology and Oncology. The Association of the Nordic Cancer Registries. *Int J Cancer* 2000; **88**:672–678.

♦22. Hawkins MM, Wilson LM, Burton HS, *et al.* Radiotherapy, alkylating agents, and risk of bone cancer after childhood cancer. *J Natl Cancer Inst* 1996; **88**:270–278.

23. Tucker MA, D'Angio GJ, Boice JD Jr, *et al.* Bone sarcomas linked to radiotherapy and chemotherapy in children. *N Engl J Med* 1987; **317**:588–593.

●24. Boice JD Jr. Radiation and breast carcinogenesis. *Med Pediatr Oncol* 2001; **36**:508–513.

♦25. Hancock SL, Tucker MA, Hoppe RT. Breast cancer after treatment of Hodgkin's disease. *J Natl Cancer Inst* 1993; **85**:25–31.

26. Metayer C, Lynch CF, Clarke EA, *et al.* Second cancers among long-term survivors of Hodgkin's disease diagnosed in childhood and adolescence. *J Clin Oncol* 2000; **18**:2435–2443.

♦27. Kaste SC, Hudson MM, Jones DJ, *et al.* Breast masses in women treated for childhood cancer: incidence and screening guidelines. *Cancer* 1998; **82**:784–792.

28. Travis LB, Curtis RE, Boice JD Jr. Late effects of treatment for childhood Hodgkin's disease [letter; comment]. *N Engl J Med* 1996; **334**:745–751.

29. Tucker MA, Jones PH, Boice JD Jr, *et al.* Therapeutic radiation at a young age is linked to secondary thyroid cancer. The Late Effects Study Group. *Cancer Res* 1991; **51**:2885–2888.

30. De Vathaire F, Hardiman C, Shamsaldin A, *et al.* Thyroid carcinomas after irradiation for a first cancer during childhood. *Arch Intern Med* 1999; **159**:2713–2719.

31. Sklar C, Whitton J, Mertens A, *et al.* Abnormalities of the thyroid in survivors of Hodgkin's disease: Data from the Childhood Cancer Survivor Study. *J Clin Endocrinol Metab* 2000; **85**:3227–3232.

32. Kimball Dalton VM, Gelber RD, Li F, *et al.* Second malignancies in patients treated for childhood acute lymphoblastic leukemia. *J Clin Oncol* 1998; **16**:2848–2853.

33. Nygaard R, Garwicz S, Haldorsen T, *et al.* Second malignant neoplasms in patients treated for childhood leukemia. *Acta Paediatr Scand* 1991; **80**:1220–1228.

34. Pratt CB, George SL, Hannock ML, *et al.* Second malignant neoplasms in survivors of childhood acute lymphocytic leukemia. *Pediatr Res* 1988; **23**(Suppl.):345a.

♦35. Loning L, Zimmermann M, Reiter A, *et al.* Secondary neoplasms subsequent to Berlin–Frankfurt–Munster therapy of acute lymphoblastic leukemia in childhood: significantly lower risk without cranial radiotherapy. *Blood* 2000: **95**:2770–2775.

36. Bhatia S, Sather HN, Trigg ME, *et al.* Low incidence of second malignant neoplasms (SMN) following childhood acute lymphoblastic leukemia (ALL): follow-up of the Childrens Cancer Group (CCG) Cohort. *Blood* 2000; **96**:465a.

●37. Smith MA, McCaffrey RP, Karp JE. The secondary leukemias: challenges and research directions. *J Natl Cancer Inst* 1996; **88**:407–418.

38. Hawkins MM, Wilson LM, Stovall MA, *et al.* Epipodophyllotoxins, alkylating agents, and radiation and risk of secondary leukaemia after childhood cancer. *Br Med J* 1992; **304**:951–958.

39. Pedersen-Bjergaard J, Erbsoll J, Hansen VL, *et al.* Carcinoma of the urinary bladder after treatment with cyclophosphamide for non-Hodgkin's lymphoma. *N Engl J Med* 1988; **318**:1028–1032.

40. Blayney DW, Longo DL, Young RC, *et al.* Decreasing risk of leukemia with prolonged follow-up after chemotherapy and radiotherapy for Hodgkin's disease. *N Engl J Med* 1987; **316**:710–714.

♦41. Neugut AI, Robinson E, Nieves J, *et al.* Poor survival of treatment-related acute non-lymphocytic leukemia. *JAMA* 1990; **264**:1006–1008.

♦42. Wolden SL, Lamborn KR, Cleary SF, *et al.* Second cancers following pediatric Hodgkin's disease. *J Clin Oncol* 1998; **16**:536–544.

43. Sankila R, Garwicz S, Olsen JH, *et al.* Risk of subsequent malignant neoplasms among 1,641 Hodgkin's disease patients diagnosed in childhood and adolescence: a population-based cohort study in the five Nordic countries. Association of the Nordic Cancer Registries and the Nordic Society of Pediatric Hematology and Oncology. *J Clin Oncol* 1996; **14**:1442–1446.

44. Schellong G, Riepenhausen M, Creutzig U, *et al.* Low risk of secondary leukemia after chemotherapy without mechlorethamine in childhood Hodgkin's disease: German–Austrian Pediatric Hodgkin's Disease Group. *J Clin Oncol* 1997; **15**:2247–2253.

45. Tucker MA, Meadows AT, Boice JD, *et al.* Leukemia after therapy with alkylating agents for childhood cancer. *J Natl Cancer Inst* 1987; **78**:459–464.

◆46. Pui C-H, Ribeiro R, Hancock ML, *et al.* Acute myeloid leukemia in children treated with epipodophyllotoxins for acute lymphocytic leukemia. *N Engl J Med* 1991; **325**:1682–1687.

47. Winick NJ, Mckenna RW, Shuster JJ, *et al.* Secondary acute myeloid leukemia in children with acute lymphoblastic leukemia treated with etoposide. *J Clin Oncol* 1993; **11**:209–217.

48. Sugita K, Furukawa T, Tsuchida M, *et al.* High frequency of etoposide (VP-16)-related secondary leukemia in children with non-Hodgkin's lymphoma. *Am J Pediatr Hematol Oncol* 1993; **15**:99–104.

49. Krishnan A, Bhatia S, Slovak ML, *et al.* Predictors of therapy-related leukemia and myelodysplasia following autologous transplantation for lymphoma: an assessment of risk factors. *Blood* 2000; **95**:1588–1593.

●50. Bhatia S, Davies SM, Robison LL. Leukemia. In: Neugut AI, Meadows AT, Robinson E (eds) *Multiple primary cancers.* Philadelphia: Lippincott Williams and Wilkins, 1999:257–275.

◆51. Smith MA, Rubinstein L, Anderson JR, *et al.* Secondary leukemia or myelodysplastic syndrome after treatment with epipodophyllotoxins. *J Clin Oncol* 1999; **17**:569–577.

52. Felix CA. Secondary leukemias induced by topoisomerase targeted drugs. *Biochim Biophys Acta* 1998; **1400**:233–235.

53. Relling MV, Rubnitz JE, Rivera GK, *et al.* High incidence of secondary brain tumors after radiotherapy and antimetabolites. *Lancet* 1999; **354**:34–39.

◆54. Relling MV, Yanishevski Y, Nemec J, *et al.* Etoposide and antimetabolite pharmacology in patients who develop secondary acute myeloid leukemia. *Leukemia* 1998; **12**:346–352.

◆55. Naoe T, Takeyama K, Yokozawa T, *et al.* Analysis of genetic polymorphism in NQO1, GST-M1, GST-T1, and CYP3A4 in 469 Japanese patients with therapy-related leukemia/myelodysplastic syndrome and de novo acute myeloid leukemia. *Clin Cancer Res* 2000; **6**:4091–4095.

◆56. Felix CA, Walker AH, Lange BJ, *et al.* Association of CYP3A4 genotype with treatment-related leukemia. *Proc Natl Acad Sci USA* 1998; **95**:13176–13181.

◆57. Allan JM, Wild CP, Rollinson S, *et al.* Polymorphism in glutathione S-transferase P1 is associated with susceptibility to chemotherapy-induced leukemia. *Proc Natl Acad Sci USA* 2001; **98**:11592–11597.

58. Woo MH, Shuster JJ, Chen CL, *et al.* Glutathione S-transferase genotypes in children who develop treatment-related acute myeloid malignancies. *Leukemia* 2000; **14**:232–237.

59. van Leeuwen FE, Klokman WJ, Stovall M, *et al.* Roles of radiotherapy and smoking in lung cancer following Hodgkin's disease. *J Natl Cancer Inst* 1995; **87**:1530–1537.

60. van Leeuwen FE, Klokman WJ, Stovall M, *et al.* Roles of radiotherapy and smoking in lung cancer following Hodgkin's disease. *J Natl Cancer Inst* 1995; **87**:1530–1537.

61. Rothman K, Keller AZ. The effect of joint exposure to alcohol and tobacco on risk of cancers of the mouth and pharynx. *J Chronic Dis* 1972; **25**:711–716.

62. Flanders WD, Rothman KJ. Interaction of alcohol and tobacco in laryngeal cancer. *Am J Epidemiol* 1982; **115**:371–379.

63. LaVecchia C, Negri E. The role of alcohol in esophageal cancer in nonsmokers, and the role of tobacco in nondrinkers. *Int J Cancer* 1989; **43**:784–785.

64. Moll AC, Imhof SM, Schouten-Van Meeteren AY, *et al.* Second primary tumors in hereditary retinoblastoma: is there an age effect on radiation-related risk? *Ophthalmology* 2001; **108**:1109–1114.

65. Abramson DH, Melson MR, Dunkel IJ, Frank CM. Third (fourth and fifth) nonocular tumors in survivors of retinoblastoma. *Ophthalmology* 2001; **108**:1868–1876.

66. Eng C, Li FP, Abramson DH, Ellsworth RM, *et al.* Mortality from second tumors among long-term survivors of retinoblastoma. *J Natl Cancer Inst* 1993; **85**:1121–1128.

67. Meadows AT, Obringer AC, Marrero O, *et al.* Second malignant neoplasms following childhood Hodgkin's disease: treatment and splenectomy as risk factors. *Med Pediatr Oncol* 1989; **17**:477–484.

68. Tucker MA. Solid second cancers following Hodgkin's disease. *Hematol Oncol Clin North Am* 1993; **7**:389–400.

69. Green DM, Hyland A, Barcos MP, *et al.* Second malignant neoplasms after treatment for Hodgkin's disease in childhood and adolescence. *J Clin Oncol* 2000; **18**:1492–1499.

70. Bhatia S, Robison L, Meadows A. High risk of second malignant neoplasms (SMN) continues with extended follow-up of childhood Hodgkin's disease (HD) cohort: Report from the Late Effects Study Group. *Blood* 2001; **98**:275a.

71. Breslow NE, Takashima JR, Whitton JA, *et al.* Second malignant neoplasms following treatment for Wilm's tumor: a report from the National Wilm's Tumor Study Group. *J Clin Oncol* 1995; **13**:1851–1859.

72. Shearer P, Kapoor G, Beckwith JB, *et al.* Secondary acute myelogenous leukemia in patients previously treated for childhood renal tumors: a report from the National Wilms Tumor Study Group. *J Pediatr Hematol Oncol* 2001; **23**:109–111.

73. Janjan NA, Zellmer DL. Calculated risk of breast cancer following mantle irradiation determined by measured dose. *Cancer Detect Prev* 1992; **16**:273–282.

74. Chung CT, Bogart JA, Adams JF, *et al.* Increased risk of breast cancer in splenectomized patients undergoing radiation therapy for Hodgkin's disease. *Int J Radiat Oncol Biol Phys* 1997; **37**:405–409.

75. Tinger A, Wasserman TH, Klein EE, *et al.* The incidence of breast cancer following mantle field radiation therapy as a function of dose and technique. *Int J Radiat Oncol Biol Phys* 1997; **37**:865–870.

76. Aisenberg AC, Finkelstein DM, Doppke KP, *et al.* High risk of breast carcinoma after irradiation of young women with Hodgkin's disease. *Cancer* 1997; **79**:1203–1210.

77. Prior P, Pope DJ. Hodgkin's disease: subsequent primary cancers in relation to treatment. *Br J Cancer* 1988; **58**:512–517.

78. Carey RW, Lingood RM, Wood W, *et al.* Breast cancer developing in four women cured of Hodgkin's disease. *Cancer* 1984; **54**:2234–2236.

79. Cook KL, Adler DD, Lichter AS, *et al.* Breast carcinoma in young women previously treated for Hodgkin's disease. *Am J Roentgenol* 1990; **155**:39–42.

80. Yahalom J, Petrek JA, Biddinger PW, *et al.* Breast cancer in patients irradiated for Hodgkin's disease: a clinical and pathologic analysis of 45 events in 37 patients. *J Clin Oncol* 1992; **10**:1674–1681.

The vast majority of patients with LFS-L syndrome lack TP53 mutations in the coding region and, although rare families have been described with mutations of an upstream effector of p53, hCHK2, the exact molecular pathology has yet to be determined.[27,28]

RETINOBLASTOMA (OMIM 180200)

Retinoblastoma occurs in approximately 1:20 000 liveborn children. A small majority of them are non-hereditary (60 per cent) and usually unilateral. The remaining 40 per cent are hereditary and, among them, 15 per cent are unilateral and 25 per cent bilateral. Knudson proposed in 1971 that both hereditary and non-hereditary retinoblastomas occurred because of mutations involving both alleles of a susceptibility gene. When one of these mutations occurs in the germline, it is transmitted to the next generation, and the offspring can, therefore, develop the tumor more frequently.[5] In 1986, Friend et al. cloned and identified mutations in the 180 kb RB1 gene, which is located on the long arm of chromosome 13 (13q14).[29] RB1 is implicated in the negative regulation of cell growth, and inactivating alterations include large or small deletions and point mutations distributed throughout the gene.

Survivors of hereditary retinoblastomas are at increased risk to develop other subsequent tumors, particularly osteosarcomas (risk increased by 500-fold compared to the general population),[30] soft tissue sarcomas, melanomas and pinealoblastomas (trilateral retinoblastoma). This increased risk is not specifically associated with therapy, as the second primary tumors will frequently occur outside the radiation field of treatment to the primary tumor.

WILMS' TUMOR [OMIM 194070 (WT1), 194071 (WT2), 194090 (WT3)]

Wilms' tumor (WT), or nephroblastoma, was described by several authors at the end of the nineteenth century, including Max Wilms, a German surgeon.[31] This embryonal tumor affects approximately 1:10 000 liveborn children, and is often associated with various congenital anomalies in several syndromes (Table 3b.1). Different genes are implicated for each syndrome (Table 3b.2). Wilms' tumor, aniridia, genitourinary malformations, mental retardation (WAGR) and Denys–Drash syndromes are due to mutations in the WT1 gene, located on the short arm of chromosome 11 (11p13).[32] WT1 is involved in the down regulation of a transcription factor, Pax-2, which is implicated in the differentiation of renal epithelium during nephrogenesis.[33] Deletions in a zinc finger domain in this gene and subsequent generation of a truncated protein product usually lead to WAGR syndrome[34] in which Wilms' tumor can develop in up to 50 per cent of the cases, whereas specific point mutations give rise to Denys–Drash syndrome,[35] which is

Table 3b.1 Syndromes associated with Wilms' tumors

WAGR syndrome	Wilms' tumor, aniridia, genitourinary malformations and mental retardation
Denys–Drash syndrome	Wilms' tumor, severe nephropathy, dysgenetic male pseudohermaphroditism
Beckwith–Wiedemann syndrome	Wilms' tumor, prenatal and postnatal gigantism, macroglossia, abdominal wall defects, visceromegaly, muscular hypertrophy, advanced bone age, craniofacial and ear anomalies, and neonatal hypoglycemia

Table 3b.2 Genes in Wilms' tumor (WT)

WT1 (11p13)-related	WT2 (11p15)-related	WT3 (17q and 19q) related	Sporadic (unilateral)
Unilateral or bilateral nephroblastomas, no other anomalies WAGR syndrome Denys–Drash syndrome	Beckwith–Wiedemann syndrome	Familial, not linked to WT1 & WT2	

WAGR, Wilms' tumor, aniridia, genitourinary malformations, mental retardation.

commonly associated with severe genitourinary malformations, pseudohermaphroditism and mesangial sclerosis of the kidney leading to renal failure in childhood.

The gene(s) responsible for Beckwith–Wiedemann (BWS) syndrome has not been defined yet, but the locus (WT2) is located at 11p15.5.[36] In patients with BWS, 8 per cent will develop tumors, among which WT is the most common, especially if the mutation occurs within the telomeric domain.[37] Rhabdomyosarcomas, neuroblastomas, hepatoblastomas and adrenocortical carcinomas are also reported.[38–41]

A third locus (WT3) is suggested by familial cases not linked to WT1 or WT2. The exact location is not clear, but seems to be at 19q and 17q.[42,43]

Several studies have showed that children having developed a Wilms' tumor are at increased risk of developing a second malignant tumor, especially if treatment includes irradiation. Contralateral tumors, hepatocellular carcinomas, Hodgkin's disease, and basal or squamous cell carcinomas have been reported.[44]

MULTIPLE ENDOCRINE NEOPLASIA [OMIM 131100 (MEN1), 171400 (MEN2)]

Multiple endocrine neoplasia (MEN) syndromes are divided into three broad types: MEN1, MEN2a and MEN2b.

◆46. Pui C-H, Ribeiro R, Hancock ML, et al. Acute myeloid leukemia in children treated with epipodophyllotoxins for acute lymphocytic leukemia. N Engl J Med 1991; 325:1682–1687.

47. Winick NJ, Mckenna RW, Shuster JJ, et al. Secondary acute myeloid leukemia in children with acute lymphoblastic leukemia treated with etoposide. J Clin Oncol 1993; 11:209–217.

48. Sugita K, Furukawa T, Tsuchida M, et al. High frequency of etoposide (VP-16)-related secondary leukemia in children with non-Hodgkin's lymphoma. Am J Pediatr Hematol Oncol 1993; 15:99–104.

49. Krishnan A, Bhatia S, Slovak ML, et al. Predictors of therapy-related leukemia and myelodysplasia following autologous transplantation for lymphoma: an assessment of risk factors. Blood 2000; 95:1588–1593.

●50. Bhatia S, Davies SM, Robison LL. Leukemia. In: Neugut AI, Meadows AT, Robinson E (eds) Multiple primary cancers. Philadelphia: Lippincott Williams and Wilkins, 1999:257–275.

◆51. Smith MA, Rubinstein L, Anderson JR, et al. Secondary leukemia or myelodysplastic syndrome after treatment with epipodophyllotoxins. J Clin Oncol 1999; 17:569–577.

52. Felix CA. Secondary leukemias induced by topoisomerase targeted drugs. Biochim Biophys Acta 1998; 1400:233–235.

53. Relling MV, Rubnitz JE, Rivera GK, et al. High incidence of secondary brain tumors after radiotherapy and antimetabolites. Lancet 1999; 354:34–39.

◆54. Relling MV, Yanishevski Y, Nemec J, et al. Etoposide and antimetabolite pharmacology in patients who develop secondary acute myeloid leukemia. Leukemia 1998; 12:346–352.

◆55. Naoe T, Takeyama K, Yokozawa T, et al. Analysis of genetic polymorphism in NQO1, GST-M1, GST-T1, and CYP3A4 in 469 Japanese patients with therapy-related leukemia/myelodysplastic syndrome and de novo acute myeloid leukemia. Clin Cancer Res 2000; 6:4091–4095.

◆56. Felix CA, Walker AH, Lange BJ, et al. Association of CYP3A4 genotype with treatment-related leukemia. Proc Natl Acad Sci USA 1998; 95:13176–13181.

◆57. Allan JM, Wild CP, Rollinson S, et al. Polymorphism in glutathione S-transferase P1 is associated with susceptibility to chemotherapy-induced leukemia. Proc Natl Acad Sci USA 2001; 98:11592–11597.

58. Woo MH, Shuster JJ, Chen CL, et al. Glutathione S-transferase genotypes in children who develop treatment-related acute myeloid malignancies. Leukemia 2000; 14:232–237.

59. van Leeuwen FE, Klokman WJ, Stovall M, et al. Roles of radiotherapy and smoking in lung cancer following Hodgkin's disease. J Natl Cancer Inst 1995; 87:1530–1537.

60. van Leeuwen FE, Klokman WJ, Stovall M, et al. Roles of radiotherapy and smoking in lung cancer following Hodgkin's disease. J Natl Cancer Inst 1995; 87:1530–1537.

61. Rothman K, Keller AZ. The effect of joint exposure to alcohol and tobacco on risk of cancers of the mouth and pharynx. J Chronic Dis 1972; 25:711–716.

62. Flanders WD, Rothman KJ. Interaction of alcohol and tobacco in laryngeal cancer. Am J Epidemiol 1982; 115:371–379.

63. LaVecchia C, Negri E. The role of alcohol in esophageal cancer in nonsmokers, and the role of tobacco in nondrinkers. Int J Cancer 1989; 43:784–785.

64. Moll AC, Imhof SM, Schouten-Van Meeteren AY, et al. Second primary tumors in hereditary retinoblastoma: is there an age effect on radiation-related risk? Ophthalmology 2001; 108:1109–1114.

65. Abramson DH, Melson MR, Dunkel IJ, Frank CM. Third (fourth and fifth) nonocular tumors in survivors of retinoblastoma. Ophthalmology 2001; 108:1868–1876.

66. Eng C, Li FP, Abramson DH, Ellsworth RM, et al. Mortality from second tumors among long-term survivors of retinoblastoma. J Natl Cancer Inst 1993; 85:1121–1128.

67. Meadows AT, Obringer AC, Marrero O, et al. Second malignant neoplasms following childhood Hodgkin's disease: treatment and splenectomy as risk factors. Med Pediatr Oncol 1989; 17:477–484.

68. Tucker MA. Solid second cancers following Hodgkin's disease. Hematol Oncol Clin North Am 1993; 7:389–400.

69. Green DM, Hyland A, Barcos MP, et al. Second malignant neoplasms after treatment for Hodgkin's disease in childhood and adolescence. J Clin Oncol 2000; 18:1492–1499.

70. Bhatia S, Robison L, Meadows A. High risk of second malignant neoplasms (SMN) continues with extended follow-up of childhood Hodgkin's disease (HD) cohort: Report from the Late Effects Study Group. Blood 2001; 98:275a.

71. Breslow NE, Takashima JR, Whitton JA, et al. Second malignant neoplasms following treatment for Wilm's tumor: a report from the National Wilm's Tumor Study Group. J Clin Oncol 1995; 13:1851–1859.

72. Shearer P, Kapoor G, Beckwith JB, et al. Secondary acute myelogenous leukemia in patients previously treated for childhood renal tumors: a report from the National Wilms Tumor Study Group. J Pediatr Hematol Oncol 2001; 23:109–111.

73. Janjan NA, Zellmer DL. Calculated risk of breast cancer following mantle irradiation determined by measured dose. Cancer Detect Prev 1992; 16:273–282.

74. Chung CT, Bogart JA, Adams JF, et al. Increased risk of breast cancer in splenectomized patients undergoing radiation therapy for Hodgkin's disease. Int J Radiat Oncol Biol Phys 1997; 37:405–409.

75. Tinger A, Wasserman TH, Klein EE, et al. The incidence of breast cancer following mantle field radiation therapy as a function of dose and technique. Int J Radiat Oncol Biol Phys 1997; 37:865–870.

76. Aisenberg AC, Finkelstein DM, Doppke KP, et al. High risk of breast carcinoma after irradiation of young women with Hodgkin's disease. Cancer 1997; 79:1203–1210.

77. Prior P, Pope DJ. Hodgkin's disease: subsequent primary cancers in relation to treatment. Br J Cancer 1988; 58:512–517.

78. Carey RW, Lingood RM, Wood W, et al. Breast cancer developing in four women cured of Hodgkin's disease. Cancer 1984; 54:2234–2236.

79. Cook KL, Adler DD, Lichter AS, et al. Breast carcinoma in young women previously treated for Hodgkin's disease. Am J Roentgenol 1990; 155:39–42.

80. Yahalom J, Petrek JA, Biddinger PW, et al. Breast cancer in patients irradiated for Hodgkin's disease: a clinical and pathologic analysis of 45 events in 37 patients. J Clin Oncol 1992; 10:1674–1681.

Genetic susceptibility and familial cancer syndromes

MANUEL DIEZI AND DAVID MALKIN

HISTORICAL BACKGROUND AND GENERAL CONSIDERATIONS

Hereditary susceptibility to develop cancer was documented as early as the eighteenth century by John Hunter, a British surgeon ('The predisposing Causes of Cancer are three, ... viz. age, parts, and hereditary disposition; perhaps climate ...').[1] and by French chemist Bernard Peyrilhe at the beginning of the nineteenth century.[2] The hypothesis was developed further at the beginning of the twentieth century by several scientists including, among many others, Kaiser ('la prédilection pour un certain organe au cancer comme un lieu de moindre résistance transmis par l'hérédité'),[3] and later the American pathologist Maud Slye ('There are apparently two factors necessary to induce cancer. ... These factors are (1) an inherited local susceptibility to the disease, and (2) irritation of the appropriate kind and the appropriate degree applied to the cancer-susceptible tissues').[4] Since then, Knudson[5] developed the basis for the understanding of the genetic causes of some hereditary cancers caused by mutations in tumor suppressor genes (whereby one mutation is inherited through the germline and the other acquired in the somatic cell), Varmus and Bishop described the role of proto-oncogenes,[6,7] and a number of familial syndromes leading to an increased risk to develop cancer have been described. We will discuss the most common of these syndromes in this subchapter.

As pointed out by Birch,[8] consideration of the following four points should be made with respect to discussion of the genetic predisposition to develop cancer:

1 highly penetrant genes lead to classical familial cancer clusters with clear patterns of inheritance;
2 lower penetrant genes, with most carriers unaffected, could explain some diagnoses of cancer in siblings, or less clearly defined familial cancer cluster phenotypes;
3 various syndromes, where other congenital anomalies represent the primary phenotypic manifestation, confer an increased risk for childhood cancer;
4 normal polymorphic variants of genes confer an increased risk of developing childhood cancer by modifying cellular responses to environmental factors.

Genetic susceptibility to develop cancer arises from alterations in the genome, affecting either large parts of one or more chromosomes, which are sometimes visible by cytogenetic analysis (such as the first genetic anomaly to be described that was linked to cancer, viz. the Philadelphia chromosome or reciprocal translocation of chromosome 9 and 22 leading to a fusion transcript of two genes, *bcr* and *abl*[9]), from point mutations of specific genes, leading to an aberrant or absent expression of a transcript, or from epigenetic events, such as methylation that leads to aberrant expression of a gene product.

These alterations can affect genes that are 'dominant' at the cellular level, such as proto-oncogenes. These are genes involved in normal cellular regulation, in which

mutations, translocations or amplifications of one allele lead to the aberrant expression of an oncogene and subsequent deregulation of cell growth, malignant transformation and tumor development. The alterations can also affect genes 'recessive' at the cellular level, such as tumor suppressor genes, for which both alleles must be functionally inactivated to allow eventual tumor development.[10]

Mutations affecting such genes are very frequent at the somatic level in human cancers. Less commonly, they occur in the germ cells, leading to genetic susceptibility to an increased risk of cancer, which may then be transmitted to the next generation. These observations have led to the now widely accepted premise of cancer as a genetic disease. Sometimes, a difference in penetrance (the proportion of mutation carriers that actually develop cancer in their lifetime) for similar mutations in different individuals might be due to additional genetic or environmental factors (risk modifiers) that these individuals have been exposed to, thus reinforcing the multifactorial theory of cancer development.

Genetic predisposition as a cause of tumor development is likely to account for only a small proportion of all cancer diagnoses (5–10 per cent) but is important to recognize, as affected individuals may benefit from preventive screening. Being aware of their predisposition, they may also avoid certain other risk factors, and make informed choices regarding their own future and that of their potential offspring.

Hereditary cancer should be strongly suspected whenever the following clinical clues are present:[11]

1 a cancer occurring at an unusually young age compared with the usual presentation of that type of cancer in the general population;
2 multifocal development of cancer in a single organ or bilateral development of cancer in paired organs;
3 development of more than one primary tumor of any type in a single individual;
4 family history of cancer of the same type in close relative(s);
5 a high rate of cancer within a family;
6 occurrence of cancer in an individual or a family exhibiting congenital anomalies or birth defects.

MAJOR FAMILY CANCER SYNDROMES BY MODE OF INHERITANCE

Autosomal dominant

LI–FRAUMENI SYNDROME (OMIM 151623)

In 1969, Li and Fraumeni described four families in which several individuals developed sarcomas at an early age.[12,13] Other cancers were also reported in the affected families including premenopausal breast cancer, acute leukemia, osteosarcomas, and an excess of brain tumors and adrenocortical carcinomas compared to the general population.[14]

Based on prospective follow-up of 24 families, a classical definition of Li–Fraumeni syndrome (LFS) was proposed that includes the following criteria:[15] a proband diagnosed with sarcoma <45 years of age who has at least one first-degree relative with any cancer diagnosed <45 years of age, and a first- or second-degree relative with either any cancer diagnosed <45 years of age or a sarcoma at any age.

Subsequently, 60–80 per cent of LFS cases have been associated with germline mutations in the gene TP53.[16,17] TP53 is a tumor suppressor gene located on the short arm of chromosome 17 (17p13.1) and encodes a protein that is involved in several cellular pathways including DNA repair, genomic stability, cell-cycle control and apoptosis. Although germline or somatic mutations occur at various locations in the gene, most of them (75 per cent) are missense point mutations involving highly conserved regions in exons 5–8, the DNA-binding domain, leading to inactivation of the protein. Sporadic p53 mutations are very frequent (>50 per cent) in human cancers[18] but the population frequency of germline p53 mutations is only approximately 1:50 000.

In addition to the wide spectrum of primary tumors present in LFS, gene carriers are at increased risk for subsequent tumors, with an overall relative risk of second cancer of 5.3 [95 per cent confidence interval (95%CI) 2.8–7.8] and a cumulative probability of second cancer occurrence of 57 per cent (±10 per cent) at 30 years after diagnosis of the first cancer, with a lifetime risk of 73 per cent for males and up to 100 per cent for females.[19] Moreover, carriers usually develop their tumors at a younger age than the general population[20] and the younger a gene carrier is diagnosed with a first cancer, the greater is the probability of being diagnosed with a second cancer.[21,22] The most frequent second malignancies in LFS patients include sarcomas, brain tumors, breast cancer, osteosarcomas and lymphomas.

Inherited mutations of the p53 gene have been found as well in children with tumors who lacked the classical family history of LFS.[23–25] The Li–Fraumeni-like syndrome (LFS-L) has subsequently been described,[26] which has the following criteria:

1 a proband diagnosed <45 years of age with any childhood cancer or sarcoma, brain tumor or adrenocortical carcinoma;
2 a first- or second-degree relative with a typical LFS cancer diagnosed at any age;
3 a first- or second-degree relative in the same parental lineage with any cancer diagnosed <60 years of age.

The vast majority of patients with LFS-L syndrome lack TP53 mutations in the coding region and, although rare families have been described with mutations of an upstream effector of p53, hCHK2, the exact molecular pathology has yet to be determined.[27,28]

RETINOBLASTOMA (OMIM 180200)

Retinoblastoma occurs in approximately 1:20 000 liveborn children. A small majority of them are non-hereditary (60 per cent) and usually unilateral. The remaining 40 per cent are hereditary and, among them, 15 per cent are unilateral and 25 per cent bilateral. Knudson proposed in 1971 that both hereditary and non-hereditary retinoblastomas occurred because of mutations involving both alleles of a susceptibility gene. When one of these mutations occurs in the germline, it is transmitted to the next generation, and the offspring can, therefore, develop the tumor more frequently.[5] In 1986, Friend et al. cloned and identified mutations in the 180 kb RB1 gene, which is located on the long arm of chromosome 13 (13q14).[29] RB1 is implicated in the negative regulation of cell growth, and inactivating alterations include large or small deletions and point mutations distributed throughout the gene.

Survivors of hereditary retinoblastomas are at increased risk to develop other subsequent tumors, particularly osteosarcomas (risk increased by 500-fold compared to the general population),[30] soft tissue sarcomas, melanomas and pinealoblastomas (trilateral retinoblastoma). This increased risk is not specifically associated with therapy, as the second primary tumors will frequently occur outside the radiation field of treatment to the primary tumor.

WILMS' TUMOR [OMIM 194070 (WT1), 194071 (WT2), 194090 (WT3)]

Wilms' tumor (WT), or nephroblastoma, was described by several authors at the end of the nineteenth century, including Max Wilms, a German surgeon.[31] This embryonal tumor affects approximately 1:10 000 liveborn children, and is often associated with various congenital anomalies in several syndromes (Table 3b.1). Different genes are implicated for each syndrome (Table 3b.2). Wilms' tumor, aniridia, genitourinary malformations, mental retardation (WAGR) and Denys–Drash syndromes are due to mutations in the WT1 gene, located on the short arm of chromosome 11 (11p13).[32] WT1 is involved in the down regulation of a transcription factor, Pax-2, which is implicated in the differentiation of renal epithelium during nephrogenesis.[33] Deletions in a zinc finger domain in this gene and subsequent generation of a truncated protein product usually lead to WAGR syndrome[34] in which Wilms' tumor can develop in up to 50 per cent of the cases, whereas specific point mutations give rise to Denys–Drash syndrome,[35] which is

Table 3b.1 *Syndromes associated with Wilms' tumors*

WAGR syndrome	Wilms' tumor, aniridia, genitourinary malformations and mental retardation
Denys–Drash syndrome	Wilms' tumor, severe nephropathy, dysgenetic male pseudohermaphroditism
Beckwith–Wiedemann syndrome	Wilms' tumor, prenatal and postnatal gigantism, macroglossia, abdominal wall defects, visceromegaly, muscular hypertrophy, advanced bone age, craniofacial and ear anomalies, and neonatal hypoglycemia

Table 3b.2 *Genes in Wilms' tumor (WT)*

WT1 (11p13)-related	WT2 (11p15)-related	WT3 (17q – and 19q) related	Sporadic (unilateral)
Unilateral or bilateral nephroblastomas, no other anomalies WAGR syndrome Denys–Drash syndrome	Beckwith–Wiedemann syndrome	Familial, not linked to WT1 & WT2	

WAGR, Wilms' tumor, aniridia, genitourinary malformations, mental retardation.

commonly associated with severe genitourinary malformations, pseudohermaphroditism and mesangial sclerosis of the kidney leading to renal failure in childhood.

The gene(s) responsible for Beckwith–Wiedemann (BWS) syndrome has not been defined yet, but the locus (WT2) is located at 11p15.5.[36] In patients with BWS, 8 per cent will develop tumors, among which WT is the most common, especially if the mutation occurs within the telomeric domain.[37] Rhabdomyosarcomas, neuroblastomas, hepatoblastomas and adrenocortical carcinomas are also reported.[38–41]

A third locus (WT3) is suggested by familial cases not linked to WT1 or WT2. The exact location is not clear, but seems to be at 19q and 17q.[42,43]

Several studies have showed that children having developed a Wilms' tumor are at increased risk of developing a second malignant tumor, especially if treatment includes irradiation. Contralateral tumors, hepatocellular carcinomas, Hodgkin's disease, and basal or squamous cell carcinomas have been reported.[44]

MULTIPLE ENDOCRINE NEOPLASIA [OMIM 131100 (MEN1), 171400 (MEN2)]

Multiple endocrine neoplasia (MEN) syndromes are divided into three broad types: MEN1, MEN2a and MEN2b.

MEN1 was first described in the mid 1950s by several authors as polyglandular adenomatosis[45,46] and subsequently redefined.[47] Prevalence is approximately 0.02–0.2:1000 and affects mainly Caucasian families, although it has also been described in families from other ethnic or racial backgrounds.[48] MEN1 is characterized by parathyroid (95 per cent), pancreatic (73 per cent) and pituitary (44 per cent) gland tumors,[49] and is due to mutations in the small 10 exons of the 2.9/4.9 kb gene MEN1, located on the long arm of chromosome 11 (11q13). This gene acts as a tumor suppressor and follows Knudson's two-hit theory, yet its precise function is not clear.[50] The penetrance of the gene is high, with 28 per cent of gene carriers affected at age 15, and 80 per cent at age 50. Carriers are at risk of developing duodenal, thymic and bronchial carcinoids, bronchial carcinoma, malignant schwannoma, ovarian tumors, pancreatic carcinomas and adrenocortical carcinomas. Several benign tumors may also develop.

MEN2a and MEN2b present in the pediatric age group. They are characterized by medullary thyroid carcinomas, parathyroid adenomas and pheochromocytomas. In MEN2b, tumors may develop at a younger age, tend to be more aggressive and are associated with skeletal anomalies. Both MEN2a and MEN2b are due to specific mutations in the RET proto-oncogene, located on the long arm of chromosome 10 (10q11.2).[51,52] Genetic mutations in MEN2a and MEN2b are not explained by Knudson's two-hit theory with a subsequent loss of function, but rather by an overactivation of RET, leading to the cellular proliferation and the malignant phenotype.

The incidence of MEN1 is 1:100 000 and that of MEN2 around 1:500 000. Overall, a family history is found in 1–3 per cent of all patients with a primary diagnosis of an endocrine tumor, and increases to 10 per cent for second primary endocrine cancer. Thus, gene carriers appear to have an increased risk of developing a second tumor compared to the general population.[53]

NEUROFIBROMATOSIS [OMIM 162200 (NF1), 101000 (NF2)]

Neurofibromatosis (NF) is divided in two major classes: NF1 and NF2. NF1 syndrome was first described in 1882 by von Recklinghausen.[54] It is caused by a wide spectrum of mutations involving the NF1 tumor suppressor gene, which contains 59 exons and is located at 17q11.2.[55,56] A large majority of mutations (70–80 per cent) lead to the production of a truncated protein. The incidence of NF1 is around 1:3000 and the clinical picture is characterized by café-au-lait macules, neurofibromas, axillary and inguinal freckles, bone anomalies, optic nerve gliomas and iris hamartomas (Lisch nodules). Beside benign tumors, affected individuals are at risk for neurofibrosarcomas (3–15 per cent), astrocytomas, pheochromocytomas, neuroblastomas, rhabdomyosarcomas, Wilms' tumor and

leukemias.[11] This risk of developing malignant tumors is 6–8 times that of the general population.[57]

Children affected by this disease, particularly those who had an embryonic tumor as a first cancer, are at risk of developing a second cancer. These probably arise through mechanisms related to the therapy they received for their first tumor, although an underlying genetic predisposition has not been ruled out.[58]

NF2 is much less common than NF1, with an incidence of approximately 1:35 000. It is due to various mutations along the NF2 gene, located at 22q12.2, which encodes the protein schwannomin. Clinically, NF2 is characterized by bilateral acoustic neuromas, with weak or absent café-au-lait spots; clinical manifestations usually appear in adulthood. The most common malignant tumors associated with NF2 are gliomas. Once the diagnosis is confirmed, regular clinical surveillance is recommended to detect new similar tumors.[59]

VON HIPPEL–LINDAU DISEASE (OMIM 193300)

First described by von Hippel and subsequently by Lindau, this syndrome is characterized by cerebellar hemangiomas, retinal angiomas, renal cell carcinomas (35– 75 per cent) and pheochromocytomas (3.5–17 per cent), as well as pancreatic carcinomas (7.5–25 per cent).[60,61] The incidence is approximately 1:36 000.[62] Von Hippel–Lindau disease (VHL) is divided into four clinical subtypes, VHL 1, 2A, 2B and 3. VHL2 families are prone to develop pheochromocytomas with (2B) or without (2A) associated renal cell carcinomas. Each of these clinical subtypes is correlated to different mutations described in the VHL gene.[63] The VHL gene, which was cloned in 1993,[64] is located at chromosome 3p25.5 and encodes a 213 amino-acid protein, which has a role in transduction of growth signals and acts as a tumor suppressor. The peak incidence of pheochromocytoma is during the second decade but it has also been reported in childhood. Renal cell carcinoma occurs primarily during the third and fourth decade; screening should thus be initiated early and continued as the risk for one or the other tumor is lifelong.[65] Beside VHL disease, several other renal cancers seem to have a familial predisposition in a number of families. As reviewed by Zbar, these groups of familial tumors seem to have involvement of parts of chromosome 3 in common, although specific predisposing genes have not been identified.[66]

FAMILIAL BREAST/OVARIAN CANCERS [OMIM 113705 (BRCA1), 600185 (BRCA2)]

Familial breast cancer was originally described by Broca in 1866.[67] In addition to its association with Li–Fraumeni, Cowden, Peutz–Jeghers and ataxia-telangiectasia syndromes, predisposition to breast cancer is associated with germline mutations in two genes, BRCA1 and BRCA2.

Overall, these two genes may account for up to 80 per cent of hereditary breast cancers, and 6–10 per cent of all breast and ovarian cancers.[68] The carrier rate ranges from 1:100 to 1:2500.[69] The lifetime risk for breast cancer in mutation carriers ranges from 40 per cent to 90 per cent.[69] Beside other known risk factors, positive family history is frequently found in women who have been diagnosed with breast cancer.[70] The overall relative risk (RR) for breast cancer associated with a positive family history has been reported by Egan *et al.* in 1998 to be 1.70 (95%CI 1.55–1.87) and 2.34 (95%CI 1.80–3.02), if the breast cancer was diagnosed younger than 45 years of age.[71]

BRCA1, a tumor suppressor gene localized in 1990 by King *et al.* at chromosome 17q21,[72] has been implicated in as many as 39 per cent (with extremes from 9 to 79 per cent depending on the populations studied) of breast cancers diagnosed when three or more cases have been identified in a family.[73] In most cases, mutations of this gene lead to the production of a truncated protein.[74] The functions of this protein are still being elucidated, although several studies suggest that it may be involved in DNA repair.[75,76] Owing to the high risk of developing breast or ovarian cancers at a younger age than the general population, breast self-examination is recommended for women aged 18–21 years and then beginning at 25 years, clinical, biological (CA-125) and radiological (mammographies, transvaginal ultrasounds) examinations should be performed on a regular basis. Also, owing to the increased risk of colon and prostate cancer, rectal and sigmoidoscopic examinations should be performed regularly starting at 50 years of age.[77]

BRCA2 was described in 1994 and localized to chromosome 13q12.5.[78] Similar to BRCA1, BRCA2 acts as a tumor suppressor gene and synthesizes a nuclear protein. Expression of this protein is cyclic, and thus it may have a role in growth and proliferation of the cell.[79] In addition to female breast cancer, mutations in BRCA2 are responsible for a great proportion of male breast cancers, accounting for up to 40 per cent of these in certain populations.[80]

BRCA1 and BRCA2 mutation carriers are also at increased risk of developing other neoplasms (Table 3b.3).[81]

COWDEN SYNDROME (OMIM 158350)

Cowden syndrome is another syndrome that confers an increased risk of developing male[82] or female breast cancer, as well as thyroid and endometrial cancer.[83] It is very difficult to diagnose, as the clinical picture is subtle. It was first described by Lloyd and Dennis in 1963,[84] and identified in the family of a patient named Rachel Cowden who had an autosomal dominant pattern of inheritance of a multiple hamartoma syndrome. Diagnosis of Cowden syndrome is mainly one of exclusion and should be considered whenever characteristic tumors appear in clusters.[85] It is caused by mutations in the PTEN gene,[86]

a tumor suppressor gene located at 10q23.3, which has been implicated in a number of other cancer susceptibility syndromes[87] and in which mutations are very often found in sporadic tumors.[88] There are three major cancers associated with Cowden syndrome: breast, thyroid and endometrium.

HEREDITARY MELANOMA (OMIM 155600, 155601, 123829, 155755)

Melanoma was first described by William Norris in 1820,[89] who, at the time, described a familial pattern. Hereditary transmission of germline mutations may account for up to 10 per cent of all melanoma cases and the condition has an incidence of approximately 1:5000. Several genes are involved and, among them, the most frequent (31–50 per cent of cases) is CDKN2A, also known as p16, INK4A or CMM2. It is located at 9p21 and implicated in cell-cycle control. The remaining genes implicated in melanoma-prone families are still unknown. Several terms are used to describe this condition: FAMMM (familial atypical multiple mole melanoma), DNS (dysplastic nevus syndrome) and AMS (atypical mole syndrome).[90] Members of affected families have an 89-fold increased melanoma risk (at a younger age than the general population) and up to a 229-fold risk of developing a second primary tumor.[91] CDKN2A mutations have been involved especially in pancreatic carcinoma, but also in breast, colon, gastric and nasopharyngeal cancers.[92] Beside the basic protection against ultraviolet (UVA) and UVB, and avoidance of sunburns, regular skin self- and medical examinations should be performed with the use of photography to detect any change in the configuration of a nevus.[93–95]

COLON CANCER SYNDROME [OMIM 120435 (HNPCC1), 120436 (HNPCC2), 600258 (HNPCC3), 600259 (HNPCC4), 158320 (MTS), 600678 (HNPCC5)]

Several hereditary colon cancer syndromes have been described, some associated with polyps [familial adenomatous polyposis (FAP), Peutz–Jeghers syndrome (PJS)], and others not (hereditary non polyposis colon cancer; HNPCC), and each of them linked to specific genes.[96] Among these genes, the most frequent, accounting for more than 90 per cent of the germline mutations in susceptible families, are hMLH1 and hMSH2, located respectively at 3p21.3 and 2p22-p21 for HNPCC, APC, located at 5q for FAP, and LKB1 located at 19p13.3 for PJS. HNPCC may account for up to 10 per cent of all colorectal cancers and polyposis syndromes for 1 per cent. Associated malignancies include endometrial carcinomas, ovarian cancers, urinary tract, stomach, small bowel, hepatobiliary tract,[97,98] thyroid[99] and pancreatic cancers, as well as basal cell cancer, sebaceous carcinomas (Muir–Torre syndrome;

Table 3b.3 *Second tumors: relative and cumulative risks in autosomal dominant syndromes*

Cancer syndrome	Primary tumors	Relative risk of second cancer	Cumulative risk of second cancer	Second primary tumors	Reference number
Li–Fraumeni syndrome	Sarcomas, breast cancer, brain neoplasms	5.3 (2.8–7.8)	47–67% at 30 years	Sarcomas, brain tumors, breast cancer, osteosarcomas, lymphomas, ovarian cancer, thyroid cancer, lung cancer, bladder cancer	21
	Sarcomas		64% at 20 years, 100% at 30 years		
Retinoblastoma	Retinoblastomas	8.9 (2.4–22.8)	26.1% at 30 years	Osteosarcoma, fibro-, chondro- and Ewing's sarcomas, leukemias, lymphomas, brain tumors, pinealoblastoma	30, 156
Wilms' tumor	Nephroblastoma	14.7 (4–37.7)	0% at 10 years, 18% at 30 years	Contralateral tumor, hepatocellular carcinomas, Hodgkin's disease, skin carcinomas	44
MEN1	Pituitary	9.1 (2.9–18.8)		Parathyroid	53
		7.8 (1.5–19.1)		Pituitary	
	Parathyroid	4.8 (1.2–10.6)		Parathyroid	
MEN2			65–70% at 70 years	All tumors	85
	Pheochromocytoma		52% at 12 years	Contralateral pheochromocytoma	157
NF1			10–75%	Myelodyplastic syndrome, leukemia, neurofibrosarcoma, osteosarcoma	58
Breast/ovarian cancer, BRCA1	Breast, ovarian		10–40% at 70 years	Ovarian	67, 68, 141
			40–85% at 70 years	Breast	
			6% at 70 years	Colon	158
			8% at 70 years	Prostate	
Breast/ovarian cancer, BRCA2	Breast, ovarian	4.65 (3.48–6.22)		Prostate	81
		3.51 (1.87–6.58)		Pancreas	
		4.97 (1.5–16.52)		Gallbladder, bile duct	
		2.59 (1.46–4.61)		Stomach	
		2.58 (1.28–5.17)		Melanoma	
			52.3% at 70 years	Breast, contralateral	
			15.9% at 70 years	Ovarian	
Cowden syndrome			20–50% lifetime	Breast	83, 85
			10% lifetime	Non-medullary thyroid cancer	
		?	?	Endometrial carcinoma, renal-cell carcinoma, melanoma	
Familial testicular cancer	Testis, seminoma	5.4 (1.4–14.1)		Thyroid	119
		3.8 (2.1–6.4)		Pancreas	
		2.5 (1.3–4.1)		Lymphomas	
	Testis, teratoma	6.4 (1.2–19)		Connective tissue	
		3.3 (0.3–12.1)		Myeloma	
		2.6 (0.7–6.8)		Leukemia	
Melanoma CDKN2A	Melanoma	13		Pancreatic carcinoma	91
		229		All	
Colon cancer syndromes (FAP)	Colon	600?		Hepatoblastoma	97–99
		160		Thyroid carcinoma	

FAP, familial adenomatous polyposis.

MTS) and glioblastomas (Turcot's syndrome). It is suggested that individuals at risk should have a colonoscopy every 2 years beginning at age 25, as well as endometrial and urinary tract assessments.[96,100,101]

Autosomal recessive

The following syndromes are not characterized by cancer as the first event, but rather by several primary

hematological, constitutional, neurologic or dermatologic anomalies. Tumors usually arise later in life, but are still more common and occur at an earlier age compared to the general population.

FANCONI'S ANEMIA [OMIM 227650 (FA-A), 227660 (FA-B), 227645 (FA-C), 605724 (FA-D1), 227646 (FA-D2), 600901 (FA-E), 603467 (FA-F), 602956 (FA-G)]

Fanconi's anemia (FA), an autosomal recessive disease, is characterized by a progressive pancytopenia, a number of different congenital anomalies and chromosomal fragility, especially when cells are exposed to alkylating agents. The incidence is approximately 1:100 to 1:600, being more frequent in Ashkenazi Jews. FA has been linked to different mutations in specific genes, depending on the complementation group: 16q24.3 for FA-A, 9q22.3 for FA-C, 3p25.3 for D2, 6p22-p21 for FA-E, 11p15 for FA-F and 9p13 for FA-G. The chromosomal locations of FA-B and FA-D1 have not yet been described. The condition is associated with a number of neoplasms, including leukemia (10 per cent), hepatocellular carcinoma (5 per cent) and myelodysplastic syndrome.[102]

BLOOM SYNDROME (OMIM 210900)

Bloom syndrome was first described in 1966 by Bloom[103] and is due to mutations involving the BLM gene located at 15q26.1. It is characterized by growth-deficiency, malar hypoplasia, small mandible and dolichocephalic skull, and is associated with increased risk of leukemias and lymphomas during childhood and young adulthood, and

carcinomas of the ear, nose and throat region, digestive tract, skin, breast and cervix later in life.[104] One case report describes hepatocellular carcinoma and Wilms' tumor in two siblings.[105] Affected individuals often develop tumors at a younger age than the general population.[106]

ATAXIA TELANGIECTASIA (OMIM 208900)

Ataxia telangiectasia is a syndrome characterized by cerebellar ataxia, initially truncal, then gradually generalized, by telangiectasia in sun-exposed areas, by endocrine dysfunction in 50 per cent of the cases, and by a quantitative immunodeficiency with decreased levels of IgA, IgE and IgG2. Associated neoplasms are mainly non-Hodgkin's lymphomas and leukemias.[107] Patients also have an increased risk of gastric carcinomas, medulloblastoma and gliomas,[108] and breast carcinomas in heterozygotes, and leukemia and lymphoma in homozygotes[109,110] (Table 3b.4).

XERODERMA PIGMENTOSUM [OMIM 278700 (XP-A), 133510 (XP-B), 278720 (XP-C), 278730 (XP-D), 278740 (XP-E), 278760 (XP-F), 278780 (XP-G)]

Xeroderma pigmentosum (XP) is a condition with dermatologic and neurologic symptoms, which is due to mutations, usually point mutations, in several genes (9q34.1 for XP-A, 2q21 for XP-B, 3p25.1 for XP-C, 19q13.2 for XP-D, 11p12-p11 for XP-E, 16p13.2-p13.1 for XP-F and 13q32-q33 for XP-G) involved in DNA excision repair when damaged by UV light. The incidence varies from 1:40 000 to 1:10[6]. Affected individuals are at great risk of developing basal cell and squamous

Table 3b.4 *Secondary tumors: relative and cumulative risks for autosomal recessive syndromes*

Syndrome	Primary manifestations	Relative risk	Cumulative risk	Tumors associated	Reference number
Fanconi's anemia	Bone marrow failure		52% at 40 years	AML	102
			?	Squamous cell carcinomas	
			?	Hepatocellular carcinomas	
Bloom	Growth deficiency Malar hypoplasia		100% at 50 years	All cancers Leukemias, lymphomas Carcinomas	104
Ataxia-telangiectasia, homozygote	Cerebellar ataxia	37		Leukemia, lymphoma	110
	Telangiectasia	70		Gastric cancer	
Ataxia-telangiectasia, heterozygote	Endocrine dysfunction	1.54 (0.95–2.36) 1.19 (1.01–1.40)		Breast All	
Xeroderma pigmentosum	Progressive neurologic degeneration	2000		Melanomas, basal and squamous cell carcinomas	111
		10–20		Other neoplasms	
Familial Hodgkin's disease		3–9		Hodgkin's disease	113

AML, acute myelogenous leukemia.

cell carcinomas (2000-fold increased frequency),[111] as well as other non-cutaneous neoplasms (10–20-fold).

Uncertain mode of inheritance

FAMILIAL HODGKIN'S DISEASE (OMIM 236000)

The incidence of familial Hodgkin's disease (HD) is rare (3:100 000) but some sibling cases have been reported by Grufferman in 1977 and others.[112] Familial Hodgkin's disease represents approximately 4.5 per cent of all Hodgkin's disease diagnoses and confers a 3–9-fold increase in the risk of developing HD. Its mode of inheritance is uncertain but may be linked to a gene locus on chromosome 6p in the major histocompatibility complex area.[113] The exact explanation for the familial clustering is not clear however, and environmental factors, such as Epstein–Barr or other viruses, have been suggested to play a role.[114] These considerations have been reviewed by Ferraris et al. in 1997.[115] This condition is not thought to increase the risk for any neoplasm other than HD.

FAMILIAL PANCREATIC CANCER (OMIM 260350)

Hereditary pancreatic cancer, whose diagnosis should be considered only when other genetic causes of pancreatic cancer (Von Hippel–Lindau, BRCA2, ataxia-telangiectasia, MEN1, as discussed earlier) have been excluded, is extremely rare. Its genetics have been reviewed by Lynch et al.[116] Familial pancreatic cancer accounts for approximately 3 per cent of all newly diagnosed pancreatic carcinomas[117] but affected individuals do not seem to have increased risk for neoplasms other than pancreatic adenocarcinomas.

FAMILIAL TESTICULAR CANCER (OMIM 273300)

Familial testicular cancer is linked to different loci depending on the histologic subtype (teratoma, seminoma, germ cell or carcinoma).[118] The relative risk is approximately 8.3 for the brother of a proband, 3.8 for his father and 3.9 for his son. Certain histologies of testicular cancers (i.e. seminomas or teratomas) increase the risk of having a second primary cancer, such as endocrinological (pancreatic, thyroid), hematological (leukemia, lymphoma, myeloma) or other types (connective tissue), as reviewed by Dong in 2001 and summarized in Table 3b.3.[119,120]

OTHER CAUSES OF 'FAMILIAL' CANCER SYNDROMES

In this subchapter we have noted that familial transmission of clearly abnormal genes is one cause of multiple primary cancers. Certain other genes may also confer a propensity to develop tumors in certain circumstances without being functionally abnormal. These represent genetic polymorphisms.

Thus, beside exposure to exogenous factors, inherited genetic particularities might influence the likelihood that an individual will develop a tumor. There are several ways by which individual polymorphisms may influence the susceptibility to develop a cancer. Variations in enzymes involved in carcinogen detoxification or DNA repair, for example, may explain the great variation in risk after being exposed to similar environmental agents.

Some polymorphic forms of enzymes involved in polycyclic aromatic hydrocarbon carcinogen detoxification may increase susceptibility to certain forms of cancer. Enzymes of the phase I cytochrome P450 group, such as CYP1A1, are such an example. One genotype of this enzyme, present in 10 per cent of the population, leads to an increased risk of lung cancer[121] and another increases the risk of childhood acute lymphoblastic leukemia.[122] Phase I enzymes act by oxidizing carcinogens, whereas Phase II enzymes generally detoxify carcinogens by making them more hydrophilic. In approximately 50 per cent of Caucasians, the gene of one enzyme of the Phase II group, $GSTM_1$, is entirely deleted. This deletion has been linked to increased risk of bladder and lung cancers, especially when exposed to tobacco smoke.[123] Other carcinogens, such as aromatic amines, are detoxified by N-acetyltranferases. Certain individuals (50–60 per cent of Caucasians, 30–40 per cent African–Americans) have a genotype deficient in the ability to N-acetylate aromatic amines (slow acetylators), conferring an increased risk of bladder or breast cancer to the carriers.[124] Interestingly, people with an increased efficacy of this acetylating ability (fast acetylators) seem to have, for unknown reasons, an increased risk of colon cancer. In addition to these detoxifying enzymes, other polymorphisms in enzymes involved in DNA repair have been linked to cancer risk variations. This is the case for certain polymorphisms in the XPD nucleotide excision-repair gene, which may increase the risk of lung cancer[125] or basal cell carcinomas in patients with psoriasis.[126] Combinations of such metabolic polymorphisms are multiple and increase the complexity of such interactions between inherited specificity and exposure to certain products.[127]

In addition to these very specific metabolic polymorphisms, it is well known that ethnic, racial, gender and age differences significantly influence susceptibility to develop certain types of cancer.[128]

Molecular epidemiology is a rapidly evolving field enhanced by recent advances in techniques such as cDNA microarrays through which we may soon be able to evaluate individual risk and develop prevention strategies to reduce exposure to potentially harmful environmental factors for genetically susceptible individuals.

Apart from known germline genetic anomalies leading to an increased risk of developing tumors, some conditions

may also confer to their carriers a particular susceptibility to cancer. This is the case in Down syndrome, or trisomy 21, where there is a well-described risk of developing childhood leukemias, especially acute megakaryocytic leukemias, or AML M7.

IDENTIFICATION OF FAMILIES, GENETIC COUNSELING AND TUMOR SCREENING

The rapidly evolving field of molecular genetics has brought to families and health care providers increasingly powerful diagnostic tools to identify both individuals and families prone to specific neoplasms. In order to use these tools effectively, it is important to attempt to attain three goals:

1 identification of individuals or families;
2 genetic education, counseling and psychological support for these individuals;
3 specific tumor screening once a diagnosis of cancer predisposition has been established.

Identification of families at risk for hereditary cancer relies almost exclusively on two criteria: obtaining an accurate family history[129,130] and a careful physical assessment. A recent study by Sweet *et al.* reported, however, that a proper family history could be found in only 69 per cent of medical records and that family history was not updated regularly.[131] Recent advances in the development of new molecular tools, such as DNA microarrays, have introduced potentially new and encouraging perspectives for extensive population screening, thus theoretically removing the subjectivity and possible lack of accuracy of clinical screening. However, such techniques rely on comprehension of the underlying molecular mechanisms of the diseases and identification of implicated genes, which is not always possible. Good clinical and relational skills of general practitioners and specialists will therefore continue to be necessary, not only to identify affected families, but also to be able to explain to them in a comprehensive manner the beneficial aspects of referring to specialists.[132,133]

Cancer genetics consultants and counselors specially trained for this purpose[134] will provide these families with the basic knowledge necessary to understand all aspects and implications of genetic testing. Once informed and able to make a decision, families and individuals are taught the plans for follow-up, including screening for the tumors they are at risk for, avoidance of certain environmental risk factors that may precipitate the appearance of the neoplasms and how to recognize certain clinical signs.[135,136]

Guidelines to evaluate, manage and follow families and individuals at risk have been drawn from previous studies of affected families and have been published for almost each familial cancer syndrome.[11,77,137–141]. The obvious interests of preventive screening, such as early surgical intervention, preventive chemotherapy treatments, such as acetyl salicylic acid (ASA), estrogen receptor modulators or retinoids, will ensure that these 'weapons' will become more available with time. New understanding of underlying mechanisms will be made, providing more reasons to detect at-risk families and individuals as early as possible.[85,142–144]

PSYCHOSOCIAL ISSUES

One of the main issues of counseling and testing in cancer genetics is the psychological impact, which may affect families already distressed by the diagnosis of a cancer affecting one of their members. Several studies about psychological impact of heredity and cancer have been reported.[145] Experience from general genetic clinics is certainly useful in understanding such impacts and general psychological sequelae are found in this particular setting as well. Individuals may have to face learning about their own carrier state when their children are tested or learn of the possibility of transferring the disease to their children. They may be distressed by practical considerations, such as the uncertainty about reactions of employers or insurance companies. They may receive only partial information of their chances of developing cancer because of incomplete penetrance of affected genes or because of the lack of scientific understanding of the mechanisms of their condition. Unaffected members may also exhibit psychological sequelae, such as feelings of 'survivor guilt', disbelief in test results, etc.[146,147] These significant sequelae may be minimized if tested individuals receive adequate pre- and post-testing genetic education, counseling and support by a team of experienced geneticists, oncologists, psychologists and social workers. Diagnostic consultation seems to be particularly important because, when patients felt they had explicit information[148] about their particular disease, prognosis and treatment, they were more likely to have an appropriate psychological adjustment.

ETHICAL, INSURANCE AND LEGAL ISSUES

As for all diseases, but perhaps more particularly for cancer syndromes, informed consent is an essential component of genetic testing. Some genetic counseling teams use the age of 12 years as an indication for direct consent, but this can vary according to individual psychological development and has to be evaluated by the counselors for each patient. Otherwise, parents are generally

accorded the authority to decide about the medical interventions their child receives. One problem that may arise is that the child then loses the right to decide whether or not he/she would like to know his/her genetic status and risk. A study about attitudes of mothers of pediatric oncology patients regarding genetic testing has been published by Patenaude *et al.* in 1996 and shows that nearly half of them (42 per cent) would test their children, even if no medical benefit would be obtained, and 33 per cent would wait until the child reaches the age of majority and can decide for himself or herself.[149]

Privacy and confidentiality about genetic test results is an issue not only concerning insurance companies or employers but also other members of the family: should they be contacted to be tested? Whose role is it? Another question that may arise is whether to identify the final goal of the genetic testing. Is it worthwhile to test a patient if there is no treatment available or if preventive management does not change the outcome?[150,151]

In addition to these psychological risks, a great concern about genetic testing is that the use of such information by insurance companies or employers could influence levels of insurance premiums or employment decisions.[152] From the medical perspective, one concern is that the fear of such use of genetic information may prevent potentially affected individuals from getting tested, thus delaying proper management. The way of handling such potential misuses differs from one country to another. Commissions composed of geneticists, insurance companies and patients' representatives have been created, and diverse legislations have been passed in different countries. A number of recommendations have been generated, but these are likely to change as new scientific progress is made.[153,154]

Finally, to complement these ethical and insurance considerations, legal issues have arisen and several courts have had to make decisions in lawsuits for medical negligence regarding genetic counseling in hereditary cancer syndromes. Physicians now have to face claims of failure to identify at-risk individuals, and warn progeny and siblings. Not establishing a genealogy survey of a patient to identify cancer-prone families is considered as a failure to meet the standard of care.[155]

In light of the continuously evolving field of cancer genetics and familial cancer predisposition syndromes, it behooves all physicians to pay close attention to family history and be aware of the varied spectrum of conditions associated with cancer risk.

KEY POINTS

- Familial cancer syndromes are rare but clearly recognized.
- Clinical expression and the subsequent risk of developing a tumor depends on the syndrome and its mode of transmission.
- Affected individuals are at risk of developing multiple tumors during their life.
- This risk depends on the underlying genetic defect as well as on the treatments used for prior tumors.
- Genetic testing for familial cancer syndromes raises important issues about ethical, insurance and psychosocial aspects.

ACKNOWLEDGEMENTS

We would like to thank Hooman Ganjavi for kindly reviewing the manuscript.

MD is supported by grants from the FORCE and SICPA foundations, the Société Académique Vaudoise, the Centre Hospitalier Universitaire Vaudois and the University of Lausanne, Switzerland. This work is supported in part by a grant from the National Cancer Institute of Canada with funds from the Canadian Cancer Society.

REFERENCES

1. Hunter J. Of poisons. In: *The complete works of John Hunter*, Philadelphia: Barrington & Haswell, **1841**:376–385.
2. Darmon P. *Les cellules folles: histoire du cancer de l'antiquité ános jours.* Paris: Plon, 1993.
3. Kaiser JH. Zum vererblichen Vorkommen von Krebsformen. *Dtsche med Woch* 1924; **50**:909.
4. Slye M. Cancer and heredity. *Ann Intern Me.* 1928; **12**:951–976.
5. Knudson AG. Mutation and cancer: statistical study of retinoblastoma, *Proc Natl Acad Sci USA* 1971; **68**:820–823.
6. Bishop JM. Cellular oncogenes and retroviruses. *Annu Rev Biochem* 1983; **52**:301–354.
7. Varmus HE. The molecular genetics of cellular oncogenes. *Annu Rev Genet* 1984; **18**:553–612.
8. Birch JM. Genes and cancer. *Arch Dis Child* 1999; **80**:1–3.
9. Nowell PC, Hungerford DA. Minute chromosome in human chronic granulocytic leukemia, *Science* 1960, **132**.1497.
10. Haber DA, Fearon ER. The promise of cancer genetics. *Lancet* 1998; **351** (Suppl. 2):SII1–SII8.
11. Lindor NM, Greene MH. The concise handbook of family cancer syndromes. Mayo Familial Cancer Program. *J Natl Cancer Inst* 1998; **90**:1039–1071.
12. Li FP, Fraumeni JF. Soft-tissue sarcomas, breast cancer, and other neoplasms: a familial syndrome?, *Ann Intern Med* 1969; **71**:747–752.
13. Li FP, Fraumeni JF. Rhabdomyosarcoma in children: an epidemiologic study and identification of a familial cancer syndrome. *J Natl Cancer Inst* 1969; **43**:1364–1373.
14. Li FP, Fraumeni JF Jr, Mulvihill JJ, *et al.* A cancer family syndrome in twenty-four kindreds. *Cancer Res* 1988; **48**:5358–5362.

15. Garber JE, Goldstein AM, Kantor AF, *et al.* Follow-up study of twenty-four families with Li–Fraumeni syndrome. *Cancer Res* 1991; **51**:6094–6097.

◆16. Malkin D, Li FP, Strong LC, *et al.* Germ line p53 mutations in a familial syndrome of breast cancer, sarcomas, and other neoplasms, *Science* 1990; **250**:1233–1238.

17. Varley JM, McGown G, Thorncroft M, *et al.* Germ-line mutations of TP53 in Li–Fraumeni families: an extended study of 39 families. *Cancer Res* 1997; **57**:3245–3252.

●18. Harris CC. Structure and function of the p53 tumor suppressor gene: clues for rational cancer therapeutic strategies. *J Natl Cancer Inst* 1996; **88**:1442–1455.

19. Chompret A, Brugieres L, Ronsin M, *et al.* P53 germline mutations in childhood cancers and cancer risk for carrier individuals. *Br J Cancer* 2000; **82**:1932–1937.

20. Nichols KE, Malkin D, Garber JE, *et al.* Germ-line p53 mutations predispose to a wide spectrum of early-onset cancers *Cancer Epidemiol Biomarkers Prevention* 2001; **10**:83–87.

21. Hisada M, Garber JE, Fung CY. Multiple primary cancers in families with Li–Fraumeni syndrome. *J Natl Cancer Inst* 1998; **90**:606–611.

22. Birch JM, Blair V, Kelsey AM. Cancer phenotype correlates with constitutional TP53 genotype in families with the Li–Fraumeni syndrome. *Oncogene* 1998; **17**:1061–1068.

◆23. Malkin D, Jolly KW, Barbier N, *et al.* Germline mutations of the p53 tumor-suppressor gene in children and young adults with second malignant neoplasms. *N Engl J Med* 1992; **326**:1309–1315.

24. Diller L, Sexsmith E, Gottlieb A, *et al.* Germline p53 mutations are frequently detected in young children with rhabdomyosarcoma. *J Clin Invest* 1995; **95**:1606–1611.

25. Wagner J, Portwine C, Rabin K, *et al.* High-frequency of germline p53 mutations in childhood adrenocortical cancer. *J Natl Cancer Inst* 1994; **86**:1707–1710.

26. Varley JM, Evans DG, Birch JM. Li–Fraumeni syndrome – a molecular and clinical review. *Br J Cancer* 1997; **76**:1–14.

27. Barel D, Avigad S, Mor C, *et al.* A novel germline mutation in the noncoding region of the p53 gene in a Li–Fraumeni family. *Cancer Genet Cytogenet* 1998; **103**:1–6.

28. Foti A, Bareli M, Ahuja HG, Cline MJ. A splicing mutation accounts for the lack of p53 gene expression in a CML blast crisis line: a novel mechanism of p53 gene inactivation. *Br J Haematol* 1990; **76**:143–145.

29. Friend SH, Bernards R, Rogelj S, *et al.* A human DNA segment with properties of the gene that predisposes to retinoblastoma and osteosarcoma. *Nature* 1986; **323**:643–646.

30. Roarty JD, McLean IW, Zimmerman LE. Incidence of second neoplasms in patients with bilateral retinoblastomas. *Ophthalmology* 1988; **95**:1583–1587.

31. Wilms M. Die Mischgeschwülste der Niere. In: *Die Mischgeschwülste.* Leipzig: A. Georgi, 1899.

32. Rose EA, Glaser T, Jones C, *et al.* Complete physical map of the WAGR region of 11p13 localizes a candidate Wilms tumor gene. *Cell* 1990; **60**:495–508.

33. Dressler GR. Pax-2, kidney development, and oncogenesis. *Med Pediatr Oncol* 1996; **27**:440–444.

34. Miller RW, Manning MD, Fraumeni JF. Association of Wilms' tumor with aniridia hemihypertrophy + other congenital malformations. *N Engl J Med* 1964; **270**:922–927.

35. Huff V. Genotype/phenotype correlations in Wilms' tumor. *Med Pediatr Oncol* 1996; **27**:408–414.

36. Weksberg R, Squire JA. Molecular biology of Beckwith–Wiedemann syndrome. *Med Pediatr Oncol* 1996; **27**:462–469.

37. Weksberg R, Nishikawa J, Caluseriu O, *et al.* Tumor development in the Beckwith–Wiedemann syndrome is associated with a variety of constitutional molecular 11p15 alterations including imprinting defects of KCNQ1OT1. *Hum Molec Genet* 2001; **10**:2989–3000.

38. Thavaraj V, Sethi A, Arya LS. Incomplete Beckwith–Wiedemann syndrome in a child with orbital rhabdomyosarcoma. *Indian Pediatr* 2002; **39**:299–304.

39. Yoon G, Graham G, Weksberg R, *et al.* Neuroblastoma in a patient with the Beckwith–Wiedemann syndrome (BWS). *Med Pediatr Oncol* 2002; **38**:193–199.

40. Debaun MR, Tucker MA. Risk of cancer during the first four years of life in children from The Beckwith–Wiedemann Syndrome Registry. *J Pediatr* 1998; **132**:398–400.

41. Tsai SY, Jeng YM, Hwu WL, *et al.* Hepatoblastoma in an infant with Beckwith–Wiedemann Syndrome. *J Formosan Med Assoc* 1996; **95**:180–183.

42. McDonald JM, Douglass EC, Fisher R, *et al.* Linkage of familial Wilms' tumor predisposition to chromosome 19 and a two-locus model for the etiology of familial tumors. *Cancer Res* 1998; **58**:1387–1390.

43. Rahman N, Arbour L, Tonin P, *et al.* Evidence for a familial Wilms' tumour gene (FWT1) on chromosome 17q12-q21. *Nature Genet* 1996; **13**:461–463.

44. Hartley AL, Birch JM, Blair V, *et al.* Second primary neoplasms in a population-based series of children diagnosed with renal tumours in childhood. *Med Pediatr Oncol* 1994; **22**:318–324.

45. Wermer P. Genetic aspects of adenomatosis of endocrine glands. *Am J Med* 1954; **16**:363–371.

46. Zollinger RM, Ellison EH. Primary peptic ulcerations of the jejunum associated with islet cell tumors of the pancreas. *Ann Surg* 1955; **142**:709–728.

47. Underwood LE, Jacobs NM. Familial endocrine adenomatosis. *Am J Dis Child* 1963; **106**:218–223.

48. Teh BT, Hii SI, David R, *et al.* Multiple endocrine neoplasia type-1 (Men1) in 2 Asian families. *Hum Genet* 1994; **94**:468–472.

49. Pang JT, Thakker RV. Multiple endocrine neoplasia type 1 (MEN1). *Eur J Cancer* 1994; **30A**:1961–1968.

50. Wong FK, Burgess J, Nordenskjold M, *et al.* Multiple endocrine neoplasia type 1. *Semin Cancer Biol* 2000; **10**:299–312.

51. Carlson KM, Dou S, Chi D, *et al.* Single missense mutation in the tyrosine kinase catalytic domain of the RET protooncogene is associated with multiple endocrine neoplasia type 2B. *Proc Natl Acad Sci USA* 1994; **91**:1579–1583.

52. Mulligan LM, Kwok JB, Healey CS, *et al.* Germ-line mutations of the RET proto-oncogene in multiple endocrine neoplasia type 2A. *Nature* 1993; **363**:458–460.

53. Hemminki K, Jiang Y. Second primary neoplasms after 19281 endocrine gland tumours: aetiological links? *Eur J Cancer* 2001; **37**:1886–1894.

54. von Recklinghausen FD. *Über die multiplen Fibrome der Haut und ihre Beziehung zu den multiplen Neuromen.* Berlin: 1882.

55. Cawthon RM, Weiss R, Xu GF, *et al.* A major segment of the neurofibromatosis type 1 gene: cDNA sequence, genomic structure, and point mutations. *Cell* 1990; **62**:193–201.

56. Cichowski K, Jacks T. NF1 tumor suppressor gene function: narrowing the GAP. *Cell* 2001; **104**:593–604.

57. Matsui I, Tanimura M, Kobayashi N, *et al.* Neurofibromatosis type-1 and childhood-cancer. *Cancer* 1993; **72**:2746–2754.

58. Maris JM, Wiersma SR, Mahgoub N, *et al.* Monosomy 7 myelodysplastic syndrome and other second malignant neoplasms in children with neurofibromatosis type 1. *Cancer* 1997; **79**:1438–1446.

59. Evans DG, Birch JM, Ramsden RT. Paediatric presentation of type 2 neurofibromatosis, *Arch Dis Child* 1999; **81**:496–499.

60. Lindau A. Studien über Kleinhirncysten. Bau, Pathogenese und Beziehungen zur Angiomatosis retinae, Doctoral thesis. *Acta Path Microbiol Scand* 1926; **3**(Suppl.):1–128.

61. von Hippel E. Vorstellung eines Patienten mit einem sehr ungewöhnlicher Netzhaut beziehungsweise Aderhautleiden. *[Reports of the 24th Meeting of the Ophthalmic Society, Heidelberg]* 1895:269.

Chemotherapy — **LONG TERM SIDE EFFECTS OF** — **Radiation**

Radiation

Cornea
- Epithelial defects
- Keratitis
- Epithelial desquamation
- Corneal neovascularization
- Corneal edema
- Corneal melting
- Corneal drying
- Corneal perforation
- → Corneal sensation
- Keratinization
- Ulceration

Conjunctiva
- Conjunctivitis
- Prolonged injection
- Telangiectasia
- Symblepharon
- Keratinization
- Loss of goblet cells
- Necrosis
- Subconjunctival hemorrhage
- Conjunctival shrinkage

Iris
- Iritis
- Neovascularization
- Closed < glaucoma

Lens
- Cataract

Vitreous
- Vitreous traction
- Vitreous hemorrhage

Macula
- Macula edema
- Macula exudates
- Macula detachment

Lacrimal gland
- Atrophy with → tear production

Sclera
- Scleral thinning
- Scleral melting
- Scleral atrophy
- Scleral perforation

Eyelids/periorbital skin
- Erythema
- Dermatitis
- Ulceration
- Telangiectasia
- Necrosis
- Epilation
- Pigment changes
- Entropion
- Ectropion

Orbital bone/tissue
- Retarded bone growth
- Temporal bone suppression
- Osteonecrosis
- Orbital infection
- Soft tissue atrophy
- Contracture of socket

Retina
- Retinal edema
- Radiation retinopathy
- Neovascularization
- Infarcts
- Exudates
- Hemorrhages
- RPE mottling/atrophy
- Microaneurysms
- Cottonwool spots
- Telangiectasia
- Retinal detachment

Optic nerve
- Optic nerve swelling
- Optic neuropathy
- Optic disc swelling
- Optic atrophy
- Infarcts

Supported in part by the May and Samuel Rudin Family Foundation, Inc.

©Abramson, Ober, Beaverson, 2001

Chemotherapy

Cornea
- Bone marrow transplant
- Busulfan
- Carmustine
- Corticosteroids
- Cyclophosphamide
- Nitrogen mustard
- Retinoids
- Tamoxifen
- Vincristine

Pupil
- Corticosteroids
- Cyclophosphamide
- Nitrosurea
- Vincristine

Conjunctiva
- Bone marrow transplant
- Corticosteroids
- Cyclophosphamide
- Mitomycin C
- Retinoids

Ciliary body
- Corticosteroids
- Nitrosureas

Lacrimal gland
- Busulfan
- Cyclophosphamide

Sclera
- Corticosteroids
- Mitomycin C

Orbital bone/tissue
- Carboplatin
- Chlorambucil
- Etoposide
- 5FU
- Interferon
- Mithramycin
- Nitrosurea
- Vincristine

Retina
- Bone marrow transplant
- Carboplatin
- Carmustine
- Cisplatin
- Corticosteroids
- Cyclosporine
- Interferon
- Mechlorethamine
- Methotrexate
- Nitrogen mustard
- Tamoxifen

Choroid
- Busulfan
- Carboplatin
- Corticosteroids
- Nitrogen mustard

Lens
- Bone marrow transplant
- Busulfan
- Corticosteroids
- Tamoxifen

Vitreous
- Bone marrow transplant
- Carmustine

Macula
- Carboplatin
- Cisplatin
- Corticosteroids
- Methotrexate
- Tamoxifen

Optic nerve
- Bone marrow transplant
- Carboplatin
- Cisplatin
- Corticosteroids
- Cytosine arabinoside
- Nitrosurea

(Optic nerve — additional)
- Cyclosporine
- 5FU
- Fludarabine
- Interferon
- Methotrexate
- Paclitaxel
- Retinoids
- Tamoxifen
- Vincristine
- Nirtogen mustard

Plate 1 *Long-term side effects of chemotherapy and radiation. 5FU, 5-fluorouracil; RPE, retinal pigment epithelium.*

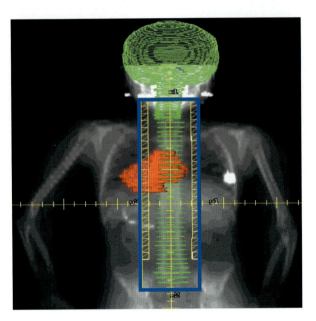

Plate 2 *A radiograph that has been digitally reconstructed from the planning computed tomography (CT) scan for a patient with medulloblastoma. On each CT slice, the cerebrospinal fluid-bearing areas of the brain and spinal cord (green), and the heart (red) have been outlined. The spine field component of the craniospinal irradiation (blue) has its width limited with shielding (yellow) for most of its upper length to reduce unnecessary irradiation of normal tissue. Despite this, a major portion of the heart still receives radiation exiting from the spinal field.*

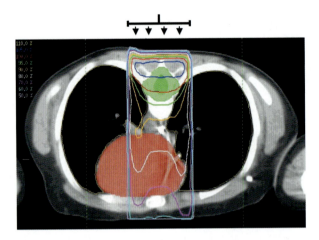

Plate 3 *A mid-thoracic transverse section from the planning computed tomography scan as displayed on the planning computer for a patient with medulloblastoma lying in the prone position for craniospinal irradiation. Radiation from the spinal field (black arrows) enters posteriorly and aims to encompass the target (green) with at least 95 per cent of the prescribed dose as shown by the green isodose line. A significant proportion of the heart (red) receives between 90 per cent of dose to its posterior wall and 70 per cent of dose to its anterior wall as the radiation exits anteriorly through the patient.*

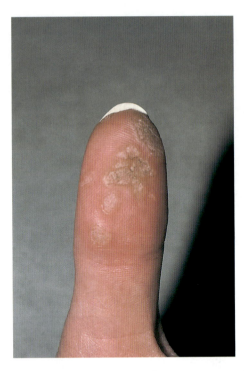

Plate 4 *Persistent mosaic viral wart in a young woman after treatment for Hodgkin's disease.*

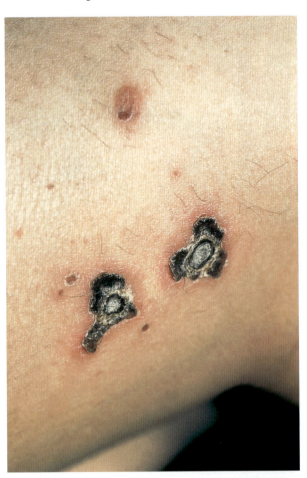

Plate 5 *Indolent ulcers caused by persistent Herpes zoster infection in an immunosuppressed patient.*

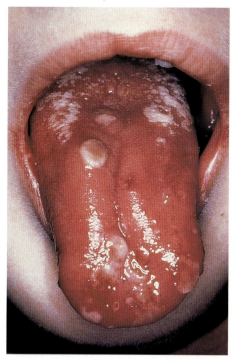

Plate 6 *Oral candidiasis in a leukemic child. (Photograph courtesy of Dr H. Wallace.)*

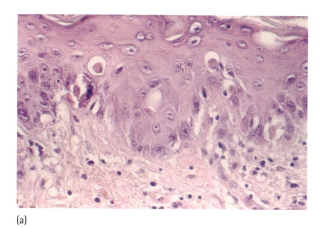

(a)

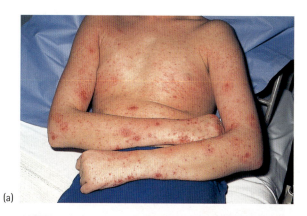

(a)

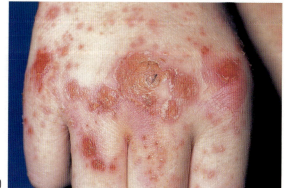

(b)

Plate 7 *(a) Impetiginized scabies infestation in an immunosuppressed child. (b) Close up of hands showing multiple burrows. (Photographs courtesy of Dr H. Wallace.)*

(b)

Plate 8 *(a) Grade 2 graft-versus-host disease (GvHD) with basal cell vacuolation and single death together with a lymphocytic infiltrate. (b) Grade 3/4 GvHD showing subepidermal split and necrosis of the overlying epidermis. (Photographs courtesy of Dr K. McLaren.)*

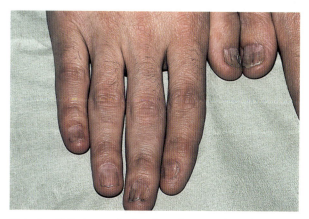

Plate 9 *Nail changes in chronic graft-versus-host disease.*

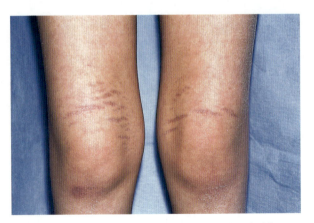

Plate 10 *Striae distensae over the knees associated with long-term corticosteroid therapy. (Photograph courtesy of Dr H. Wallace.)*

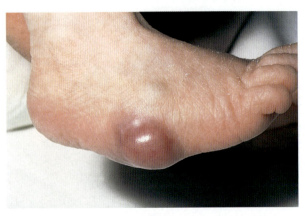

Plate 11 *Cutaneous metastatic deposit from a neuroblastoma. (Photograph courtesy of Dr H. Wallace.)*

62. Maher ER, Iselius L, Yates JR, *et al.* Von Hippel–Lindau disease: a genetic study. *J Med Genet* 1991; **28**:443–447.

63. Zbar B, Kishida T, Chen F, *et al.* Germline mutations in the Von Hippel–Lindau disease (VHL) gene in families from North America, Europe, and Japan. *Hum Mutation* 1996; **8**:348–357.

64. Latif F, Tory K, Gnarra J, *et al.* Identification of the Von Hippel–Lindau disease tumor-suppressor gene. *Science* 1993; **260**:1317–1320.

65. Friedrich CA. Von Hippel–Lindau syndrome – a pleomorphic condition. *Cancer* 1999; **86**:2478–2482.

66. Zbar B. Inherited epithelial tumors of the kidney: old and new diseases. *Semin Cancer Biol* 2000; **10**:313–318.

67. Arver B, Du Q, Chen JD, *et al.* Hereditary breast cancer: a review. *Semin Cancer Biol* 2000; **10**:271–288.

68. Greene MH. Genetics of breast cancer. *Mayo Clinic Proc* 1997; **72**:54–65.

69. Chang-Claude J. Inherited genetic susceptibility to breast cancer. *IARC Scientific Publications (Lyon)* 2001; **154**:177–190.

70. Hemminki K, Vaittinen P. Familial risks in second primary breast cancer based on a family cancer database. *Eur J Cancer* 1999; **35**:455–458.

71. Egan KM, Stampfer MJ, Rosner BA, *et al.* Risk factors for breast cancer in women with a breast cancer family history. *Cancer Epidemiol Biomarkers Prevention* 1998; **7**:359–364.

72. Hall JM, Lee MK, Newman B, *et al.* Linkage of early-onset familial breast-cancer to chromosome-17Q21, *Science* 1990; **250**:1684–1689.

73. Szabo CI, King MC. Population genetics of BRCA1 and BRCA2. *Am J Hum Genet* 1997; **60**:1013–1020.

74. Szabo CI, King MC. Inherited breast and ovarian cancer. *Hum Molec Genet* 1995; **4**(Spec. No.):1811–1817.

75. Abbott DW, Thompson ME, Robinson-Benion C, *et al.* BRCA1 expression restores radiation resistance in BRCA1-defective cancer cells through enhancement of transcription-coupled DNA repair. *J Biol Chem* 1999; **274**:18808–18812.

76. Gowen LC, Avrutskaya AV, Latour AM, *et al.* BRCA1 required for transcription-coupled repair of oxidative DNA damage. *Science* 1998; **281**:1009–1012.

77. Burke W, Petersen G, Lynch P, *et al.* Recommendations for follow-up care of individuals with an inherited predisposition to cancer. I. Hereditary nonpolyposis colon cancer. Cancer Genetics Studies Consortium. *JAMA* 1997; **277**:915–919.

78. Wooster R, Neuhausen SL, Mangion J, *et al.* Localization of a breast-cancer susceptibility gene, BRCA2, to chromosome 13q12–13. *Science* 1994; **265**:2088–2090.

79. Vaughn JP, Cirisano FD, Huper G, *et al.* Cell cycle control of BRCA2. *Cancer Res* 1996; **56**:4590–4594.

80. Csokay B, Udvarhelyi N, Sulyok Z, *et al.* High frequency of germ-line BRCA2 mutations among Hungarian male breast cancer patients without family history. *Cancer Res* 1999; **59**: 995–998.

◆81. Anonymous. Cancer risks in BRCA2 mutation carriers. The Breast Cancer Linkage Consortium. *J Natl Cancer Inst* 1999; **91**:1310–1316.

82. Fackenthal JD, Marsh DJ, Richardson AL, *et al.* Male breast cancer in Cowden syndrome patients with germline PTEN mutations. *J Med Genet* 2001; **38**:159–164.

83. Eng C. Genetics of Cowden syndrome: through the looking glass of oncology. *Int J Oncol* 1998; **12**:701–710.

84. Lloyd K, Dennis M. Cowden's disease: a possible new symptom complex with multiple system involvement. *Ann Intern Med* 1963; **58**:136–142.

●85. Eng C, Hampel H, de la Chapelle A. Genetic testing for cancer predisposition. *Annu Rev Med* 2001; **52**:371–400.

86. Liaw D, Marsh DJ, Li J, *et al.* Germline mutations of the PTEN gene in Cowden disease, an inherited breast and thyroid cancer syndrome. *Nature Genet* 1997; **16**:64–67.

87. Marsh DJ, Dahia PLM, Zheng ZM, *et al.* Germline mutations in PTEN are present in Bannayan–Zonana syndrome. *Nature Genet* 1997; **16**:333–334.

88. Dahia PLM, Marsh DJ, Zheng ZM, *et al.* Somatic deletions and mutations in the Cowden disease gene, PTEN, in sporadic thyroid tumors. *Cancer Res* 1997; **57**:4710–4713.

89. Norris W. Case of fungoid disease. *Edinburgh Med Surg J* 1820; **16**:562–565.

90. Platz A, Ringborg U, Hansson J. Hereditary cutaneous melanoma. *Semin Cancer Biol* 2000; **10**:319–326.

91. Tucker MA, Fraser MC, Goldstein AM, *et al.* Risk of melanoma and other cancers in melanoma-prone families. *J Invest Dermatol* 1993; **100**:S350–S355.

92. Foulkes WD, Flanders TY, Pollock PM, Hayward NK. The CDKN2A (p16) gene and human cancer. *Molec Med* 1997; **3**:5–20.

93. DiFronzo LA, Wanek LA, Elashoff R, Morton DL. Increased incidence of second primary melanoma in patients with a previous cutaneous melanoma. *Ann Surg Oncol* 1999; **6**:705–711.

94. Gruis NA, van der Velden PA, Bergman W, Frants RR. Familial melanoma; CDKN2A and beyond. *J Invest Dermatol* 1999; Symposium Proceedings **4**:50–54.

95. Greene MH. The genetics of hereditary melanoma and nevi. 1998 update. *Cancer* 1999; **86**:2464–2477.

96. Aaltonen LA. Hereditary intestinal cancer. *Semin Cancer Biol* 2000; **10**:289–298.

97. Garber JE, Li FP, Kingston JE, *et al.* Hepatoblastoma and familial adenomatous polyposis. *J Natl Cancer Inst* 1988; **80**:1626–1628.

98. Garber JE, Finegold MJ, Kingston JE, *et al.* Familial adenomatous polyposis in hepatoblastoma survivors (abstract). *Proc Am Assoc Cancer Res* 1988; **29**:257–257.

99. Plail RO, Bussey HJR, Glazer G, Thomson JPS. Adenomatous polyposis – an association with carcinoma of the thyroid. *Br J Surg* 1987; **74**:377–380.

100. Schoen RE. Families at risk for colorectal cancer: risk assessment and genetic testing. *J Clin Gastroenterol* 2000; **31**:114–120.

101. Syngal S, Fox EA, Li C, *et al.* Interpretation of genetic test results for hereditary nonpolyposis colorectal cancer: implications for clinical predisposition testing. *JAMA* 1999; **282**:247–253.

102. Alter BP. Fanconi's anemia and malignancies *Am J Hematol* 1996; **53**:99–110.

103. Bloom D. Syndrome of congenital telangiectatic erythema and stunted growth. *J Pediatr* 1966; **68**:103–113.

104. German J. Bloom's syndrome. The first 100 cancers. *Cancer Genet Cytogenet* 1997; **93**:100–106.

105. Jain D, Hui P, McNamara J, *et al.* Bloom syndrome in sibs: first reports of hepatocellular carcinoma and Wilms tumor with documented anaplasia and nephrogenic rests. *Pediatr Dev Pathol* 2001; **4**:585–589.

106. Sullivan NF, Willis AE. Cancer predisposition in Bloom's syndrome. *Bioessays* 1992; **14**:333–336.

107. Takeuchi S, Koike M, Park S, *et al.* The ATM gene and susceptibility to childhood T-cell acute lymphoblastic leukaemia. *Br J Haematol* 1998; **103**:536–538.

108. Gatti RA, Boder E, Vinters HV, *et al.* Ataxia-telangiectasia – an interdisciplinary approach to pathogenesis. *Medicine* 1991; **70**:99–117.

109. Geoffroy-Perez B, Janin N, Ossian K, *et al.* Cancer risk in heterozygotes for ataxia-telangiectasia. *Int J Cancer* 2001; **93**:288–293.

110. Olsen JH, Hahnemann JM, Borresen-Dale AL, *et al.* Cancer in patients with ataxia-telangiectasia and in their relatives in the Nordic countries. *J Natl Cancer Inst* 2001; **93**:121–127.

111. Cleaver JE, Thompson LH, Richardson AS, States JC. A summary of mutations in the UV-sensitive disorders: xeroderma pigmentosum, Cockayne syndrome, and trichothiodystrophy. *Hum Mutation* 1999; **14**:9–22.

112. Grufferman S, Cole P, Smith PG, Lukes RJ. Hodgkins-disease in siblings. *N Engl J Med* 1977; **296**:248–250.

113. Lynch HT, Marcus JN, Lynch JF. Genetics of Hodgkin's and non-Hodgkin's lymphoma: a review. *Cancer Invest* 1992; **10**:247–256.

114. Lin AY, Kingma DW, Lennette ET, *et al.* Epstein–Barr virus and familial Hodgkin's disease. *Blood* 1996; **88**:3160–3165.

115. Ferraris AM, Racchi O, Rapezzi D, *et al.* Familial Hodgkin's disease: a disease of young adulthood? *Ann Hematol* 1997; **74**:131–134.

116. Lynch HT, Fusaro L, Smyrk TC, *et al.* Medical genetic-study of 8 pancreatic cancer-prone families, *Cancer Investigation* 1995; **13**:141–149.

117. Fernandez E, Lavecchia C, Davanzo B, *et al.* Family history and the risk of liver, gallbladder, and pancreatic-cancer. *Cancer Epidemiol Biomarkers Prevention* 1994; **3**:209–212.

118. Anonymous. Candidate regions for testicular cancer susceptibility genes. The International Testicular Cancer Linkage Consortium. *Acta Pathol Microbiol Immunol Scand* 1998; **106**:64–70.

119. Dong C, Lonnstedt I, Hemminki K. Familial testicular cancer and second primary cancers in testicular cancer patients by histological type. *Eur J Cancer* 2001; **37**:1878–1885.

120. Nicholson PW, Harland SJ. Inheritance and testicular cancer. *Br J Cancer* 1995; **71**:421–426.

121. Bartsch H, Nair U, Risch A, *et al.* Genetic polymorphism of CYP genes, alone or in combination, as a risk modifier of tobacco-related cancers. *Cancer Epidemiol Biomarkers Prevention* 2000; **9**:3–28.

122. Krajinovic M, Labuda D, Richer C, *et al.* Susceptibility to childhood acute lymphoblastic leukemia: influence of CYP1A1, CYP2D6, GSTM1, and GSTT1 genetic polymorphisms, *Blood* 1999; **93**:1496–1501.

123. Houlston RS. Glutathione S-transferase M1 status and lung cancer risk: a meta-analysis. *Cancer Epidemiol Biomarkers Prevention* 1999; **8**:675–682.

124. Ambrosone CB, Freudenheim JL, Graham S, *et al.* Cigarette smoking, N-acetyltransferase 2 genetic polymorphisms, and breast cancer risk. *JAMA* 1996; **276**:1494–1501.

125. Hou SM, Falt S, Angelini S, *et al.* The XPD variant alleles are associated with increased aromatic DNA adduct level and lung cancer risk. *Carcinogenesis* 2002; **23**:599–603.

126. Dybdahl M, Vogel U, Frentz G, *et al.* Polymorphisms in the DNA repair gene XPD: correlations with risk and age at onset of basal cell carcinoma. *Cancer Epidemiol Biomarkers Prevention* 1999; **8**:77–81.

127. Perera FP, Weinstein IB. Molecular epidemiology: recent advances and future directions. *Carcinogenesis* 2000; **21**:517–524.

128. Perera FP. Environment and cancer: who are susceptible? *Science* 1997; **278**:1068–1073.

●129. Cornelisse CJ, Devilee P. Facts in cancer genetics. *Patient Educ Counseling* 1997; **32**:9–17.

130. Tinley ST, Lynch HT. Integration of family history and medical management of patients with hereditary cancers. *Cancer* 1999; **86**:2525–2532.

◆131. Sweet KM, Bradley TL, Westman JA. Identification and referral of families at high risk for cancer susceptibility. *J Clin Oncol* 2002; **20**:528–537.

132. Worthen HG. Inherited cancer and the primary care physician. Barriers and strategies. *Cancer* 1999; **86**:2583–2588.

133. Bleiker EM, Aaronson NK, Menko FH, *et al.* Genetic counseling for hereditary cancer: a pilot study on experiences of patients and family members. *Patient Educ Counseling* 1997; **32**:107–116.

◆134. Weitzel JN. Genetic cancer risk assessment – putting it all together. *Cancer* 1999; **86**:2483–2492.

●135. National Cancer Institute Familial Cancer Risk Counseling and Genetic Testing Information Search Database, 2002: http://www.cancer.gov/cancer_information

◆136. Anonymous. Statement of the American Society of Clinical Oncology: genetic testing for cancer susceptibility, adopted on February 20, 1996. *J Clin Oncol* 1996; **14**:1730–1736.

137. Debaun MR, Brown M, Kessler L. Screening for Wilms' tumor in children with high-risk congenital syndromes: considerations for an intervention trial. *Med Pediatr Oncol* 1996; **27**:415–421.

138. Kodish ED. Testing children for cancer genes: the rule of earliest onset. *J Pediatr* 1999; **135**:390–395.

◆139. Lynch HT, Watson P, Shaw TG, *et al.* Clinical impact of molecular genetic diagnosis, genetic counseling, and management of hereditary cancer. Part I: Studies of cancer in families. *Cancer* 1999; **86**:2449–2456.

140. Emery J, Lucassen A, Murphy M. Common hereditary cancers and implications for primary care. *Lancet* 2001; **358**:56–63.

141. Burke W, Daly M, Garber J, *et al.* Recommendations for follow-up care of individuals with an inherited predisposition to cancer. II. BRCA1 and BRCA2. *JAMA* 1997; **277**:997–1003.

◆142. Laxova R. Testing for cancer susceptibility genes in children. *Adv Pediatr* 1999; **46**:1–40.

143. Petersen GM. Genetic testing. *Hematol Oncol Clinics North Am* 2000; **14**:939–952.

144. Visser A, Bleiker E. Genetic education and counseling. *Patient Educ Counseling* 1997; **32**:1–7.

145. Hopwood P. Psychological issues in cancer genetics: current research and future priorities. *Patient Educ Counseling* 1997; **32**:19–31.

146. Grosfeld FJ, Lips CJ, Beemer FA, *et al.* Psychological risks of genetically testing children for a hereditary cancer syndrome. *Patient Educ Counseling* 1997; **32**:63–67.

147. Grosfeld FJ, Beemer FA, Lips CJ, *et al.* Parents' responses to disclosure of genetic test results of their children. *Am J Med Genet* 2000; **94**:316–323.

148. Fallowfield L. Giving sad and bad news. *Lancet* 1993; **341**:476–478.

149. Patenaude AF, Basili L, Fairclough DL. Li FP. Attitudes of 47 mothers of pediatric oncology patients toward genetic testing for cancer predisposition. *J Clin Oncol* 1996; **14**:415–421.

150. Wilfond BS, Rothenberg KH, Thomson EJ, Lerman C. Cancer genetic susceptibility testing: ethical and policy implications for future research and clinical practice. Cancer Genetic Studies Consortium, National Institutes of Health. *J Law Med Ethics* 1997; **25**:243–251.

151. MacDonald DJ. Genetic predisposition testing for cancer: effects on families' lives. *Holist Nurs Pract* 1998; **12**:9–19.

152. Lynch HT, Watson P, Shaw TG, *et al.* Clinical impact of molecular genetic diagnosis, genetic counseling, and management of hereditary cancer, Part II: Hereditary nonpolyposis colorectal carcinoma as a model. *Cancer* 1999; **86**:2457–2463.

153. Morrison PJ, Steel CM, Vasen HF, *et al.* Insurance implications for individuals with a high risk of breast and ovarian cancer in Europe. *Dis Markers* 1999; **15**:159–165.

◆154. Malkin D, Knoppers BM. Genetic predisposition to cancer – issues to consider. *Semin Cancer Biol* 1996; **7**:49–53.

155. Severin MJ. Genetic susceptibility for specific cancers – medical liability of the clinician. *Cancer* 1999; **86**:2564–2569.

4

Cardiovascular complications

Cardiotoxicity caused by chemotherapy

ANDREA S HINKLE, CINDY B PROUKOU, SAMPADA S DESHPANDE, SARAH A DUFFY,
AMY M KOZLOWSKI, CAROL A FRENCH AND STEVEN E LIPSHULTZ

INTRODUCTION

Cardiotoxicity is a well-recognized late effect of therapy for childhood and adolescent malignancies and is a serious problem for long-term survivors. Cardiotoxicity may be caused by chemotherapy, radiation therapy or the combined use of both modalities. A survey of pediatric cardiology centers in North America found that more than 12 per cent of all patients with cardiomyopathy had been treated for cancer during childhood or adolescence.[1] In a large cohort of American patients who had survived at least 5 years from a diagnosis of pediatric cancer, the standardized mortality ratio (SMR) for overall mortality was 10.8, and the SMR for cardiac mortality was 8.2.[2] A study from the Nordic countries produced similar findings (overall mortality SMR, 10.8; cardiac and circulatory system death SMR, 5.8).[3] The SMR for sudden or ill-defined deaths was 3.9; some of these deaths were probably attributable to cardiac causes.[3]

Mortality from anthracycline-induced cardiac failure is substantial, with some large studies reporting rates higher than 20 per cent.[4,5] A study of 474 15-year survivors of childhood cancer found overall SMRs of 3.78 for men and 4.84 for women, with a cardiac mortality SMR for men of 7.91.[6] Exposure to doxorubicin was associated with higher risk of death from cardiac disease.

Cardiotoxicity can present as acute, early onset or late onset. It may be subclinical and asymptomatic or progressive with the development of clinical symptoms. Clinical presentation and relationship to known risk factors for chemotherapy-induced cardiotoxicity differ, particularly between acute cardiotoxicity and other categories (Table 4a.1).[7] Acute cardiotoxicity may occur with or without subsequent development of other forms of cardiotoxicity.

Anthracyclines are the most common class of chemotherapeutic agents associated with adverse effects on the heart. Anthracyclines were introduced as chemotherapeutic agents in the late 1960s (daunorubicin) and early 1970s (doxorubicin).[8] They are highly effective against a wide range of malignancies and survival from pediatric cancers has increased from 45 to 77 per cent since their introduction (although some of the improvement can be attributed to other agents and improvements in supportive care).[9] Protocols from the former Pediatric Oncology Group (POG) show that more than 50 per cent of 12 680 patients treated between 1974 and 1990 received anthracycline chemotherapy.[10] Thus, the benefits of anthracyclines currently outweigh their cardiotoxicity. The most commonly used drugs in this class are doxorubicin (Adriamycin), daunorubicin (Cerubidine), and idarubicin (Idamycin).[7]

Other chemotherapeutic agents that may cause cardiac abnormalities include alkylating agents, antimetabolites, and antimicrotubule agents (Table 4a.2).[11,12] Some factors that influence the development of cardiotoxicity can be modified to decrease patient risk. These factors include the type of anthracycline, the cumulative dose of anthracycline, the rate of administration, the use of cardioprotectants and concomitant mantle radiation.[7] Other factors that affect the potential for the development of cardiomyopathy cannot be altered. These factors include such

Table 4a.1 *Characteristics of different types of anthracycline cardiotoxicity. (Reprinted from Giantris A et al. Anthracycline-induced cardiotoxicity in children and young adults.* Crit Rev Oncol Hematol *27:53–68, copyright 1998, with permission from Elsevier Science.)*

Characteristic	Acute cardiotoxicity	Early-onset chronic progressive cardiotoxicity	Late-onset chronic progressive cardiotoxicity
Onset	Within the first week of anthracycline treatment	<1 year after the completion of anthracycline treatment	≤1 year after the completion of anthracycline treatment
Risk-factor dependence	Unknown	Yes	Yes
Clinical features in adults	Transient depression of myocardial contractility	Dilated cardiomyopathy	Dilated cardiomyopathy
Clinical features in children	Transient depression of myocardial contractility	Restrictive cardiomyopathy or dilated cardiomyopathy	Restrictive cardiomyopathy or dilated cardiomyopathy
Course	Potentially reversible on discontinuation of anthracycline	Can be progressive	Can be progressive

patient characteristics as age at time of treatment, gender, race and length of follow-up. Additional patient characteristics that may influence the development of cardiomyopathy include pre-existing or concomitant medical conditions and treatments.

This subchapter will review patient characteristics and treatment factors that place survivors at risk for the development of cardiomyopathy (Table 4a.3 and Figure 4a.1).[7] Preventive strategies, appropriate monitoring and interventions will also be presented.

PATIENT CHARACTERISTICS INFLUENCING CARDIOTOXICITY

Age

Patients who receive treatment at a younger age appear to be more vulnerable to anthracycline-induced myocardial impairment (Figure 4a.1).[13–17] In one study, age under 4 years at the time of exposure was a significant risk factor for abnormal cardiac function.[16] A retrospective study of children and adults who had received cumulative doxorubicin doses of 244–550 mg/m^2 for acute lymphoblastic leukemia (ALL) or osteosarcoma during childhood showed that younger age at diagnosis was associated with, and predictive of, ventricular dysfunction.[17] Left ventricular contractility, posterior wall thickness and fractional shortening were reduced in many patients, and left ventricular afterload was increased.

Gender

Girls appear to be more vulnerable to the cardiotoxic effects of anthracycline therapy (Figure 4a.1). In a review of 6493 patients who received anthracycline chemotherapy on POG protocols from 1974 to 1990, Krischer *et al.*

report that being female was an independent risk factor for cardiotoxicity.[18] Lipshultz *et al.* also found that female patients were more likely to have depressed contractility than male patients.[17] The cohort of 120 children and adults had been treated with bolus doxorubicin with cumulative doses of at least 244 mg/m^2 for ALL (73 per cent) or non-metastatic osteogenic sarcoma (27 per cent). Forty-five per cent of the female patients (28 of 62) had contractility more than 2 standard deviations below normal, compared to 12 per cent of male patients (7 of 58; $p < 0.001$). In addition, the higher the cumulative dose, the greater the difference in contractility between male and female patients.

The findings of Silber *et al.* also show the association with female sex.[19] In this study, 150 patients underwent resting and gated nuclear angiography, exercise testing using standard cycle ergometry with electrocardiographic (ECG) monitoring, or both tests. Approximately 38 per cent (32 of 85) of the male patients had abnormalities in one or both of the cardiac function tests compared to 64 per cent (42 of 66) of the female patients. The reason for the sex difference is unclear. One hypothesis is that anthracyclines may be distributed differently in the male and female bodies. Doxorubicin does not concentrate in fat tissue and is metabolized more slowly in the obese.[20] Because females have more body fat than males of the same body surface area and because anthracyclines do not distribute into fat, equal doses of anthracycline given to males and females may lead to higher dose exposure in the hearts of females. This hypothesis is supported by Silber's study, which found that the association between cardiac dysfunction and female sex was particularly strong in children older than age 12, when puberty began to produce larger differences in fat distribution between boys and girls.[19] Similar results were found in a study by Green *et al.* in patients treated on the National Wilms' Tumor Studies where, with the same level of cumulative doxorubicin dose and radiation to the lung and

Table 4a.2 *Cardiac toxicities of chemotherapeutic agents*

Drug	Risk factors	Manifestations of acute toxicity	Manifestations of chronic toxicity
Cytostatic antibiotics			
Doxorubicin, Daunoribicin	Cumulative dose, rate and schedule of anthracycline administration, age, mediastinal radiation therapy, female gender, history of cardiac disorders	*Acute or subacute* ECG changes, sinus tachycardia, arrhythmias, pericarditis/myocarditis, MI, sudden cardiac death, CHF, cardiomyopathy	Early and late onset chronic CHF, cardiomyopathy
Epirubicin	Unknown	CHF	CHF
Idarubicin	Unknown	CHF, arrhythmias, angina, MI	
Mitoxantrone	Cumulative doses, prior anthracycline therapy, pre-existing cardiovascular disorders	Arrhythmias, CHF, MI, ECG changes, decreases in LVEF	
Alkylating agents			
Cyclophosphamide	Total dose/cycle or daily dose, prior anthracycline or mitoxantrone therapy, mediastinal radiation	CHF, chest pain, pleural and pericardial effusions, pericardial friction rub, cardiomegaly, loss of QRS voltage on ECG, hemorrhagic cardiac necrosis, reversible systolic dysfunction, ECG changes	
Ifosfamide	Total dose	CHF, pleural effusion, re-entrant ventricular tachycardia, pulseless tachycardia, ST or T wave abnormalities, decreased QRS complex, arrhythmias	
Cisplatin	Unknown	Palpitations, left-sided chest pain, nausea, vomiting, dyspnea, hypotension, arrhythmias, interventricular block, MI, ST segment/T-wave changes, T-wave inversions, Raynaud's phenomenon	
Mitomycin	Cumulative dose, prior doxorubicin therapy, chest irradiation	CHF	CHF
Carmustine	Unknown	Chest pain, hypotension, sinus tachycardia, ECG changes	
Busulfan	Unknown	CHF, palpitations, cardiac tamponade, pulmonary congestion, cardiomegaly, pericardial effusion, ECG changes, endocardial/pulmonary fibrosis, pulmonary hypertension	
Mechlorethanine	Unknown	Persistent tachycardia, pulse irregularity, junctional or atrial ectopic beats	
Antimetabolites			
Fluorouracil	History of cardiovascular disorders, prior mediastinal radiation, concurrent use of other cardiotoxic chemotherapy, rate of administration, higher dose	Angina, MI, hypotension, cardiogenic shock/sudden death, ECG changes, dilated cardiomyopathy	
Cytarabine	Definitive information unknown, possibly cytarabine dose	Pericarditis with dyspnea, chest pain, pericardial friction rub, pulsus paradoxus, CHF, pleural/pericardial effusions, arrhythmias	

(continued)

Table 4a.2 *(continued)*

Drug	Risk factors	Manifestations of acute toxicity	Manifestations of chronic toxicity
Antimicrotubule agents			
Paclitaxel	Definitive information unknown, possibly history of cardiovascular disorders	Sinus bradycardia/bradyarrhythmias, atrial and ventricular arrhythmias, MI, supraventricular tachycardia, AV or left bundle branch block, sudden death, myocardial dysfunction	
Etoposide	Definitive information unknown, possibly history of cardiac disease, mediastinal radiation, prior cardiotoxic chemotherapy	Hypotension, acute MI, ECG changes	
Teniposide	Unknown	Arrhythmia, hypotension	
Vinblastine	Unknown	Acute MI, dyspnea, tachypnea, pulmonary edema, ECG changes, T-wave inversion, ST-segment changes, atrial fibrillation, Raynaud's phenomenon	
Vincristine	Mediastinal radiation, coexisting ischemic heart disease	Acute MI, dyspnea, tachypnea, pulmonary edema, ECG changes, T-wave inversion, ST-segment changes, atrial fibrillation, acute CHF, hypotension, cardiovascular autonomic neuropathy	
Miscellaneous			
Amasacrine	Hypokalemia, prior anthracycline therapy	Atrial and ventricular tachyarrhythmias, CHF, hypotension, cardiopulmonary arrest	Cardiomyopathy
Cladribine	Unknown	CHF	
Asparaginase	Unknown	Acute MI, ECG changes	
Tretinoin	Unknown	Retinoic acid syndrome (fever, respiratory distress, body weight gain, peripheral edema, pleural–pericardial effusions), MI	
Pentostatin	Definite information unknown, possibly underlying cardiovascular disorders	Angina and MI, CHF, acute arrhythmias	CHF
Trastuzumab	Prior or concomitant anthracycline use	Ventricular dysfunction, CHF	Cardiomyopathy
Arsenic trioxide	Unknown	Arrhythmias, pericardial effusion	
Interferon α-2A	Unknown	Exacerbation of underlying cardiac disease, hypotension, arrhythmias	Cardiomyopathy
Interleukin-2	Unknown	Myocardial injury/myopericarditis, ventricular arrhythmias, hypotension, sudden death	Dilated cardiomyopathy

AV, atrioventricular; CHF, congestive heart failure; ECG, electrocardiogram; LVEF, left ventricular ejection fraction; MI, myocardial infarction.

Table 4a.3 *Risk factors for anthracycline-induced cardiotoxicity. (Reprinted from Giantris A et al. Anthracycline-induced cardiotoxicity in children and young adults. Crit Rev Oncol Hematol 27:53–68, copyright 1998, with permission from Elsevier Science.)*

Risk factor	Features
Total cumulative dose	Most significant risk factor
Rate of anthracycline administration	Higher rate may predispose to cardiotoxicity
Age	For cumulative doses, younger age predisposes to cardiotoxicity
Length of follow-up	Longer follow-up results in higher prevalence of myocardial impairment
Gender	Females more vulnerable than males for comparable doses
Concomitant mantle irradiation	Evidence of enhanced cardiotoxicity is suggestive but not conclusive
Others	Concomitant exposure to cyclophosphamide, bleomycin, vincristine, amsacrine or mitoxantrone may predispose to cardiotoxicity. Trisomy 21 and black race have been associated with a higher risk of early clinical cardiotoxicity

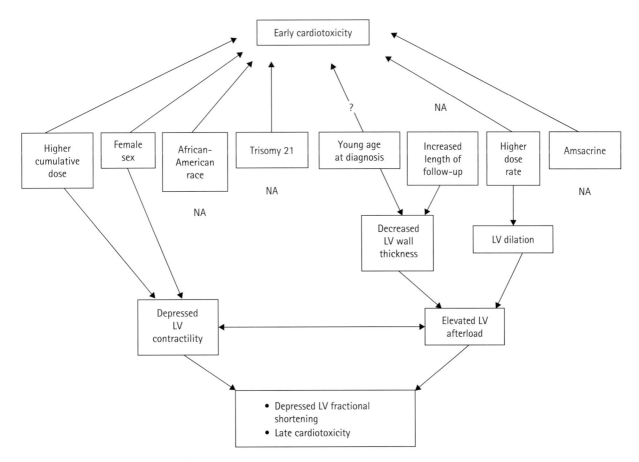

Figure 4a.1 *Risk factors for the development of anthracycline-associated pediatric ventricular dysfunction. LV, left ventricular. (Reprinted from Lipshultz SE. Ventricular dysfunction clinical research in infants, children and adolescents. Prog Pediatr Cardiol 12:1–28, copyright 2000, with permission from Elsevier Science.)*

left abdomen, the risk of developing congestive heart failure for girls is about four times greater than for boys.[21]

Race

Few studies have examined the effect of racial differences. In the previously discussed review of children treated on POG protocols from 1974 to 1990, African-American race was associated with a higher risk of early cardiotoxicity.[22]

Trisomy 21

In the same review, an increased risk of early clinical cardiotoxicity was seen in children with trisomy 21 without

congenital cardiovascular malformations.[22] Those children with both conditions were excluded from the study.

Non-cardiotoxic effects of cancer therapy that may potentiate cardiotoxicity

Chemotherapy and radiation therapy in children can produce other long-term sequelae that may also affect the development of cardiotoxicity (Table 4a.4).[23]

Growth hormone insufficiency or deficiency is a prevalent late effect that deserves special mention. Stunted

Table 4a.4 *Late effects of therapy and complications that may alter cardiac function or injure myocardium. (Reprinted from Hinkle AS et al. Cardiotoxicity related to cancer therapy.* Prog Pediatr Cardiol *8:145–155, copyright 1998, with permission from Elsevier Science.)*

Uncompensated hypothyroidism
Decreased heart rate, stroke volume, pulses, blood pressure,
    ECG voltage
Conduction disturbances
Increased cholesterol and/or triglyceride levels
Pericardial effusion
Peripheral edema
Increased sensitivity to digoxin

Hyperthyroidism
Increased heart rate, systolic blood pressure, pulses,
    QRS voltages
Palpitations
Mitral valve prolapse
Abnormal rhythms including heart block, interventricular
    conduction delay, notched P waves, peaked T waves
CHF

Obesity
Increased cholesterol and/or triglyceride levels
Systemic and/or pulmonary hypertension
Insulin resistance with subsequent glucose dysregulation
Hypoventilation and sleep apnea
Prolongation of the QTc interval on ECG
Left ventricular dysfunction
Ventricular dilatation or hypertrophy
CHF

Ovarian failure
Decreased HDL and increased LDL levels
Earlier onset of coronary artery disease with subsequent
    decreased coronary blood flow and exercise-induced
    coronary artery dilatation

Renal dysfunction
Hypertension

Pulmonary fibrosis
Tricuspid insufficiency
Pulmonary hypertension
Right heart failure

CHF, congestive heart failure; ECG, electrocardiogram; HDL, high-density lipoprotein; LDL, low-density lipoprotein.

growth after radiation therapy is common; in one cohort of radiation-treated ALL survivors, 74 per cent achieved an adult height of only 1 standard deviation or more below the mean, and 32 per cent were 2 standard deviations or more below the mean.[24]

Although growth impairment may be caused by non-hormonal factors that do not affect cardiac function, it may also be caused by impaired growth hormone production. Growth hormone may act indirectly on the heart through the action of insulin-like growth factor 1 (IGF-1). In the rat, IGF-1 appears to stimulate myocardial hypertrophy and increase myocyte contractility.[25] In humans, numerous studies confirm that growth hormone deficiency impairs cardiac function. In a cohort of 333 Swedish adults with treated hypopituitarism and untreated growth hormone deficiency, there were 60 deaths attributed to cardiovascular disorders when only 31 deaths would have been expected.[26] Growth hormone treatment improves cardiac indices at rest and during exercise.[27,28] Growth hormone deficiency is also associated with dyslipidemia. In a case-control study, patients with growth hormone deficiency had higher total cholesterol and low-density lipoprotein (LDL) and lower high-density lipoprotein (HDL) than matched controls.[29] Patients who received 6 months of treatment with growth hormone had lower total cholesterol and LDL levels with no changes in HDL levels.[29] Growth hormone treatment in deficient patients also decreases amounts of adipose tissue, particularly the amount of visceral fat.[30]

Children with idiopathic growth hormone deficiency who are treated with growth hormone do not differ from their peers in cardiovascular mortality.[31] Children treated with growth hormone who do not have any underlying cardiac abnormalities do not differ significantly from controls in blood pressure, left ventricular function, cardiac output or systemic vascular resistance.[32] Growth hormone therapy in children is generally safe, with only two adverse events related to the heart among 20 000 children followed since 1985.[25] For some growth hormone-deficient survivors of childhood cancer with left ventricular dysfunction due to thin left ventricular walls, we observed rapid cardiac deterioration, in some cases requiring cardiac transplantation, owing to the inability of the myocardium to grow further. However, owing to the potential long-term benefits in improving body composition, lipid profiles and cardiac indices in adults, the use of growth hormone therapy in adult survivors of childhood cancer deserves further investigation.

Pregnancy

Pregnancy may pose an additional challenge to women who have been treated with potentially cardiotoxic therapy.

Case reports have described women who have experienced cardiac decompensation during the peripartum period[33,34] but additional research is needed to delineate actual risk. We have had a selected referral population of over 40 pregnant anthracycline-treated survivors of childhood cancer with cardiac concerns. In this non-representative population, 30 per cent developed symptomatic heart disease, including heart failure and ventricular tachycardia. The third trimester and first two postpartum months were the window of onset of symptoms. Two patients died and one was referred for a cardiac transplantation. Current recommendations include baseline echocardiography with repeat testing during the third trimester, and a team approach with cardiology and a high-risk obstetrical team. Occasionally, invasive hemodynamic monitoring and controlled deliveries are indicated.

LENGTH OF FOLLOW-UP

The importance of longer follow-up has become apparent. Both prevalence and severity of cardiac abnormalities increase over time (Figure 4a.1).[17,35] In serial follow-up of 120 doxorubicin-treated patients, those with longer follow-up were more likely to have reduced left ventricular wall thickness and secondary increased left ventricular afterload.[17] The authors suggest that changes may develop as somatic growth outstrips myocardial growth.

Asymptomatic cancer survivors are at increasing risk for cardiac dysfunction later in life. Patients may develop cardiomyopathy with congestive heart failure (CHF) after years of latency.[7,16,17,22,36,37] Although acute episodes can often be treated successfully, cardiac function generally shows a progressive decline even with long-term medication. Sixty-five per cent of childhood cancer survivors treated with anthracyclines have subclinical cardiac dysfunction 6 years after completion of therapy, and the dysfunction is often progressive.[7,16,17,37]

Heart failure may develop after an added stress on the heart, such as pregnancy, infection, an unsupervised exercise program or cocaine use. Monitoring cardiac function is thus extremely important during pregnancy or other events that can increase stress on the heart.[38]

Early-onset versus late-onset cardiotoxicity

Heart damage from anthracycline therapy can be divided into two categories: early onset and late onset. Early-onset cardiotoxicity occurs during therapy or within the first year after treatment. Late toxicity occurs at least 1 year after the completion of therapy. The development of new cases of late-onset cardiotoxicity together with the progressive worsening of early-onset cases probably accounts for the overall increase in severity and prevalence of anthracycline-induced cardiotoxicity with time.[2]

Krischer et al. reported that 1.6 per cent of a cohort of 6493 childhood cancer patients treated with anthracycline developed early clinical cardiotoxicity.[22] No clinical cardiotoxicity was reported in the 6187 newly diagnosed childhood cancer patients who did not receive anthracycline therapy. Early-onset cardiotoxicity was defined as CHF not attributable to other known causes or changes in cardiac function that prompted permanent discontinuation of anthracycline therapy.

Late-onset cardiotoxicity is described by Lipshultz et al. in more than half of a cohort of 115 children treated for ALL with doxorubicin from 1 to 15 years earlier.[16] Patients were evaluated by history, 24-hour ambulatory ECG recording, exercise testing and echocardiography. Fifty-seven per cent had abnormal end-systolic wall stress (afterload) or contractility. Patients with excess afterload at the initial evaluation showed less increase in left ventricular wall thickness than expected for somatic growth. In addition, there was a significant increase in age-adjusted afterload during the follow-up, with 24 of 34 patients (71 per cent) having higher values on the last study. Thus, clinical cardiac decompensation may develop in only a small subset of the patients with subclinical cardiac damage. Similar results were found among patients in the National Wilms' Tumor Study who received doxorubicin for their initial treatment: two out of three cases of CHF occurred late.[21]

Steinherz et al. reported progressive deterioration of systolic function measurements in 15 of 300 patients (5 per cent) who had been treated with anthracyclines at least 4 years earlier (median dose 540 mg/m^2; range 285–870 mg/m^2).[39]

Five patients who had had cardiomyopathy and improvement experienced reappearance of cardiac failure 6–10 years after therapy.[35] In two of them, CHF recurred within 3 months after they began lifting heavy objects at work or for exercise. All five developed progressive dysrhythmias and abnormal conduction patterns. One underwent a successful heart transplant, three died suddenly from dysrhythmia and one patient was stabilized under medical management with activity restrictions.

The remaining ten patients had no signs of cardiac dysfunction during therapy or the year following treatment, but developed congestive heart failure and life-threatening dysrhythmias from 8 to 19 years after treatment.[35] Seven of them had begun or intensified a weight-lifting program during the previous 6 months, two had increased their alcohol consumption and one reported abusing cocaine. All improved with intensive medical management.

TREATMENT FACTORS INFLUENCING CARDIOTOXICITY

Cumulative dose

A high cumulative anthracycline dose is well established as a risk factor for cardiac damage (Figure 4a.1). In 6493 children who received anthracycline chemotherapy on POG protocols from 1974 to 1995, higher cumulative doses were significantly associated with the development of cardiotoxicity.[22] The risk of cardiotoxicity in children treated with 550 mg/m^2 or more was five times higher than the risk in children treated with lower cumulative doses. In fact, a high cumulative dose of anthracycline was the strongest predictor of cardiotoxicity. In this study, cardiotoxicity was defined as clinical CHF, a documented change in cardiac function by echocardiography or radionuclide scanning serious enough to prompt discontinuation of anthracycline therapy, or sudden death from presumed cardiac causes.[22]

Lipshultz et al. found a similar relationship among 115 children treated for ALL with doxorubicin in the previous 1 to 15 years (Figure 4a.1).[16] Patients receiving 45 mg/m^2 in a single dose were compared to patients receiving 228 mg/m^2 or more in multiple doses. Left ventricular posterior wall thickness adjusted for body surface was lower in patients who received doxorubicin than in normal controls. In patients in the higher dose group, the left ventricular posterior wall thickness was significantly lower than normal. Children who received a single dose of doxorubicin had less impaired function than children who received 228 mg/m^2 or more.

Fractional shortening and left ventricular contractility were significantly reduced, and afterload was significantly elevated in all patients in the high-dose group.[16] Afterload is a function of blood pressure, the size of the ventricular cavity and wall thickness, but in these patients, blood pressure and size of the left ventricular cavity were normal. Thus, increased afterload was attributable to reduced left ventricular wall thickness.

Higher cumulative dose of anthracyclines was a significant predictor for both increased afterload and decreased contractility.[16] In an earlier study of serial measurements, Lipshultz et al. reported an increasing disproportion between wall thickness and ventricular size with time, especially in children who had substantial somatic growth.[40]

Although the risk of cardiotoxicity increases with the cumulative dose of anthracyclines administered, the relationship is complex and far from linear.[7] Some studies have reported heart failure incidence of 0.15 per cent or less among patients with cumulative doses of 400 mg/m^2 or less, and 7 per cent incidence among patients with cumulative doses of 550 mg/m^2.[4] The doses of anthracyclines associated with the development of chronic cardiomyopathy among children are probably lower than the doses tolerated by adults.[7] Although cumulative doses in excess of 1000 mg/m^2 have been well tolerated by some patients,[41,42] there are reports of cardiac dysfunction in patients treated with less than 300 mg/m^2.[43,44] Individuals vary in their susceptibility and the risk may increase over time. It is, therefore, important to note that there is no absolutely safe dose of anthracycline. A study of the National Wilms' Tumor Study Group found that cumulative dose of doxorubicin increased the patient's relative risk of CHF by a factor of 3.3 for every 100 mg/m^2 of doxorubicin.[21]

Rate of administration

The rate of administration (continuous infusion versus bolus doses) may also affect the risk of developing cardiotoxicity during or after treatment.[7]

Continuous infusion methods reduce peak anthracycline levels but they prolong the exposure period. Many investigators are concerned about the potential effects of this longer exposure time in children because the risk to children may be significantly higher than the risk to adults. Lipshultz et al. recently reported that serum measurements of cardiac troponin T were elevated in children who received doxorubicin for ALL by either a continuous or bolus infusion, suggesting that the lower peak doxorubicin concentrations in continuous infusions failed to prevent cardiac damage.[45] In both groups, multiple echocardiographic measurements showed abnormalities, including a significant decrease in median left ventricular (LV) fractional shortening and LV contractility, and a significant increase in LV peak systolic wall stress. The median follow-up period in this study was only 1.5 years. Levitt et al. found that late subclinical cardiotoxicity after moderate doses of anthracycline is not alleviated by 6-hour infusions [fractional shortening (FS) <28 per cent, end systolic wall stress (ESWS) >2SD].[46]

Use of cardioprotectants

Ideally, any alteration to an antineoplastic regimen that is aimed at minimizing cardiotoxicity should not affect the regimen's antineoplastic efficacy. One approach to preventing or minimizing chemotherapy-induced cardiotoxicity is to add a cardioprotectant.[11] One such cardioprotectant is dexrazoxane (Zinecard; Pharmacia & Upjohn, Peapack, NJ, USA). A randomized clinical trial of women with advanced breast cancer showed that dexrazoxane provided significant protection against doxorubicin-induced cardiac toxicity without reducing its antineoplastic effect.[47] The 92 women in the trial were on a regimen of fluorouracil, doxorubicin and cyclophosphamide (FDC). Cardiac toxicity

was assessed by clinical examination, multigated radio-nuclide angiography (MUGA) scans and endomyocardial biopsy. Results showed 11 episodes of clinical cardiac toxicity in the control arm and two in the dexrazoxane arm. In a follow-up study, Speyer et al. concluded that adding dexrazoxane could also allow patients to receive higher cumulative doses of doxorubicin.[48]

Swain et al. found similar results in a randomized double-blind study of 534 patients with advanced breast cancer.[49] Patients received fluorouracil, doxorubicin and cyclophosphamide with either dexrazoxane (at 1/10 the dose of doxorubicin) or placebo every 3 weeks. Dexrazoxane had a significant cardioprotective effect, as shown by serial physical examinations, ECGs and MUGA scans. Chances of developing a cardiac event were 2.0–2.6 times higher in the group that did not receive dexrazoxane. The most substantial cardioprotective effect was seen at the higher cumulative doses of doxorubicin. However, there was a decreased response rate seen in one of the trials utilizing dexrazoxane.

Wexler et al. conducted an open-label randomized trial that showed that dexrazoxane reduced the incidence of short-term subclinical doxorubicin-induced cardiotoxicity in pediatric sarcoma patients.[50] Thirty-eight patients received an intravenous bolus of doxorubicin; half were randomized to receive dexrazoxane. Resting left ventricular ejection fraction (LVEF) was monitored with MUGA scans at baseline and at 6–12 weeks after the 210, 310, 360 and 410 mg/m^2 doses of doxorubicin. The two groups were compared on incidence and degree of cardiotoxicity, response rates to four cycles of chemotherapy, event-free and overall survival, and incidence and severity of non-cardiac toxicities. Eighteen dexrazoxane-treated and 15 control patients were assessable for cardiac toxicity. Dexrazoxane-treated patients were less likely to develop subclinical cardiotoxicity (22 per cent vs. 67 per cent, $p < 0.01$), had a smaller decline in LVEF per 100 mg/m^2 of doxorubicin (1.0 vs. 2.7 percentage points, $p = 0.02$), and received a higher median cumulative dose of doxorubicin (410 vs. 310 mg/m^2, $p < 0.05$) than did control patients. There were no significant differences in response rate, event-free survival and overall survival.

This study suggests that dexrazoxane reduces the risk of developing short-term subclinical cardiotoxicity in pediatric sarcoma patients who receive up to 410 mg/m^2 of doxorubicin. Dexrazoxane is being used more frequently in multiple treatment regimens, but additional clinical trials with more patients are needed to determine if the short-term cardioprotection provided by dexrazoxane will reduce the incidence of late cardiac complications in long-term survivors of childhood cancer.

We have recently reported that in a randomized prospective multicentered study of dexrazoxane in newly diagnosed childhood ALL patients treated with doxorubicin that there is a 50 per cent reduction in cardiac troponin, indicating significant reduced acute myocardial injury during therapy, and no difference in event-free survival or toxicities at 2–3 years of follow-up.[51]

Another approach to minimizing chemotherapy-induced cardiotoxicity would be to combine antineoplastic therapy with agents that reduce oxidative stress, such as probucol,[7] vitamin E, glutathione, amifostine and mesna. These agents may offer promise in reducing or preventing cardiomyopathy,[11] but unfortunately the mechanism that protects against oxidative stress injury may also limit antineoplastic efficacy.

Use of analogues

Another emerging approach to reducing cardiomyopathy is to replace conventional anthracyclines with less cardiotoxic analogues or new formulations, such as epirubicin hydrochloride, idarubicin hydrochloride and liposomal anthracyclines.[11]

Concomitant mantle radiation

Radiation therapy is frequently used in combination with multidrug chemotherapy regimens in the treatment of various hematologic cancers and solid tumors.[7] Although it is widely accepted that the concomitant exposure of the mantle (mediastinum) to radiation and anthracycline enhances the risk of cardiotoxicity, the evidence is suggestive rather than conclusive. Praga et al. found more severe histologic changes in endomyocardial biopsy specimens obtained from 12 patients who had received mediastinal radiation before anthracycline therapy than in specimens from patients who had received mediastinal radiation only.[5] There are other reports in the literature that suggest that radiation exposure worsens the cardiotoxic effects of anthracyclines.[52,53] In a study by the National Wilms' Tumor Study Group, the risk of CHF was estimated to increase by a factor of 1.6 for every 10 Gy of lung irradiation and by 1.8 for every 10 Gy of left abdominal irradiation independent of other factors assessed in the analysis.[21]

ASSESSMENT OF CARDIAC INJURY DURING AND AFTER THERAPY

Appropriate methods for monitoring and detecting chemotherapy-induced cardiotoxicity has been a topic of intense focus, discussion and even controversy.[54,55] No well-accepted criteria have been established for reducing or withholding cardiotoxic chemotherapy in response to changes on echocardiograms. In addition, the predictive value of these on-therapy changes for long-term or

progressive cardiotoxicity has not been definitively determined. Although most patients who manifest cardiotoxicity will do so within the first year of therapy, some may develop late cardiotoxicity, either subclinical or symptomatic. Monitoring has not reached the point at which it can be used to predict or prevent subacute or late-onset cardiotoxicity. It is reasonable to believe that accurate prediction of cardiotoxicity could reduce the incidence of late complications. However, long-term monitoring, potentially with different modalities, may remain necessary.

Electrocardiography and echocardiography

Most of the changes on ECGs that are associated with cardiomyopathy (e.g. decreased QRS voltage or ST segment/T-wave changes) may occur too late to be useful for monitoring. However, prolonged QTc has been identified as a potentially useful measure of myocardial injury and indicator of increased risk of cardiotoxicity.[56]

Echocardiograms have the advantage of being non-invasive and, in children, good windows can usually be obtained that provide adequate pictures and measurements. A decrease in ejection fraction or fractional shortening, the preferred measurement in children, represents potential anthracycline cardiotoxicity. The drawback to measurement of fractional shortening is that it is dependent on loading conditions, which may vary considerably, particularly during chemotherapy.[2] Helpful information about myocyte health and myocardial function can be provided by measurements of wall stress, contractility and the relationship between wall stress and velocity of circumferential fiber shortening (contractility), as well as by anatomic measurements, such as posterior wall thickness.[7,37,57]

Current monitoring recommendations include obtaining echocardiograms with these measurements at regular intervals after therapy. The monitoring interval depends on cumulative anthracycline dose, other therapies received, the detection of any abnormalities, symptoms and coexistent stressors, such as growth or participation in competitive athletics.

Radiologic imaging

Contrast radionuclide angiography has good specificity and results correlate with pathologic changes, but it measures ejection fraction.[58] Exercise radionuclide angiography has excellent sensitivity and specificity for detecting coronary disease, but its application to detecting anthracycline cardiomyopathy is not adequately studied.[54] Radionuclide angiography has several distinct drawbacks in that it is semi-invasive and involves radiation exposure.

Several other imaging modalities have been explored for monitoring anthracycline toxicity but remain investigational. These include indium-111 antimyosin scintigraphy for the detection of myocardial cell injury, and iodine-123 metaiodobenzylguanidine (MIBG) scintigraphy to assess cardiac adrenergic innervation, which is disrupted by anthracycline toxicity.[8,58–60] A study of iodine-123 beta-methyl-iodophenyl-pentadecanoic acid (^{123}I-BMIPP) dynamic single photon emission computed tomography (SPECT) detected early evidence of doxorubicin cardiomyopathy. Magnetic resonance spectroscopy (MRS) and positron emission tomography (PET) scanning are also being investigated to evaluate anthracycline cardiac damage.[61,62] These imaging modalities have been studied in animals and adults, but data on children are not available.

Biopsy

Endomyocardial biopsy data can be obtained for adults, but abnormalities that may correlate with increased dose are not necessarily predictive of symptomatic cardiomyopathy.[7] As an invasive and expensive test with no evidence of improving outcome, it cannot be recommended for routine monitoring in children, but may be useful in selected cases.

Laboratory testing, including cardiac troponin monitoring

Accurate laboratory detection of anthracycline-induced myocyte injury and cardiomyopathy would be very useful. Multiple studies have examined the potential usefulness of atrial natriuretic peptides (ANP) and brain natriuretic peptides (BNP) in detecting anthracycline-induced damage. In one study in children, both BNP and ANP were significantly elevated in children with echocardiographic evidence of left ventricular dysfunction, and the elevations were associated with systolic function but not diastolic function.[63] Another study demonstrated an increase in natriuretic peptides above a doxorubicin dose of 400 mg/m^2 after decreases in LVEF were noted on echocardiogram. The increase in plasma ANP was correlated with the decrease in LVEF.[64] An additional study in children found variation in ANP during chemotherapy with a persistent increase following chemotherapy. Bone marrow transplant patients and patients treated with cardiac irradiation had the highest levels.[65] Further study will be necessary to determine whether natriuretic peptides offer advantages over current monitoring modalities to predict cardiomyopathy and detect subclinical disease.

One of the most promising areas of laboratory monitoring is the use of troponin T and I levels to detect

anthracycline-induced cardiac injury. Testing cardiac troponin levels can detect myocardial injury even during periods of latency because it is highly sensitive and specific.

Troponins are contractile protein components of the tropomyosin complex that regulate the interaction of actin and myosin. They are thin-filament associated complexes of the myocyte.[66] The three components in the complex of troponin are named after their functions. Troponin T binds the complex to tropomyosin; troponin C binds calcium then undergoes conformational changes that induce change in the troponin I molecule, which inhibits actin and myosin in the absence of calcium.[67] Troponin T and I exist in three isoforms: one for slow-twitch skeletal muscle, one for fast-twitch skeletal muscle and one for cardiac muscle.[68,69] The troponins are localized in at least two intracellular compartments. Small quantities of cardiac troponin T (cTnT) and cardiac troponin I (cTnI) are found in the cytoplasm, most of it (96 per cent) in the myofibrillar bound state.[70] Cardiac troponin can be detected in serum approximately 4–8 hours after myocardial injury and levels remain elevated for 1–14 days.[71] The quantity of protein released is in direct proportion to the extent of myocardial injury.[72]

Measurements of cardiac troponin offer the potential to detect cardiotoxicity accurately in the following settings: (1) during front-line chemotherapy; (2) during anthracycline therapy for relapse or second malignancy to children previously treated with anthracyclines; (3) during bone marrow transplantation; (4) when using experimental therapy that might potentiate cardiotoxicity; and (5) in the setting of intercurrent illness that may potentiate cardiotoxicity.[70] Examples of these illnesses would be viral infections, graft vs. host disease, renal disease and hypertension, autonomic and hormonal derangements, anemia, and interstitial lung disease.

In a study of 15 children with acute lymphoblastic leukemia, cTnT levels were frequently elevated during anthracycline therapy.[73] In seven of the children, cTnT levels were measured at diagnosis, before doxorubicin therapy. One of these children had a low-level elevation. In the remaining eight, cTnT was measured during chemotherapy. Four had elevations after the first dose of doxorubicin, and two out of three patients had elevations mid-therapy. No elevations were observed after doxorubicin therapy was completed. The magnitude of the cTnT elevations correlated with the degree of left ventricular dysfunction. Patients with high cTnT levels after the first dose of doxorubicin had a significantly thinner and more dilated left ventricle than did patients with lower-level cTnT elevations.

Similar results were observed in a prospective study of 202 children with newly diagnosed ALL.[74] Approximately 15–18 per cent of the patients had elevated cTnT levels at diagnosis, prior to receiving any doxorubicin. These patients may have been acutely ill when they were diagnosed with cancer and may have had conditions that contributed to myocardial injury. About 35 per cent had cTnT elevations during doxorubicin therapy. The cTnT elevations were significantly more frequent in patients who received cumulative doxorubicin doses of more than 60 mg/m^2 than in patients who received less than 60 mg/m^2. Higher dose was also associated with chronically elevated cTnT for a period of 5 months.

The ability to detect myocardial injury accurately through serum cTnT levels in cancer patients receiving cardiotoxic therapy may be integral to targeting cardioprotective interventions. The degree of elevation may suggest the extent of myocardial injury previously sustained. It may also be useful in individualizing therapy by altering the dosing, schedule or approach to drug delivery to maximize oncologic efficacy while minimizing cardiotoxicity. It may identify patients who would benefit most from the addition of a cardioprotectant to the antineoplastic regimen or who require treatment of asymptomatic left ventricular dysfunction to prevent disease progression.

Lipid monitoring

Lipid tests are useful in monitoring the cardiac health of anthracycline-treated cancer patients. Patients who have received anthracyclines, 5-fluoracil, cisplatin, vinblastine, vincristine, asparaginase or irradiation to the chest or central nervous system should undergo screening for and treatment of dyslipidemia. The National Cholesterol Education Program guidelines provide a minimum standard for lipid levels.[75] Children should receive serial screenings for coronary artery disease (CAD) risk factors including lipid level measurements. Screenings should begin soon after the completion of therapy and continue into young adulthood.[11]

INTERVENTIONS TO IMPROVE CARDIAC FUNCTION

Lifestyle

Simbre et al. reported that heart-healthy lifestyles should be encouraged in all survivors of cancer treated with potentially cardiotoxic therapies.[11] All patients should also be educated about the cardiotoxic risks of their treatments and, when appropriate, about the need for lifelong monitoring of heart function and coronary artery disease risks. Alcohol consumption, cigarette smoking and illicit drug use should be discouraged in patients at risk for cardiomyopathy, and especially in patients with left ventricular dysfunction because these behaviors may further impair left ventricular function.

Diet

Restricting salt intake to 2.5 g per day and minimizing fluctuations in sodium intake may be beneficial in patients with symptomatic CHF.[11] A heart-healthy diet low in saturated fat is appropriate, but no specific evidence is available for recommending any particular follow-up diet and lifestyle regimen in patients exposed to anthracyclines. Efforts to maintain an ideal body weight should be encouraged, as obesity is a major preventable coronary risk factor and its prevalence is increased in survivors of pediatric malignancy, especially ALL.[23] However, the impact of obesity on chemotherapy-induced cardiomyopathy is not known.

Exercise

Aerobic exercise can produce symptomatic, physiologic and psychological benefits.[76,77] However, it is important for patients to be monitored under maximal or submaximal exercise testing to ensure they have stable cardiac function before exercise programs are recommended. Isometric exercises, such as weight lifting, should be pursued only under the direct supervision of a cardiologist and exercise physiologist.[11]

Pharmacologic treatment of subclinical abnormalities

Patients with subclinical monitoring abnormalities should be referred to a cardiologist for intervention and subsequent follow-up testing. Current treatment for subclinical chemotherapy-induced cardiomyopathy focuses on correcting the underlying abnormalities, such as increased afterload and decreased contractility.[36] There is no specific therapy for chemotherapy-related cardiomyopathy, and thus treatment is guided by the type of cardiomyopathy (dilated, restrictive, etc.).

Therapy with angiotensin-converting enzyme (ACE) inhibitors and/or beta-blockers may delay subclinical abnormalities from deteriorating to symptomatic heart failure.[11]

ANGIOTENSIN–CONVERTING ENZYME INHIBITORS

Afterload reduction with enalapril may alter the course of progressive ventricular dysfunction for patients with or without heart failure. In one group of doxorubicin-treated long-term survivors of childhood cancer, enalapril therapy resulted in improvement, lasting 6–10 years in patients with asymptomatic left ventricular dysfunction and 2–6 years in patients with CHF (Lipshultz, unpublished data). In another randomized study, captopril was given to patients with some systolic dysfunction but without severe

left ventricular dilatation. Overall mortality in the captopril group was 19 per cent lower than in the placebo group.[78]

Although enalapril may have short-term benefits, it is unclear whether chronic use in children with doxorubicin-induced thinning of left ventricular walls will be beneficial. Enalapril may also limit cardiac growth potential by inhibiting cardiac growth factors. This could result to further thinning of left ventricular walls relative to body surface area, with a subsequent increase in afterload.[11]

The absolute contraindications of ACE inhibitor therapy are a known hypersensitivity to the drug class, pregnancy and symptomatic hypotension. Some of the relative contraindications are renal insufficiency, systolic blood pressure less than 90 mm Hg, hyperkalemia and breast-feeding.[10] ACE inhibitors may also interact with other medications. Blood pressure may fall drastically after initiation of ACE inhibitor therapy in some patients on diuretic therapy; ACE inhibitors may attenuate potassium loss caused by thiazide-type diuretics. Patients taking lithium may develop lithium toxicity.

BETA–BLOCKERS

One study has shown that the LVEF of patients with doxorubicin-induced cardiomyopathy improved from 28 per cent to 41 per cent after treatment with beta-blockers.[79] The effect was similar to the effect in idiopathic cardiomyopathy patients.[79] The mechanism by which beta-blockers improve myocardial function may include reducing oxidative stress and the rate of apoptosis.[11]

The absolute contraindications to beta-blocker therapy include a known hypersensitivity to this drug class, sinus bradycardia, second- and third-degree atrioventricular (AV) heart block, and cardiogenic shock.[11] Some relative contraindications are fatigue, dizziness, fainting, asthma and overt cardiac failure. Beta-blockers may interact with catecholamine-depleting drugs (e.g. reserpine), resulting in hypotension or marked bradycardia.

Treatments for clinical cardiomyopathy

Current treatment for clinical chemotherapy-induced cardiomyopathy focuses on providing symptomatic relief and continuing to correct the underlying abnormalities.[11] Many anthracycline-treated long-term survivors with late CHF have a restrictive cardiomyopathy. These patients are often more severely affected and refractory than their history and physical examination suggest.[38] Careful early invasive assessment of hemodynamics, followed by aggressive tailored pharmacologic therapy and early heart transplantation has been beneficial. Before transplantation is considered, all reversible factors should be treated and the medical regimen should be optimized.[11]

Heart transplantation is an option for patients with end-stage cardiac failure. The goal of transplantation is to

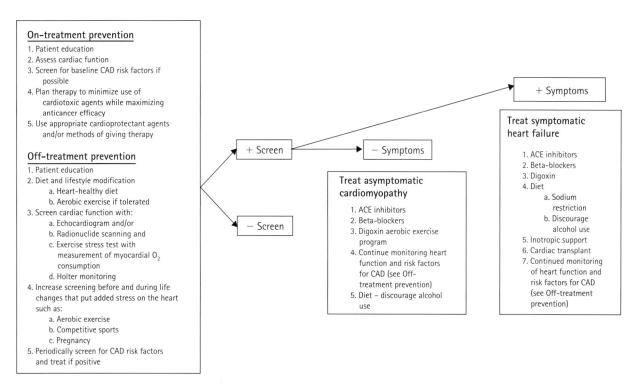

On-treatment prevention
1. Patient education
2. Assess cardiac funtion
3. Screen for baseline CAD risk factors if possible
4. Plan therapy to minimize use of cardiotoxic agents while maximizing anticancer efficacy
5. Use appropriate cardioprotectant agents and/or methods of giving therapy

Off-treatment prevention
1. Patient education
2. Diet and lifestyle modification
   a. Heart-healthy diet
   b. Aerobic exercise if tolerated
3. Screen cardiac function with:
   a. Echocardiogram and/or
   b. Radionuclide scanning and
   c. Exercise stress test with measurement of myocardial O_2 consumption
   d. Holter monitoring
4. Increase screening before and during life changes that put added stress on the heart such as:
   a. Aerobic exercise
   b. Competitive sports
   c. Pregnancy
5. Periodically screen for CAD risk factors and treat if positive

+ Screen

− Screen

− Symptoms

+ Symptoms

Treat asymptomatic cardiomyopathy
1. ACE inhibitors
2. Beta-blockers
3. Digoxin aerobic exercise program
4. Continue monitoring heart function and risk factors for CAD (see Off-treatment prevention)
5. Diet – discourage alcohol use

Treat symptomatic heart failure
1. ACE inhibitors
2. Beta-blockers
3. Digoxin
4. Diet
   a. Sodium restriction
   b. Discourage alcohol use
5. Inotropic support
6. Cardiac transplant
7. Continued monitoring of heart function and risk factors for CAD (see Off-treatment prevention)

Figure 4a.2 *Recommended screening and treatment of cardiomyopathy in patients treated with cardiotoxic cancer therapy. ACE, angiotensin-converting enzyme; CAD, coronary artery disease. (Reproduced with permission from Simbre et al. Current Treatment Options in Cardiovascular Medicine 2001; 3:493–505.)*

improve functional capacity, quality of life and length of life. Rejection is no more likely in cancer survivors than in other transplant recipients.[73] Cancer survivors require no significant modification of immunosuppression and their 2-year survival rate is similar to that of other recipients. Absolute contraindications to this approach are active rheumatologic disease, any major systemic condition with the potential to further deteriorate on immunosuppression and active oncologic disease. The relative contraindications are active infection, active ulcer disease, severe diabetes mellitus, recently treated cancer (not yet reaching 5-year event-free survival) and any condition that would limit the potential for full rehabilitation, such as cognitive impairment, psychiatric instability, alcohol or drug abuse, and repeated noncompliance.[11]

The extended prognosis for patients with advanced CHF treated medically remains worse than the extended prognosis for those who undergo transplantation. Unfortunately, the inadequate supply of donor organs, the cost of post-transplant care and the finite lifespan after transplantation require that indications for transplantation be based on the 1–2-year prognosis (Figure 4a.2).[11,80] As further information regarding troponin, other biochemical markers and imaging modalities is obtained, the recommendations for screening for transplantation may change. Additional research into cardiotoxicity in long-term survivors should also allow evidence-based studies

of lifestyle and medical interventions for preventing and treating cardiomyopathy.

CONCLUSION

Advances in chemotherapy have significantly increased the number of children cured of childhood cancer. However, the toxicities associated with chemotherapy affect the quality of the cure. Curing childhood cancers remains the priority but measures can be taken to minimize the development of cardiotoxicity. Treatment protocols should be adjusted on the basis of knowledge about cardiotoxicity, which is affected by cumulative dose, dosing regimens, concomitant therapy and strategies to reduce cardiotoxicity (dose adjustments, use of cardioprotectants and use of less cardiotoxic analogues).

Long-term cancer survivors need ongoing monitoring. Patients with early evidence of cardiac damage are at greatest risk for cardiomyopathy but many patients may also develop late cardiotoxicity. Predicting individual risk for the development and progression of cardiotoxicity is difficult. Ongoing study is needed to further refine detection and monitoring strategies. Echocardiography is a widely available, non-invasive test appropriate for children and advances in this technology have allowed

the detection of subclinical changes. Laboratory tests, particularly for cardiac troponins, also show promise in identifying patients at higher risk. Radiologic techniques that detect the biochemical changes in cardiac injury may allow more sophisticated imaging and detection of permanent and potentially progressive heart damage. The goal of each of these assessments is to identify patients at risk and allow appropriate monitoring schedules. Further study and longer follow-up will define which evaluations are most useful.

There have been many advances in the area of pediatric oncology, but further investigation is needed to eliminate the cost of the cure.

KEY POINTS

- Youth at time of treatment, female sex and growth hormone deficiency are among the patient characteristics that increase the cardiotoxic potential of anthracyclines.
- Most cases of anthracycline-induced cardiotoxicity develop within the first year after therapy, but the prevalence and severity of cardiac abnormalities both increase with longer follow-up.
- Although continuous infusion of anthracyclines reduces peak concentration, it does not appear to be cardioprotective in children.
- Higher cumulative dose of anthracyclines increases the risk of cardiotoxicity and concomitant radiation therapy may also do so.
- Adding cardioprotectant drugs to an anthracycline regimen and substituting anthracyclines with analogues are two ways to reduce the risk of cardiotoxicity.
- Echocardiography and cardiac troponin testing are among the most useful methods of assessing cardiac injury.
- Long-term cancer survivors should be encouraged to adopt heart-healthy diets and lifestyles with aerobic exercise, if not contraindicated by cardiac impairment.
- Angiotensin-converting enzyme inhibitors and beta-blockers are beneficial for both clinical and subclinical cardiac abnormalities.
- Heart transplantation may be necessary when pharmacologic therapy fails.

REFERENCES

1. Lipshultz SE. Ventricular dysfunction clinical research in infants, children, and adolescents. *Prog Pediatr Cardiol 2000*; **12**:1–28.
2. Mertens AC, Yasui Y, Neglia JP, *et al.* Late mortality experience in five-year survivors of childhood and adolescent cancer: The Childhood Cancer Survivor Study. *J Clin Oncol* 2001; **19**:3163–3172.
3. Moller TR, Garwicz S, Barlow L, *et al.* Decreasing late mortality among five-year survivors of cancer in childhood and adolescence: a population-based study in the Nordic countries. *J Clin Oncol* 2001; **19**:3173–3181.
4. Von Hoff DD, Layard MW, Basa P, *et al.* Risk factors for doxorubicin-induced congestive heart failure. *Ann Intern Med* 1979; **97**:710–717.
5. Praga C, Beretta G, Vigo PL, *et al.* Adriamycin cardiotoxicity: a survey of 1273 patients. *Cancer Treat Rep* 1979; **63**:827–834.
♦6. Green DM, Hyland A, Chung CS, *et al.* Cancer and cardiac mortality among 15-year survivors of cancer diagnosed during childhood or adolescence. *J Clin Oncol* 1999; **17**:3207–3215.
♦7. Giantris A, Abdurrahman L, Hinkle A, *et al.* Anthracycline-induced cardiotoxicity in children and young adults. *Crit Rev Oncol Hematol* 1998; **27**:53–68.
8. Steinherz LJ, Wexler LH. The prevention of anthracycline cardiomyopathy. *Prog Pediatr Cardiol* 1998; **8**:97–108.
9. Jemal A, Thomas A, Murray T, Thun M. Cancer Statistics 2002. *CA* 2002; **52**:23–47.
10. Tracy RP, Lemaitre RN, Psaty BM, *et al.* Relationship of C-reactive protein to risk of cardiovascular disease in the elderly. Results from the Cardiovascular Health Study and the Rural Health Promotion Project. *Arterioscler Thromb Vasc Biol* 1997; **17**:1121–1127.
♦11. Simbre VC, Adams MJ, Deshpande SS, *et al.* Cardiomyopathy caused by antineoplastic therapies. *Curr Treat Options Cardiovasc Med* 2001; **3**:493–505.
12. Pai VB, Nahata MC. Cardiotoxicity of chemotherapeutic agents. *Drug Safety* 2000; **22**:263–302.
13. Von Hoff DD, Rozencweig M, Layard M, *et al.* Daunomycin-induced cardiotoxicity in children and adults: a review of 110 cases. *Am J Med* 1977; **62**:200–208.
14. Dearth J, Osborn R, Wilson E, *et al.* Anthracycline-induced cardiomyopathy in children: a report of six cases. *Med Pediatr Oncol* 1984; **12**:54–58.
15. Pratt CB, Ransom JL, Evans WE. Age-related adriamycin cardiotoxicity in children. *Cancer Treat Rep* 1978; **62**:1381–1385.
16. Lipshultz SE, Lipsitz SR, Mone SM, *et al.* Late cardiac effects of doxorubicin therapy for acute lymphoblastic leukemia in childhood. *N Engl J Med* 1991; **324**:808–815.
♦17. Lipshultz SE, Lipsitz SR, Mone SM, *et al.* Female sex and higher drug dose as risk factors for late cardiotoxic effects of doxorubicin therapy for childhood cancer. *N Engl J Med* 1995; **332**:1738–1743.
♦18. Krischer JP, Cuthbertson DD, Epstein S, *et al.* Risk factors for early anthracycline clinical cardiotoxicity in children: the Pediatric Oncology Group experience. *Prog Pediatr Cardiol* 1998; **8**:83–90.
19. Silber JH, Jakacki RI, Larsen RL, *et al.* Increased risk of cardiac dysfunction after anthracyclines in girls. *Med Pediatr Oncol* 1993; **21**:477–479.
20. Rodvold KA, Rushing DA, Tewksbury DA. Doxorubicin clearance in the obese. *J Clin Oncol* 1988; **6**:1321–1327.
21. Green DM, Grigoriev YA, Nan B, *et al.* Congestive heart failure after treatment for Wilms' tumor: a report from the National Wilms' Tumor Study Group. *J Clin Oncol* 2001; **19**:1926–1934.
22. Krischer JP, Epstein S, Cuthbertson DD, *et al.* Clinical cardiotoxicity following anthracycline treatment for childhood cancer: the Pediatric Oncology Group experience. *J Clin Oncol* 1997; **15**:1544–1552.
23. Hinkle AS, Truesdell SC, Proukou CB, Constine LS. Cardiotoxicity related to cancer therapy. *Prog Pediatr Cardiol* 1998; **8**:145–155.
24. Schriock EA, Schell MJ, Carter M, *et al.* Abnormal growth patterns and adult short stature in 115 long-term survivors of childhood leukemia. *J Clin Oncol* 1991; **9**:400–405.

25. Silverman BL, Friedlander JR. Is growth hormone good for the heart? *J Pediatr* 1997; **131**:S70–S74.

26. Rosen T, Bengtsson BA. Premature mortality due to cardiovascular disease in hypopituitarism. *Lancet* 1990; **336**:285–288.

27. Cittadini A, Cuocolo A, Merola B, *et al.* Impaired cardiac performance in GH-deficient adults and its improvement after GH replacement. *Am J Physiol* 1994; **267**:E219–E225.

28. Johannsson G, Bengtsson BA, Andersson B, *et al.* Long-term cardiovascular effects of growth hormone treatment in GH-deficient adults: preliminary data in a small group of patients. *Clin Endocrinol* 1996; **45**:305–314.

29. Cuneo RC, Salomon F, Watts GF, *et al.* Growth hormone treatment improves serum lipids and lipoproteins in adults with growth hormone deficiency. *Metabolism* 1993; **42**:1519–1523.

30. Bengtsson BA, Eden S, Lonn L, *et al.* Treatment of adults with growth hormone (GH) deficiency with recombinant human GH. *J Clin Endocrinol Metab* 1993; **76**:309–317.

31. Taback SP, Dean HJ, members of the Canadian Growth Hormone Advisory Committee. Mortality in Canadian children with growth hormone (GH) deficiency receiving GH therapy 1967–1992. *J Clin Endocrinol* 1996; **81**:1693–1696.

32. Crepaz R, Pitscheider W, Radetti G, *et al.* Cardiovascular effects of high-dose growth hormone treatment in growth hormone-deficient subjects. *Pediatr Cardiol* 1995; **16**:223–227.

33. Katz A, Goldenberg I, Maoz C, *et al.* Peripartum cardiomyopathy occurring in a patient previously treated with doxorubicin. *Am J Med Sci* 1997; **314**:399–400.

34. Davis LE, Brown CE. Peripartum heart failure in a patient treated previously with doxorubicin. *Obstet Gynecol* 1988; **71**(3 Pt 2): 506–508.

35. Postma A, Bink-Boelkens MTE, Beaufort-Krol GCM, *et al.* Late cardiotoxicity after treatment for a malignant bone tumor. *Med Pediatr Oncol* 1996; **26**:230–237.

36. Nysom K, Holm K, Lipsitz SR, *et al.* The relation between cumulative anthracycline dose and late cardiotoxicity in survivors of childhood leukemia. *J Clin Oncol* 1998; **16**:545–550.

◆37. Grenier MA, Lipshultz SE. Epidemiology of anthracycline cardiotoxicity in children and adults. *Semin Oncol* 1998; **25**(Suppl. 10):72–85.

38. Lipshultz SE, Sanders SP, Goorin A, *et al.* Monitoring for anthracycline cardiotoxicity. *Pediatrics* 1994; **93**:433–437.

39. Steinherz LJ, Steinherz PG, Tan C. Cardiac failure and dysrhythmias 6–19 years after anthracycline therapy: a series of 15 patients. *Med Pediatr Oncol* 1995; **24**:352–361.

40. Lipshultz, SE, Colan, SD, Sanders, SP, Sallan SE. Cardiac mechanics after growth hormone therapy in pediatric adriamycin recipients [abstract]. *Pediatr Res* 1989; **25**(Suppl):153A.

41. Henderson IC, Allegra JC, Woodcock T, *et al.* Randomized clinical trial comparing mitoxantrone with doxorubicin in previously treated patients with metastatic breast cancer. *J Clin Oncol* 1989; **7**:560–571.

42. Bristow MR, Thompson PD, Martin R, *et al.* Early anthracycline cardiotoxicity. *Am J Med* 1978; **65**:823–832.

43. Bristow MR, Mason JW, Billingham ME, *et al.* Doxorubicin cardiomyopathy: evaluation by phonocardiography, endomyocardial biopsy and cardiac catheterization. *Ann Intern Med* 1978; **88**:168–175.

44. Cortes EP, Lutman G, Wanka J, *et al.* Adriamycin (NSC-123127) cardiotoxicity: a clinicopathologic correlation. *Cancer Chemother Rep* 1975; **6**:215–225.

45. Lipshultz SE, Giantris AL, Lipsitz SR, *et al.* Doxorubicin administration by continuous infusion is not cardioprotective: The Dana–Farber 91-01 Acute Lymphoblastic Leukemia Protocol. *J Clin Oncol* 2002; **20**:1677–1682.

46. Levitt GA, Sorenson K, Dorup I, Bull C, Sullivan I. Duration of anthracycline administration: does it affect late cardiac outcome? *Med Pediatr Oncol* 2001; **37**:307 (abstract).

47. Speyer JL, Green MD, Kramer E, *et al.* Protective effect of the bispiperazinedione ICRF-187 against doxorubicin-induced cardiac toxicity in women with advanced breast cancer. *N Engl J Med* 1988; **319**:745–752.

48. Speyer JL, Green MD, Zeleniuch-Jacquotte A, *et al.* ICRF-187 permits longer treatment with doxorubicin in women with breast cancer. *J Clin Oncol* 1992; **10**:117–127.

49. Swain SM, Whaley FS, Gerber MC, *et al.* Cardioprotection with dexrazoxane for doxorubicin-containing therapy in advanced breast cancer. *J Clin Oncol* 1997; **15**:1318–1332.

◆50. Wexler LH, Andrich MP, Venzon D, *et al.* Randomized trial of the cardioprotective agent ICRF-187 in pediatric sarcoma patients treated with doxorubicin. *J Clin Oncol* 1996; **14**:362–372.

51. Lipshultz SE, Colan SD, Silverman LB, *et al.* Dexrazoxane reduces incidence of doxorubicin-associated acute myocardiocyte injury in patients with acute lymphoblastic leukemia (ALL). *Proc Am Soc Clin Oncol* 2002; **21**:390a (#1557).

52. Bu'Lock FA, Mott MG, Oakhill A, *et al.* Left ventricular diastolic function after anthracycline chemotherapy in childhood: relation with systolic function, symptoms, and pathophysiology. *Br Heart J* 1995; **73**:340–350.

53. Pihkala J, Saarinen UM, Lundstrom U, *et al.* Myocardial function in children and adolescents after therapy with anthracyclines and chest irradiation. *Eur J Cancer* 1996; **32A**:97–103.

54. Steinherz LJ, Graham T, Hurwitz R, *et al.* Guidelines for cardiac monitoring of children during and after anthracycline therapy: Report of the Cardiology Committee of the Children's Cancer Study Group. *Pediatrics* 1992; **89**:942–949.

55. Lipshultz SE, Sanders SP, Goorin AM, *et al.* Monitoring for anthracycline cardiotoxicity. *Pediatrics* 1994; **93**:433–437.

56. Schwartz CL, Hovvie WI, Truesdell S, *et al.* Corrected QT interval prolongation in anthracycline-treated survivors of childhood cancer. *J Clin Oncol* 1993; **11**:1906–1910.

57. Druck MN, Gulenchyn KY, Evans WK, *et al.* Radionuclide angiography and endomyocardial biopsy in the assessment of doxorubicin cardiotoxicity. *Cancer* 1998; **53**:1667–1674.

◆58. Kremer LCM, van Dalen EC, Offringa M, *et al.* Anthracycline-induced clinical heart failure in a cohort of 607 children: long-term follow-up study. *J Clin Oncol* 2001; **19**:191–196.

59. Nousiainen T, Vanninen E, Jantunen E, *et al.* Anthracycline-induced cardiomyopathy: long-term effects on myocardial cell integrity, cardiac adrenergic innervation and fatty acid uptake. *Clin Physiol* 2001; **21**:123–128.

60. Jeon TJ, Lee JD, Ha JW, *et al.* Evaluation of cardiac adrenergic neuronal damage in rats with doxorubicin-induced cardiomyopathy using iodine-131 MIBG autoradiography and PGP 9.5 immunohistochemistry. *Eur J Nucl Med* 2000; **27**:686–693.

61. Nony P, Guastalla JP, Rebattu P, *et al.* In vivo measurement of myocardial oxidative metabolism and blood flow does not show changes in cancer patients undergoing doxorubicin therapy. *Cancer Chemother Pharmacol* 2000; **45**:375–380.

62. Schaefer S. Magnetic resonance spectroscopy in human cardiomyopathies. *J Cardiovasc Mag Res* 2000; **2**:151–157.

63. Hayakawa H, Komada Y, Hirayama M, *et al.* Plasma levels of natriuretic peptides in relation to doxorubicin-induced cardiotoxicity and cardiac function in children with cancer. *Med Pediatr Oncol* 2001; **37**:4–9.

64. Nousiainen T, Jantunen E, Vanninen E, Remes J, Vuolteenaho O, Hartikainen J. Natriuretic peptides as markers of cardiotoxicity during doxorubicin treatment for non-Hodgkin's lymphoma. *Eur J Haematol* 1999; **62**:135–141.

65. Tikanoja T, Riikonen P, Perkkio M, Helenius T. Serum N-terminal atrial natriuretic peptide (NT-ANP) in the cardiac follow-up in children with cancer. *Med Pediatr Oncol* 1998; **31**:73–78.

66. Katus HA, Scheffold T, Remppis A, Zehlein J. Proteins of the troponin complex. *Lab Med* 1992; **23**:311–317.

67. Guyton AC. *Textbook of medical physiology*, 7th edn. Philadelphia; Saunders, 1986.
68. Bodor GZ. Cardiac troponin I: a highly specific biochemical marker for myocardial infarction. *J Clin Immunoassay* 1994; **17**:40–44.
69. Wu AH. Cardiac troponin T: biochemical, analytical, and clinical aspects. *J Clin Immunoassay* 1994; **17**:45–48.
70. Ottlinger ME, Pearsall L, Rifai N, Lipshultz SE. New developments in the biochemical assessment of myocardial injury in children: troponins T and I as highly sensitive and specific markers of myocardial injury. *Progr Pediatr Cardiol* 1998; **8**:71–81.
71. Storrow AB, Gibler WB. The role of cardiac markers in the emergency department. *Clin Chim Acta* 1999; **284**:187–196.
72. Gerhardt W, Katus H, Ravkilde J, *et al.* S-troponin T in suspected ischemic myocardial injury compared with mass and catalytic concentrations of S-creatine kinase isoenzyme MB. *Clin Chem* 1991; **37**:1405–1411.
73. Lipshultz SE, Rifai N, Sallan SE, *et al.* Predictive value of cardiac troponin T in pediatric patients at risk for myocardial injury. *Circulation* 1997; **96**:2641–2648.
74. Lipshultz SE, Sallan SE, Dalton V, *et al.* Elevated serum cardiac troponin-T as a marker for active cardiac injury during therapy for childhood acute lymphoblastic leukemia (ALL). *Proc ASCO* 1999; **18**:568A.
75. Executive summary of the third report of the National Cholesterol Education Program (NCEP) expert panel on detection, evaluation, and treatment of high blood cholesterol in adults (Adult Treatment Panel III). *JAMA* 2001; **285**:2486–2497.
76. Heart Failure Guideline Panel: Heart failure: evaluation and care of patients with left ventricular systolic dysfunction. *Clinical Practice Guideline No 11*. Rockville, MD: US Department of Health and Human Services, Agency for Health Care Policy and Research, 1994. ACCPR Publication **94**:6012.
77. Guidelines for the evaluation and management of heart failure. Report of the American College of Cardiology/American Heart Association Task Force on Practice Guidelines (Committee on Evaluation and Management of Heart Failure). *Circulation* 1995, **92**:2764–2784.
78. Pfeffer MA, Braunwald E, Moye LA, *et al.* Effect of captopril on mortality and morbidity in patients with left ventricular dysfunction after myocardial infarction. Results of the survival and ventricular enlargement trial. The SAVE Investigators. *N Engl J Med* 1992; **327**:669–677.
79. Lipshultz SE. Dexrazoxane for protection against cardiotoxic effects of anthracyclines in children. *J Clin Oncol* 1996; **14**:328–331.
◆80. Herman EH, Zhang J, Lipshultz SE, *et al.* Correlation between serum levels of cardiac troponin-T and the severity of chronic cardiomyopathy induced by doxorubicin. *J Clin Oncol* 1999; **17**:2237–2243.

4b

Radiation damage

GILL A LEVITT AND FRANK H SARAN

INTRODUCTION

Radiotherapy is the therapeutic use of γ-rays or X-rays to treat malignancies mediated by direct DNA damage or by the creation of free intracellular radicals. Radiotherapy is predominantly a local and locoregional treatment modality, which forms together with surgery and chemotherapy the backbone of modern oncological management strategies. Radiation-induced acute or late effects have been well documented. As early as 1899, Gassman described radiodermatitis and vascular lesions in association with radiation.[1] The prevalence of radiotherapy-induced late effects has increased. This is due to the continuous improvement in overall survival of pediatric and adolescent patients and, in turn, this has exposed the long gestation for the development of clinically important sequelae.

The mainstay of radiotherapy in the early part of the last century was either with orthovoltage or cobalt-60 (^{60}Co) megavoltage treatment machines. Orthovoltage machines deliver a maximum dose to the skin and lose their energy rapidly in depth. The delivery of therapeutically useful doses in deeper seated tumors, as for example required in the treatment for Hodgkin's disease, became available with the introduction of ^{60}Co megavoltage machines. A further improvement was achieved by the introduction of high-energy linear accelerators (LINACs) employing photons with a therapeutic range of 4–25 MV into routine clinical service. These treatment machines became commonly available in the latter part of the last century and today form the backbone of any department of radiotherapy worldwide.

The degree of differentiation, cell turnover and renewal potential of normal tissues determines the radiosensitivity of organs and the ability to recover from radiation-induced injuries. Today radiobiologists divide normal tissues into acute- and late-responding tissues. For acute-responding tissues (such as mucosal membranes or intestine), the late morbidity is closely related to total dose and overall treatment time. In contrast, in late-responding tissues, such as the heart or brain, the likelihood of late effects is closely related to the dose per fraction and to a lesser extent to the total dose given.

With the growing knowledge of radiation-induced morbidity and the increasing number of long-term survivors, radiation oncologists changed 'standard' fractionation regimens to reduce late sequelae. Fractionation schemes changed from four fractions per week with daily fraction sizes of 2.25–2.5 Gy to five fractions per week of 1.6–1.8 Gy. This went hand in hand with a continuous reduction in total doses of radiation delivered in many pediatric malignancies. This fractionation related benefit was further enhanced by a change in practice to daily parallel opposing fields instead of alternating anterior–posterior fields. This led to a more homogenous dose delivery, avoiding excess dose peaks to organs encompassed in the radiation volume.[2] An additional change of practice occurred in the treatment of Hodgkin's disease that significantly influenced cardiac late morbidity and mortality. After a total dose of 30 Gy, subcarinal blocks were positioned in 'mantle fields', limiting the total dose to the heart.

Most data on radiation-induced late effects reported between the 1960s and 1980s are from cohorts treated as

early as 1940. These are predominantly based on retrospective reviews of single-institution series employing radiation techniques and fractionation schemes, which no longer represent current standard of care. It is, therefore, important to observe closely the era of treatment and techniques of radiation employed when reviewing and interpreting the literature on radiation-induced morbidity.

PATHOPHYSIOLOGY

Many radiation-associated late effects are probably mediated by damage to the vasculature.[3] The capillaries are considered the most susceptible structure with the endothelial cells being the most radiosensitive cells within the vessel walls. The endothelium reacts to radiation in a number of ways, by cell swelling, increasing cell membrane permeability,[4] apoptosis[5] and increased leukocyte adhesiveness.[6] This results in loss of endothelial cells from the basement membrane leading to thrombosis and cell pyknosis. The viable endothelial cells have the capacity to repair radiation-induced damage, but it may cause intimal hyperplasia and occlusion of the lumen in the process. Damage to large vessels is less frequently seen and is thought in part to be secondary to injury of the vasa vasorum.[7] The histopathological findings of lipid deposits and fibrosis are very similar to those of atheroma and, therefore, non-specific.[4] High-dose radiation can rarely cause 'spontaneous' ruptures of major blood vessels, usually carotid arteries, and is commonly in association with local surgical complications, such as infection.[8]

One hypothesis to explain the difference in tissue tolerance to therapeutic irradiation may relate to the ability of tissues to develop collateral blood vessels and to the density of the vaso vasorum. The varying findings after brain and cardiac radiation may be explained by this theory. Cerebral vessels, in particular, are lacking in the latter but have the ability to form a collateral blood supply.[9,10] The human heart lacks anastomoses between major arteries and there are no redundant vessels for recruitment in the damaged cardiac areas.[11]

Radiation damage of large veins is rare, but damage can occur to small and medium vessels in the liver and intestine. Veno-occlusive disease is an end-point for vascular damage as a result of radiation alone or in association with chemotherapy to the liver. Histopathologically the organ shows focal parenchymal congestion, with centrilobular necrosis from collagen fiber obstruction of the central sublobar and small portal veins.[12]

Heart

In the early parts of last century, the heart was believed to be an organ system resistant to radiotherapy-induced toxicity, as it represents an organ without high cell turnover and, therefore, was believed not to be affected by fractionated radiotherapy.

The first description of heart toxicity associated with radiotherapy was described as early as 1924.[13] The term radiation-induced heart disease (RIHD) was established following a systematic report of a series of long-term survivors treated with high-dose mediastinal irradiation, particularly for Hodgkin's disease.[14] RIHD is defined as the clinical and pathological conditions derived from radiotherapy-induced injuries to the heart.

Radiation-induced heart disease may manifest itself primarily in the pericardium, the myocardium or in the coronary arteries as an early or delayed reaction to therapeutic irradiation. Most commonly, early reactions occur within the first few weeks or months after the start of radiotherapy, while late sequelae usually require several years to manifest. The majority of acute injuries to the heart are transient and short lived. Improved understanding of RIHD is derived from animal models of the New Zealand White rabbit. This experimental animal system is closely related to the human heart structure and pathophysiology. Sequential studies of New Zealand White rabbits demonstrated a transient acute granulocytic infiltration of the heart following 6–8 hours after the start of mediastinal irradiation. Histopathologically, an extensive exudate of granulocytes was visible throughout the entire heart (parietal pericardium, epicardium, myocardium, endocardium and valves).[15] This cellular infiltrate disappears spontaneously after 48 hours. Electron microscopy performed a few days later revealed damage to the myocardial endothelium.

The late changes in humans are predominately seen in the pericardium with variable development of fibrosis and pericardial fluid, but rarely associated with an inflammatory cellular infiltrate. The exudate is a protein rich fluid (up to 6 g/dl) and approximately 30 per cent of pericardial effusions disappear spontaneously within 2–5 months.[16] The induced pericardial fibrosis can be progressive leading to constrictive pericarditis.[11]

The histopathological correlate to delayed myocardial damage induced by irradiation is myocyte death and cell replacement with diffuse patchy fibrosis without an inflammatory reaction and never involving the entire myocardium.[17] The myocardial damage has been shown to be secondary to radiation damage to the capillary bed in rats and rabbits.[18,19] Any morphological and functional myocardial damage is preceded by a severe reduction of the capillary network. The clinical effect is dictated by the remodeling potential of the heart. By the postnatal age of 6 months, the heart is composed of a defined number of myocytes, which remain constant throughout life. Cardiac development during infancy and childhood, required to keep pace with the increasing functional demands, occurs solely from myocyte hypertrophy and hyperplasia.

If substantial damage occurs at this stage, there will come a point where no further improvement in function can be achieved by cell hypertrophy and cardiac failure ensues.[20] It may be difficult to distinguish between the constrictive and restrictive components of myocardial damage in patients who have coexistent pericardial disease. To relate the etiology of myocardial disease solely to irradiation becomes even more difficult in modern series, as many patients are likely to receive cardiotoxic chemotherapy, particularly anthracyclines, as part of their management (see Chapter 4a).

Coronary artery disease (CAD) is a potentially life-threatening form of late sequel to radiation therapy. Radiation as a direct cause of the development of CAD was controversial for many years.[21] The reason for the controversy was the morphological similarity between radiation-induced CAD and other causes of CAD, such as atherosclerosis. Two mechanisms are implicated in the pathogenesis of CAD: as a result of microvasculopathy, or the development of atheromatous plaques. In small coronary arteries, the major cause for CAD is probably microvasculopathy.[18] In the New Zealand White rabbit model, ultrastructural damages of the capillaries were observed during the asymptomatic phase of the disease. This was accompanied by swelling of the endothelial cytoplasm and obliteration of the capillary lumen. The end-result was a significant reduction of the capillary/myocyte ratio with subsequent insufficient microcirculation and ischemia. This type of capillary damage may explain the sudden cardiac deaths observed in patients treated with mediastinal irradiation without abnormalities on previous angiography.[22]

In larger coronary arteries, atheromatous plaques occur. Animals studies imply the need for concomitant cofactors, such as high-cholesterol diets to induce atherosclerosis in radiated vessels.[23] This may not be relevant for humans as studies have noted young patients suffering from severe CAD.[22] Researchers have noted that in radiation-induced CAD, the media is more severely destroyed and there is increased thickening and fibrosis of the adventitia.[24] Boivin observed that, in a population of patients treated with mediastinal radiation for Hodgkin's disease, that there was a stronger association for death *from* CAD than death from other causes *with* ischaemic heart disease, implying that radiation causes more severe CAD than that seen in other causes of CAD.[21] Additionally, other coexisting risk factors (e.g. lifestyle toxins, such as smoking) precipitate RIHD further.

Thickening of the valvular endocardium has been described in a post mortem study.[22] It is currently unproven whether radiotherapy causes valvular disease. Most delayed cardiac late sequelae related to radiotherapy are mediated through vascular damage. Given that the cardiac valves do not contain blood vessels, it is difficult to establish a causal link between valvular disease

and radiotherapy. Furthermore, in large series of New Zealand White rabbits irradiated at various dose levels, no valvular disease has been reported.[15]

CLINICAL IMPACT

Recent reports on the causes of late deaths in patients treated during childhood or adolescence for cancer in both hospital- and population-based studies found that 10 per cent of patients died 5–35 years post-treatment.[25–28] The majority of late deaths were due to recurrent disease (67–70 per cent).[25,26] Treatment-related deaths account for 18–21 per cent with approximately 20 per cent of those being due to cardiotoxicity. It is impossible from these data to ascertain the exact contribution from radiation-induced cardiovascular injury to deaths in remission. Cardiac mortality is due to both radiation- and/or anthracycline-induced damage with standardized mortality ratios (SMRs) ranging from 8.2 to 5.8.[25,26] The relative risk (RR) of cardiac deaths from cardiac radiation compared with no radiation was increased [RR 2.2, 95% CI, 1.2–4.4].[25] As mentioned above, this risk has to be seen in the context of the era of treatment (1970–86). The RR was highest for Hodgkin's disease and Wilms' tumors, and many of the deaths occurred in patients requiring retreatment for relapse.[27]

The contribution of cerebrovascular disease to late mortality is more problematical to establish. This is in part due to the common practice of combining cerebrovascular disease with other central nervous system (CNS) causes. In the reported studies, the percentage of CNS tumors within the population varies from 3 to 25 per cent and, therefore, as a group, they may not be reliably represented owing to differing referral patterns and registration definitions.[26,29] In a population-based series, a SMR of 4.6 (95% CI, 3.3–6.2) due to CNS diseases was found when combining all causes.[27]

While mortality is well reported, there is little useful information on incidence of morbidity and severity of vascular damage in the literature. Two large epidemiological studies are currently being performed on long-term survivors (>14 000 survivors) in America[30] and the UK, which are addressing these questions.[31]

To date, only single-center studies or those consisting of particular diagnoses have reported on treatment-related morbidity.[32,33]

CLINICAL MANIFESTATIONS

Clinical manifestations of radiation-induced toxicity relate to the type of organs and/or the areas supplied by the irradiated blood vessels. The degree and type of

damage is dependent on the dose, fractionation, vessel-wall anatomy and genetic abnormalities, e.g. neurofibromatosis type1 (NF1), ataxia telangiectasia.[34,35] Vessel rupture is rarely seen in adults and has not been reported in children, in part because the radiotherapy doses required to treat carcinomas (50–70 Gy) are usually not required in the treatment of the majority of extracranial childhood malignancies. In adults, the risk factors for vascular damage are associated with timing of surgery and concomitant infection, particularly with the development of fistula formation.[36]

The following section will be divided into the effects on the heart and coronary vessels, cerebral and carotid vessels, and other vessels within radiation fields.

Heart and coronary vessels

Any radiation involving the thorax or chest wall potentially may include the heart, and thus may give rise to radiation-induced cardiac toxicity. There are few reports on long-term sequelae in children who have received radiation alone to the heart. As previously indicated, it is difficult to disentangle the effects of additional chemotherapy and lifestyle on late sequelae.

The majority of the literature relevant to this area is derived from adult cohorts treated for breast cancer and Hodgkin's disease, the latter containing a proportion of children and adolescents. The largest comprehensive study assessing late sequelae reported 635 patients less than 21 years at diagnosis treated for Hodgkin's disease between 1961 and 1991.[37] Of those, only 57 had received no mediastinal radiation. The remainder received radiation alone or in combination with chemotherapy, only 56 received anthracycline-containing chemotherapy regimes. Of the cohort, 12 patients died from cardiac causes with a RR of 29.6 (95% CI, 16.0–49.3) and an actuarial risk of death of 8.8 per cent at 22 years. The absolute risk was 17.7 excess cases in 10 000 person years. There was no gender preference, although there was a trend for a higher risk in males and those receiving combination treatment (actuarial risk in the radiation alone group was 10 per cent compared with 12 per cent in combination group; $p = 0.03$).[38]

The most common acute radiation-induced toxicity is transient asymptomatic pericardial effusions. The risk of radiation-induced pericarditis follows a sigmoid curve and increases steeply with higher doses to the whole pericardium. It has been estimated that the risk is low at doses below 40 Gy, rising to 10 per cent at 50 Gy and 50 per cent at 60 Gy.[39] There is good evidence of a dose–response relationship between the incidence of pericarditis and the dose per fraction delivered.

Diagnosis can be established either by chest X-ray or echocardiography. Conventional posterior–anterior chest

X-rays will detect pericardial effusions of 250–500 ml and is a non-sensitive technique, whereas echocardiography can detect effusions as low as 20 ml. The clinical relevance of very small effusions is unknown. Most reports on pericardial toxicity are in children and adolescents treated with mediastinal radiation for Hodgkin's disease. The incidence of clinically relevant pericarditis in patients treated since the mid-1970s varies between 0 and 8 per cent,[40,41] but is rarely life threatening. The Stanford group reported two deaths in 635 survivors related to pericardial damage. One patient died at 2.6 years post-treatment owing to pericarditis and the other at 19 years after diagnosis from pancardities.[37] Clinically identified acute pericarditis based on positional chest pain, pericardial friction rub, cardiomegaly and/or effusions on chest X-ray or echocardiography was noted in 32 patients (0.3–18 years post-radiation). Constrictive pericarditis requiring pericardiectomy occurred in 2 per cent of patients at a mean interval of 7 years with the earliest intervention required after 10 months. All patients received a radiation dose larger than 38 Gy to the mediastinum. In a retrospective echocardiographic study of 28 asymptomatic children, pericardial thickening was found in 43 per cent at a median follow-up of 7.5 years. All received mediastinal radiation doses of 20–40 Gy by equally weighted anterior/posterior fields between 1968 and 1981. The risk of subclinical abnormalities increased with longer follow-up.[42]

Late myocardial damage occurs after direct radiation damage on myocytes and/or ischaemia from capillary damage causing secondary myocyte loss. The myocardium is prone to acute toxicity manifesting as flattening or inversion of the T wave on electrocardiogram (ECG).[43] This phenomenon usually resolves within the first year after treatment. In adults, measurably reduced ventricular function 5–15 years after radiotherapy could be demonstrated in 10–20 per cent of patients receiving 30–36 Gy to the heart, as measured by radionuclide angiography or heart catheterization.[44,45] Mean organ doses of 50 Gy lead to a reduced ejection fraction in approximately one-third of patients.[46]

Currently, a number of treatment regimens for children and adolescents incorporate radiation to the heart and anthracycline-based chemotherapy. Anthracylines are well known to cause myocardial damage with diffuse focal myocyte loss and replacement fibrosis.[47] Anthracycline cardiomyopathy is dose dependent and progressive with lengthening follow-up interval (see Chapter 4a). There is evidence of a synergistic effect when high doses of anthracyclines are given in conjunction with cardiac irradiation.[48] The children and adolescents at most risk are those treated for mediastinal Hodgkin's disease and Wilms' tumor with pulmonary metastases, or a left-sided abdominal tumor requiring flank irradiation.[49] Estimations of radiation doses to the heart from left-flank

radiation can vary between 25 and 100 per cent of the tumor dose involving varying volumes of the ventricles.[50,51]

Patients treated on the American national Wilms' tumor studies (NWTS 1–4) showed an increased risk of congestive cardiac failure if they received anthracyclines and left-flank irradiation (RR $= 1.8/$ Gy; $p = 0.037$). For patients receiving anthracyclines and whole-lung irradiation, the RR was $1.6/10$ Gy ($p = 0.013$).[33] An earlier study found mediastinal radiation as a dichotomous variable in a regression analysis for cardiac disease.[52] Two other studies were unable to confirm this relationship. Using cardiac failure as an end-point in a diverse patient cohort, radiation was not correlated with the incidence of cardiomyopathy.[53] A further study using subclinical echocardiographic abnormalities in asymptomatic Wilms' tumor survivors as an end-point was also unable to confirm a causal relationship.[50]

Radiation fields not specifically targeting the heart or lungs may, because of the close anatomical proximity, radiate areas of the heart and cause RIHD. Subclinical cardiac dysfunction was reported in a group of patients receiving spinal radiation through a single posterior field.[51] The authors hypothesize that cardiotoxicity was related to the asymmetric radiation dose to the posterior left ventricular wall with a mean dose of 25.77 Gy (range 9.6–36 Gy). Although a number of patients received anthracycline-containing chemotherapy, the dose to the posterior wall predicted increased end-wall stress in a multiple regression analysis ($p = 0.007$). Figures 4b.1–4b.3 (and Plates 2 and 3) demonstrate cardiac radiation dose and volume in a patient treated for medulloblastoma with craniospinal radiation.

Isolated case reports have highlighted the possibility of radiation damage involving the conducting system. Conduction defects have been reported in patients undergoing mediastinal irradiation usually detected at least 5 years after completion of treatment.[39] This occurred predominately in patients treated for Hodgkin's disease without a subcarinal block and at higher doses than commonly applied today in association with other forms of RIHD.[54] The incidence of conduction defects in two screened childhood and adolescent Hodgkin's disease population varied from no cases in patients receiving parallel opposed fields treated daily with a median fraction size of 1.5 Gy (total dose range 25–40 Gy) to 6 of 28 patients (21 per cent) receiving 34–47 Gy.[55] In the large record extraction study from Stanford, 4 of 635 patients had conductive defects. All four patients received more than 40 Gy to the mediastinum.[38] The defects varied from incomplete to very rare complete bundle branch blocks, usually right sided, to first- to third-degree atrioventricular blocks. Most commonly, the level of an atrioventricular block is infranodal and is associated with patchy fibrosis on pathologic examination.

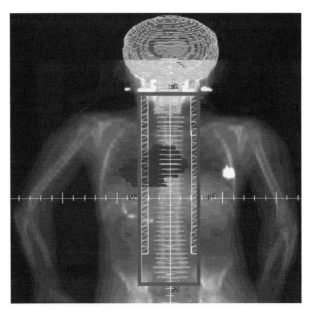

Figure 4b.1 *A radiograph that has been digitally reconstructed from the planning computed tomography (CT) scan for a patient with medulloblastoma. On each CT slice, the cerebrospinal fluid-bearing areas of the brain and spinal cord (green), and the heart (red) have been outlined. The spine field component of the craniospinal irradiation (blue) has its width limited with shielding (yellow) for most of its upper length to reduce unnecessary irradiation of normal tissue. Despite this, a major portion of the heart still receives radiation exiting from the spinal field. See plate for colour.*

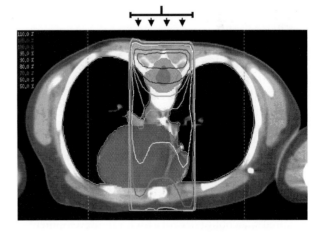

Figure 4b.2 *A mid-thoracic transverse section from the planning computed tomography scan as displayed on the planning computer for a patient with medulloblastoma lying in the prone position for craniospinal irradiation. Radiation from the spinal field (black arrows) enters posteriorly and aims to encompass the target (green) with at least 95 per cent of the prescribed dose as shown by the green isodose line. A significant proportion of the heart (red) receives between 90 per cent of dose to its posterior wall and 70 per cent of dose to its anterior wall as the radiation exits anteriorly through the patient. See plate for colour.*

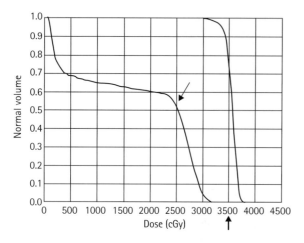

Figure 4b.3 *A dose–volume histogram of the above patient with medulloblastoma treated with craniospinal axis (CSA) irradiation. The x-axis represents the dose received and the y-axis the cumulative volume of a tissue as outlined on the planning computed tomography scan. The line on the right represents the entire cerebrospinal fluid space and it receives the prescribed dose of 35 Gy (bottom arrow) relatively homogeneously. The line on the left depicts the dose received by the heart and the dose–volume histogram demonstrates that more than 50 per cent of the cardiac volume receives up to 25 Gy (top arrow), a dose associated with potential cardiac late morbidity.*

Valvular disease has been reported in a few cases, but in association with other features of RIHD or as an observation on screening.[55] In Hancock's series, two deaths were attributed to valvular disease. Three patients underwent surgery for abnormal valves but no comment is made as to whether these patients underwent pretreatment screening.[38] In an autopsy study, valvular endocardial fibrosis was found in 12 of 16 patients, treated with medastinal radiation.[24]

Repeated publications on coronary artery disease have emphasized the similarity between typical atherosclerosis and radiation-induced coronary athersclerosis. The main difference is the appearance of disease occurring at a younger age and in vessels confined to the radiation field. There has been a suggestion that hyperlipidemia is required as an obligatory cofactor for the development of atherosclerosis.[38]

A 'standard' mediastinal/mantle field for the treatment of Hodgkin's disease encompasses in the first phase approximately 50–70 per cent of the heart. Following subcarinal blocking, the cardiac volume is reduced by approximately 20–40 per cent. Despite the reduction in cardiac volume exposed to high-dose radiation, the proximal coronary arteries will receive the full dose of radiotherapy prescribed. All reported series on CAD relate to patients treated with such an approach. In the Stanford series, the relative risk of myocardial infarction was 41.5

(95% CI, 18.1–82.1) with an actuarial risk of 6 per cent at 22 years. In patients receiving radiation alone the RR was 52.2 (95% CI, 21–108.7) and 21.1 (95% CI, 0–104.4) for those receiving combined modality treatment. Of the 13 patients, seven died from acute myocardial infarction and three required coronary revascularization.[37] All received total radiation doses of 42–45 Gy. Green reviewed the causes of death in a cohort of 15-year survivors of childhood cancer with a mean follow-up interval of 24 ± 6.13 years and an actuarial survival of 88 ± 2 per cent at 35 years.[27] Of the 9 per cent of patients who died (25/275), only three patients died as a result of CAD following irradiation. Two patients received 21 Gy to the mediastinum. The third patient was treated with 36 Gy to the mediastinum combined with a moderate dose of doxorubicin. He died after a mitral valve replacement and arterial bypass grafting. Postradiation CAD has a characteristic pattern on coronary angiography with tendancy for proximal lesions involving the left main and ostium of the right coronary artery.[56] In these patients coronary artery bypass surgery is less successful owing to other comorbidities (diffuse mediastinal scarring, pulmonary dysfunction). Internal mammary arteries are often used as an arterial conduit and may be at risk of early restenosis. Preoperative normal selective angiography does not guarantee long-term patency.[57,58]

Cerebral and carotid vessels

Radiation damage to vessels of all sizes has been reported. The extent of the clinical manifestation depends on the distribution, size of the vessels and the remodeling.[7]

The commonest clinicopathological finding is mineralizing microangiopathy. Diagnosis is made on computed tomography (CT) imaging as calcification in small blood vessels typically located at the gray/white matter junction. This pathology is predominantly seen in survivors of acute lymphoblastic leukemia with an incidence of up to 30 per cent in patents who received radiation and/or intrathecal methotrexate.[59,60] Mineralizing microangiopathy is rarely documented in patients who receive less than 20 Gy.[61] The prevalence and severity of CT/ magnetic resonance imaging (MRI) findings probably decreases with increasing length of follow-up.[62] Many patients with mineralizing microangiopathy have no symptoms. Others present with cognitive deficits, headache, focal seizures or ataxia.[63] The radiological findings do not correlate with clinical presentation and severity of symptoms.

Cerebrovascular accidents (CVAs) can present as a result of radiation-induced localized atherosclerosis, intracranial or extracranial arterial occulsion/stenosis, moyamoya syndrome, cerebral hemorrhage or aneursymal formation.[64–70] Vasculopathies tend to be reported in

young children with brain tumors treated with high radiation doses, although there are rare reports of patients who received low-dose cranial radiation (10–24 Gy) or neck radiation.[66,67] A single institution case-note review of CNS malignancies identified strokes in 1.6 per cent of the cohort (equivalent to 4.03 strokes/1 000 patient years[69]). Ascertainment of data was available for 84 per cent of all patients treated at the center. To put this in perspective, the incidence of CVAs is comparable to patients with sickle cell disease. Of the 13 patients diagnosed with a vasculopathy, ten were diagnosed with a thrombosis of the internal carotid or major cerebral arteries. The remainder had infarctions in the watershed distribution. The only significant risk factor identified on stepwise logistic analysis was previous radiotherapy ($p = 0.007$), although type of primary tumor approached significance. This relationship is supported by other reports of centrally placed tumors, particularly optic pathway gliomas, being at an increased risk of CVAs.[69–71] Radiation dose in the affected patients varied between 27 and 70 Gy. Median onset of symptoms was 2.3 years (range 0.3–15.8 years).[69]

Coexisting NF1 has also been recognized as risk factor. Grill identified vasculopathy in 13 of 69 optic pathway gliomas with a significantly higher incidence in patients with NF1.[72] Of the NF1 cohort, 11 out of 37 (30 per cent) developed vasculopathies during follow-up compared with 2 out of 32 (5 per cent) without NF1 ($p = 0.015$). Similarly, Kestle found an association in a NF1 population with 60 per cent of patients developing a moyamoya syndrome following a radical course of radiotherapy.[71]

Cerebrovascular abnormalities can occur after any radiotherapy involving either the whole or parts of the brain for non-CNS malignancies. Laitt reports two cases of asymptomatic vasculopathy identified on magnetic resonance angiography (MRA) in acute lymphoblastic leukemia survivors who received cranial radiation at doses of 18 Gy.[67] Currently there are no reports on vasculapathies in patients treated for paramenigeal soft tissue sarcoma, although they maybe at certain risk.

The moyamoya syndrome (the term originating from the Japanese description of the angiographic abnormalities 'puff of smoke') is another documented manifestation of radiation-induced vascular damage. It is characterized by progressive bilateral intracranial carotid artery stenosis, resulting in the development of a collateral circulation in response to the occluded internal carotid and/or the proximal parts of the anterior and middle cerebral arteries.[73] This syndrome has been well documented by case histories and small series of children who have received cranial radiation.[71,74–76] Moyamoya syndrome can coexist with NF1 with or without identifiable tumors and untreated central brain tumors.[34,77,78] Bitzer reviewed the literature on progressive cerebral occlusive disease in 1995 and described 30 children with a range of ages at diagnosis from birth up to 15 years with a median

age of 3 years.[79] The underlying tumor was most frequently located parasellar with 50 per cent of the children diagnosed with optic pathway gliomas followed by craniopharyngioma (30 per cent). In the majority of cases, symptoms appeared within 8 years of completion of radiotherapy. The author suggests that dose and technique of radiation regime were not related to the appearance of vascular changes, but the radiation dose was high in the majority of case reports. Yet a few cases have been identified with radiation doses as low as 10–20 Gy.[7,66,79]

Complicated migraine-type episodes have been reported after cranial radiation with doses ranging from 40 to 60 Gy. Radiological imaging studies revealed no evidence of vasculopathy.[80] The author suggested this may represent radiation-induced transient vascular instability and noted that it can be provoked by angiography.

The presentation of radiation-induced CVA is similar to those due to other causes and is dependent on the area of ischemia. Headaches, seizures, hemiparesis and aphasia are common symptoms.

In moyamoya disease, the majority of patients present with focal neurological deficits with 25 per cent of them manifesting initially as transient ischemic attacks. Less frequent symptoms are seizures, headaches, dizziness, speech disturbances and altered consciousness. Intellectual impairment is the initial presentation in 15 per cent of cases and increases during the course of the disease to 29 per cent.[79] Carotid angiography or MRA is essential for diagnosis of radiation-induced vasculopathies. The ability to form collaterals in response to stenoses is more common in children or adolescents compared to adults, and is related to a better prognosis.

Cerebral aneuysms are a rare manifestation of radiation damage. Less than 20 cases are recorded in the literature between 1984 and 2001. Seven (35 per cent) occurred after radiation treatment in childhood between the age of 0.6 and 13 years. Diagnoses were medulloblastoma (4), astrocytoma (2) and germinoma.[9,65,81–83] All patients had received high radiation doses of 47–110 Gy with three receiving colloidal gold as part of their treatment. In all three cases the saccular aneurysms had developed at the site where the intrathecal gold was likely to have pooled.[81] Five suffered fatal subarachnoid hemorrhages.[9,65,82] The interval between radiation treatment and presentation was wide 0.8–19 years. Clipping was performed in the three most recent cases with good results, although the youngest patient died subsequently from cardiac failure.[9,82]

Lacunar lesions, detected on MRI as small white-matter cavities with signals on T1- and T2-weighted images characteristic of cerebrospinal fluid, are well described in the adult literature. They are thought to be the result of ischemic infarcts. They have recently been described for the first time in children with brain tumors treated with radiotherapy with or without chemotherapy. In a series of 421 pediatric brain-tumor patients, Fouladi described

these lesions in 6 per cent of cases. Of clinical importance is that all lesions were asymptomatic. The number of lesions may increase with follow-up, but is not associated with neuropsychological decline.[84]

Carotid artery disease has been reported in patients receiving radiation for head and neck malignancies. Elderding examined in 1981 a Hodgkin's disease population with a mean age of 28 years (range 6–58 years) and a mean follow-up interval of 10 years for cerebrovascular symptoms.[85] Patients were prospectively studied for cerebrovascular symptoms defined as transient attacks of monocular blindness, hemiparesis or aphasia or a fixed neurological deficit lasting more than 24 hours. Symptoms were found in 10 out of 77 patients (13 per cent). A total of 12 patients had significant hemodynamic carotid lesions on oculoplethysmography, including the youngest patient.

A small series of laryngeal rhabdomyosarcoma survivors who received radiotherapy reported bilateral internal carotid stenosis in one out of five patients.[68] The boy presented 13 years after the end of treatment with left-sided hemiparesis following combined modality treatment with vincristine, cyclophosphamide and actinomycin. Actinomycin was given concomitantly with radiation of 48 Gy over 6 weeks to the larynx and regional lymph nodes. King et al. used carotid arterial ultrasonography to assess carotid arterial disease in a cohort of asymptomatic Hodgkin's survivors, age 18–37 years, treated at an age range of 4–29 years (median 13 years).[86] Treatment doses received ranged between 22.5 and 40 Gy in 15–25 fractions using a standard mantle radiation therapy field up to the base of skull. Results were compared with matched controls with an age range of 23–36 years. There was no significant difference in blood pressure, lipid profile, gender, smoking, or family history of hypercholesterolemia or cerebrovascular or cardiovascular disease between the controls and study group. Twenty six per cent of the study group had abnormal scans with evidence of significant increase in intima-media thickness compared with 3 per cent of the controls ($p = 0.01$). The older patients (30–39 years) were more likely to have detectable abnormalities than the younger patient group (20–29 years): 64 per cent and 13 per cent, respectively.

Aorta and main branches

The occurrence of arterial injury in children is rare, with less then 30 cases reported, although Ganry suggested that some children may have undiagnosed asymptomatic stenosis.[87] The reports relate to radiation given for treatment of Hodgkin's disease, non-Hodgkin lymphoma, abdominal neuroblastoma, Wilms' tumor, hepatoblastoma and sarcomas with abdominal, pelvic or limb primaries.[87–95] The radiation fields in these cases have not

been well described but include flank, hemiabdominal, pelvic, inguinal or lower limb fields. The majority of patients received abdominal radiation between the ages of 4 months and 16 years with a mean dose of 38 Gy. The dose varied from as high as 66 Gy in an 11-year-old down to 20 Gy in a 3-year-old both with neuroblastoma.[87,89] The latent period between treatment and presentation varied from 4 to 20 years but 80 per cent presented beyond 10 years. All the nine patients with renal artery stenosis presented with hypertension (five with a primary diagnosis of Wilms' tumor). Other patients presented with abdominal pain, intermittent claudication or syncope. Ganry also cites two asymptomatic patients in his series identified by serial Doppler ultrasound. Radiological findings described included stenosis of renal, perioneal, splenic, celiac, iliac and popiteal arteries. Hypoplasia of different regions of the abdominal aorta, including the bifurcation, was noted. Arterial hypertension may occur as a result of radiation-induced intrarenal vascular damage.[94]

An increase risk of miscarriages, premature births and small-for-dates infants has been reported following total body (TBI) and pelvic irradiation in females. It has been postulated that the uterine vasculature may have been damaged by radiation, leading to an inability to provide the required increased blood supply to the pregnant uterus.[96,97]

Bone

Femoral avascular necrosis has been reported in cancer patients as a result of chemotherapy, particularly steroid treatment and as a consequence of total body radiation or focal radiation, including the femoral head. Radiation damages the small blood vessels, thereby affecting chondrogenesis and calcification.[98] St Jude's reported 15 cases in patients with various malignant diagnoses. Nine received steroid treatment and four had focal radiation at a dose range of 35–65 Gy.[99] The remaining patient received TBI (12 Gy) in combination with high-dose steroids. The median interval from treatment in the irradiated group was 7 years (range 0.6–11 years). The time to development of avascular necrosis is shorter after high-dose steroids than radiation alone.

Venous vessels

Venous vessel damage related to radiotherapy is extremely rare[4] and has only been reported with exceptionally high radiation doses, which are unlikely to be used in the treatment of childhood malignancies. Veno-occlusive disease (VOD) is the only reported radiation-induced complication of small venous vessels. VOD is more commonly reported after actinomycin-based chemotherapy or combined modality treatment.[100] Radiation alone can

cause VOD, but usually requires radiation doses above 30 Gy to the whole liver and rarely leads to cirrhosis.[101]

IMPLICATIONS AND SURVEILLANCE

The development of more refined radiotherapy techniques has most likely increased the latent period for the appearance of late effects. This has to be taken into account when planning long-term follow-up strategies for current patients. Synergistic effects between radiotherapy and chemotherapy must be acknowledged as in the case of the heart and anthracyclines[102] or methotrexate and the brain.[63]

Unfortunately, there are no evidence-based cardiovascular long-term follow-up guidelines, and there continues to be controversy regarding the type and timing of late effects surveillance. Two important factors must be considered. First, can screening be predictive for identification of abnormalities? Are these abnormalities amenable to corrective treatment and, if not, is the information gained of benefit to the patient? Second, by continually investigating these survivors, are we making them into unnecessary 'patients' adversely affecting their quality of life? We have presented papers reporting on asymptomatic abnormalities, but none of these reports have determined the natural history and potential benefit of interventional treatments. Maybe careful history taking and clinical examination rather than exhaustive imaging is sufficient to enable appropriate investigations and interventions to be performed. Particularly attention should be paid to lifestyle, family history and correction of endocrine deficiencies, as these may adversely affect radiation-induced cardiovascular late effects.[103] Smoking, high lipid diets, hypertension, growth hormone, thyroid or sex-hormone deficiencies increase the risks of late sequelae. Genetic counseling may also be appropriate, for example, in families with a history of hypercholesteremia or neurofibromatosis.[69]

To relate possible late cardiovascular sequelae to the radiotherapy received, individual review of the radiation planning films needs to be performed. This allows the accurate assessment of radiation dose and vessel involvement, and the relationship between the signs and symptoms experienced by the patient.

In practice, patients who have received radiation involving the heart in the USA are recommended to receive 3–5-yearly echocardiograms or electrocardiograms.[20] In Britain (United Kingdom Children's Cancer Study Group long-term follow-up guidelines) and in Germany (German Late Effects Study Group Late Effects Surveillance system), the guidelines do not lay down specific timing for investigations.[104,105]

Clinical review should include direct questioning for the presence of chest pain, exercise tolerance, palpitations and syncopal attacks. Particularly sedentary patients should be encouraged to take more exercise. Smokers should be advised of the additional risks inherent in smoking after radiation. If chest pain is reported, the underlying cause must be clarified (cardiac or pleuritic) and exclude the more common costochondritis (Tietze's syndrome) as seen in adolescence. Blood pressure monitoring is mandatory in all patients. Screening for abnormal lipid profiles in patients with predisposing factors for CAD may also be considered.[106]

If coronary bypass surgery is indicated, then the surgeon must be advised of the applied radiation field to assist in planning surgery.[58]

In patients who have received cranial radiation, the importance of reporting new symptoms suggestive of vasculopathies or progression of previous symptoms must be emphasized. Particularly symptoms such as unilateral blindness, paralysis, convulsions, severe headaches, abnormal transient episodes or cognitive decline need to be verified and further investigated to identify occlusion/stenosis with the appropriate tool. It must also be kept in mind that, at present, more patients die late from relapse of their malignancy than due to late treatment sequelae. There is no evidence that regular long-term CNS imaging would be useful.

A subsection of patients at particular risk of vasculopathy are those with primary CNS tumors in association with NF1. Intervention may be required; reports have suggested a good clinical outcome in the pediatric age group.[107] Again, attention to correction of hormonal deficiencies may reduce the risk of developing cerebrovascular disease.[103]

Screening for hypertension and proteinuria is important in patients who have received abdominal radiation, particularly if the kidneys were in the field, as this may herald arterial renal stenosis or intrarenal disease.[86,93] Confirmation with Doppler ultrasound and angiography may be required. Renal artery stenosis is usually associated with reduced glomerular filtration rate. Revascularization by angioplasty can be performed, although this does not reduce the hypertension, but it may prevent progressive renal dysfunction.[95]

Rarely, symptoms of intermittent claudication are elicited and should be investigate with ultrasound/Doppler and/or MRI to identify arterial stenosis.

CONCLUSION

Vascular damage is one of the main causes of radiation-mediated late effects. With modern treatment techniques and increased attention to detail when planning children and adolescents, radiotherapy-associated late sequelae of heart and vessels should be minimized. Additionally,

potential reductions of dose and volumes further contribute to improved quality of life without compromising event-free and overall survival. In the light of the complex modern pediatric treatment protocols, which incorporate both multiagent chemotherapy and radiation, there is a risk that the anticipated reduction in late sequelae may not be realized, owing to a potential synergism with the chemotherapy.

Radiation oncologists should be encouraged to provide clinically useful details of radiotherapeutic treatment techniques employed. This will enable other specialities involved in the long-term care for these patients to predict radiation-induced late sequelae more accurately. It is equally important to feed back to the radiation oncologist to inform his practice.

To date, the knowledge of the natural history of subclinical abnormalities is unknown, but is vital for the prediction of clinically significant disease and to educate follow-up practices. Therefore, prospective surveillance of subclinical damage to obtain this knowledge should be encouraged in the context of properly conducted studies. These studies should be carried out in the full knowledge of the patients and not under the guise of surveillance. Until these data are available, clinicians must be vigilant and patients encouraged to report any cardiac- or vascular-related symptoms.

KEY POINTS

- The degree of differentiation, cell turnover and renewal potential of normal tissues determines the tissue radiosensitivity.
- The majority of radiation-induced toxicities are mediated by damage to the vasculature.
- The late effects of radiation are dependent on the radiation field, total dose, fractionation, vessel-wall anatomy and genetic predisposition to radiation damage.
- The delivery of radiation has become more accurate over time and there has been a reduction of total dose and daily fraction sizes. Therefore, prevalence of abnormalities in past studies may not be relevant to present-day patients.
- Radiation-induced heart disease affects all layers of the heart, the most important clinically is early-onset coronary artery disease, particularly in patients receiving >40 Gy to the heart.
- Cerebrovascular accidents can present as a result of cranial/carotid radiation. Mainly seen in association with centrally placed brain tumors, particularly in the presence of neurofibromatosis type 1.
- The occurrence of other arterial damage is rare in children.

- Long-term follow-up planning is dependent on the detailed knowledge of radiation treatment. To date, there are no evidence-based guidelines for surveillance. Careful history taking and examination with appropriate imaging is important.

REFERENCES

1. Gassman A. Zur Histlogie der Rontgenulcere. *Fortsch Roentgenstr* 1899; **2**:199–207.
2. Gagliardi G, Lax I, Rutqvist LE. Partial irradiation of the heart. *Semin Radiat Oncol* 2001; **11**:224–233.
3. Hopewell JW. The importance of vascular damage in the development of late radiation effects in normal tissues. In: Meyn RE, Withers HR (ed.) *Radiation biology in cancer research*. New York: Raven Press, 1980:449–459.
4. Fajardo LF. Is the pathology of radiation injury different in small vs large blood vessels? *Cardiovasc Radiat Med* 1999; **1**:108–110.
5. Langley RE, Bump EA, Quartuccio SG, *et al.* Radiation-induced apoptosis in microvascular endothelial cells. *Br J Cancer* 1997; **75**:666–672.
6. Gajdusek C, Onoda K, London S, *et al.* Early molecular changes in irradiated aortic endothelium. *J Cell Physiol* 2001; **188**:8–23.
◆7. O'Connor MM, Mayberg MR. Effects of radiation on cerebral vasculature: a review. *Neurosurgery* 2000; **4**:138–149.
8. Fajardo LF, Lee A. Rupture of major vessels after radiation. *Cancer* 1975; **36**:904–913.
9. Aichholzer M, Gruber A, Haberler C, *et al.* Intracranial hemorrhage from an aneurysm encased in a pilocytic astrocytoma – case report and review of the literature. *Childs Nerv Syst* 2001; **17**:173–178.
10. Azzarelli B, Moore J, Gilmor R, *et al.* Multiple fusiform intracranial aneurysms following curative radiation therapy for suprasellar germinoma. Case report. *J Neurosurg* 1984; **61**:1141–1145.
11. Stewart JR, Fajardo LF, Gillette SM, Constine LS. Radiation injury to the heart. *Int J Radiat Oncol Biol Phys* 1995; **31**:1205–1211.
12. Fajardo LF, Colby TV. Pathogenesis of veno-occlusive liver disease after radiation. *Arch Pathol Lab Med* 1980; **104**:584–588.
13. Schweizer E. Ueber spezifische Roentgenschaedigungen des Herzmuskels. *Strahlentherapie* 1924; **18**:812–828.
14. Cohn KE, Stewart JR, Fajardo LF, Hancock EW. Heart disease following radiation. *Medicine (Baltimore)* 1967; **46**:281–298.
15. Fajardo LF, Stewart JR. Experimental radiation-induced heart disease. I. Light microscopic studies. *Am J Pathol* 1970; **59**:299–316.
16. Pierce RH, Haferman MD, Kagan AR. Changes in the traverse cardiac diameter following irradiation for Hodgkin's disease. *Radiology* 1960; **93**:619–624.
17. Fajardo LF, Stewart JR, Cohn KE. Morphology of radiation-induced heart disease. *Arch Pathol* 1986; **186**:512–519.
18. Fajardo LF, Stewart JR. Capillary injury preceding radiation-induced myocardial fibrosis. *Radiology* 1971; **101**:429–433.
19. Lauk S. Endothelial alkaline phosphatase activity loss as an early stage in the development of radiation-induced heart disease in rats. *Radiat Res* 1987; **110**:118–128.
●20. Truesdell SC, Schwartz CL, Conroy T, *et al.* Cardiovascular effects of cancer. In: Schwartz CL, Hobbie WL, Constine LS, Ruccione KS (eds) *Survivors of childhood cancer*. St Louis: Mosby, 1994:159–175.

21. Boivin JF, Hutchison GB, Lubin JH, Mauch P. Coronary artery disease mortality in patients treated for Hodgkin's disease. *Cancer* 1992; **69**:1241–1247.

22. Brosius FC III, Waller BF, Roberts WC. Radiation heart disease. Analysis of 16 young (aged 15 to 33 years) necropsy patients who received over 3,500 rads to the heart. *Am J Med* 1981; 70:519–530.

23. Benoff LJ, Schweitzer P. Radiation therapy-induced cardiac injury. *Am Heart J* 1995; **129**:1193–1196.

24. Virmani R, Farb A, Carter A, Jones RM. Pathology of radiation-induced coronary artery disease in human and pig. *Cardiovasc Radiat Med* 1999; **1**:98–101.

25. Mertens AC, Yasui Y, Neglia JP, *et al.* Late mortality experience in five-year survivors of childhood and adolescent cancer: the Childhood Cancer Survivor Study. *J Clin Oncol* 2001; **19**:3163–3172.

◆26. Moller TR, Garwicz S, Barlow L, *et al.* Decreasing late mortality among five-year survivors of cancer in childhood and adolescence: a population-based study in the Nordic countries. *J Clin Oncol* 2001; **19**:3173–3181.

◆27. Green DM, Hyland A, Chung CS, *et al.* Cancer and cardiac mortality among 15-year survivors of cancer diagnosed during childhood or adolescence. *J Clin Oncol* 1999; **17**:3207–3215.

28. Robertson CM, Hawkins MM, Kingston JE. Late deaths and survival after childhood cancer: implications for cure. *Br Med J* 1994; **309(6948)**:162–166.

29. Hudson MM, Jones D, Boyett J, *et al.* Late mortality of long-term survivors of childhood cancer. *J Clin Oncol* 1997; **15**:2205–2213.

30. Robison LL, Mertens AC, Boice JD, *et al.* Study design and cohort characteristics of the Childhood Cancer Survivor Study: a multi-institutional collaborative project. *Med Pediatr Oncol* 2002; **38**:229–239.

31. Hawkins MM. Commentary to second tumours. *Eur J Cancer* 2001; **37**:2079–2081.

32. Stevens MC, Mahler H, Parkes S. The health status of adult survivors of cancer in childhood. *Eur J Cancer* 1998; **34**: 694–698.

33. Green DM, Grigoriev YA, Nan B, *et al.* Congestive heart failure after treatment for Wilms' tumor: a report from the National Wilms' Tumor Study group. *J Clin Oncol* 2001; **19**:1926–1934.

34. Biller J, Mathews KD, Love B. Stroke in neonates and children: Overview. In: Biller J (ed.) *Stroke in children and young adults.* Newton: Butterworth-Heinemann, 1994: 15–30.

35. Tamminga RY, Dolsma WV, Leeuw JA, Kampinga HH. Chemo- and radiosensitivity testing in a patient with ataxia telangiectasia and Hodgkin disease. *Pediatr Hematol Oncol* 2002; **19**:163–171.

36. McCready RA, Hyde GL, Bivins BA, *et al.* Radiation-induced arterial injuries. *Surgery* 1983; **93**:306–312.

◆37. Hancock SL, Donaldson SS, Hoppe RT. Cardiac disease following treatment of Hodgkin's disease in children and adolescents. *J Clin Oncol* 1993; **11**:1208–1215.

●38. Hancock SL, Donaldson SS. Radiation-related heart disease: risks after treatment of Hodgkin's disease during childhood and adolescence. In: Bricker JT, Green DM, D'Angio G (eds) *Cardiac toxicity after treatment for childhood cancer.* New York: Wiley-Liss, 1993:35–43.

●39. Lauk S. Radiation injury to the heart. In: Scherer E, Streffer C, Trott KR (eds) *Radiation pathology of organs and tissues.* Springer: Heidelberg, 1990.

40. Mauch PM, Weinstein H, Botnick L, *et al.* An evaluation of long-term survival and treatment complications in children with Hodgkin's disease. *Cancer* 1983; **51**:925–932.

41. Jenkin D, Freedman M, McClure P, *et al.* Hodgkin's disease in children: treatment with low dose radiation and MOPP without staging laparotomy: a preliminary report. *Cancer* 1979; **44**:80–86.

42. Green DM, Gingell RL, Pearce J, *et al.* The effect of mediastinal irradiation on cardiac function of patients treated during childhood and adolescence for Hodgkin's disease. *J Clin Oncol* 1987; **5**:239–245.

43. Catterall M, Evans W. My ocardial injury from therapeutic irradiation. *Br Heart J* 1960; **22**:168–174.

44. Gomez GA, Park JJ, Panahon AM, *et al.* Heart size and function after radiation therapy to the mediastinum in patients with Hodgkin's disease. *Cancer Treat Rep* 1983; **67**:1099–1103.

45. Morgan GW, Freeman AP, McLean RG, *et al.* Late cardiac, thyroid, and pulmonary sequelae of mantle radiotherapy for Hodgkin's disease. *Int J Radiat Oncol Biol Phys* 1985; **11**:1925–1931.

46. Gottdiener JS, Katin MJ, Borer JS, *et al.* Late cardiac effects of therapeutic mediastinal irradiation. Assessment by echocardiography and radionuclide angiography. *N Engl J Med* 1983; **308**:569–572.

47. Billingham ME, Masek MA. The pathology of anthracycline cardiotoxicity in children, adolescents and adults. In: Bricker JT, Green DM, D'Angio GJ (eds) *Cardiac toxicity after anthracycline treatment for childhood cancer.* New York: Wiley-Liss, 1993:17–24.

48. Billingham ME. Endomyocardial changes in anthracycline-treated patients with and without irradiation. *Front Radiat Ther Oncol* 1979; **13**:67–81.

49. Pinkel D, Camitta B, Kun L, *et al.* Doxorubicin cardiomyopathy in children with left-sided Wilms tumor. *Med Pediatr Oncol* 1982; **10**:483–488.

50. Sorensen K, Levitt G, Sebag-Montefiore D, *et al.* Cardiac function in Wilms' tumor survivors. *J Clin Oncol* 1995; **13**:1546–1556.

51. Jakacki RI, Goldwein JW, Larsen RL, *et al.* Cardiac dysfunction following spinal irradiation during childhood. *J Clin Oncol* 1993; **11**:1033–1038.

52. Steinherz LJ, Steinherz PG, Tan CT, *et al.* Cardiac toxicity 4 to 20 years after completing anthracycline therapy. *JAMA* 1991; **266**:1672–1677.

53. Krischer JP, Epstein S, Cuthbertson DD, *et al.* Clinical cardiotoxicity following anthracycline treatment for childhood cancer: the Pediatric Oncology Group experience. *J Clin Oncol* 1997; **15**:1544–1552.

54. Orzan F, Brusca A, Conte MR, *et al.* Severe coronary artery disease after radiation therapy of the chest and mediastinum: clinical presentation and treatment. *Br Heart J* 1993; **69**:496–500.

55. Pohjola-Sintonen S, Totterman KJ, Salmo M, Siltanen P. Late cardiac effects of mediastinal radiotherapy in patients with Hodgkin's disease. *Cancer* 1987; **60**:31–37.

56. McEniery PT, Dorosti K, Schiavone WA, *et al.* Clinical and angiographic features of coronary artery disease after chest irradiation. *Am J Cardiol* 1987; **60**:1020–1024.

57. Khan MH, Ettinger SM. Post mediastinal radiation coronary artery disease and its effects on arterial conduits. *Catheter Cardiovasc Interv* 2001; **52**:242–248.

58. Van Son JA, Noyez L, van Austen WN. Use of internal mammary artery in myocardial revascularization after mediastinal irradiation. *J Thorac Cardiovasc Surg* 1992; **104**:1539–1544.

59. Valk PE, Dillon WP. Radiation injury of the brain. *AJNR Am J Neuroradiol* 1991; **12**:45–62.

60. Kingma, A Mooyaart EL, Kamps WA, *et al.* Magnetic resonance imaging of the brain and neurophysiological evaluation in children treated for acute lymphoblastic leukaemia at a young age. *Am J Pediatr Hematol Oncol* 1993; **15**:231–238.

61. Price RA, Birdwell DA. The central nervous system in childhood leukemia. III. Mineralizing microangiopathy and dystrophic calcification. *Cancer* 1978; **42**:717–728.

62. Paakko E, Talvensaari K, Pyhtinen J, Lanning M. Late cranial MRI after cranial irradiation in survivors of childhood cancer. *Neuroradiology* 1994; **36**:652–655.

63. Packer RJ, Meadows AT, Rorke LB, *et al.* Long-term sequelae of cancer treatment on the central nervous system in childhood. *Med Pediatr Oncol* 1987; **15**:241–253.

64. Mitchell WG, Fishman LS, Miller JH, *et al.* Stroke as a late sequela of cranial irradiation for childhood brain tumors. *J Child Neurol* 1991; **6**:128–133.

65. Casey AT, Marsh HT, Uttley D. Intracranial aneurysm formation following radiotherapy. *Br J Neurosurg* 1993; **7**:575–579.

66. Foreman NK, Laitt RD, Chambers EJ, *et al.* Intracranial large vessel vasculopathy and anaplastic meningioma 19 years after cranial irradiation for acute lymphoblastic leukaemia. *Med Pediatr Oncol* 1995; **24**:265–268.

67. Laitt RD, Chambers EJ, Goddard PR, *et al.* Magnetic resonance imaging and magnetic resonance angiography in long term survivors of acute lymphoblastic leukemia treated with cranial irradiation. *Cancer* 1995; **76**:1846–1852.

68. Kato MA, Flamant F, Terrier-Lacombe MJ, *et al.* Rhabdomyosarcoma of the larynx in children: a series of five patients treated in the Institut Gustave Roussy (Villejuif, France). *Med Pediatr Oncol* 1991; **19**:110–114.

◆69. Bowers DC, Mulne AF, Reisch JS, *et al.* Nonperioperative strokes in children with central nervous system tumors. *Cancer* 2002; **94**:1094–1101.

70. Brada M, Burchell L, Ashley S, Traish D. The incidence of cerebrovascular accidents in patients with pituitary adenoma. *Int J Radiat Oncol Biol Phys* 1999; **45**:693–698.

71. Kestle JR, Hoffman HJ, Mock AR. Moyamoya phenomenon after radiation for optic glioma. *J Neurosurg* 1993; **79**:32–35.

72. Grill J, Couanet D, Cappelli C, *et al.* Radiation-induced cerebral vasculopathy in children with neurofibromatosis and optic pathway glioma. *Ann Neurol* 1999; **45**:393–396.

73. Suzuki J, Kodama N. Moyamoya disease – a review. *Stroke* 1983; **14**:104–109.

74. Rajakulasingam K, Cerullo LJ, Raimondi AJ. Childhood moyamoya syndrome. Postradiation pathogenesis. *Childs Brain* 1979; **5**:467–475.

75. Servo A, Puranen M. Moyamoya syndrome as a complication of radiation therapy. Case report. *J Neurosurg* 1978; **48**:1026–1029.

76. Okuno T, Prensky AL, Gado M. The moyamoya syndrome associated with irradiation of an optic glioma in children: report of two cases and review of the literature. *Pediatr Neurol* 1985; **1**:311–316.

77. Kitano S, Sakamoto H, Fujitani K, Kobayashi Y. Moyamoya disease associated with a brain stem glioma. *Childs Nerv Syst* 2000; **16**:251–255.

78. Tsuji N, Kuriyama T, Iwamoto M, Shizuki K. Moyamoya disease associated with craniopharyngioma. *Surg Neurol* 1984; **21**:588–592.

◆79. Bitzer M, Topka H. Progressive cerebral occlusive disease after radiation therapy. *Stroke* 1995; **26**:131–136.

80. Shuper A, Packer RJ, Vezina LG, *et al.* 'Complicated migraine-like episodes' in children following cranial irradiation and chemotherapy. *Neurology* 1995; **45**:1837–1840.

81. Benson PJ, Sung JH. Cerebral aneurysms following radiotherapy for medulloblastoma. *J Neurosurg* 1989; **70**:545–550.

82. Maruyama K, Mishima K, Saito N, *et al.* Radiation-induced aneurysm and moyamoya vessels presenting with subarachnoid haemorrhage. *Acta Neurochir (Wien)* 2000; **142**:139–143.

83. Jensen FK, Wagner A. Intracranial aneurysm following radiation therapy for medulloblastoma. A case report and review of the literature. *Acta Radiol* 1997; **38**:37–42.

84. Fouladi M, Langston J, Mulhern R, *et al.* Silent lacunar lesions detected by magnetic resonance imaging of children with brain tumors: a late sequela of therapy. *J Clin Oncol* 2000; **18**:824–831.

85. Elerding SC, Fernandez RN, Grotta JC, *et al.* Carotid artery disease following external cervical irradiation. *Ann Surg* 1981; **194**:609–615.

86. King LJ, Hasnain SN, Webb JA, *et al.* Asymptomatic carotid arterial disease in young patients following neck radiation therapy for Hodgkin lymphoma. *Radiology* 1999; **213**:167–172.

◆87. Ganry O, Habrand JL, Lemerle J, *et al.* Arterial lesions after radiotherapy in children. Apropos of 16 cases. *Arch Fr Pediatr* 1993; **50**:9–14.

88. Lee KF, Hodes PJ. Intracranial ischemic lesions. *Radiol Clin North Am* 1967; **5**:353–360.

89. Coquhoun J. Hypoplasia of the abdominal aorta following therapeutic irradiation in infancy. *Radiology* 1966; **86**:454–456.

90. Butler P, Chalhal P, Hudson NM, Hubner PJ. Pulmonary hypertension after lung irradiation in infancy. *Br Med J* 1981; **283**:1365.

91. Gerlock AJ Jr, Goncharenko VA, Ekelund L. Radiation-induced stenosis of the renal artery causing hypertension: case report. *J Urol* 1977; **118**:1064–1065.

92. McGill CW, Holder TM, Smith T, Ashcraft KW. Post-radiation renovascular hypertension. *J Pediatr Surg* 1979; **14**:831–833.

93. Stanley P, Gyepes MT, Olson DL, Gates GF. Renovascular hypertension in children and adolescents. *Radiology* 1978; **129**:123–131.

94. Koskimies O. Arterial hypertension developing 10 years after radiotherapy for Wilms's tumour. *Br Med J (Clin Res Ed)* 1982; **285**:996–998.

95. Fakhouri F, La Batide AA, Rerolle JP, *et al.* Presentation and revascularization outcomes in patients with radiation-induced renal artery stenosis. *Am J Kidney Dis* 2001; **38**:302–309.

96. Critchley HO, Wallace WH, Shalet SM, *et al.* Abdominal irradiation in childhood; the potential for pregnancy. *Br J Obstet Gynaecol* 1992; **99**:392–394.

97. Sanders, JE. Effects of bone marrow transplantation on reproductive function. In: Green DM, D'Angio G (ed.) *Late effects of treatment for childhood cancer.* New York: Wiley-Liss, 1992:95–102.

98. Silverman CL, Thomas PR, McAlister WH, *et al.* Slipped femoral capital epiphyses in irradiated children: dose, volume and age relationships. *Int J Radiat Oncol Biol Phys* 1981; **7**:1357–1363.

99. Hanif I, Mahmoud H, Pui CH. Avascular femoral head necrosis in pediatric cancer patients. *Med Pediatr Oncol* 1993; **21**:655–660.

100. Raine J, Bowman A, Wallendszus K, Pritchard J. Hepatopathy-thrombocytopenia syndrome – a complication of dactinomycin therapy for Wilms' tumor: a report from the United Kingdom Childrens Cancer Study Group. *J Clin Oncol* 1991; **9**:268–273.

101. Halperin EC, Constine LS, Tarbell NJ, Kun L. Late effects of cancer treatment. *Pediatric radiation oncology.* Philadelphia: Lippincott Williams and Wilkins, 1999:457–537.

102. Billingham ME, Bristow MR, Glatstein E, *et al.* Adriamycin cardiotoxicity: endomyocardial biopsy evidence of enhancement by irradiation. *Am J Surg Pathol* 1977; **1**:17–23.

103. Heikens J, Ubbink MC, van der Pal HP, *et al.* Long term survivors of childhood brain cancer have an increased risk for cardiovascular disease. *Cancer* 2000; **88**:2116–2121.

104. Kissen GDN, Wallace WHD. *Therapy based guidelines for long-term follow up of children treated for cancer.* Published on behalf of the Late Effects Group of the UKCCSG. Milton Keynes, UK: Pharmacia, 1995.

105. Langer T, Henze G, Beck JD. Basic methods and the developing structure of a late effects surveillance system (LESS) in the long-term follow-up of pediatric cancer patients in Germany. For the German Late Effects Study Group in the German Society Pediatric Oncology and Hematology (GPOH). *Med Pediatr Oncol* 2000; **34**:348–351.

106. Lipshultz SE, Sallan SE. Cardiovascular abnormalities in long-term survivors of childhood malignancy. *J Clin Oncol* 1993; **11**:1199–1203.

107. Houkin K, Kuroda S, Nakayama N. Cerebral revascularization for moyamoya disease in children. *Neurosurg Clin N Am* 2001; **12**:575–584, ix.

5

Respiratory complications

NEYSSA MARINA, CHRISTINE SHARIS AND NANCY TARBELL

INTRODUCTION

With the use of multimodality therapy, the survival for childhood cancer has steadily improved over the last three decades.[1] The improved survival has increased our concerns regarding the impact of late sequelae on survivors. Therefore, an increasing number of studies have investigated the incidence and consequences of these complications.[2–14] This chapter will focus on the respiratory complications resulting from the use of combined modality therapy on survivors of childhood malignancies.

The first part of the chapter will focus on the respiratory complications resulting from the use of radiotherapy for patients with pediatric malignancies. Radiation therapy has been an important treatment modality for childhood cancers for many years. In light of the decades of experience and the improvement in long-term survival, we have a better understanding of the potential for early and late radiation complications. Children treated with radiation therapy to their chests may develop pulmonary injury or respiratory compromise from a variety of mechanisms. Depending on several factors, there may be direct damage to type II pneumocytes, developmental inhibition of new alveoli, and/or bone growth abnormalities in the ribs, sternum, muscles and cartilage.[15] The second part of the chapter will discuss respiratory complications resulting from chemotherapy administration in the context of adjuvant therapy or in the bone marrow transplant setting. Since the number of bone marrow transplant studies in children is somewhat limited, some of the data presented are from reports pertaining to the use of bone marrow transplantation in patients with adult malignancies.

RADIATION PNEUMONITIS

Radiation pneumonitis is a clinical syndrome of cough, dyspnea, chest pain/pleuritis and low-grade fever, which may occur after radiation to the lungs.[15] Cough may be non-productive initially and then turn productive, sometimes with pink sputum. Computed tomography (CT) scans of the lungs during this time may show a ragged infiltrate within the radiation fields; chest X-rays may show volume loss as well as linear densities corresponding to the radiation fields.[15] Radiographic changes alone in the absence of clinical symptoms and signs do not make the diagnosis of pneumonitis. Indeed, the frequency of clinical radiation pneumonitis ranges from 0 to 18 per cent in several studies; however, asymptomatic radiographic abnormalities may occur in 27–92 per cent of all treated patients in those studies.[16–21]

Laboratory tests are not diagnostic, although abnormal levels of serum surfactant apoprotein and plasma transforming growth factor (TGFβ) seem to correspond to the clinical signs and symptoms, and are subjects of further study.[22,23] Lung function test abnormalities are not typically seen at this early stage. Laboratory and other quantitative tests, however, are important to help rule out other diagnoses.

Radiation pneumonitis is a diagnosis of exclusion; tumor recurrence, metastases, lymphangitic spread of tumor and infection must be ruled out.[24] Acute radiation pneumonitis may occur 1–3 months after radiation therapy, if radiation is given alone.[24] However, if it is combined with chemotherapy, then the syndrome may occur earlier and as early as during radiation treatments. Treatment

for acute radiation pneumonitis often includes steroids at relatively high doses (prednisone 50 mg daily or dexamethasone 16–20 mg daily[24]) and, if necessary, supplemental oxygen. A slow taper of steroids is needed, often over several months. With these measures, the clinical symptoms often clear within 1 or 2 days.[24] If the syndrome persists, biopsy of the area showing radiographic changes may be necessary to rule out other etiologies.

Acute radiation pneumonitis may be due to injury of type II pneumocytes, endothelial cells, fibroblasts and macrophages.[15] Within minutes to hours after radiation is given, type II alveolar cells are injured and surfactant is released into alveoli.[25] This is called the exudative phase of radiation injury.[24] Intra-alveolar edema also occurs. Penney *et al.* described several changes including type II pneumocyte alterations within 1–7 days, changes in endothelial cells within 1–15 days, decrease in the number of macrophages in alveoli within 1–3 weeks, and increase in numbers of fibroblasts between 2 and 6 months of radiotherapy administration.[26] Alveolar epithelial cell desquamation may also occur and, as a result of this, impaired gas exchange may result. Rubin *et al.* have shown that radiation causes changes in the cytokine cascades; interleukin (IL)-1, IL-6, tumor necrosis factor α (TNFα), TGFβ and platelet-derived growth factor (PDGF) have been shown to be released by type II pneumocytes, endothelial cells and macrophages, causing the expression of fibronectin and collagens I, III and IV.[27–29] In the clinic, Anscher *et al.* have shown that increased TGFβ levels correspond to increased risk of pneumonitis and hepatic veno-occlusive disease in patients undergoing radiation during bone marrow transplant.[22,30]

At 2–4 months after radiation, the fibrotic phase of radiation pneumonitis may occur. Often during this phase the patient is asymptomatic but dyspnea, cyanosis and chronic cor pulmonale/heart failure may occur.[15] On chest X-ray or chest CT, retraction of the irradiated lung and elevation of the corresponding hemidiaphragm may be seen. Linear densities may now extend outside the originally irradiated volume.[15] In addition, the hilum may retract, causing overinflation of the contralateral lung. Decreased pulmonary blood flow in the affected area and decreased pulmonary function tests with a restrictive picture may result. Chronic fibrosis may be seen up to many years after radiation but most changes are apparent within 1 or 2 years.[15] In general, symptoms from chronic fibrosis are minimal if the fibrosis involves <50 per cent of one lung.[31]

At the cellular level, type II pneumocyte proliferation may occur at 1–3 months, causing lamellar body hypertrophy.[24] At approximately 3–6 months following radiotherapy treatment, alveolar wall sclerosis and thickening may occur from interstitial edema consolidating into collagen, and alveolar space collapse, causing volume loss and restrictive changes.[24] Because of radiation damage

to the capillary endothelial cells, platelet thrombi and capillary obstruction may occur, leading to capillary loss and thus decreased pulmonary blood flow.[32]

What radiation factors are important in the development, or avoidance, of radiation pneumonitis and fibrosis? The dose of radiation, overall treatment time, volume of lung treated, type of chemotherapy and the age of the patient are all important factors.

Dose

Doses of radiation are usually fractionated, or divided among several days to weeks, to increase the tolerance of the irradiated organ by allowing the normal tissues adequate time to heal. If radiation is given in a large single dose, there is a much greater risk of causing injury. This is illustrated in a study that showed a single dose of 8.2 Gy to the whole lung resulted in lethal radiation pneumonitis in 5 per cent, a single dose of 9.3 Gy to the whole lung resulted in a lethal pneumonitis rate of 50 per cent, and a single dose of 11 Gy resulted in an 80 per cent mortality.[33] In contrast, after fractionating the whole lung radiation, one study showed that the lethal radiation pneumonitis estimate for 26.5 Gy in 20 fractions was 5 per cent, and 50 per cent after 30.5 Gy in 20 fractions.[23]

Children with metastatic Wilms' tumor to the lung are often treated with fractionated whole-lung radiation. The acute risk of pneumonitis is low when doses are limited to less than 12 Gy at 1.5 Gy per day or lower. However, long-term studies have shown that total doses of 12–14 Gy decreased total lung capacity and vital capacity to about 70 per cent of the predicted value.[34–36] If the child had also undergone thoracotomy, the pulmonary capacities were even lower.

Time

Increasing the time intervals between small radiation doses also seems to decrease the risk of lung injury. Siemann *et al.* showed this effect when comparing once a day, twice a day and once a week radiation therapy schedules.[37] In general, radiation therapy today is given daily, although twice a day regimens with 6–8 hours interfraction times are occasionally used.

Volume

The volume of lung treated is also important. A small volume of lung can tolerate a relatively high dose of radiation, while the whole organ cannot. Generally, in an adult, up to one-third of a lung can tolerate doses >50 Gy at 1.5–1.8 Gy/fraction. This is thought to be similar in a child. In adults, Choi *et al.* noted decreases in pulmonary

function tests to be related to the relative fraction of lung receiving radiation.[38]

Chemotherapy

As will be discussed in the next section, the addition of certain chemotherapies, such as bleomycin, actinomycin D, cyclophosphamide, vincristine and Adriamycin, all can produce radiation pneumonitis at much lower doses.[15] For example, while doses of 25 Gy to the whole lung in 20 fractions or 18 Gy in ten fractions without actinomycin may be safe, many radiation oncologists would not give more than 12–15 Gy to the whole lung in 10–12 fractions when actinomycin D is administered concomitantly.[15]

Age

There is also reason to believe that younger children who have had pulmonary radiation may be more affected than older children or adults. Radiation can prevent the development of new alveoli, which are necessary as the child grows, as well as preventing the adequate growth of ribs, cartilage and muscle.[15]

CHEMOTHERAPY-INDUCED PULMONARY TOXICITY

Bleomycin-containing regimens

Multiple chemotherapeutic agents, including bleomycin, the alkylating agents and the nitrosureas, have the capacity to produce some degree of pulmonary toxicity.[39,40] The symptomatology produced by any of these agents is similar to that produced by radiotherapy and usually consists of dyspnea, fever and cough associated with rales, cyanosis on physical examination and the presence of bibasilar infiltrates on chest radiographs.[39–41] Perhaps the most studied of the agents producing pulmonary toxicity is bleomycin, an antineoplastic antibiotic isolated from *Streptomyces verticillus*.[41] Bleomycin is attractive as a therapeutic alternative because, unlike other chemotherapeutic agents, its dose-limiting toxicity is not myelosuppression but rather the development of interstitial pneumonitis and skin toxicity.[39,41,42]

The pulmonary toxicity associated with bleomycin appears to be dose-related, since it is rare when doses are limited to <500 mg.[39,41,42] At doses <450 mg there is a relatively constant incidence of 3–5 per cent with a sharp increase up to about 20 per cent at doses >450 mg.[39–41] The symptoms associated with bleomycin-induced interstitial pneumonitis are similar to those produced by any other pulmonary toxin.

Although the radiographic findings usually include the presence of interstitial infiltrates, bleomycin toxicity can occasionally manifest as the presence of pulmonary nodules, which might be difficult to differentiate from metastatic tumor.[43,44] Risk factors associated with increased pulmonary toxicity include the use of high concentrations of oxygen,[45] older age,[39,46] and the use of concomitant radiotherapy.[46–48] Another risk factor for increased toxicity appears to be the development of renal dysfunction as may occur with the administration of cisplatin. The presence of renal dysfunction in these instances can lead to altered clearance of bleomycin and higher drug levels resulting in increased toxicity.[49,50] There is some controversy as to whether the method of administration of the drug (continuous infusion versus bolus administration) influences the development of pulmonary toxicity. There are reports of continuous-infusion bleomycin producing lower toxicity;[51] however, this has not been studied in a randomized controlled trial and, therefore, no firm conclusions can be drawn.

Histologically, the features of bleomycin pulmonary toxicity include the presence of intra-alveolar exudates with subsequent organization, hyaline membrane formation, interstitial fibrosis, atypical proliferation of alveolar cells and squamous metaplasia with dysplasia of distal air-space epithelium.[40,41,46]

Bleomycin has clinical activity against various squamous cell carcinomas, lymphomas and testicular germ cell tumors.[41] Since carcinomas are uncommon in children, we will now discuss the pulmonary toxicity associated with the use of bleomycin in children with either Hodgkin's disease[52–54] or germ cell tumors.[55–58]

PULMONARY TOXICITY FOR PATIENTS WITH GERM CELL TUMORS

The use of bleomycin-containing multiagent chemotherapy has dramatically improved the outcome for adults with testicular germ cell tumors, especially those with metastatic disease.[59,60] Therefore, clinical investigation has focused on the identification of subclinical markers for lung toxicity in an effort to minimize the number of patients with this complication.[61–66]

Comis and coworkers first identified the diffusion capacity of carbon monoxide (DLco) as measured on pulmonary function studies as a reliable indicator of early bleomycin-induced pulmonary toxicity.[65] Subsequently, the utility of the DLco as a predictor of lung toxicity has been questioned,[61,62,64] and a recent publication suggests that the decrease in DLco encountered during treatment for testicular germ cell tumors might be a result of the effect of cisplatin and etoposide rather than bleomycin.[50] These authors suggest that the vital capacity and the pulmonary capillary blood volume rather than the DLco

should be used as markers of bleomycin toxicity because they more accurately reflect the effects of bleomycin on lung function. Other investigators previously suggested that vascular damage was an important feature of bleomycin-induced lung toxicity and that vital capacity was indeed the more prominent finding in bleomycin-induced lung toxicity.[61] At this point, it is not clear what the best marker for bleomycin-induced lung toxicity is and, in most instances, DLco will be used to determine whether or not there is pulmonary damage.

The use of bleomycin in children with germ cell tumors has significantly lagged behind the adult experience secondary to the significant concerns regarding pulmonary toxicity. Investigators at St Jude Children's Research Hospital[58] and the UK Children's Cancer Study Group[67] pioneered studies of bleomycin-containing regimens in pediatric germ cell tumors. Subsequently, bleomycin has become part of the standard of care for children with malignant germ cell tumors and the concerns regarding pulmonary toxicity have decreased.[55–57,68]

PULMONARY TOXICITY FOR PATIENTS WITH HODGKIN'S DISEASE

Although Hodgkin's disease is curable with the use of radiotherapy alone, the number of late sequelae[69,70] associated with its use in pediatric patients prompted early investigation of the use of multimodality therapy.[71] Since then, the outcome for patients with Hodgkin's disease has dramatically improved and current 5-year survivals are reported to be over 85 per cent.[52–54,72] For patients with such a good outcome, the incidence and impact of late sequelae have become increasingly important. Thus, bleomycin-induced lung toxicity has been extensively studied.[72–79] Although it is clear that there is a decrease in pulmonary function tests, more specifically, DLco and forced vital capacity during therapy for Hodgkin's disease, it is difficult to determine which component of therapy (bleomycin or radiotherapy) has the greatest impact. For this reason, some investigators suggest that the changes in pulmonary function tests are a result of treatment with radiotherapy.[75] Nevertheless, it has become standard to monitor pediatric patients receiving bleomycin with pulmonary function tests and to hold bleomycin when there is a significant decrease in DLco.[53,79]

Role of other chemotherapeutic agents in pulmonary toxicity

There are a number of other chemotherapeutic agents that can produce pulmonary toxicity,[39,40] such as the nitrosoureas,[80] cyclophosphamide,[81] melphalan, busulfan, chlorambucil[39] and some antimetabolites, including methotrexate.[82]

ALKYLATING AGENTS

Nitrosoureas

The nitrosoureas are one of the groups of chemotherapeutic agents with significant antitumor activity in patients with malignant brain tumors.[83,84] The potential side effects associated with administration of nitrosoureas include delayed myelosuppression, nausea, vomiting, liver toxicity and renal impairment.[85] Pulmonary toxicity has also been described particularly in patients receiving carmustine.[80,85–88] This toxicity is usually manifested by a fibrosing alveolitis and interstitial pneumonitis.[80] Carmustine-induced pulmonary toxicity was originally described by Durant[89] in nine patients for an overall incidence of 1.1 per cent. Subsequently, Aronin et al.[86] described pulmonary toxicity in approximately 20 per cent of patients receiving carmustine for malignant brain tumors. The pulmonary toxicity appears to be dose related because it is more common in patients receiving doses over $1500 \, mg/m^2$ and in those receiving more prolonged treatment. Two subsequent publications[87,88] described delayed pulmonary toxicity in a significant number of survivors of malignant brain tumors treated with carmustine. The overall mortality was up to 47 per cent and age at the time of treatment appeared to be a significant factor affecting survival but cumulative dose was not.[88] The available literature would suggest that patients receiving carmustine, particularly if younger than 5 years of age, should have monitoring with pulmonary function tests for many years following treatment completion because there appears to be a continuous gradual decline in forced vital capacity and total lung capacity over time.

Carmustine is also used as part of the preparative regimen for stem cell transplants.[90–94] It is noted in one of those studies that doses in excess of $450 \, mg/m^2$ produced unacceptable extramedullary toxicity, including hepatic and cardiac necrosis,[93] although when used as a single agent in a different study, doses were escalated up to $1200 \, mg/m^2$,[91] and other authors have described administration of $600 \, mg/m^2$ with tolerable toxicity.[92] It is likely that the ability to escalate carmustine as part of the preparative regimen in various malignancies is related to the patient's prior exposure to pulmonary toxins and the other agents included in the preparative regimen.

Busulfan

Busulfan was the first chemotherapeutic agent identified as producing pulmonary toxicity.[39] The drug is primarily used in the management of chronic myelogenous leukemia and thus lung toxicity has been mainly described in these patients. In pediatric patients, busulfan is mostly used as part of the preparative regimen for patients with leukemias and lymphomas.[95–99] Since transplant is usually reserved for children with recurrent disease, determining the role of busulfan therapy on lung toxicity in this setting is difficult.

Melphalan

Melphalan is another agent known to produce pulmonary toxicity.[39] However, other than in the transplant setting,[93,100,101] this drug is rarely used in the pediatric population.

Cyclophosphamide

Cyclophosphamide is the alkylating agent most widely used in the management of pediatric malignancies. It has significant antitumor activity in several malignancies and, although it can cause pulmonary toxicity,[81] this is rarely reported at standard doses. Pulmonary toxicity appears to be a more common problem when cyclophosphamide is used as part of any pretransplant conditioning regimen. However, in those circumstances, it is usually combined with other agents also known to cause pulmonary toxicity, making it difficult to determine the impact of cyclophosphamide on lung toxicity.[95–99]

OTHER AGENTS

Other chemotherapy drugs are rarely associated with the development of pulmonary toxicity. Among these, hydroxyurea has been reported to produce a hypersensitivity pneumonitis,[102] which, although unusual, can be life threatening. In this report, the patient responded to elimination of the offending agent and the use of corticosteroids. Cytarabine is another agent known to cause pulmonary toxicity, particularly non-cardiogenic pulmonary edema.[39,40] Alveolar hemorrhage has additionally been reported in two patients treated with cytarabine and fludarabine.[103] The use of corticosteroids resulted in clinical improvement in at least one of the patients. Furthermore, gemcitabine, a new antineoplastic drug structurally related to cytarabine has produced pulmonary toxicity.[104,105] Finally, etoposide[106] and irinotecan[107] have been reported to induce lung toxicity. As with any other drug-induced lung toxicity, elimination of the presumed offending agent and consideration of the use of corticosteroids might be useful.

BONE MARROW TRANSPLANT-INDUCED PULMONARY TOXICITY

Pulmonary toxicity is a common complication of a number of pretransplant regimens.[95–99] The transplant-associated lung toxicity can manifest as interstitial pneumonitis,[108,109] idiopathic pneumonia syndrome,[109,110] bronchiolitis obliterans organizing pneumonia (BOOP), bronchiolitis obliterans,[111] pulmonary hemorrhage[112] and pulmonary edema.[109,110] In fact, interstitial pneumonitis accounts for over 40 per cent of transplant-related mortality. Interstitial pneumonitis typically occurs within 90 days after bone marrow transplant and, in this setting, it is extremely important to eliminate infectious agents as a cause of the process. However, no organisms are identified in up to 60 per cent of cases. It appears that, in the transplant setting, multiple factors contribute to the occurrence of interstitial pneumonitis but prompt evaluation is essential so that appropriate therapy can be initiated.[108]

The post-transplant course can be complicated by the occurrence of BOOP and bronchiolitis obliterans. BOOP is a restrictive lung disorder characterized by the presence of organizing exudates with plugs of granulation and connective tissue.[109,113] While its pathogenesis in transplant patients is unclear, it is associated with the presence of graft-versus-host disease (GvHD). Patients present with a flu-like illness, crackles, cough and dyspnea and, with the use of corticosteroids, it has a benign clinical course. In contrast, bronchiolitis obliterans is a post-transplant complication also associated with GvHD. Clinical presentation includes expiratory wheezing, cough and dyspnea. Histopathologically the lesion is characterized by bronchiolar inflammation, scarring, obliteration and the presence of obstruction on lung function studies. Unlike patients with BOOP, patients with bronchiolitis obliterans have progressive deterioration despite treatment with corticosteroids.[109] The presence of obstructive lung disease post-transplant has been identified as a serious complication associated with a mortality up to 75 per cent and with the presence of GvHD.[111]

RECOMMENDATIONS FOR FOLLOW-UP

As a general rule, children who have received whole lung radiation may be evaluated in follow-up with baseline chest X-rays, oxygen saturation, pulmonary function tests including DLco, every 3–5 years, or as clinically indicated.[15] Children and adult survivors of childhood cancer treated with thoracic radiation are also strongly advised to avoid smoking and consider having the influenza vaccine and Pneumovax.[15]

Although there are no firm guidelines defining optimal follow-up for children treated with potential pulmonary toxins, it is essential to monitor these patients. It appears that children treated with bone marrow transplantation are at higher risk for pulmonary complications. These may be associated with the preparative regimen, the presence of GvHD and/or previous history of exposure to pulmonary toxins. It seems prudent to perform pulmonary function tests in these patients at 6-month intervals for the first 2 years and yearly until 5 years from the procedure. If, at that time, the pulmonary function tests are stable, they could be performed less frequently, i.e. every 2–3 years.

For children who received potential pulmonary toxins without the use of a bone marrow transplant, the potential pulmonary toxicity should be manifested earlier during

treatment so that by 1–2 years following treatment completion,[79] their lung function will have likely stabilized and they could be followed every 2–3 years.

CONCLUSIONS

Radiotherapy and a significant number of chemotherapeutic agents can produce lung toxicity. The most studied of these agents appear to be bleomycin and radiation therapy, but the nitrosoureas and other alkylating agents have the potential of producing similar toxicities. It is important that each care provider remain updated regarding the agents associated with lung toxicity so that they will be able to perform appropriate follow-up and adjust therapy as necessary for the disease process.

KEY POINTS

- Radiotherapy and chemotherapeutic agents can produce lung toxicity characterized by injury of type II pneumocytes, endothelial cells, fibroblasts and macrophages.
- Clinical symptoms include cough, dyspnea, chest pain/pleuritis and a low-grade fever.
- Physical signs include the presence of rales and cyanosis on physical examination.
- Chest radiographs may reveal bibasilar infiltrates or the presence of volume loss as well as linear densities.
- Laboratory tests are not diagnostic.
- The most studied of these agents are bleomycin and radiation therapy; however, nitrosureas and other alkylating agents have been shown to produce similar toxicities.
- The authors review the factors associated with the development of this toxicity as well as the therapeutic alternatives and prognosis.
- Care providers must remain updated on the agents associated with lung toxicity so that they will be able to perform appropriate follow-up and adjust therapy as necessary for the disease process.

REFERENCES

1. Miller RW, Young JL Jr, Novakovic B. Childhood cancer. *Cancer* 1995; **75**(1 Suppl.):395–405.
2. Byrne J, Fears TR, Steinhorn SC, *et al*. Marriage and divorce after childhood and adolescent cancer. *JAMA* 1989; **262**:2693–2699.
3. Garre ML, Gandus S, Cesana B, *et al*. Health status of long-term survivors after cancer in childhood. Results of an uniinstitutional study in Italy. *Am J Pediatr Hematol Oncol* 1994; **16**:143–152.
4. Green DM, Zevon MA, Hall B. Achievement of life goals by adult survivors of modern treatment for childhood cancer. *Cancer* 1991; **67**:206–213.
5. Hays DM, Landsverk J, Sallan SE, *et al*. Educational, occupational, and insurance status of childhood cancer survivors in their fourth and fifth decades of life. *J Clin Oncol* 1992; **10**:1397–1406.
6. Lansky SB, List MA, Ritter-Sterr C. Psychosocial consequences of cure. *Cancer* 1986; **58**(2 Suppl.):529–533.
●7. Marina N. Long-term survivors of childhood cancer. The medical consequences of cure. *Pediatr Clin North Am* 1997; **44**:1021–1042.
8. Meadows AT, Hobbie WL. The medical consequences of cure. *Cancer* 1986; **58**(2 Suppl.):524–528.
9. Mulhern RK, Wasserman AL, Friedman AG, Fairclough D. Social competence and behavioral adjustment of children who are long-term survivors of cancer. *Pediatrics* 1989; **83**:18–25.
10. Mulhern RK, Friedman AG, Stone PA. Acute lymphoblastic leukemia: long-term psychological outcome. *Biomed Pharmacother* 1988; **42**:243–246.
11. Neglia JP, Nesbit ME. Care and treatment of long-term survivors of childhood cancer. *Cancer* 1993; **71**(10 Suppl.):3386–3391.
12. Teta MJ, Del Po MC, Kasl SV, *et al*. Psychosocial consequences of childhood and adolescent cancer survival. *J Chronic Dis* 1986; **39**:751–759.
13. Zeltzer LK, Chen E, Weiss R, *et al*. Comparison of psychologic outcome in adult survivors of childhood acute lymphoblastic leukemia versus sibling controls: a cooperative Children's Cancer Group and National Institutes of Health study. *J Clin Oncol* 1997; **15**:547–556.
14. Zevon MA, Neubauer NA, Green DM. Adjustment and vocational satisfaction of patients treated during childhood or adolescence for acute lymphoblastic leukemia. *Am J Pediatr Hematol Oncol* 1990; **12**:454–461.
15. Halperin EC, Constine LS, Tarbell NJ, Kun LE. *Pediatric radiation oncology*, 3rd edn. Philadelphia: Lippincott Williams & Wilkins, 1999.
16. Marks LB, Spencer D, Bentel G, *et al*. The utility of SPECT lung perfusion scans in minimizing and assessing the physiologic consequences of thoracic irradiation. *Int J Radiat Oncol Biol Phys* 1993; **26**:659–668.
◆17. Mah K, van Dyke J, Keane T, Poon P. Acute radiation-induced pulmonary damage: a clinical study on the response of fractionated radiation therapy. *Int J Radiat Oncol Biol Phys* 1987; **13**:736–743.
18. Polansky S, Ravin C, Prosnitz L. Pulmonary changes after primary radiation for early breast carcinoma. *Am J Roentgenol* 1980; **134**:101–105.
19. Gross N. Pulmonary effects of radiotherapy. *Ann Intern Med* 1977; **86**:81–92.
20. Morgan G, Freeman A, McLean R, *et al*. Late cardiac, thyroid, and pulmonary sequelae of mantle radiotherapy for Hodgkin's disease. *Int J Radiat Oncol Biol Phys* 1985; **11**:1925–1931.
21. Shapiro S, Shapiro S, Mill W, Campbell E. Prospective study of long-term pulmonary manifestations of mantle irradiation. *Int J Radiat Oncol Biol Phys* 1990; **19**:707–714.
22. Anscher MS, Peters W, Reisenbichler H, *et al*. Transforming growth factor-β as a predictor of liver and lung fibrosis after autologous bone marrow transplantation for advanced breast cancer. *N Engl J Med* 1993; **328**:1592–1598.
23. McDonald S, Rubin P, Marks LB. Injury to the lung from cancer therapy: clinical syndromes, measurable endpoints, and potential scoring systems. *Int J Radiat Oncol Biol Phys* 1995; **31**:1187–1203.
24. Rubin P, Constine LS, Williams JP. Late effects of cancer treatment: radiation and drug toxicity. In: Perez CA, Brady LW (eds) *Principles and practice of radiation oncology*, 3rd edn. Philadelphia: Lippincott-Raven, 1997:155–211.

25. Rubin P, Siemann D, Shapiro D, *et al.* Surfactant release as an early measure of radiation pneumonitis. *Int J Radiat Oncol Biol Phys* 1983; **9**:1669–1673.

26. Penney D, Shapiro D, Rubin P, *et al.* Effects of radiation on the mouse lung and potential induction of radiation pneumonitis. *Virchows Arch B Cell Pathol Mol Pathol* 1981; **37**:327–336.

27. Johnston C, Piedboeuf B, Baggs R, *et al.* Differences in correlation of mRNA gene expression in mice sensitive and resistant to radiation-induced pulmonary fibrosis. *Radiat Res* 1995; **142**:197–203.

28. Johnston C, Piedboeuf B, Rubin P, *et al.* Early and persistent alterations in the expression of IL-1α, IL-1β, and TNFα mRNA levels in fibrosis-resistant and sensitive mice following thoracic irradiation. *Radiat Res* 1996; **145**:762–767.

29. Finkelstein J, Johnston C, Baggs R, Rubin P. Early alterations in extracellular matrix and transforming growth factor β gene expression in mouse lung indicative of late radiation fibrosis. *Int J Radiat Oncol Biol Phys* 1994; **28**:621–631.

30. Anscher MS, Murase T, Prescott D, *et al.* Changes in plasma transforming growth factor-β levels during pulmonary radiotherapy as a predictor or the risk of developing radiation pneumonitis. *Int J Radiat Oncol Biol Phys* 1994; **30**:671–676.

31. Rubin P. Quantitative radiation pathology for predicting effects. *Cancer* 1977; **39**(Suppl. 21):729–736.

32. Penney D. Ultrastructural organization of the distal lung and potential target cells of ionizing radiation. In: *International Conference on New Biology of Lung and Lung Injury and Their Implications for Oncology*, Porvoo, Finland, 1987.

33. Keane T, van Dyke J, Rider W. Idiopathic interstitial pneumonia following bone marrow transplantation: the relationship with total body irradiation. *Int J Radiat Oncol Biol Phys* 1981; **7**:1365–1370.

34. Wara W, Phillips T, Margolis L, *et al.* Radiation pneumonitis: a new approach to the derivation of time-dose factors. *Cancer* 1973; **32**:547–552.

35. Wohl M, Griscom N, Traggis D, *et al.* Effects of therapeutic irradiation delivered in early childhood upon subsequent lung function. *Pediatrics* 1975; **55**:507–516.

◆36. McDonald S, Rubin P, Maasilta P. Response of normal lung to irradiation tolerance doses/tolerance volumes in pulmonary radiation syndromes. *Front Radiat Ther Oncol* 1989; **23**:255–276.

37. Siemann D, Rubin P, Penney D. Pulmonary toxicity following multi-fraction radio-therapy. *Br J Cancer* 1986; **53**(Suppl.):365–367.

38. Choi N, Kanarek D, Kazemi H. Physiologic changes in pulmonary function after thoracic radiotherapy for patients with lung cancer and role of regional pulmonary function studies in predicting post-radiotherapy pulmonary function before radiotherapy. *Cancer Treat Symp* 1985; **2**:119–130.

◆39. Ginsberg SJ, Comis RL. The pulmonary toxicity of antineoplastic agents. *Semin Oncol* 1982; **9**:34–51.

◆40. Cooper JA Jr, White DA, Matthay RA. Drug-induced pulmonary disease. Part 1: Cytotoxic drugs. *Am Rev Respir Dis* 1986; **133**:321–340.

◆41. Blum RH, Carter SK, Agre K. A clinical review of bleomycin – a new antineoplastic agent. *Cancer* 1973; **31**:903–914.

◆42. Van Barneveld PW, Sleijfer DT, van der Mark TW, *et al.* Natural course of bleomycin-induced pneumonitis. A follow-up study. *Am Rev Respir Dis* 1987; **135**:48–51.

43. Zucker PK, Khouri NF, Rosenshein NB. Bleomycin-induced pulmonary nodules: a variant of bleomycin pulmonary toxicity. *Gynecol Oncol* 1987; **28**:284–291.

◆44. Ben Arush MW, Roguin A, Zamir E, *et al.* Bleomycin and cyclophosphamide toxicity simulating metastatic nodules to the lungs in childhood cancer. *Pediatr Hematol Oncol* 1997; **14**:381–386.

45. Donat SM, Levy DA. Bleomycin associated pulmonary toxicity: is perioperative oxygen restriction necessary? *J Urol* 1998; **160**:1347–1352.

◆46. Samuels ML, Johnson DE, Holoye PY, Lanzotti VJ. Large-dose bleomycin therapy and pulmonary toxicity. A possible role of prior radiotherapy. *JAMA* 1976; **235**:1117–1120.

47. Einhorn L, Krause M, Hornback N, Furnas B. Enhanced pulmonary toxicity with bleomycin and radiotherapy in oat cell lung cancer. *Cancer* 1976; **37**:2414–2416.

◆48. Catane R, Schwade JG, Turrisi AT III, *et al.* Pulmonary toxicity after radiation and bleomycin: a review. *Int J Radiat Oncol Biol Phys* 1979; **5**:1513–1518.

49. Rabinowits M, Souhami L, Gil RA, Andrade CA, Paiva HC. Increased pulmonary toxicity with bleomycin and cisplatin chemotherapy combinations. *Am J Clin Oncol* 1990; **13**:132–138.

◆50. Sleijfer S, van der Mark TW, Schraffordt Koops H, Mulder NH. Decrease in pulmonary function during bleomycin-containing combination chemotherapy for testicular cancer: not only a bleomycin effect. *Br J Cancer* 1995; **71**:120–123.

51. Gerson R, Tellez Bernal E, Lazaro Leon M, *et al.* Low toxicity with continuous infusion of high-dose bleomycin in poor prognostic testicular cancer. *Am J Clin Oncol* 1993; **16**:323–326.

52. Fryer CJ, Hutchinson RJ, Krailo M, *et al.* Efficacy and toxicity of 12 courses of ABVD chemotherapy followed by low-dose regional radiation in advanced Hodgkin's disease in children: a report from the Children's Cancer Study Group. *J Clin Oncol* 1990; **8**:1971–1980.

53. Hudson MM, Greenwald C, Thompson E, *et al.* Efficacy and toxicity of multiagent chemotherapy and low-dose involved-field radiotherapy in children and adolescents with Hodgkin's disease. *J Clin Oncol* 1993; **11**:100–108.

54. Hunger SP, Link MP, Donaldson SS. ABVD/MOPP and low-dose involved-field radiotherapy in pediatric Hodgkin's disease: the Stanford experience. *J Clin Oncol* 1994; **12**:2160–2166.

55. Cushing B, Giller R, Lauer S, *et al.* Comparison of high dose or standard dose cisplatin with etoposide and bleomycin (HDPEB vs. PEB) in children with stage I–IV extragonadal malignant germ cell tumors (MGCT): a Pediatric Intergroup report (POG9049/CCG8882). *Proc Am Soc Clin Oncol* 1998; **17**:525.

56. Giller R, Cushing B, Lauer S, *et al.* Comparison of high-dose or standard-dose cisplatin with etoposide and bleomycin (HDPEB vs. PEB) in children with stage III and IV malignant germ cell tumors (MGCT) at gonadal primary sites: a pediatric intergroup (POG9049/CCG8882). *Proc Am Soc Clin Oncol* 1998; **17**:525.

57. Mann JR, Raafat F, Robinson K, *et al.* The United Kingdom Children's Cancer Study Group's second germ cell tumor study: carboplatin, etoposide, and bleomycin are effective treatment for children with malignant extracranial germ cell tumors, with acceptable toxicity. *J Clin Oncol* 2000; **18**:3809–3818.

58. Marina N, Fontanesi J, Kun L, *et al.* Treatment of childhood germ cell tumors. Review of the St. Jude experience from 1979 to 1988. *Cancer* 1992; **70**:2568–2575.

◆59. Einhorn LH, Donohue J. Cis-diamminedichloroplatinum, vinblastine, and bleomycin combination chemotherapy in disseminated testicular cancer. *Ann Intern Med* 1977; **87**:293–298.

60. Einhorn LH. Testicular cancer: an oncological success story. *Clin Cancer Res* 1997; **12**:2630–2632.

◆61. Luursema PB, Star-Kroesen MA, van der Mark TW, *et al.* Bleomycin-induced changes in the carbon monoxide transfer factor of the lungs and its components. *Am Rev Respir Dis* 1983; **128**:880–883.

62. Bell MR, Meredith DJ, Gill PG. Role of carbon monoxide diffusing capacity in the early detection of major bleomycin-induced pulmonary toxicity. *Aust NZ J Med* 1985; **15**:235–240.

63. Pagnoni A, Riboldi G, Valagussa P. Evaluation of lung ventilation and carbon monoxide-diffusing capacity in patients with

nonseminomatous testicular tumors treated with bleomycin. *Tumori* 1982; **68**:85–89.

64. Lucraft HH, Wilkinson PM, Stretton TB, Read G. Role of pulmonary function tests in the prevention of bleomycin pulmonary toxicity during chemotherapy for metastatic testicular teratoma. *Eur J Cancer Clin Oncol* 1982; **18**:133–139.

65. Comis RL, Kuppinger MS, Ginsberg SJ, *et al.* Role of single-breath carbon monoxide-diffusing capacity in monitoring the pulmonary effects of bleomycin in germ cell tumor patients. *Cancer Res* 1979; **39**:5076–5080.

66. Sorensen PG, Rossing N, Rorth M. Carbon monoxide diffusing capacity: a reliable indicator of bleomycin-induced pulmonary toxicity. *Eur J Respir Dis* 1985; **66**:333–340.

67. Mann JR, Pearson D, Barrett A, *et al.* Results of the United Kingdom Children's Cancer Study Group's malignant germ cell tumor studies. *Cancer* 1989; **63**:1657–1667.

68. Baranzelli MC, Kramar A, Bouffet E, *et al.* Prognostic factors in children with localized malignant nonseminomatous germ cell tumors. *J Clin Oncol* 1999; **17**:1212–1218.

69. Probert JC, Parker BR. The effects of radiation therapy on bone growth. *Radiology* 1975; **114**:155–162.

70. Donaldson SS, Kaplan HS. Complications of treatment of Hodgkin's disease in children. *Cancer Treat Rep* 1982; **66**:977–989.

71. Donaldson SS, Link MP. Combined modality treatment with low-dose radiation and MOPP chemotherapy for children with Hodgkin's disease. *J Clin Oncol* 1987; **5**:742–749.

72. Brusamolino E, Lunghi F, Orlandi E, *et al.* Treatment of early-stage Hodgkin's disease with four cycles of ABVD followed by adjuvant radio-therapy: analysis of efficacy and long-term toxicity. *Haematologica* 2000; **85**:1032–1039.

73. Salloum E, Tanoue LT, Wackers FJ, *et al.* Assessment of cardiac and pulmonary function in adult patients with Hodgkin's disease treated with ABVD or MOPP/ABVD plus adjuvant low-dose mediastinal irradiation. *Cancer Invest* 1999; **17**:171–180.

74. Allavena C, Conroy T, Aletti P, Bey P, Lederlin P. Late cardiopulmonary toxicity after treatment for Hodgkin's disease. *Br J Cancer* 1992; **65**:908–912.

75. Horning SJ, Adhikari A, Rizk N, Hoppe RT, Olshen RA. Effect of treatment for Hodgkin's disease on pulmonary function: results of a prospective study. *J Clin Oncol* 1994; **12**:297–305.

76. Villani F, De Maria P, Bonfante V, *et al.* Late pulmonary toxicity after treatment for Hodgkin's disease. *Anticancer Res* 1997; **17**(6D):4739–4742.

77. Brice P, Tredaniel J, Monsuez JJ, *et al.* Cardiopulmonary toxicity after three courses of ABVD and mediastinal irradiation in favorable Hodgkin's disease. *Ann Oncol* 1991; **2**(Suppl. 2): 73–76.

78. Hirsch A, Vander Els N, Straus DJ, *et al.* Effect of ABVD chemotherapy with and without mantle or mediastinal irradiation on pulmonary function and symptoms in early-stage Hodgkin's disease. *J Clin Oncol* 1996; **14**:1297–1305.

79. Marina NM, Greenwald CA, Fairclough DL, *et al.* Serial pulmonary function studies in children treated for newly diagnosed Hodgkin's disease with mantle radiotherapy plus cycles of cyclophosphamide, vincristine, and procarbazine alternating with cycles of doxorubicin, bleomycin, vinblastine, and dacarbazine. *Cancer* 1995; **75**:1706–1711.

◆80. Weiss RB, Poster DS, Penta JS. The nitrosoureas and pulmonary toxicity. *Cancer Treat Rev* 1981; **8**:111–125.

81. Patel AR, Shah PC, Rhee HL, *et al.* Cyclophosphamide therapy and interstitial pulmonary fibrosis. *Cancer* 1976; **38**: 1542–1549.

82. Sostman HD, Matthay RA, Putman CE, Smith GJ. Methotrexate-induced pneumonitis. *Medicine (Baltimore)* 1976; **55**:371–388.

83. Friedman HS, Pluda J, Quinn JA, *et al.* Phase I trial of carmustine plus 0-6-benzylguanine for patients with recurrent or progressive malignant glioma. *J Clin Oncol* 2000; **18**:3522–3528.

84. Grossman SA, Wharam M, Sheidler V, *et al.* Phase II study of continuous infusion carmustine and cisplatin followed by cranial irradiation in adults with newly diagnosed high-grade astrocytoma. *J Clin Oncol* 1997; **15**:2596–2603.

85. Gaetani P, Silvani V, Butti G, *et al.* Nitrosourea derivatives-induced pulmonary toxicity in patients treated for malignant brain tumors. Early subclinical detection and its prevention. *Eur J Cancer Clin Oncol* 1987; **23**:267–271.

◆86. Aronin PA, Mahaley MS Jr, Rudnick SA, *et al.* Prediction of BCNU pulmonary toxicity in patients with malignant gliomas: an assessment of risk factors. *N Engl J Med* 1980; **303**:183–188.

◆87. O'Driscoll BR, Hasleton PS, Taylor PM, *et al.* Active lung fibrosis up to 17 years after chemotherapy with carmustine (BCNU) in childhood. *N Engl J Med* 1990; **323**:378–382.

◆88. O'Driscoll BR, Kalra S, Gattamaneni HR, Woodcock AA. Late carmustine lung fibrosis. Age at treatment may influence severity and survival. *Chest* 1995; **107**:1355–1357.

89. Durant JR, Norgard MJ, Murad TM, *et al.* Pulmonary toxicity associated with bischloroethylnitrosourea (BCNU). *Ann Intern Med* 1979; **90**:191–194.

90. Carlson K, Backlund L, Smedmyr B, *et al.* Pulmonary function and complications subsequent to autologous bone marrow transplantation. *Bone Marrow Transplant* 1994; **14**:805–811.

91. Phillips GL, Fay JW, Herzig GP, *et al.* Intensive 1,3-bis(2-chloroethyl)-1-nitrosourea (BCNU), NSC #4366650 and cryopreserved autologous marrow transplantation for refractory cancer. A phase I–II study. *Cancer* 1983; **52**:1792–1802.

92. Bhalla KS, Wilczynski SW, Abushamaa AM, *et al.* Pulmonary toxicity of induction chemotherapy prior to standard or high-dose chemotherapy with autologous hematopoietic support. *Am J Respir Crit Care Med* 2000; **161**:17–25.

93. Ager S, Mahendra P, Richards EM, *et al.* High-dose carmustine, etoposide and melphalan ('BEM') with autologous stem cell transplantation: a dose-toxicity study. *Bone Marrow Transplant* 1996; **17**:335–340.

94. Seiden MV, Elias A, Ayash L, *et al.* Pulmonary toxicity associated with high dose chemotherapy in the treatment of solid tumors with autologous marrow transplant: an analysis of four chemotherapy regimens. *Bone Marrow Transplant* 1992; **10**:57–63.

95. Prince DS, Wingard JR, Saral R, *et al.* Longitudinal changes in pulmonary function following bone marrow transplantation. *Chest* 1989; **96**:301–306.

96. Hartsell WF, Czyzewski EA, Ghalie R, Kaizer H. Pulmonary complications of bone marrow transplantation: a comparison of total body irradiation and cyclophosphamide to busulfan and cyclophosphamide. *Int J Radiat Oncol Biol Phys* 1995; **32**:69–73.

97. Santos GW, Tutschka PJ, Brookmeyer R, *et al.* Marrow transplantation for acute nonlymphocytic leukemia after treatment with busulfan and cyclophosphamide. *N Engl J Med* 1983; **309**:1347–1353.

98. Rosenthal MA, Grigg AP, Sheridan WP. High dose busulphan/cyclophosphamide for autologous bone marrow transplantation is associated with minimal non-hemopoietic toxicity. *Leuk Lymphoma* 1994; **14**(3–4):279–283.

99. Shaw PJ, Hugh-Jones K, Hobbs J, *et al.* Busulphan and cyclophosphamide cause little early toxicity during displacement bone marrow transplantation in fifty children. *Bone Marrow Transplant* 1986; **1**:193–200.

100. Matthay KK. Intensification of therapy using hematopoietic stem-cell support for high-risk neuroblastoma. *Pediatr Transplant* 1999; **3**(Suppl. 1):72–77.

101. Ladenstein R, Lasset C, Pinkerton R, *et al.* Impact of megatherapy in children with high-risk Ewing's tumours in complete remission: a report from the EBMT Solid Tumour Registry. *Bone Marrow Transplant* 1995; **15**:697–705.

102. Sandhu HS, Barnes PJ, Hernandez P. Hydroxyurea-induced hypersensitivity pneumonitis: a case report and literature review. *Can Respir J* 2000; **7**:491–495.

103. Salvucci M, Zanchini R, Molinari A, *et al.* Lung toxicity following fludarabine, cytosine arabinoside and mitoxantrone (flan) treatment for acute leukemia. *Haematologica* 2000; **85**:769–770.

104. Linskens RK, Golding RP, van Groeningen CJ, Giaccone G. Severe acute lung injury induced by gemcitabine. *Neth J Med* 2000; **56**:232–235.

105. Briasoulis E, Froudarakis M, Milionis HJ, *et al.* Chemotherapy-induced noncardiogenic pulmonary edema related to gemcitabine plus docetaxel combination with granulocyte colony-stimulating factor support. *Respiration* 2000; **67**:680–683.

106. Gurjal A, An T, Valdivieso M, Kalemkerian GP. Etoposide-induced pulmonary toxicity. *Lung Cancer* 1999; **26**:109–112.

107. Madarnas Y, Webster P, Shorter AM, Bjarnason GA. Irinotecan-associated pulmonary toxicity. *Anticancer Drugs* 2000; **11**:709–713.

◆108. Weiner RS, Bortin MM, Gale RP, *et al.* Interstitial pneumonitis after bone marrow transplantation. Assessment of risk factors. *Ann Intern Med* 1986; **104**:168–175.

◆109. Quabeck K. The lung as a critical organ in marrow transplantation. *Bone Marrow Transplant* 1994; **14**(Suppl. 4):S19–S28.

110. Rubio C, Hill ME, Milan S, *et al.* Idiopathic pneumonia syndrome after high-dose chemotherapy for relapsed Hodgkin's disease. *Br J Cancer* 1997; **75**:1044–1048.

111. Clark JG, Crawford SW, Madtes DK, Sullivan KM. Obstructive lung disease after allogeneic marrow transplantation. Clinical presentation and course. *Ann Intern Med* 1989; **111**:368–376.

112. Robbins RA, Linder J, Stahl MG, *et al.* Diffuse alveolar hemorrhage in autologous bone marrow transplant recipients. *Am J Med* 1989; **87**:511–518.

113. Epler GR, Colby TV, McLoud TC, *et al.* Bronchiolitis obliterans organizing pneumonia. *N Engl J Med* 1985; **312**:152–158.

6

Urological complications

6a

Renal damage

RODERICK SKINNER

This subchapter describes the nature and consequences of chronic renal impairment caused by the treatment of malignant disease in children and adolescents. Most episodes of clinically important chronic nephrotoxicity are due to ifosfamide or cisplatin.[1,2] Although the clinical features of and risk factors for renal toxicity due to these drugs are well documented, the mechanisms of toxicity remain unclear, hindering efforts at prediction or prevention.

WHAT IS NEPHROTOXICITY AND WHY IS IT IMPORTANT?

Nephrotoxicity may be defined as the ability of a treatment to specifically impair renal function or cause pathological renal lesions. It may occur acutely or insidiously, and may be reversible, or progressive and irreversible. Its severity is very variable, ranging from subclinical impairment of renal function detectable only by sensitive investigations, to life-threatening disease.

Chronic nephrotoxicity is important for several reasons. It may cause significant morbidity, impairing the quality of both short- and long-term survival. Its consequences may necessitate complex treatment, and reduce the ability to deliver the best possible antineoplastic treatment. Even in patients with subclinical toxicity only, the potential for serious morbidity in later life is worrying, especially in children. Therefore, attempts to reduce the frequency and severity of nephrotoxicity are very important.

WHAT CAUSES CHRONIC NEPHROTOXICITY?

There are many potential causes of chronic renal impairment in patients treated for cancer or leukemia, including the malignant process itself and complications of its treatment, which may include chemotherapy, radiotherapy, surgery, immunotherapy or supportive treatment.[1] Features of the malignant disease itself may contribute to chronic renal impairment, e.g. damage to normal renal tissue owing to tumor infiltration or urinary tract obstruction.

The high renal blood flow across a large endothelial surface area enables the kidneys to perform their excretory functions but renders them particularly vulnerable to toxic damage. Furthermore, the reabsorptive and secretory capabilities of proximal tubular cells expose them to toxic substances, which may accumulate or undergo further metabolism in these metabolically highly active cells.

The most important cytotoxic drugs likely to cause chronic renal toxicity are cisplatin and ifosfamide (Table 6a.1), both of which are used extensively owing to their efficacy in many solid tumors, but may cause chronic nephrotoxicity in 30–60 per cent of children.[3,4] Nephrotoxicity due to other cytotoxic drugs is less frequent, but

Table 6a.1 *Nephrotoxic treatments in children with cancer*

Chemotherapy
- Frequent and potentially severe nephrotoxicity
  - Cisplatin
  - Ifosfamide
- Infrequent but potentially severe nephrotoxicity
  - Carboplatin
  - Methotrexate (especially high-dose)
  - Nitrosoureas (especially semustine)
- Rare reports of nephrotoxicity
  - Anthracyclines (daunorubicin, doxorubicin)
  - 5-Azacytidine[a]
  - Cyclophosphamide
  - Cytosine arabinoside
  - Melphalan
  - Mithramycin[a]
  - Mitomycin C[a]
  - Streptozotocin[a]
  - 6-Thioguanine

Radiotherapy
Surgery
Immunotherapy
Bone marrow transplantation
Supportive treatment

[a]Rarely used in children.

carboplatin, methotrexate and nitrosoureas may cause serious damage.[1] Rarely, significant renal damage may occur after cytotoxic drugs not usually regarded as major nephrotoxins.

Radiotherapy may lead to chronic 'radiation nephritis', which may have a delayed onset yet progress to chronic renal failure (CRF). Late hypertension, sometimes severe, may also occur.[5] Surgical removal of significant amounts of renal tissue (e.g. a unilateral nephrectomy) may result in glomerular hyperfiltration, which may occasionally lead to hypertension, and more rarely to glomerular impairment.[6] However, most survivors of contemporary treatment for Wilms' tumor do not suffer from clinically significant renal dysfunction.[7] Although some immunotherapeutic agents (e.g. interleukin-2) may cause reversible acute renal failure owing to capillary leak syndrome and intravascular hypovolemia, chronic renal damage is not generally recognized.[8] Several drugs used in supportive care (e.g. aminoglycosides, amphotericin B) may contribute to renal toxicity, which may occasionally be persistent.[9] Episodes of acute tubular necrosis owing to severe sepsis or hemorrhage are not infrequent, and renal function may not recover fully. Likewise, it is theoretically possible that recovery of renal function may be incomplete after severe uric acid nephropathy due to tumor lysis syndrome, although this appears to be very rare in practice.

In many clinical situations, chronic renal damage may be multifactorial, for example after bone marrow transplantation (BMT). The conditioning treatment used prior to BMT may include high doses of potentially nephrotoxic chemotherapy (e.g. carboplatin, melphalan), and/or total body irradiation (TBI). Early transplant-related complications, e.g. septicemia, hepatic veno-occlusive disease, may lead to prerenal failure owing to hemodynamic factors, with incomplete renal recovery. Frequent use of potentially nephrotoxic antibiotics, and often prolonged immunosuppressive treatment with cyclosporin A or tacrolimus, perpetuate renal impairment. Unsurprisingly, chronic renal damage is frequent after BMT, occurring in up to 50 per cent of children. Glomerular toxicity is usually predominant and, although radiotherapy is generally held to be primarily responsible, it is clear that other causative factors are also involved.[10] In contrast, tubular impairment is probably mainly due to conditioning chemotherapy.[11]

HOW IS CHRONIC NEPHROTOXICITY MEASURED?

The traditional evaluation of nephrotoxicity using the Common Toxicity Criteria depends on insensitive tests (e.g. serum creatinine concentration, which only becomes abnormal when much renal function has already been lost), or non-specific measures (e.g. proteinuria). Even measurement of glomerular filtration rate (GFR) by the creatinine clearance method has considerable limitations, especially in children, and gives an incomplete picture of, for example, ifosfamide or cisplatin nephrotoxicity.[12]

Meaningful evaluation of nephotoxicity requires an understanding of the renal regulation of fluid and electrolyte balance, and excretion of metabolic and toxic waste products. The human kidney has about one million nephrons, each comprising a glomerulus, proximal tubule, loop of Henle and distal tubule, draining into a collecting duct (Figure 6a.1). In functional terms, the

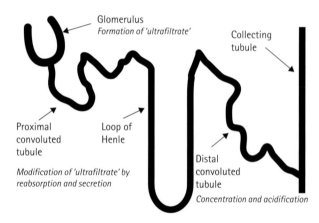

Figure 6a.1 *Structure and functions of the nephron.*

proximal nephron can be considered to include both the proximal convoluted tubule and the loop of Henle, and the distal nephron to comprise the distal convoluted tubule, the collecting tubule and collecting duct. Unless separate evaluation of glomerular, proximal and distal tubular function is performed, it is easy to underestimate or even overlook nephrotoxicity, especially tubular toxicity. Viewed simplistically, *glomerular filtration* leads to the formation of an 'ultrafiltrate', which then enters the *proximal nephron* where it is progressively modified by tubular reabsorption and secretion of electrolytes and other small molecules. Tubular secretion eliminates endogenous and exogenous toxic substances. Acidification and concentration of the ultrafiltrate occur in the *distal nephron*, with the formation of urine. Finally, the kidney has several non-excretory functions. Bone homeostasis is maintained, not just by regulating the urinary excretion

of calcium and phosphate, but also through the production of 1,25 dihydroxy vitamin D_3 in proximal tubular mitochondria. Other important roles include blood pressure regulation, production of erythropoietin, prostaglandin synthesis and drug metabolism.

The ideal investigation protocol for use in children should be simple, yet sensitive and comprehensive, providing functionally and clinically meaningful information. For example, a standardized investigation protocol (Table 6a.2) has been validated in a large number of children.[12] Investigations with varying levels of sensitivity may be chosen to allow assessment of clinically relevant toxicity, subtler degrees of subclinical dysfunction, or both.

Grading systems have the potential to improve reporting of the nature, severity and reversibility of nephrotoxicity, and to facilitate evaluation of risk factors, but many fail to describe renal toxicity adequately, e.g. by failing to assess tubular function. It is important to evaluate clinically significant toxicity, preferably by measuring the underlying abnormalities of renal function. Specific grading systems are required to reflect the distinct nephrotoxic profiles of different drugs.

Table 6a.2 *Protocol for investigation of nephrotoxicity in children*

Glomerular function
- Serum creatinine concentration
- Glomerular filtration rate (GFR; ideally measured by radioisotope plasma clearance method)

Proximal tubular function
- Blood and urine concentrations of sodium, potassium, chloride, bicarbonate, creatinine, (ionized) calcium, magnesium, phosphate, glucose
  - with calculation of fractional excretion of sodium[a,b], calcium[b], magnesium[a,b], phosphate[c], glucose[c]; and of renal tubular threshold of phosphate (Tm_p/GFR)[c]
- *Urine excretion of low-molecular-weight proteins (e.g. RBP), amino acids*

Distal tubular function[c]
- Early morning urine osmolality
- Assessment of renal control of acid–base balance (in patients with RTA)
- DDAVP test (in patients with consistently low urine osmolalities)

Bone chemistry
- Blood alkaline phosphatase activity
- Radiological assessment (in patients with hypophosphataemic rickets)[c]

General aspects of renal function
- Blood concentrations and urine excretion of albumin, protein
- *Urine excretion of renal tubular enzymes (e.g. NAG)*
- Blood pressure
- Height and weight
- Growth

Investigations in italics will detect subclinical nephrotoxicity.
[a,b,c]These investigations are most helpful in evaluating nephrotoxicity owing to [a]carboplatin, [b]cisplatin or [c]ifosfamide.
DDAVP, desmopressin; NAG, *N*-acetylglucosaminidase; RBP, retinol-binding protein; RTA, renal tubular acidosis.

WHAT ARE THE CLINICAL CONSEQUENCES OF CHRONIC NEPHROTOXICITY?

The clinical consequences of chronic nephrotoxicity may be categorized according to the functional segments of the nephron. Glomerular damage may lead to CRF and its potential complications, e.g. renal osteodystrophy. Proximal tubular impairment reduces reabsorption of a variety of electrolytes (e.g. phosphate, magnesium) and small molecules; extensive damage may lead to the Fanconi syndrome, with a wide range of severe clinical manifestations, e.g. hypophosphatemic rickets (HR), proximal renal tubular acidosis (RTA). Distal tubular dysfunction impairs urinary concentration and acidification; when severe, this results in nephrogenic diabetes insipidus (NDI) and distal RTA, respectively. Additionally, it is important to recognize other potential consequences of renal damage, including reduced production of 1,25 dihydroxy vitamin D_3,[13] hypertension, anemia, growth impairment, and the risk of impaired renal drug metabolism and excretion.

CAN NEPHROTOXICITY BE TREATED?

Ideally, nephrotoxicity should be treated before the development of chronic damage by withdrawal of the causative agent, but often this is not possible owing to the delayed onset of detectable renal damage. Therefore, management

is frequently supportive, comprising correction of established biochemical abnormalities and occasionally renal replacement treatment. Rarely, specific treatment may be possible, e.g. steroids for drug-induced interstitial nephritis.

CAN CHRONIC NEPHROTOXICITY BE PREDICTED?

Since early acute nephrotoxicity is often progressive,[14] it is feasible that early subclinical renal dysfunction may predict later nephrotoxicity. A small study in eight adults suggested a relationship between the cumulative increase in retinol-binding protein (RBP) excretion (a marker of subclinical proximal tubular toxicity) during the first 4 days after cisplatin treatment and the serum creatinine concentration 3 weeks later,[15] but no later follow-up data were available. Preliminary observations in 12 children treated with ifosfamide suggested that early acute reductions in the urine excretion of Tamm-Horsfall protein, which is produced in the loop of Henle in healthy subjects, may be more common in those who subsequently develop chronic nephrotoxicity.[16] However, the marked inter- and intra-individual variability in measures of subclinical tubular toxicity during ifosfamide treatment in children suggests that reliable prediction of chronic toxicity may be difficult (Font de Mora and Skinner, unpublished observations). Alternatively, it has been suggested that measurement of pharmocokinetic parameters during treatment may enable prediction of the risk of later nephrotoxicity. An analysis in 12 adults receiving cisplatin suggested a relationship between the peak plasma concentration of ultrafilterable platinum and glomerular toxicity after four treatment courses.[17] However, no simple relationship has been identified between the pharmacokinetics of ifosfamide and its acute or chronic nephrotoxicity in children.[18] In summary, reliable prediction of significant chronic nephrotoxicity has not been achieved yet.

CAN CHRONIC NEPHROTOXICITY BE PREVENTED?

Several general strategies may be investigated with the aim of reducing the risk and severity of chronic nephrotoxicity.[19] Clinical risk factors for the development of chronic ifosfamide or cisplatin nephrotoxicity have been established (see below), and this knowledge may be used to identify high-risk patients or design less nephrotoxic chemotherapy protocols. However, such approaches do not prevent all instances of significant renal toxicity and, since they often involve reducing the dose of the nephrotoxic drug, they may reduce the curative potential of treatment. A more attractive approach seeks to identify the molecular events underlying nephrotoxicity, allowing design of less toxic analogues. Several new platinum drugs have been developed but it is important to ensure that their cytotoxic efficacy is not inferior to the parent compound. Improved methods of drug delivery are under development (e.g. using liposomes).

Specific protective measures may be adopted, such as renal shielding, where feasible in abdominal radiotherapy, and vigorous hydration regimens during administration of cisplatin, ifosfamide or methotrexate. The potential use of subtotal nephrectomy for Wilms' tumor, to reduce loss of normal renal tissue, is under investigation. Several protective drugs have been studied, especially for cisplatin nephrotoxicity, but none has found general acceptance yet in pediatric practice.

CHRONIC NEPHROTOXICITY DUE TO CHEMOTHERAPY

Unless stated otherwise, only chronic nephrotoxicity is described below, although it is important to recognize that recovery from acute damage may be incomplete, thereby causing or contributing to chronic renal impairment.

CHRONIC IFOSFAMIDE NEPHROTOXICITY

Clinical features (Table 6a.3)

Ifosfamide may cause any combination of chronic glomerular, proximal or distal tubular toxicity, with a very wide range of severity.[3] The reported incidence of significant chronic glomerular toxicity in children has ranged from 1.4 per cent[20] to about 30 per cent,[21,22] depending on the patient group and the measures of toxicity studied. Chronic proximal tubular toxicity is very common, ranging from subclinical glycosuria in about 90 per cent of children in a large multicenter study[23] to HR and/or proximal RTA in over 25 per cent in smaller single-center studies.[22,24] Although apparent reductions in urinary concentrating ability may occur in 30 per cent of children after ifosfamide,[22] their clinical significance is dubious.[25]

Although there is much interindividual variability in the onset, nature and severity of chronic ifosfamide nephrotoxicity in children, proximal tubular damage is usually predominant. Chronic subclinical proximal tubular toxicity may lead to glycosuria, aminoaciduria and increased urine excretion of low-molecular-weight proteins [including RBP, α_1-microglobulin and

Table 6a.3 *Clinical features of ifosfamide nephrotoxicity*

Glomerular toxicity
- Elevated blood creatinine concentration
- Reduced glomerular filtration rate
- *Acute renal failure*
- *Chronic renal failure*

Proximal tubular toxicity
- Aminoaciduria
- Glycosuria
- Increased urinary excretion of
  - low-molecular-weight proteins (e.g. RBP)
  - proximal tubular antigens (e.g. ADBP)
- Fanconi syndrome (as above, plus phosphaturia, bicarbonaturia, kaluria), leading to
  - *hypophosphatemia and hypophosphatemic rickets (HR)*
  - *proximal renal tubular acidosis (RTA)*
  - *hypokalemia*
- Calciuria, magnesuria, natriuria (rarely)

Distal tubular toxicity
- Subclinical impairment of urinary acidification
- Subclinical impairment of urinary concentration
- *Distal RTA*
- *Nephrogenic diabetes insipidus*

Tubular toxicity (not specific of proximal or distal tubular localization)
- Increased urinary excretion of renal tubular enzymes (e.g. NAG)

Renal toxicity (not specific of glomerular or tubular localization)
- Proteinuria
- *Hypertension*
- *Growth failure* (related to chronic HR and/or RTA)

Clinically relevant features of toxicity are listed in italics.
ADBP, adenosine deaminase binding protein; NAG, N-acetylglucosaminidase; RBP, retinol-binding protein.

β_2-microglobulin (β_2-M)], or of the proximal tubular antigen adenosine deaminase-binding protein (ADBP).[14,24,26–28] More severe failure of proximal tubular reabsorption leads to a Fanconi syndrome, with phosphaturia, kaluria, bicarbonaturia and, more rarely, calciuria and magnesuria. Tubular damage may be accompanied by chronic glomerular impairment,[21,22,29] manifest by an elevated serum creatinine concentration and a reduced GFR. In some patients, particularly adolescents, glomerular toxicity may be the major feature of toxicity.[30] However, CRF is rare. Clinically relevant distal RTA and NDI are well described but uncommon.[22,31–33] Raised urinary excretion of renal tubular enzymes (RTEs)[14,34] reflects chronic tubular damage in general. Proteinuria may be a non-specific consequence of glomerular and/or tubular damage.

The clinical consequences of chronic ifosfamide-induced nephrotoxicity in children include HR, RTA and NDI.[22,29,33,35] Rarely, hypertension may occur.[36] CRF, HR and RTA may cause growth impairment in children.[37]

Clinical management

The prevention or treatment of manifestations of established severe tubular toxicity, especially HR and RTA in growing children, may necessitate prolonged supplementation with high doses of phosphate or bicarbonate, or less commonly other electrolytes. 1α-hydroxy vitamin D_3 is used occasionally, but the risk of metastatic calcification and nephrocalcinosis necessitates careful monitoring especially in normocalcaemic patients.

Reversibility

The degree of reversibility of chronic ifosfamide nephrotoxicity appears unpredictable. Although some recovery may occur after acute nephrotoxicity, both glomerular[30,38] and tubular function[39] may deteriorate after the end of treatment. Subsequently, partial recovery from severe renal damage may occur[40] but complete resolution appears to be rare.[41] There are no published very long-term follow-up data; however, anecdotal reports suggest that the outcome is variable with nephrotoxicity persisting relatively unchanged in most children, but either deteriorating or improving considerably in some.

Risk factors

Risk factors suggested for the development of nephrotoxicity after ifosfamide include higher cumulative ifosfamide dose, younger patient age at treatment, the administration schedule, previous or concurrent cisplatin (or other potential nephrotoxins), and pre-existing renal impairment or tumor invasion. Children receiving higher total doses of ifosfamide (>60–$80\,\text{g/m}^2$) appear to be at greater risk,[23,42] but extensive damage may still occur after much lower doses.[33] Likewise, although ifosfamide may cause severe renal damage at any age, most published reports of severe toxicity have been in infants and young children, who may be more vulnerable both to proximal tubular toxicity and its consequences, especially growth failure.[42,43] There is no convincing evidence that the duration of intravenous administration of ifosfamide (bolus, short or continuous infusion) influences the risk of acute or chronic nephrotoxicity.[18,44] Ifosfamide nephrotoxicity appears to be increased by prior cisplatin therapy,[20,45] whilst combination with very high-dose carboplatin may cause severe toxicity.[46] Severe renal damage has been reported in patients with prior unilateral nephrectomy, renal impairment or tumor infiltration,[29,47] but the relative risk of toxicity in such patients is unknown. However, these factors are of less predictive value in individual patients. It is attractive to speculate that differences in ifosfamide pharmacokinetics may explain some of the interindividual variability in the severity of

nephrotoxicity, but there is no direct evidence to support this hypothesis.

Pathogenesis

The few reported renal biopsies have described focal proximal tubular changes with relatively little or no glomerular damage.[48] The balance of evidence suggests a toxic, rather than immunopathological, lesion but the pathogenesis is still poorly understood. Studies in rats and *in vitro* proximal renal tubular cell cultures have demonstrated direct cellular toxicity owing to the drug or, more likely, a metabolite.[49–51] The nature of this toxicity is not clear, but disruption of tubular cell energy pathways and membrane function have been implicated.[50,52] Although the metabolism of ifosfamide and its non-nephrotoxic structural isomer cyclophosphamide are qualitatively similar, quantitative differences provide possible clues.[3] Ifosfamide is activated by ring-hydroxylation to 4-hydroxyifosfamide/aldoifosfamide, which may either decompose to isophosphoramide mustard (the active alkylating metabolite) and acrolein, or undergo oxidation to inactive carboxyifosfamide. The magnitude of each of these metabolic routes varies greatly between individual patients, while the influence of ifosfamide dose and schedule is unclear.[18,53] Furthermore, side-chain dechlorethylation to chloroacetaldehyde (CAA) may account for up to 50 per cent of ifosfamide metabolism in some patients, while cyclophosphamide metabolism yields very little CAA.[54]

Unchanged ifosfamide and its metabolites are excreted in urine. After intravenous injection, mesna (a synthetic thiol capable of detoxifying reactive ifosfamide metabolites, including CAA and acrolein) is rapidly oxidized in plasma to dimesna. Both mesna and dimesna are cleared by glomerular filtration, and either excreted or alternatively taken up by renal tubular cells. The amount of mesna in tubular cells available to detoxify ifosfamide metabolites may depend on the mesna administration schedule, but the clinical importance of this is not clear.[3] CAA is highly toxic to epithelial cells, and may induce an experimental Fanconi syndrome in the LLCPK$_1$ cell line (a proximal tubular model) and in the isolated perfused rat kidney, possibly by inhibiting active transport and increasing the permeability of tubular cell membranes.[55,56] Therefore, CAA may account for the occurrence of renal toxicity after ifosfamide but not cyclophosphamide, while the considerable variability in its production and urinary excretion may lead to the variable severity seen in clinical practice. Theoretically mesna should be capable of detoxifying CAA, but this protective effect may be incomplete[57] and may be compromised further by the short plasma half-life and hence tubular 'transit time' of mesna.[3] Alternative explanations

for ifosfamide nephrotoxicity might be the production of a toxic metabolite not formed by cyclophosphamide metabolism (e.g. isophosphoramide mustard).[58]

Prevention

Until its pathogenesis is understood more completely, efforts to prevent ifosfamide nephrotoxicity depend on minimizing known risk factors. Cumulative doses over $80 \, \text{g/m}^2$ should be avoided,[23] and the drug used carefully in children younger than 5 years,[59] in those previously given cisplatin or with poor renal function. Other potentially nephrotoxic drugs should be used carefully. Separate studies using rat models have suggested that glycine or carnitine supplementation may ameliorate ifosfamide nephrotoxicity,[50,52] but the efficacy of this approach in humans has yet to be confirmed in a clinical trial.

CHRONIC CISPLATIN NEPHROTOXICITY

Clinical features (Table 6a.4)

Children treated with cisplatin may suffer substantial impairment of glomerular or tubular function, or both.[60,61] The reported incidence of glomerular toxicity has varied from about 20 per cent[62] to over 80 per cent,[61] depending on the nature and timing of investigation, and that of hypomagnesemia from about 30 per cent[4] to 100 per cent.[63]

Glomerular impairment may cause a rise in plasma creatinine concentration or fall in GFR,[4,61,64,65] and CRF may develop insidiously.[66] Plasma creatinine levels and endogenous creatinine clearance are insensitive indicators of cisplatin-induced glomerular toxicity,[67] and may underestimate the true frequency of nephrotoxicity. Magnesuria, leading to hypomagnesemia, is the commonest manifestation of chronic proximal tubular toxicity.[68] There have been no specific investigations of distal tubular function after cisplatin treatment in children. However, chronic magnesuria, hypomagnesemia, hypocalciuria, with normocalcemia or mild hypercalcemia, and mild hypokalemic metabolic alkalosis, may result from dissociation of magnesium and calcium handling due to a lesion at a distal convoluted tubular site.[60,68,69] Alternatively, it has been suggested that hypocalcemia may be due to hypomagnesemia-induced impairment of parathyroid hormone.[70] Similarly, kaluria and hypomagnesemia may both contribute to hypokalemia, while natriuria may lead to hyponatremia.[69–72] Polyuria is described, perhaps due to distal nephron resistance to vasopressin.[73]

Subclinical tubular toxicity may lead to aminoaciduria, glycosuria, phosphaturia and increased urine excretion of RBP, β_2-M, *N*-acetylglucosaminidase (NAG), alanine aminopeptidase and β-galactosidase,[15,71] but this is rarely

Table 6a.4 *Clinical features of cisplatin nephrotoxicity*

Glomerular toxicity
- Elevated blood creatinine concentration
- Reduced glomerular filtration rate
- *Acute renal failure*
- *Chronic renal failure*

Proximal tubular toxicity
- Increased urinary excretion of
  - magnesium, potassium, sodium, glucose, ?calcium
  - amino acids
  - low-molecular-weight proteins (e.g. RBP)
- The consequences of proximal tubular toxicity include
  - *hypomagnesemia*
  - *hypocalcemia*
  - *hypokalemia*
  - *hyponatremia*

Distal tubular toxicity
- Impairment of water and sodium reabsorption
- Syndrome of hypomagnesemia – hypokalemia with hypocalciuria

Tubular toxicity (not specific of proximal or distal tubular localization)
- Increased urinary excretion of renal tubular enzymes (e.g. NAG)

Renal toxicity (not specific of glomerular or tubular localization)
- Albuminuria, proteinuria
- *Hypertension*

Clinically relevant features of toxicity are listed in italics.
NAG, N-acetylglucosaminidase; RBP, retinol-binding protein.

persistent. Hypertension may occur,[74] probably due to renovascular mechanisms.[75]

The clinical consequences of chronic cisplatin nephrotoxicity include CRF, and hypomagnesemia, which may cause paraesthesiae, tremor, tetany and convulsions.[64,70] Hemolytic uremic syndrome is a rare but well-described complication of cisplatin.[76]

Clinical management

The management of cisplatin nephrotoxicity involves correction of hypomagnesemia, which may also improve the associated hypocalcemia.[70] Although frequently prescribed, it is not clear whether routine long-term magnesium supplementation is absolutely necessary. Indeed, there has been no detailed study of the long-term clinical consequences of chronic cisplatin-induced hypomagnesemia in children.

Reversibility

Although several reports have emphasized the apparent irreversibility of cisplatin nephrotoxicity, two studies in children have suggested that glomerular impairment, but not hypomagnesemia, may improve partially with time.[4,77]

Risk factors

There are relatively few data about the importance of patient- and treatment-related risk factors for cisplatin nephrotoxicity in children. These may include high total dose and dose rate, administration schedule, patient age, concurrent treatment with other potential nephrotoxins, and interindividual differences in cisplatin pharmacokinetics. The dose intensity of cisplatin may be an important determinant of risk. Daugaard found less glomerular and tubular toxicity in adults after low-dose (i.e. 20 mg/m^2 per day) than after high-dose cisplatin (i.e. 40 mg/m^2 day).[67,71] Moderate or severe glomerular impairment and/or hypomagnesemia were significantly more frequent in children receiving a high cisplatin dose rate (>40–120 mg/m^2 per day) than in those receiving a low rate (40 mg/m^2 per day).[77] The influence of total dose is uncertain; while some studies in adults and children have suggested a relationship between cumulative dose and nephrotoxicity,[68,78] others have not.[4,77] There is no clear relationship between age and GFR or hypomagnesemia in children.[4,77] Treatment with other potential nephrotoxins, including ifosfamide and methotrexate, may increase renal toxicity.[79] Interindividual variability in cisplatin pharmacokinetics may be important. As mentioned above, measurement of pharmacokinetic parameters may predict the risk of chronic nephrotoxicity[17] but there is no evidence that it allows successful reduction of this risk by subsequent treatment modification.

Pathogenesis

Platinum is still detectable in blood up to 20 years after treatment with cisplatin[80] and it is likely that the chronicity of cisplatin nephrotoxicity is related to its retention in renal tissue. Histopathological studies in adults have usually shown a variety of tubular lesions but a striking lack of glomerular abnormalities.[81] However, the precise cause of cisplatin nephrotoxicity is unknown, with uncertainty over whether a proximal or distal tubular lesion, or indeed both, is primarily responsible.

The pharmacology of cisplatin is complex.[82] After rapid distribution, substantial protein-binding of platinum occurs, predominantly to plasma proteins but also to cellular proteins, with both reversible and irreversible components.[83] The slow excretion of protein-bound platinum leads to a long terminal half-life (20–80 hours) of total platinum. The details of the renal tubular handling of cisplatin are not clear, but both reabsorption and secretion may be involved with net tubular secretion.

In plasma that has a relatively high chloride concentration the neutral dichlorocisplatin complex predominates, whereas in the low-chloride intracellular environment, formation of large amounts of the more reactive aquated species may produce nephrotoxic metabolites.[84] This is the rationale for the use of hypertonic saline hydration with cisplatin. Cisplatin nephrotoxicity may be mediated by renal tubular transport and accumulation of the drug or a (so far, unidentified) toxic metabolite.[85,86] Alternatively, renal damage may be initiated by renal arteriolar vasoconstriction,[69,87] possibly via mechanisms involving adenosine, platelet-activating factor (PAF) or thromboxane A_2, although the evidence is conflicting.[88-90] There is similar uncertainty about the subcellular basis of cisplatin nephrotoxicity. The many suggestions of biochemical events that may be involved include binding to biological nucleophiles and proteins such as glutathione, inhibition of enzymes including ATPase, reduction in cellular and nuclear synthetic activity, especially of DNA and RNA, and damage to mitochondrial DNA, glutathione or enzymes.[82,91-93] However, the relevance of these processes to nephrotoxicity is unclear.

Prevention

Given its major contribution to the successful treatment of many solid malignancies, cisplatin is likely to remain in frequent use until improved analogues are introduced. Many strategies that may prevent or reduce its nephrotoxicity have been investigated.[94,95] Prophylactic intravenous magnesium supplements in hydration fluid reduce the frequency and severity of hypomagnesemia.[96] As a result of early experience, the administration of cisplatin by prolonged continuous infusion and saline hyperhydration, with or without frusemide or mannitol osmotic diuresis, is believed to reduce nephrotoxicity,[95] but it is clear that nephroprotection is not complete.[69] However, it would appear wise to use a low dose rate of cisplatin.

Many pharmacological agents that may ameliorate cisplatin nephrotoxicity have been investigated,[94] but none has found widespread acceptance yet owing to uncertainty about the mechanism of toxicity, and the lack of clear evidence to demonstrate improvements in the therapeutic index of cisplatin. Amongst many others, the drugs studied have included a variety of sulfur-containing compounds, such as sodium thiosulphate, WR-2721 (amifostine), DDTC (sodium diethyldithiocarbamate), mesna, biotin, cephalexin and sulfathiazole, all of which probably react with nephrotoxic cisplatin metabolites to form less toxic products.[94,97] The role of amifostine in children is under investigation in a current North American trial. Based on data from adult studies, guidelines from the American Society of Clinical Oncology suggest that its use may be considered for the prevention of cisplatin nephrotoxicity.[98] A second pharmacological approach involves inhibiting tubular cisplatin transport; e.g. with probenecid (organic anion) or cimetidine (organic cation transport), but the uncertainty concerning which tubular pathways transport cisplatin has hampered the development of this strategy.[99,100] A third potential method of nephroprotection is the use of agents that may counteract possible mediators of renal vasoconstriction, including aminophylline (to block adenosine) and BN 52063 (to antagonize PAF).[88,89] Numerous cisplatin analogues (e.g. ormaplatin, oxaliplatin and zeniplatin) and complexes (e.g. with alginates, methionine, procaine hydrochloride) have been developed in the search for pharmacokinetic and pharmacodynamic properties that will reduce nephrotoxicity without losing cytotoxic efficacy. Recently, liposomal and microsphere preparations have been designed. A Phase I clinical study of liposomal cisplatin in children demonstrated reduced renal toxicity but cisplatin appeared to be retained within the liposomes, thereby compromising efficacy.[101]

CHRONIC CARBOPLATIN NEPHROTOXICITY

The use of carboplatin as an adjunct or alternative to cisplatin has increased in view of its activity in several adult and pediatric solid tumors and its lower nephrotoxic potential.[102] Preclinical and early clinical studies suggested that carboplatin causes much less renal damage than cisplatin.[103,104]

Clinical features (Table 6a.5)

Carboplatin nephrotoxicity, similar to that seen after cisplatin, may occur in children, but it is less frequent, usually milder and often reversible. The incidence of glomerular impairment has ranged from 0 per cent[105] to about 25 per cent[106] and that of hypomagnesemia from 0 per cent[107] to 10 per cent.[108] Glomerular impairment is generally absent[105] or mild with a small reduction in GFR.[106] Acute renal failure (ARF), sometimes reversible, may develop occasionally in adults.[109-111] ARF occurred after high-dose carboplatin and melphalan in four children, with resultant CRF in one,[112] and after high-dose carboplatin alone in one child, with incomplete recovery.[113] Tubular damage leading to hypomagnesemia may occur[103] but is often reversible.[114] Natriuria and hyponatremia have been reported[115] but appear to be reversible. Chronic subclinical tubular damage, manifest by increased urine RBP and RTE excretion, is reported.[114]

Table 6a.5 *Clinical features of carboplatin nephrotoxicity*

Glomerular toxicity
- Elevated blood creatinine concentration
- Reduced glomerular filtration rate
- *Acute renal failure* (very rare)

Proximal tubular toxicity
- *Hypomagnesemia* (magnesuria not yet demonstrated)
- Natriuria and *hyponatremia*
- Increased urinary excretion of
  - low-molecular-weight proteins (e.g. β2-microglobulin)

Tubular toxicity (not specific of proximal or distal tubular localization)
- Increased urinary excretion of renal tubular enzymes (e.g. *N*-acetylglucosaminidase)

Renal toxicity (not specific of glomerular or tubular localization)
- *Albuminuria, proteinuria*

Clinically relevant features of toxicity are listed in *italics*.

Clinical sequelae of carboplatin nephrotoxicity in children are rare and usually fully reversible, except for hypomagnesemia, and, rarely, CRF.

Risk factors

Adult studies have not revealed clear relationships between individual or cumulative carboplatin doses, age or sex, and nephrotoxicity.[110,111] However, a pediatric study found that the frequency and severity of hypomagnesemia was correlated with cumulative carboplatin dose.[114] Carboplatin-induced ARF has been reported in adults given prior cisplatin,[109,110] while prior ifosfamide or concomitant melphalan have been associated with ARF in children.[112,113] Indeed, glomerular clearance is the major route of carboplatin excretion and patients with pre-existing renal impairment may be more susceptible to carboplatin nephrotoxicity.[103,110]

Pathogenesis

Histopathological lesions suggesting interstitial nephritis have been decribed in two women with carboplatin nephrotoxicity, one of whom also had 'toxic' tubular changes on electron microscopy,[109] but these findings may not be truly representative of carboplatin nephrotoxicity, since both patients received the drug intraperitoneally. It is usually assumed that cisplatin and carboplatin share the same nephrotoxic mechanism, but that the greater frequency and severity of cisplatin toxicity may result from formation of increased amounts of a putative nephrotoxic metabolite. This may be due to the increased lability of the chloride ligands of cisplatin compared to the cyclobutane dicarboxylate group of carboplatin.[116]

Prevention

Hydration reduces the risk of nephrotoxicity with high-dose carboplatin[117] but appears unnecessary with conventional doses of 400–600 mg/m^2.

NEPHROTOXICITY DUE TO OTHER CYTOTOXIC DRUGS USED IN BOTH ADULTS AND CHILDREN

Methotrexate may cause glomerular or tubular toxicity, albeit uncommonly. Initial studies of low-dose intravenous methotrexate revealed tubular cell necrosis and glomerular impairment, while high-dose intravenous methotrexate regimens ($>1 g/m^2$) occasionally caused serious or even fatal systemic or renal toxicity in adults.[118] Subclinical acute nephrotoxicity is well documented in children after high-dose methotrexate administration, with considerable reductions in GFR,[119] and rises in urine excretion of RTEs and ADBP,[27] but there is a lack of information about chronic nephrotoxicity. Methotrexate may cause nephrotoxicity by several mechanisms, including changes in glomerular hemodynamics, direct tubular toxicity, and precipitation of methotrexate or a metabolite within the distal nephron, causing intrarenal obstruction and ARF. The risk of methotrexate nephrotoxicity is reduced greatly by prophylactic intravenous fluid and alkalinization regimens to prevent tubular precipitation.[118]

Melphalan has been linked with nephrotoxicity, usually when given in high doses prior to BMT, but its precise role in causing renal damage is unclear owing to the frequent presence of other concurrent nephrotoxic insults. Two of eight adults developed transient glomerular impairment, which was ameliorated by intravenous hydration in subsequent patients.[120] A later report of melphalan and TBI described chronic glomerular toxicity in a third of 27 patients. However, high-dose cyclophosphamide and TBI caused similar toxicity, and cyclosporin A may have contributed to renal damage, which was again reduced by hydration.[121] ARF and proximal tubular damage occurred after very high-dose melphalan in an adolescent who died from hemorrhage before renal recovery could be evaluated,[122] while ARF has been reported after the combination of high-dose carboplatin and melphalan in four children, with incomplete renal recovery in one of two survivors.[112]

Chronic glomerular damage has been described after doxorubicin in an elderly man, with gradual recovery,[123] and has been recognized in animal studies. Reversible proteinuria has been reported in an adult patient given intravenous and intraperitoneal cyclophosphamide.[124] An acute antidiuretic effect, owing to direct distal nephron

damage, promotes water reabsorption and may lead to inappropriate urinary concentration and potentially fatal dilutional hyponatremia.[125] Acute nephrotoxicity, sometimes severe, was reported in over half of 33 adults treated with cytosine arabinoside, probably as a component of multiorgan toxicity.[126] There are no published reports of chronic nephrotoxicity after these drugs in children.

The nitrosourea compounds, carmustine (BCNU), lomustine (CCNU) and semustine (methyl-CCNU), may all cause chronic irreversible glomerular impairment, which often develops only after completion of treatment. In six children receiving >1500 mg/m^2 of semustine, end-stage renal failure (ESRF) developed in four and CRF in one, and the authors recommended a dose limit of 1200 mg/m^2.[127] Renal histology usually reveals glomerulosclerosis, tubular loss and interstitial fibrosis.[128] Nephrotoxicity due to the other nitrosoureas is rarer. Of 89 patients given carmustine, four adults suffered from an insidious onset of mild glomerular impairment,[129] while slowly progressive ESRF may follow lomustine treatment.[130] It has been suggested that a toxic electrophilic metabolite may be responsible for nitrosourea nephrotoxicity.[127]

Nephrotoxicity has not been reported after oral 6-thioguanine in children, although acute reversible glomerular impairment was described in 12 of 66 adults, with severe toxicity in four given intravenous boluses.[131] Although direct renal toxicity has not been described, it has been suggested that actinomycin D may sensitize renal tissue to chronic damage from radiation doses that do not normally cause nephropathy,[132] and hence impair compensatory renal hypertrophy in children with Wilms' tumor.[133] Rarely, vincristine may cause acute hyponatremia owing to inappropriate vasopressin secretion.[134]

NEPHROTOXICITY DUE TO CYTOTOXIC DRUGS USED PREDOMINANTLY IN ADULTS

Certain cytotoxic drugs rarely used in children may cause chronic nephrotoxicity. Acute and chronic glomerular damage may occur after mithramycin.[135] Mitomycin C causes two clinically distinct patterns of severe, progressive and potentially lethal renal damage,[136] including cancer-associated hemolytic uraemic syndrome.

KEY POINTS

- There are many causes of nephrotoxicity in children treated for malignancy, including the disease itself, chemotherapy, radiotherapy, surgery, immunotherapy, and supportive treatment.
- Renal toxicity is common, leads to a wide range of manifestations of variable severity and may be irreversible.
- Assessment of renal toxicity should include both glomerular and tubular function.
- Ifosfamide nephrotoxicity usually affects predominantly the proximal tubule (causing a Fanconi syndrome), but may also impair glomerular function.
- Platinum nephrotoxicity (commoner after cisplatin than carboplatin) causes glomerular impairment and hypomagnesemia due to tubular damage.
- Although the development of nephrotoxicity is sometimes unpredictable, avoidance of risk factors (e.g. higher total ifosfamide dose) may allow a reduction in incidence and severity.
- However, incomplete understanding of the pathogenesis of ifosfamide or platinum nephrotoxicity has hindered attempts at developing protective treatment.

REFERENCES

●1. Rossi R, Kleta R, Ehrich JHH. Renal involvement in children with malignancies. *Pediatr Nephrol* 1999; **13**:153–162.
2. Skinner R. Strategies to prevent nephrotoxicity of anticancer drugs. *Curr Opin Oncol* 1995; **7**:310–315.
●3. Skinner R, Sharkey IM, Pearson ADJ, Craft AW. Ifosfamide, mesna and nephrotoxicity in children. *J Clin Oncol* 1993; **11**:173–190.
◆4. Brock PR, Koliouskas DE, Barratt TM, *et al*. Partial reversibility of cisplatin nephrotoxicity in children. *J Pediatr* 1991; **118**:531–534.
◆5. Luxton RW. Radiation nephritis. *Lancet* 1961; **ii**:1221–1224.
6. Welch TR, McAdams AJ. Focal glomerulosclerosis as a late sequela of Wilms tumor. *J Pediatr* 1986; **108**:105–109.
7. Bailey S, Roberts A, Brock C, *et al*. Nephrotoxicity in survivors of Wilms' tumours in the North of England. *Br J Cancer* 2002; **87**:1092–1098.
8. Mercatello A, Hadj-Aissa A, Negrier S, *et al*. Acute renal failure with preserved renal plasma flow induced by cancer immunotherapy. *Kidney Int* 1991; **40**:309–314.
9. Wu B, Atkinson SA, Halton JM, Barr RD. Hypermagnesiuria and hypercalciuria in childhood leukemia: an effect of amikacin therapy. *J Pediatr Hematol Oncol* 1996; **18**:86–89.
10. Van Why SK, Friedman AL, Wei LJ, Hang R. Renal insufficiency after bone marrow transplantation in children. *Bone Marrow Transplant* 1991; **7**:383–388.
11. Patzer L, Ringelmann F, Kentouche K, *et al*. Renal function in long-term survivors of stem cell transplantation in childhood. A prospective trial. *Bone Marrow Transplant* 2001; **27**:319–327.
●12. Skinner R, Pearson ADJ, Coulthard MG, *et al*. Assessment of chemotherapy-associated nephrotoxicity in children with cancer. *Cancer Chemother Pharmacol* 1991; **28**:81–92.
13. Gao Y, Shimizu M, Yamada S, *et al*. The effects of chemotherapy including cisplatin on vitamin D metabolism. *Endocrinol J* 1993; **40**:737–742.
14. Heney D, Wheeldon J, Rushworth P, *et al*. Progressive renal toxicity due to ifosfamide. *Arch Dis Child* 1991; **66**:966–970.

15. Verplanke AJW, Herber RFM, de Wit R, Veenhof CHN. Comparison of renal function parameters in the assessment of cis-platin induced nephrotoxicity. *Nephron* 1994; **66**:267–272.

16. MacLean FR, Skinner R, Hall AG, *et al.* Acute changes in urine protein excretion may predict chronic ifosfamide nephrotoxicity: a preliminary observation. *Cancer Chemother Pharmacol* 1998; **41**:413–416.

17. Reece PA, Stafford I, Russell J, *et al.* Creatinine clearance as a predictor of ultrafilterable platinum disposition in cancer patients treated with cisplatin: relationship between peak ultrafilterable platinum plasma levels and nephrotoxicity. *J Clin Oncol* 1987; **5**:304–309.

18. Boddy AV, English M, Pearson ADJ, *et al.* Ifosfamide nephrotoxicity: Limited influence of metabolism and mode of administration during repeated therapy in paediatrics. *Eur J Cancer* 1996; **32A**:1179–1184.

●19. Loebstein R, Koren G. Strategies to prevent drug-induced nephrotoxicity in children. *Bailliere's Clin Paediatr* 1998; **6**:471–479.

20. Pratt CB, Meyer WH, Jenkins JJ, *et al.* Ifosfamide, Fanconi's syndrome, and rickets. *J Clin Oncol* 1991; **9**:1495–1499.

21. Ashraf MS, Brady J, Breatnach F, *et al.* Ifosfamide nephrotoxicity in paediatric cancer patients. *Eur J Paediatr* 1994; **153**: 90–94.

22. Skinner R, Pearson ADJ, English MW, *et al.* Risk factors for ifosfamide nephrotoxicity in children. *Lancet* 1996; **348**:578–580.

◆23. Skinner R, Cotterill S, Stevens MCG, on behalf of the Late Effects Group of the United Kingdom Children's Cancer Study Group. Risk factors for nephrotoxicity after ifosfamide treatment in children: a UKCCSG Late Effects Group Study. *Br J Cancer* 2000; **82**:1636–1645.

24. De Schepper J, Hachimi-Idrissi S, Verboven M, *et al.* Renal function abnormalities after ifosfamide treatment in children. *Acta Paediatr* 1993; **82**:373–376.

25. Skinner R, Cole M, Pearson ADJ, *et al.* Early morning urine pH and osmolality are of limited value in assessing distal renal tubular function in children. *Br Med J* 1996; **312**:1337–1338.

26. Rossi R, Kist C, Wurster U, *et al.* Estimation of ifosfamide/cisplatinum-induced renal toxicity by urinary protein analysis. *Pediatr Nephrol* 1994; **8**:151–156.

27. Goren MP, Wright RK, Horowitz ME, Pratt CB. Cancer chemotherapy-induced tubular nephrotoxicity evaluated by immunochemical determination of urinary adenosine deaminase binding protein. *Am J Clin Pathol* 1986; **86**:780–783.

28. Al Sheyyab M, Worthington D, Beetham R, Stevens M. The assessment of subclinical ifosfamide-induced renal tubular toxicity using urinary excretion of retinol-binding protein. *Pediatr Hematol Oncol* 1993; **10**:119–128.

◆29. Burk CD, Restaino I, Kaplan BS, Meadows AT. Ifosfamide-induced renal tubular dysfunction and rickets in children with Wilms tumor. *J Pediatr* 1990; **117**:331–335.

◆30. Prasad VK, Lewis IJ, Aparicio SR, *et al.* Progressive glomerular toxicity of ifosfamide in children. *Med Pediatr Oncol* 1996; **27**:149–155.

31. Rossi R, Godde A, Kleinebrand A, *et al.* Concentrating capacity in ifosfamide-induced severe renal dysfunction. *Ren Fail* 1995; **17**:551–557.

32. DeFronzo RA, Abeloff M, Braine H, *et al.* Renal dysfunction after treatment with isophosphamide (NSC-109724). *Cancer Chemother Rep* 1974; **58**:375–382.

33. Smeitink J, Verreussel M, Schroder C, Lippens R. Nephrotoxicity associated with ifosfamide. *Eur J Paediatr* 1988; **148**:164–166.

34. Goren MP, Pratt CB, Viar MJ. Tubular nephrotoxicity during long-term ifosfamide and mesna therapy. *Cancer Chemother Pharmacol* 1989; **25**:70–72.

35. Sweeney LE. Hypophosphataemic rickets after ifosfamide treatment in children. *Clin Radiol* 1993; **47**:345–347.

36. Schwartzman E, Scopinaro M, Angueyra N. Phase II study of ifosfamide as a single drug for relapsed paediatric patients. *Cancer Chemother Pharmacol* 1989; **24**(Suppl,):S11–S12.

37. De Schepper J, Stevens G, Verboven M, *et al.* Ifosfamide-induced Fanconi's syndrome with growth failure in a 2-year-old child. *Am J Pediatr Hematol Oncol* 1991; **13**:39–41.

38. Stuart-Harris RC, Harper PG, Parsons CA, *et al.* High-dose alkylation therapy using ifosfamide infusion with mesna in the treatment of adult advanced soft-tissue sarcoma. *Cancer Chemother Pharmacol* 1983; **11**:69–72.

39. Caron HN, Abeling N, van Gennip A, *et al.* Hyperaminoaciduria identifies patients at risk of developing renal tubular toxicity associated with ifosfamide and platinate containing regimens. *Med Pediatr Oncol* 1992; **20**:42–47.

40. Van Gool S, Brock P, Wijndaele G, *et al.* Reversible hypophosphatemic rickets following ifosfamide treatment. *Med Pediatr Oncol* 1992; **20**:254–257.

41. Ashraf MS, Skinner R, English MW, *et al.* Late reversibility of chronic ifosfamide-associated nephrotoxicity in a child. *Med Pediatr Oncol* 1997; **28**:62–64.

◆42. Raney B, Ensign LG, Foreman J, *et al.* Renal toxicity of ifosfamide in pilot regimens of the Intergroup Rhabdomyosarcoma Study for patients with gross residual disease. *Am J Pediatr Hematol Oncol* 1994; **16**:286–295.

43. Shore R, Greenberg M, Geary D, Koren G. Iphosphamide-induced nephrotoxicity in children. *Pediatr Nephrol* 1992; **6**:162–165.

44. Rossi R, Schafers P, Pleyer J, *et al.* The influence of short versus continuous ifosfamide infusion on the development of renal tubular impairment. *Int J Pediatr Hematol Oncol* 1997; **4**:393–399.

45. Rossi R, Danzebrink S, Hillebrand D, *et al.* Ifosfamide-induced subclinical nephrotoxicity and its potentiation by cisplatinum. *Med Pediatr Oncol* 1994; **22**:27–32.

46. Elias AD, Ayash LJ, Eder JP, *et al.* A phase I study of high-dose ifosfamide and escalating doses of carboplatin with autologous bone marrow support. *J Clin Oncol* 1991; **9**:320–327.

◆47. Rossi R, Godde A, Kleinebrand A, *et al.* Unilateral nephrectomy and cisplatin as risk factors of ifosfamide-induced nephrotoxicity: analysis of 120 patients. *J Clin Oncol* 1994; **12**:159–165.

48. Morland BJ, Mann JR, Milford DV, *et al.* Ifosfamide nephrotoxicity in children: histopathological features in two cases. *Med Pediatr Oncol* 1996; **27**:57–61.

49. Broadhead CL, Walker D, Skinner R, Simmons NL. Differential cytotoxicity of ifosfamide and its metabolites in renal epithelial cell cultures. *Toxicol in Vitro* 1998; **12**:209–217.

50. Nissim I, Weinberg JM. Glycine attenuates Fanconi syndrome induced by maleate or ifosfamide in rats. *Kidney Int* 1996; **49**:684–695.

◆51. Mohrmann M, Ansorge S, Schmich U, *et al.* Toxicity of ifosfamide, cyclophosphamide and their metabolites in renal tubular cells in culture. *Pediatr Nephrol* 1994; **8**:157–163.

52. Schlenzig JS, Charpentier C, Rabier D, *et al.* L-carnitine: a way to decrease cellular toxicity of ifosfamide? (letter). *Eur J Pediatr* 1995; **154**:686–690.

53. Silies H, Blaschke G, Hohenlochter B, *et al.* Excretion kinetics of ifosfamide side-chain metabolites in children on continuous and short-term infusion. *Int J Clin Pharmacol Ther* 1998; **36**:246–252.

54. Tasso MJ, Boddy AV, Price L, *et al.* Pharmacokinetics and metabolism of cyclophosphamide in paediatric patients. *Cancer Chemother Pharmacol* 1992; **30**:207–211.

55. Zamlauski-Tucker MJ, Morris ME, Springate JE. Ifosfamide metabolite chloroacetaldehyde causes Fanconi syndrome in the perfused rat kidney. *Toxicol Appl Pharmacol* 1994; **129**:170–175.

56. Mohrmann M, Pauli A, Walkenhorst H, *et al.* Effect of ifosfamide metabolites on sodium-dependent phosphate transport in a model of proximal tubular cells (LLC-PK₁) in culture. *Renal Physiol Biochem* 1993; **16**:285–298.

57. Mohrmann M, Ansorge S, Schonfeld B, Brandis M. Dithio-bis-mercaptoethanesulphonate (DIMESNA) does not prevent cellular damage by metabolites of ifosfamide and cyclophosphamide in LLC-PK1 cells. *Pediatr Nephrol* 1994; **8**:458–465.

●58. Rossi R. Nephrotoxicity of ifosfamide – moving towards understanding the molecular mechanisms. *Nephrol Dial Transplant* 1997; **12**:1091–1092.

●59. Loebstein R, Koren G. Ifosfamide-induced nephrotoxicity in children: Critical review of predictive risk factors. *Pediatrics* 1998; **101**:e8.

60. Bianchetti MG, Kanaka C, Ridolfi-Luthy A, *et al.* Chronic renal magnesium loss, hypocalciuria and mild hypokalaemic metabolic alkalosis after cisplatin. *Pediatr Nephrol* 1990; **4**:219–222.

61. Womer RB, Pritchard J, Barratt TM. Renal toxicity of cisplatin in children. *J Pediatr* 1985; **106**:659–663.

62. Kamalaker P, Freeman AI, Higby DJ, *et al.* Clinical response and toxicity with cis-dichlorodiammine-platinum (II) in children. *Cancer Treat Rep* 1977; **61**:835–839.

63. Hayes FA, Green AA, Casper J, *et al.* Clinical evaluation of sequentially scheduled cisplatin and VM26 in neuroblastoma: response and toxicity. *Cancer* 1981; **48**:1715–1718.

64. Pratt CB, Hayes A, Green AA, *et al.* Pharmacokinetic evaluation of cisplatin in children with malignant solid tumors: a phase II study. *Cancer Treat Rep* 1981; **65**:1021–1026.

65. Hartmann O, Pinkerton CR, Philip T, Zucker JM, Breatnach F. Very-high-dose cisplatin and etoposide in children with untreated advanced neuroblastoma. *J Clin Oncol* 1988; **6**:44–50.

66. Madias NE, Harrington JT. Platinum nephrotoxicity. *Am J Med* 1978; **65**:307–314.

67. Daugaard G, Rossing N, Rorth M. Effects of cisplatin on different measures of glomerular function in the human kidney with special emphasis on high-dose. *Cancer Chemother Pharmacol* 1988; **21**:163–167.

68. Lam M, Adelstein DJ. Hypomagnesemia and renal magnesium wasting in patients treated with cisplatin. *Am J Kidney Dis* 1986; **8**:164–169.

●69. Daugaard G, Abildgaard U. Cisplatin nephrotoxicity. *Cancer Chemother Pharmacol* 1989; **25**:1–9.

70. Bellin SL, Selim M. Cisplatin-induced hypomagnesemia with seizures: a case report and review of the literature. *Gynecol Oncol* 1988; **30**:104–113.

71. Daugaard G, Abildgaard U, Holsten-Rathlou NH, *et al.* Renal tubular function in patients treated with high-dose cisplatin. *Clin Pharmacol Ther* 1988; **44**:164–172.

72. Kurtzberg J, Dennis VW, Kinney TR. Cisplatinum-induced renal salt wasting. *Med Pediatr Oncol* 1984; **12**:150–154.

73. Wong NLM, Walker VR, Wong EFC, Sutton RAL. Mechanism of polyuria after cisplatin therapy. *Nephron* 1993; **65**:623–627.

74. Ettinger LJ, Douglass HO, Higby DJ, *et al.* Adjuvant adriamycin and cis-diamminedichloroplatinum (cis-platinum) in primary osteosarcoma. *Cancer* 1981; **47**:248–254.

75. Harrell RM, Sibley R, Vogelzang NJ. Renal vascular lesions after chemotherapy with vinblastine, bleomycin and cisplatin. *Am J Med* 1982; **23**:429–433.

76. Canpolat C, Pearson P, Jaffe N. Cisplatin-associated hemolytic uremic syndrome. *Cancer* 1994; **74**:3059–3062.

◆77. Skinner R, Pearson ADJ, English MW, *et al.* Cisplatin dose rate as a risk factor for nephrotoxicity in children. *Br J Cancer* 1998; **77**:1677–1682.

78. Bianchetti MG, Kanaka C, Oetliker OH. Bartter-like syndrome, hypomagnesemia associated with hypocalciuria,

and isolated hypocalciuria: late sequelae after treatment with cisplatin (abstract). *Pediatr Nephrol* 1990; **4**:C33.

79. Preiss R, Brovtsyn VK, Perevodchikova NI, *et al.* Effect of methotrexate on the pharmacokinetics and renal excretion of cisplatin. *Eur J Clin Pharmacol* 1988; **34**:139–144.

80. Gietema JA, Meinardi MT, Messerschmidt J, *et al.* Circulating plasma platinum more than 10 years after cisplatin treatment for testicular cancer (letter). *Lancet* 2000; **355**:1075–1076.

81. Gonzalez-Vitale JC, Hayes DM, Cvitkovic E, Sternberg SS. The renal pathology in clinical trials of cis-platinum (II) diamminedichloride. *Cancer* 1977; **39**:1362–1371.

82. Borch RF. The platinum anti-tumor drugs. In: Powis G, Prough RA (eds) *Metabolism and action of anti-cancer drugs.* London: Taylor and Francis, 1987:163–193.

83. Daley-Yates PT, McBrien DCH. The renal fractional clearance of platinum antitumour compounds in relation to nephrotoxicity. *Biochem Pharmacol* 1985; **34**:1423–1428.

84. Daley-Yates PT, McBrien DCH. Cisplatin (cisdichlorodiammineplatinum II) nephrotoxicity. In: Bach PH, Bonner FW, Bridges JW Lock EA (eds) *Nephrotoxicity – assessment and pathogenesis.* Chichester: John Wiley and Sons, 1981:356–370.

85. Caterson R, Etheredge S, Snitch P, Duggin G. Mechanisms of renal excretion of cisdichlorodiamine platinum. *Res Commun Chem Pathol Pharmacol* 1983; **41**:255–264.

86. Williams PD, Hottendorf GH. Effect of cisplatin on organic ion transport in membrane vesicles from rat kidney cortex. *Cancer Treat Rep* 1985; **69**:875–880.

87. Barros EJG, Boim MA, Santos OFP, Schor N. Effect of cisplatin on glomerular haemodynamics. *Braz J Med Biol Res* 1989; **22**:1295–1301.

88. Heidemann HT, Muller S, Mertins L, *et al.* Effect of aminophylline on cisplatin nephrotoxicity in the rat. *Br J Pharmacol* 1989; **97**:313–318.

89. dos Santos OFP, Boim MA, Barros EJG, *et al.* Effect of platelet-activating factor antagonist BN 52063 on the nephrotoxicity of cisplatin. *Lipids* 1991; **26**:1324–1328.

90. Blochl-Daum B, Pehamberger H, Kurz C, *et al.* Effects of cisplatin on urinary thromboxane B2 excretion. *Clin Pharmacol Ther* 1995; **58**:418–424.

91. Singh G. A possible cellular mechanism of cisplatin-induced nephrotoxicity. *Toxicology* 1989; **58**:71–80.

92. Yasumasu T, Ueda T, Uozumi J, *et al.* Comparative study of cisplatin and carboplatin on pharmacokinetics, nephrotoxicity and effect on renal nuclear DNA synthesis in rats. *Pharmacol Toxicol* 1992; **70**:143–147.

93. Zhang J-G, Lindup WE. Cisplatin nephrotoxicity: Decreases in mitochondrial protein sulphydryl concentration and calcium uptake by mitochondria from rat renal cortical slices. *Biochem Pharmacol* 1994; **47**:1127–1135.

●94. Pinzani V, Bressolle F, Haug IJ, *et al.* Cisplatin-induced renal toxicity and toxicity-modulating stategies: a review. *Cancer Chemother Pharmacol* 1994; **35**:1–9.

95. Cornelison TL, Reed E. Nephrotoxicity and hydration management for cisplatin, carboplatin, and ormaplatin. *Gynecol Oncol* 1993; **50**:147–158.

96. Kibirige MS, Morris Jones PH, Addison GM. Prevention of cisplatin-induced hypomagnesemia. *Pediatr Hematol Oncol* 1988; **5**:1–6.

97. Jones MM, Basinger MA, Holscher MA. Control of the nephrotoxicity of cisplatin by clinically used sulfur-containing compounds. *Fundam Appl Toxicol* 1992; **18**:181–188.

98. Schuchter LM, Hensley ML, Meropol NJ, Winer EP, for the American Society of Clinical Oncology Chemotherapy and Radiotherapy Expert Panel. 2002 update of recommendations for the use of chemotherapy and radiotherapy protectants: Clinical

practice guidelines of the American Society of Clinical Oncology. *J Clin Oncol* 2002; **20**:2895–2903.

99. Jacobs C, Kaubisch S, Halsey J, *et al.* The use of probenecid as a chemoprotector against cisplatin nephrotoxicity. *Cancer* 1991; **67**:1518–1524.

100. Sleijfer DT, Offerman JJG, Mulder NH, *et al.* The protective potential of the combination of verapamil and cimetidine on cisplatin-induced nephrotoxicity in man. *Cancer* 1987; **60**:2823–2828.

101. Veal GJ, Griffin MJ, Price E, *et al.* A phase I study in paediatric patients to evaluate the safety and pharmacokinetics of SPI-77, a liposome encapsulated formulation of cisplatin. *Br J Cancer* 2001; **84**:1029–1035.

102. Doz F, Pinkerton R. What is the place of carboplatin in paediatric oncology? *Eur J Cancer* 1994; **30A**:194–201.

103. Foster BJ, Clagett-Carr K, Leyland-Jones B, Hoth D. Results of NCI-sponsored phase I trials with carboplatin. *Cancer Treat Rev* 1985; **12**(Suppl. A):43–49.

104. Calvert AH, Harland SJ, Newell DR, *et al.* Early clinical studies with cis-diammine-1,1-cyclobutane dicarboxylate platinum II. *Cancer Chemother Pharmacol* 1982; **9**:140–147.

105. Brandt LJ, Broadbent V. Nephrotoxicity following carboplatin use in children: is routine monitoring of renal function necessary? *Med Pediatr Oncol* 1993; **21**:31–35.

106. Pinkerton CR, Broadbent V, Horwich A, *et al.* JEB – a carboplatin based regimen for malignant germ cell tumours in children. *Br J Cancer* 1990; **62**:257–262.

107. Lewis IJ, Stevens MCG, Pearson ADJ, *et al.* Carboplatin activity in cisplatin treated neuroblastoma. *Adv Neuroblastoma Res* 1991; **3**:553–559.

108. Ettinger LJ, Siegel SE, Baum ES, *et al.* Phase I pediatric trial of cis-diammine-1, 1-cyclobutane dicarboxylate platinum II (NSC 241240, CBDCA) (abstract). *Am Soc Clin Oncol Abstracts* 1984; **1**:44.

109. McDonald BR, Kirmani S, Vasquez M, Mehta RL. Acute renal failure associated with the use of intraperitoneal carboplatin: a report of two cases and review of the literature. *Am J Med* 1991; **90**:386–391.

110. Curt GA, Grygiel JJ, Corden BJ, *et al.* A phase I and pharmacokinetic study of diamminecyclobutane-dicarboxylato-platinum (NSC 241240). *Cancer Res* 1983; **43**:4470–4473.

111. Shea TC, Flaherty M, Elias A, *et al.* A phase I clinical and pharmacokinetic study of carboplatin and autologous bone marrow support. *J Clin Oncol* 1989; **7**:651–661.

112. Gordon SJ, Pearson ADJ, Reid MM, Craft AW. Toxicity of single-day high-dose vincristine, melphalan, etoposide, and carboplatin consolidation with autologous bone marrow rescue in advanced neuroblastoma. *Eur J Cancer* 1992; **28A**: 1319–1323.

113. Frenkel J, Kool G, de Kraker J. Acute renal failure in high-dose carboplatin chemotherapy. *Med Pediatr Oncol* 1995; **25**:473–474.

◆114. English MW, Skinner R, Pearson ADJ, *et al.* Dose-related nephrotoxicity of carboplatin in children. *Br J Cancer* 1999; **81**:336–341.

115. Tscherning C, Rubie H, Chancolle A, *et al.* Recurrent renal salt wasting in a child treated with carboplatin and etoposide. *Cancer* 1994; **73**:1761–1763.

116. Siddik ZH, Dible SE, Boxall FE, Harrap KR. Renal pharmacokinetics and toxicity of cisplatin and carboplatin in animals. In: McBrien DCH, Slater TF (eds) *Biochemical*

mechanisms of platinum antitumour drugs. Oxford: IRL Press, 1986:171–198.

117. Reed E, Jacob J. Carboplatin and renal dysfunction (letter). *Ann Intern Med* 1989; **110**:409.

118. Von Hoff DD, Penta JS, Helman LJ, Slavik M. Incidence of drug-related deaths secondary to high-dose methotrexate and citrovorum factor administration. *Cancer Treat Rep* 1977; **61**:745–748.

119. Abelson HT, Fosburg MT, Beardsley GP, *et al.* Methotrexate-induced renal impairment: clinical studies and rescue from systemic toxicity with high-dose leucovorin and thymidine. *J Clin Oncol* 1983; **1**:208–216.

120. McElwain TJ, Hedley DW, Burton G, *et al.* Marrow autotransplantation accelerates haematological recovery in patients with malignant melanoma treated with high-dose melphalan. *Br J Cancer* 1979; **40**:72–80.

121. Helenglass G, Powles RL, McElwain TJ, *et al.* Melphalan and total body irradiation (TBI) versus cyclophosphamide and TBI as conditioning for allogeneic matched sibling bone marrow transplants for acute myeloblastic leukaemia in first remission. *Bone Marrow Transplant* 1988; **3**:21–29.

122. Alix JL, Swiercz P, Schaerer R, *et al.* Nephrotoxicite du melphalan utilise a haute dose. *La Presse Medicale* 1983; **12**:575–576.

123. Burke JF, Laucius JF, Brodovsky HS, Soriano RZ. Doxorubicin hydrochloride-associated renal failure. *Arch Intern Med* 1977; **137**:385–388.

124. Lopes VM. Cyclophosphamide nephrotoxicity in man (letter). *Lancet* 1967; **i**:1060.

125. Harlow PJ, DeClerck YA, Shore NA, *et al.* A fatal case of inappropriate ADH secretion induced by cyclophosphamide therapy. *Cancer* 1979; **44**:896–898.

126. Slavin RE, Dias MA, Saral R. Cytosine arabinoside induced gastrointestinal toxic alterations in sequential chemotherapeutic protocols. A clinico-pathologic study of 33 patients. *Cancer* 1978; **42**:1747–1759.

127. Weiss RB, Posada JG Jr, Kramer RA, Boyd MR. Nephrotoxicity of semustine. *Cancer Treat Rep* 1983; **67**:1105–1112.

128. Harman WE, Cohen HJ, Schneeberger EE, Grupe WE. Chronic renal failure in children treated with methyl CCNU. *N Engl J Med* 1979; **300**:1200–1203.

129. Schacht RG, Feiner HD, Gallo GR, *et al.* Nephrotoxicity of nitrosoureas. *Cancer* 1981; **48**:1328–1334.

130. Silver HKB, Morton DL. CCNU nephrotoxicity following sustained remission in oat cell carcinoma. *Cancer Treat Rep* 1979; **63**:226–227.

131. Presant CA, Denes AE, Klein L, *et al.* Phase I and preliminary phase II observations of high-dose intermittent 6-thioguanine. *Cancer Treat Rep* 1980; **64**:1109–1113.

132. Arneil GC, Emmanuel IG, Flatman GE, *et al.* Nephritis in two children after irradiation and chemotherapy for nephroblastoma. *Lancet* 1974; **i**:960–963.

133. Makipernaa A, Koskimies O, Jaaskelainen J, *et al.* Renal growth and function 11–28 years after treatment of Wilms' tumour. *Eur J Pediatr* 1991; **150**:444–447.

134. Stuart MJ, Cuaso C, Miller M, Oski FA. Syndrome of recurrent increased secretion of antidiuretic hormone following multiple doses of vincristine. *Blood* 1975; **45**:315–320.

135. Kennedy BJ. Metabolic and toxic effects of mithramycin during tumor therapy. *Am J Med* 1970; **49**:494–503.

136. Hanna WT, Krauss S, Regester RF, Murphy WM. Renal disease after mitomycin C therapy. *Cancer* 1981; **48**:2583–2588.

6b

Bladder complications

R BEVERLY RANEY, ROBIN ZAGONE AND MICHAEL RITCHEY

INTRODUCTION

Malignant tumors that involve the bladder directly or can arise adjacent to it are relatively infrequent in pediatric oncologic practice. The primary conditions are vesical and prostatic rhabdomyosarcomas as well as sarcomas of the urachus, abdominal wall, paratesticular region, vagina, uterus, retroperitoneum, pelvis and perineal–perianal region. In addition, germ-cell tumors can occur in the testis, ovary or sacrococcygeal region, and may spread to involve pelvic and retroperitoneal lymph nodes. Sometimes a lymphoma or neuroblastoma arises in soft tissues near the bladder, as can primary tumors of pelvic bones such as Ewing's sarcoma or osteosarcoma. Patients with acute leukemia can occasionally have direct involvement of the testis or, less commonly, of the ovary.[1]

Patients with soft-tissue sarcomas, neuroblastoma, Wilms' tumor, bone sarcomas and germ-cell tumors usually require systemic treatment with various chemotherapeutic agents, and some may need surgical intervention and/or therapeutic irradiation in order to control the tumor locally. The bladder can be affected by certain systemic chemotherapeutic agents, and by interactions among some of them and radiation therapy, which can augment the toxicity of the drugs and increase the severity of the damage.

TYPES OF TREATMENT FOR CHILDHOOD CANCERS AND THEIR EFFECTS ON THE BLADDER

Surgery

Surgical removal of solid tumors is often an important part of the overall therapeutic strategy. However, an intact bladder is very important to having a normal quality of life. Therefore, the usual initial approach for patients with a possible sarcoma of the bladder trigone or prostate gland is to obtain a biopsy and confirm the diagnosis. Afterward, chemotherapy and radiation therapy are administered in an attempt to eradicate the tumor and still leave the bladder in place, in the hope that continence and acceptable urinary function will be preserved. From 1984 to 1991, 87 patients with localized tumors of the bladder and prostate were treated on the third protocol of the Intergroup Rhabdomyosarcoma Study (IRS) Group. Eighty-one per cent of these patients achieved a complete response (complete disappearance of the tumor) and the bladder salvage rate was 60 per cent.[2] Thirty-eight of the 44 patients with localized prostate sarcoma (81 per cent) were cured and 64 per cent of them retained the bladder.[3] A review of 109 patients treated for bladder/prostate sarcoma on the first two IRS protocols (1972–1984) found that 38 of 52 patients with

bladders in place (73 per cent) had satisfactory bladder function. However, hydronephrosis, bacteriuria and elevated blood urea nitrogen or creatinine levels were approximately 2–4 times more frequent in patients who had undergone total cystectomy with urinary diversion.[4] Occasionally, a vesical or urachal sarcoma can arise distant from the trigone, in such a location that a partial cystectomy can be performed and still leave a sufficient amount of intravesical volume with good bladder sphincter control.[5] Methods of augmenting the available bladder volume or of producing a continent urinary diversion after total cystectomy will be discussed below.

Radiation therapy

The effects of radiation therapy (XRT) on body tissues can be acute or late. Acute effects are those that occur during treatment or soon after the XRT is completed; they consist primarily of local tissue irritation, and reddening or darkening of the overlying skin. The acute effects on the irradiated bladder may include urgency, frequency, dysuria (frequently denoted generically as cystitis) and hematuria. The amount of hematuria is variable and can occur during treatment or afterward. Late effects begin to take place at some point after any acutely detected effects have diminished or resolved, and may be progressive over months to years. The long-term effects are thought to result from progressive vascular and parenchymal cell damage, which causes bladder fibrosis and diminished bladder growth in the pre-adult child. As with acute effects, the late effects increase proportionally to the total dose delivered and the volume irradiated and are generally worse in inverse proportion to the patient's age at the time of receiving the XRT.[6,7] Thus, the late effects are of particular concern in young children with large tumors in or adjacent to the bladder. In addition, while the acute effects are expected to clear over time, the later sequelae can develop insidiously and may be progressively apparent as the patient ages. Bladder dysfunction can result from both decreased bladder capacity, and diminished compliance and contractility. The underlying etiology appears to be vascular ischemia of the muscular wall.[8,9] The risk of bladder dysfunction is related both to the total dose of XRT and to the percentage of the bladder included in the treatment volume.[10] In adults, a small volume of the bladder can tolerate relatively high total doses of XRT. But even a high dose to a small volume can cause focal bleeding and sometimes induce formation of intravesical stones.[11–13] If the entire bladder receives more than 50 Gy, severe bladder contraction and secondary dysfunction may result. Urinary dysfunction may also be related to fibrosis of the ureters or urethra.[14] Imaging studies and/or cystoscopy would be needed to elucidate their contribution to the overall problem.

Chemotherapy

Bladder damage, including cystitis, hematuria, fibrosis and occasionally bladder shrinkage, can occur following chronic administration of certain alkylating agents, notably cyclophosphamide[15–17] and ifosfamide.[18] The metabolic byproducts of these drugs include the compound acrolein, which is a mucosal irritant. Within the last 20 years, this problem has been largely prevented by the concomitant use of increased hydration during administration of the drugs along with intravenous or oral mercaptoethane sulfonate (Mesna). Mesna binds and inactivates acrolein, preventing it from causing bladder irritation. Currently, most treatment regimens incorporating cyclophosphamide for children with cancer require that it be administered intravenously. Increased hydration to twice maintenance levels or greater can also be given intravenously, which is preferable to relying on oral hydration by the patient. Cyclophosphamide has also been implicated in the development of several histologic varieties of bladder tumors and possibly of renal cell carcinoma.[19–23]

Combined chemotherapy and radiation therapy

Several chemotherapeutic agents may interact with radiation therapy in such a manner as to increase the effect of the XRT on the irradiated tissues. This augmentation of XRT is most notable when actinomycin D or doxorubicin is given.[24–27] Thus, administering either of these agents is contraindicated during the XRT treatment period itself, because the amount of enhancement is not easily quantified, and increased skin and deep tissue damage can result. The phenomenon of 'radiation recall' can also occur when either of these drugs is administered after the radiation course has been completed.[28] The oncologist is cautioned to consider a modest drug dose reduction when continuing chemotherapy in patients who have previously experienced severe mucositis or other radiation-related acute effects, especially in young children. If tolerated, drug doses can be escalated to the full amount over the next several weeks. There is also an interaction between cyclophosphamide or ifosfamide and bladder irradiation, which can increase the likelihood of hemorrhagic cystitis and subsequent bladder fibrosis. In one review of 110 children who received cyclophosphamide with or without pelvic XRT, the incidence of chronic bladder toxicity (hematuria, fibrosis and dysuria) was 18 per cent in 50 patients who had received both the alkylating agent and pelvic radiation. Only 8 per cent of the 60 patients treated with cyclophosphamide without pelvic irradiation had hematuria, and it was temporary and did not become chronic.[29] If overt hemorrhagic cystitis has

occurred after the patient has received one of these alkylating agents and bladder irradiation, particular care should be taken with subsequent administration of actinomycin D or doxorubicin. Because of the radiation recall effect, severe vesical hemorrhage may take place and require local measures to stop the bleeding and perhaps blood transfusions.

CLINICAL MANIFESTATIONS AND TREATMENT

Essential tools for detecting signs and symptoms of bladder damage include a thorough history, physical examination, and urinalysis. The history should focus on:

1 the frequency of voiding, including episodes at night;
2 whether incontinence is present;
3 whether dribbling or spotting of the underwear is noted;
4 whether the patient is experiencing urgency, discomfort on urination, or hematuria; and
5 whether there are spasmodic pains in the pelvic-bladder region.

The physical examination should include direct visualization of the urethral orifice and palpation of the pelvis to see whether pain is elicited or a mass can be felt. It may be useful to observe the patient's urinary stream during voiding. If the urinalysis shows hematuria with or without elevated protein, cystoscopy may be indicated. Ultrasonography, cystography and urodynamic studies may also be useful to determine:

1 whether there are impairments of urethral or ureteric function;
2 whether the patient's bladder capacity is sufficient for daytime continence; and
3 whether bladder compliance is adequate to prevent elevated pressures that can harm the upper tracts.

The initial management of hemorrhagic cystitis includes confirmation by urinalysis followed by increased hydration, orally or intravenously. Urine samples should be obtained in a sterile fashion and sent for bacterial and viral cultures. It is also prudent to obtain a complete blood count with white cell differential and platelet count, as well as a serum creatinine and possibly a urea nitrogen level. Transfusion of packed red blood cells and/or platelets may be needed, and a creatinine clearance may be indicated later. If the patient is receiving cyclophosphamide or ifosfamide, the drug is discontinued until the urine has been grossly and microscopically normal for at least 1–2 weeks. The drug can be reintroduced at 50 per cent dosage along with Mesna, at the discretion of the patient's pediatric oncologist, after consultation with the pediatric urologist. If the problem persists or worsens to include the passage of blood clots with dysuria or obstruction, placing an indwelling catheter for bladder irrigation may be necessary. Cystoscopy should also be considered in such instances, because occasionally a bleeding vessel can be cauterized. If the bleeding is due to diffuse mucosal damage, instillation of dilute solutions of silver nitrate may control the bleeding. Alum irrigation of the bladder is useful in older children or adults, but requires placement of a large catheter to fully irrigate the bladder. For refractory bleeding, intravesical instillation of formalin may be needed. This can result in fibrosis of the bladder and evaluation for vesicoureteral reflux is mandatory prior to formalin instillation.[30,31] Instillation of alum should be avoided in the patient with renal failure, however, because of the possibility of central nervous system toxicity.[32] In severe situations that do not respond to the above measures, complete diversion of the urinary stream may become necessary. Reconstruction of the urinary tract can be accomplished at a later date.

UROLOGIC MANAGEMENT OF A CONTRACTED OR SMALL URINARY BLADDER

As noted above, the bladder capacity may be physically reduced owing to surgical resection or functionally reduced owing to fibrosis following treatment of pelvic malignancies. The consequences of a reduced bladder capacity will vary. If there is no concomitant neurologic impairment, the only symptom may be urinary frequency and/or urgency. A greater reduction in capacity will result in urge incontinence.

While the patient and their family may likely seek treatment for these symptoms, the impact of the reduced capacity on bladder compliance may offer the strongest indication for reconstruction. The ability of the bladder to store urine at low intravesical pressures is essential to prevent upper urinary tract damage.[33] Even a capacious bladder may cause renal dysfunction if its compliance is poor. A bladder storing urine at elevated pressures may impede antegrade urine flow from the kidneys into the bladder. Even in the absence of frank reflux, these sustained pressures will result in hydronephrosis and renal damage over time.

The initial management of a patient with decreased bladder compliance is to give anticholinergic medication and to empty the bladder frequently. Failure to restore normal compliance or continence is the primary indication for reconstruction. The following section will briefly review available surgical techniques to accomplish these goals. Surgical procedures to restore continence owing to an inadequate bladder outlet (e.g. owing to damage of the urethra or sphincter) will not be addressed.

Augmentation cystoplasty

The goals of bladder augmentation are to increase bladder capacity and improve compliance. The procedure used most frequently today was described in the 1950s. The procedure has been more commonly performed after the introduction and widespread acceptance of intermittent catheterization several decades later.

All portions of the intestinal tract have been utilized for bladder augmentation.[34] Ileum is used most often owing to its ready availability and excellent compliance. Typically, a 25–35-cm length of ileum is used for this purpose. A segment is selected far enough proximal from the ileocecal valve to prevent malabsorption phenomena. The segment is based on a mobile mesenteric vascular pedicle to allow it to easily reach the bladder. It is very important to detubularize the ileal segment by incising along the antimesenteric border. The bowel segment is reconfigured into a 'U' shape and anastomosed to the bivalved native bladder. Even with a very small contracted native bladder, it is possible to restore a spherical-shaped reservoir of normal capacity and compliance. In most patients, it is not necessary to relocate the insertion of the ureters from the bladder base. Most cases of hydronephrosis and even reflux owing to elevated intravesical pressure will resolve after augmentation.[35] If reimplantation of the ureter is necessary, it can be placed into the augmented bowel segment rather than the fibrotic bladder.

If the patient has received extensive pelvic radiation, the distal ileum may not be suitable. Other options include stomach or transverse colon that would presumably have been outside of the radiation field. The stomach is also preferred in patients with renal insufficiency to avoid some of the metabolic consequences of ileal augmentation (see below).

Bladder substitution/continent urinary diversion

A complete bladder replacement is necessary if the entire bladder has been removed to achieve local tumor control. It may also be necessary in a patient with a non functional bladder outlet combined with poor bladder compliance. Many different procedures have been described for bladder replacement.[36] A larger segment of bowel is used for bladder substitution than for bladder augmentation alone. Detubularization of the bowel segment is important to create a compliant low-pressure reservoir. When the entire bladder is removed, the ureters need to be reimplanted into the new reservoir. The ureters can be implanted into any of the bowel segments. A reliable antireflux mechanism can be created with a submucosal tunnel in both the colon and stomach. Also, techniques have been described for placing the ureters into ileal reservoirs with low rates of postoperative reflux.

Continent urinary reservoirs fashioned from the ileocecal segment are commonly used in adults, but we try to avoid using this segment for reconstruction in children because of the risk of malabsorption and deleterious effects on growth. Composite reservoirs of ileum, colon and/or gastric segments work very well for reconstruction. This is often the case if the reconstruction is performed in stages in a very young child. When the bladder is removed in a young infant or toddler, a temporary cutaneous diversion is often performed. A colon conduit, usually a short segment of sigmoid colon, is generally preferred for the cutaneous diversion. The ureters can be implanted in a non-refluxing fashion into the sigmoid. After an interval of time, usually after the age of 5 years, the colon conduit can be incorporated into a composite continent reservoir.

If the urethra is spared, the bladder is replaced with a detubularized bowel segment and anastomosed directly to the urethra.[37] This has been used more extensively in adult patients following cystectomy for cancer but is applicable to male children. The advantage of preserving the urethra is the potential for the child to void spontaneously. Initially, emptying the reservoir may be incomplete, which would require intermittent catheterization. This problem is more common in very young children.

If the urethra is removed or damaged, the urinary reservoir will need to have an outlet on the abdominal wall. Creation of a continent reservoir is preferred. This will, of course, require that the reservoir be emptied by intermittent catheterization postoperatively. The preferred method of emptying the reservoir is to create a continent catheterizable channel from the reservoir to the abdominal wall.[38] Mitrofanoff described the use of the appendix as a catheterizable conduit from the skin to the bladder. However, there are many patients in whom the appendix is absent, of insufficient length or caliber, or needed for other reconstructive purposes. The Yang–Monti procedure creates a narrow channel by tubularizing a 2 cm segment of ileum.[39] Other catheterizable channels have been fashioned out of segments of ureter, fallopian tube or other tubularized bowel segments.

The basic principle of the appendicovesicostomy and the other catheterizable channels is a small-caliber tube that can be implanted into the storage reservoir. A submucosal tunnel is created in a similar manner as for ureteral reimplantation. This provides the continence mechanism. The other end of the catheterizable channel is brought up the abdominal wall to create a stoma. This stoma can be placed in the right or left lower quadrant, but the preferred location is the umbilicus. This allows concealment of the stoma. Appendicovesicostomy and the Monti procedure yield a high rate of continence with good durability. The most frequent complication is stomal stenosis requiring surgical revision.

Complications of bladder augmentation/substitution

Although continent reconstruction of the bladder has many advantages over incontinent cutaneous diversions, many late sequelae have been recognized. These include bladder stones, perforation and metabolic abnormalities. Bladder stones have been reported in 5–50 per cent of patients. It is now recognized that stones are frequently the result of incomplete removal of the mucus produced by the augmented bowel segment. This is particularly true in the continent reservoirs, where the outlet is not in a dependent location. Daily irrigation of the bladder reservoir with tap water has markedly decreased the rate of stone formation.

A more serious consequence of bladder augmentation is late perforation of the reservoir. This is most likely the result of infrequent bladder emptying in those patients requiring catheterization. Chronic distension of the bowel segment leads to ischemia and subsequent perforation. The patient often presents with abdominal pain, and signs and symptoms of an acute abdomen. However, making the diagnosis can be difficult and requires a high index of suspicion. Most patients require surgical exploration to repair the perforation and drain the infected urine from the abdominal cavity.

A number of metabolic sequelae of intestinocystoplasty have been observed.[34] The bowel mucosa, particularly ileum, can absorb urinary chlorides leading to metabolic acidosis. There is some concern that the chronic acidosis can affect bone metabolism and result in short stature.[40] The distal ileum absorbs bile acids and vitamin B_{12} and use of an excessive portion of the distal ileum for reconstruction can produce untoward effects. Use of the ileocecum for creation of a reservoir can produce intractable diarrhea from loss of the impedance of the ileocecal valve.

Occasionally a carcinoma can occur in the bladder of a patient who has previously undergone bladder augmentation.[41] One such patient had two cancers simultaneously, both a transitional cell carcinoma and an adenocarcinoma; the intestinal portion of the composite bladder was tumor-free.[42]

SUMMARY

It is evident from the above discussion that children with cancer are at risk for bladder damage if they have received certain drugs (cyclophosphamide, ifosfamide), especially if uroprotection with Mesna was not provided simultaneously. Pelvic or vesical irradiation can also cause similar problems due to changes in the bladder mucosa. The risk is increased when both forms of treatment have been

administered. Radiation damage may be increased by delivery of actinomycin D or doxorubicin subsequently. Although the likelihood of secondary cancer of the bladder is low, children cured of cancer usually have a long life span and are thus at risk for a considerable period of time. It is not known whether routine urinalyses following completion of treatment for childhood cancer would help diagnose the patient with early bladder cancer in the absence of gross hematuria. Nevertheless, the appearance of hematuria in such a patient years after cessation of cancer treatment should lead to prompt investigation by imaging studies along with cystoscopy and biopsy as indicated. Children with cancer deserve careful follow-up for many years in order to detect abnormalities related to their disease and its treatment, so that intervention can be accomplished in a timely fashion. Surgeons, internists, pediatricians, nurses and psychologists as well as other medical specialists may be necessary to provide the necessary forms of rehabilitation for the patient cured of cancer in childhood.[43]

KEY POINTS

- The goal of treatment is to preserve a functional bladder while curing the cancer.
- Radiation therapy (XRT) to the bladder can cause acute cystitis with or without hematuria, and later may cause fibrosis and diminished bladder volume. Ureters and/or urethra may be constricted if irradiated.
- Cyclophosphamide and ifosfamide can cause similar problems with bladder irritation and dysfunction, but these are usually preventable with concomitant Mesna infusions. The likelihood of bladder damage is increased when these drugs are given along with bladder irradiation.
- Actinomycin D and doxorubicin can augment the deleterious effects of XRT on the bladder.
- Treatment of cystitis includes increased hydration to minimize blood clot formation and obstruction of the bladder outflow tract. Cystoscopy, bladder catherization and perhaps instillation of certain compounds may alleviate the bleeding.
- Several ways of augmenting bladder capacity or of creating a new 'bladder' after total cystectomy are reviewed.

REFERENCES

• 1. Ries LAG, Smith MA, Gurney JG, et al. (eds). *Cancer incidence and survival among children and adolescents: United States SEER Program 1975–1995*. Bethesda, MD: National Cancer Institute, 2001:2–3.

◆2. Crist W, Gehan EA, Ragab AH, et al. The Third Intergroup Rhabdomyosarcoma Study. J Clin Oncol 1995; 13:610–630.

◆3. Lobe TE, Wiener E, Andrassy RJ, et al. The argument for conservative, delayed surgery in the management of prostatic rhabdomyosarcoma. J Pediatr Surg 1996; 31:1084–1087.

●4. Raney B Jr, Heyn R, Hays DM, et al. Sequelae of treatment in 109 patients followed for 5 to 15 years after diagnosis of sarcoma of the bladder and prostate. Cancer 1993; 71:2387–2394.

5. Hays DM, Lawrence W Jr, Crist WM, et al. Partial cystectomy in the management of rhabdomyosarcoma of the bladder: a report from the Intergroup Rhabdomyosarcoma Study. J Pediatr Surg 1990; 25:719–723.

6. Probert JC, Parker BR. The effects of radiotherapy on bone growth. Radiology 1975; 114:155–162.

◆7. Donaldson SS. Effects of irradiation on skeletal growth and development. In: Green DM, D'Angio GJ (eds) Late effects of treatment for childhood cancer. New York: Wiley-Liss, 1992:63–70.

8. Antonakopoulos GN, Hicks RM, Berry RJ. The subcellular basis of damage to the human urinary bladder induced by irradiation. J Pathol 1984; 143:103–116.

◆9. Stewart FA. Mechanism of bladder damage and repair after treatment with radiation and cytostatic drugs. Br J Cancer 1986; 53(Suppl. VII):280–291.

◆10. Dewit L, Ang KK, Van der Schueren E. Acute side effects and late complications after radiotherapy of localized carcinoma of the prostate. Cancer Treat Rev 1983; 10:79–89.

11. Montana GS, Fowler WC. Carcinoma of the cervix: analysis of bladder and rectal radiation dose and complications. Int J Radiat Oncol Biol Phys 1989; 16:95–100.

12. Perez CA, Camel HM, Kuske RR, et al. Radiation therapy alone in the treatment of carcinoma of the uterine cervix: a 20-year experience. Gynecol Oncol 1986; 23:127–140.

13. Pourquier H, Delard R, Achille E, et al. A quantified approach to the analysis and prevention of urinary complications in radiotherapeutic treatment of cancer of the cervix. Int J Radiat Oncol Biol Phys 1987; 13:1025–1033.

14. Meadows AT, Baum E, Fossati-Bellani F, et al. Second malignant neoplasms in children: an update from the Late Effects Study Group. J Clin Oncol 1985; 3:532–538.

◆15. Levine LA, Richie JP. Urological complications of cyclophosphamide. J Urol 1989; 141:1063–1069.

◆16. Stillwell TJ, Benson RC Jr. Cyclophosphamide-induced hemorrhagic cystitis: a review of 100 patients. Cancer 1988; 61:451–457.

◆17. Brugieres L, Hartmann O, Travagli JP, et al. Hemorrhagic cystitis following high-dose chemotherapy and bone marrow transplantation in children with malignancies: Incidence, clinical course, and outcome. J Clin Oncol 1989; 7:194–199.

●18. Sarosy G. Ifosfamide – pharmacologic overview. Semin Oncol 1989; 16(Suppl. 3):2–8.

◆19. Fairchild WV, Spence CR, Solomon HD, Gangai MP. The incidence of bladder cancer after cyclophosphamide therapy. J Urol 1979; 122:163–164.

20. Thrasher JB, Miller GJ, Wettlaufer JN. Bladder leiomyosarcoma following cyclophosphamide therapy for lupus nephritis. J Urol 1990; 143:119–121.

21. Kawamura J, Sakurai M, Tsukamoto K, Tochigi H. Leiomyosarcoma of the bladder eighteen years after cyclophosphamide therapy for retinoblastoma. Urol Int 1993; 51:49–53.

◆22. Pedersen-Bjergaard J, Jonsson V, Pedersen M, Hou-Jensen K. Leiomyosarcoma of the urinary bladder after cyclophosphamide. J Clin Oncol 1995; 13:532–533.

23. Travis LB, Curtis RE, Glimelius B, et al. Bladder and kidney cancer following cyclophosphamide therapy for non-Hodgkin's lymphoma. J Natl Cancer Inst 1995; 87:524–530.

◆24. Tefft M, Lattin PB, Jereb B, et al. Acute and late effects on normal tissues following combined chemo- and radiotherapy for childhood rhabdomyosarcoma and Ewing's sarcoma. Cancer 1976; 37:1201–1213.

◆25. Phillips TL, Wharam MD, Margolis LW. Modification of radiation injury to normal tissues by chemotherapeutic agents. Cancer 1975; 35:1678–1684.

26. Redpath JL, Colman M. The effect of Adriamycin and actinomycin D on radiation-induced skin reactions in mouse feet. Int J Radiat Oncol Biol Phys 1979; 5:483–486.

◆27. Cassady JR, Richter MP, Piro AJ, Jaffe N. Radiation–Adriamycin interactions: preliminary clinical observations. Cancer 1975; 36:946–949.

◆28. D'Angio GJ, Farber S, Maddock CL. Potentiation of x-ray effects by actinomycin D. Radiology 1959; 73:175–177.

◆29. Jayalakshmamma B, Pinkel D. Urinary-bladder toxicity following pelvic irradiation and simultaneous cyclophosphamide therapy. Cancer 1976; 38:701–707.

30. Donahue LA, Frank IN. Intravesical formalin for hemorrhagic cystitis: analysis of therapy. J Urol 1989; 141:809–812.

31. Ostroff EB, Chenault OW Jr. Alum irrigation for the control of massive bladder hemorrhage. J Urol 1982; 128:929–930.

32. Phelps KR, Naylor K, Brien TP, et al. Encephalopathy after bladder irrigation with alum: case report and literature review. Am J Med Sci 1999; 318:181–185.

33. McGuire EJ, Woodside JR, Borden TA, Weiss RM. Prognostic value of urodynamic testing in myelodysplastic patients. J Urol 1981; 126:205–209.

●34. Kropp BP, Cheng EY. Bladder augmentation: current and future techniques. In: Belman AB, King LR, Kramer SA (eds). Clinical pediatric urology. London: Martin Dunitz, 2002:455–491.

35. Nasrallah PF, Aliabadi HA. Bladder augmentation in patients with neurogenic bladder and vesicoureteral reflux. J Urol 1991; 146:563–566.

●36. Rink RC, Cain MP. Urinary diversion. In: Belman AB, King LR, Kramer SA (eds). Clinical pediatric urology. London: Martin Dunitz, 2002:491–529.

37. Studer UE, Ackermann D, Casanova GA, Zingg EJ. A newer form of bladder substitute based on historical perspectives. Semin Urol 1988; 6:57–65.

●38. Mitrofanoff P: Bladder reconstruction and substitution. In: Gearhart JP, Rink RC, Mouriquand PDE (eds) Pediatric urology. Philadelphia: WB Saunders, 2001;947–979.

39. Monti PR, Lara RC, Dutra MA, de Carvalho JR. New techniques for construction of efferent conduits based on the Mitrofanoff principle. Urology 1997; 49:112–115.

40. Gros DA, Dodson JL, Lopatin UA, et al. Decreased linear growth associated with intestinal bladder augmentation in children with bladder exstrophy. J Urol 2000; 164:917–920.

◆41. Filmer RB, Spencer JR. Malignancies in bladder augmentations and intestinal conduits. J Urol 1990; 143:671–678.

42. Gregoire M, Kantoff P, DeWolf WC. Synchronous adenocarcinoma and transitional cell carcinoma of the bladder associated with augmentation: case report and review of the literature. J Urol 1993; 149:115–118.

◆43. D'Angio GJ. The child cured of cancer: a problem for the internist. Semin Oncol 1982; 9:143–149.

7

Gastrointestinal, hepatic and related complications

Body composition and obesity

JOHN W GREGORY AND JOHN J REILLY

INTRODUCTION: ASSESSMENT OF OBESITY, BODY COMPOSITION AND ENERGY BALANCE

Definitions of obesity in childhood and adolescence

Obesity has been defined traditionally as a level of excess body fat associated with health risk. There is increasing evidence that central body fat distribution, independent of total body fat, is associated with cardiovascular risk factors in childhood.[1,2] This suggests that, ideally, both the amount of excess body fat and its distribution should be considered in the assessment of obesity in children. However, in clinical practice, assessment of body fatness and/or fat distribution is usually impractical (see 'Measurement of body fat') and so simpler proxy measures are required. Subjective (clinical) diagnosis of childhood obesity is unreliable, even when carried out by experienced observers and so obesity must be defined using objective body measurements (anthropometry). Body weight alone is inadequate as an index of obesity because of its association with height, so weight must be adjusted for height in some way. Several approaches to this adjustment for height are in use, but there is now an international consensus that the body mass index (BMI), weight (kg)/height^2 (m^2), is the most practical and clinically meaningful.[3–5]

The BMI cannot be used in the same way as in adults for a number of reasons. First, BMI values of children/adolescents are lower than those of adults. Second, BMI changes with age and differs between the sexes. This means that interpreting a BMI value requires comparison with population reference data. Good, accessible, population reference data now exist for many countries including the UK[5] and the USA.[6] These are usually available as centile charts on which BMI values can be plotted to assess obesity or to monitor changes over time.

The BMI is an index of weight adjusted for height. While it is highly correlated with body fatness in children, it is not a direct measure of fatness. However, when used to screen for obesity in children and adolescents, the BMI is undoubtedly useful. A number of studies have tested the ability of various BMI centile cut-offs to identify the fattest children, by measuring body fatness by a more accurate method such as total body water. These generally conclude that by using cut-offs at the top end of the BMI distribution (above about the 90th centile), the BMI can provide moderate sensitivity (low-moderate false-negative rate), but high specificity (low false-positive rate) and so the fattest children can be identified with some confidence.[7] Furthermore, cut-offs for BMI that exceed the 95th centile are predictive of obesity-related morbidity: children with BMI > 95th centile have a high probability of remaining obese and morbidity increases significantly above the 95th centile for BMI.[8,9] An additional advantage in pediatric oncology is that the ability of BMI cut-offs to define obesity appears to differ little between healthy children vs. those with disease, including malignancy.[10]

Measurement of body fat

In routine clinical practice, obesity is most easily defined using body mass index measurements (see earlier). However, in clinical research or when stature is abnormal, as may occur in growth hormone deficiency,

BMI measurements may provide inadequate estimates of adiposity and more direct measures of body fat may be required. Furthermore, annual changes in BMI of individual healthy children are more usually attributed to changes in fat-free rather than fat mass and this needs to be taken into account during longitudinal clinical monitoring for evolving obesity.[11] Many techniques for the measurement of body composition exist. The most frequently used methods that will be encountered in the pediatric literature are dual-energy X-ray absorptiometry (DEXA), simple anthropometric measurements, such as those of skinfold thickness, and bioelectrical impedance measurements. Data from the majority of these studies subdivide body composition into two compartments – fat and fat-free mass.

DUAL–ENERGY X–RAY ABSORPTIOMETRY

DEXA measurements are increasingly used for the measurement of body composition in clinical studies. DEXA is a relatively non-invasive method that allows quantification of whole-body composition into fat-free mass (bone mineral and lean tissues) and fat mass with a precision of <1–2 per cent.[12] The technique also permits the regional distribution of body composition to be assessed. DEXA is dependent on the differential attenuation of photons of two different energies passing through the body tissues. The method is particularly suitable for use in children owing to the minimal doses of radiation involved (<0.1 mSv, whole body) and the minimal cooperation required of patients undergoing these measurements in a relatively short scan time (<10 minutes).[12–14] However, although DEXA measurements of body composition are highly correlated with those derived from other methods, there are relatively large limits of agreement when results from different methods are compared with each other. This suggests that different methods for measuring body composition should not be used interchangeably.[15]

SKINFOLD THICKNESS MEASUREMENTS

The assessment of adiposity by skinfold thickness measurements is the longest established of the methods for body composition measurement in children in clinical practice. Triceps and subscapular skinfold thickness can be measured and values compared with sex- and age-specific centile charts.[16] However, the value of using these charts is limited by the changes in the nutritional state of the childhood population since these charts were published and the effect of disease processes on body fat distribution.[17,18] Alternatively, values for the total amount of body fat and fat-free mass can be calculated from skinfold thicknesses, assuming a constant relationship between subcutaneous and deep fat stores, using separate regression equations for adolescents[19] and prepubertal children.[20] The value of skinfold thickness measurements is, however, limited by the need for careful training of the observer, the difficulty of using the method in obese individuals and the relatively high interobserver and intraobserver error for the method.[15]

BIOELECTRICAL IMPEDANCE

Bioelectrical impedance measurements of body water have been widely used in clinical research to derive measures of body composition in children.[14,15,21] The method is based on the relationship between the physical dimensions and electrical properties of the body acting as a conductor. Thus, electrical resistance to a flow of current of 50 kHz in the human body is related to the amount of total body water and, assuming a constant relationship between this and fat-free mass, fat mass can be calculated. Various regression equations have been derived for this method by comparison with other techniques, such as isotope labeling of body water.[21–23] The technique is limited by its poor accuracy in certain clinical situations but has the advantage of relatively high precision and utility in children given its non-invasive nature, as the electrical current used cannot be detected by the child.[21]

In clinical practice or research, if more direct measures of adiposity are required than those provided by the measurement of the body mass index, DEXA scanning has a number of advantages over skinfold thickness and bioelectrical impedance methods.

Principles of energy balance

In healthy human beings, energy intake is remarkably closely balanced by energy expenditure, resulting in relatively stable body composition. The first law of thermodynamics defines the principle of conservation of energy. This principle means that surprisingly small differences between energy intake and expenditure on a daily basis (e.g. 25–50 kcal/day) will lead to large changes in stored energy after a few years. Obesity occurs when energy intake exceeds energy expenditure. However, in most circumstances leading to obesity, it is not known whether this is due to a decrease in energy expenditure or an increase in energy intake relative to energy needs, or the effects of both.[24]

ENERGY INTAKE

Energy intake arises from the consumption of fat, carbohydrate and protein in the diet. The measurement of energy intake is particularly difficult to do with any degree of precision. To be accurate, the technique requires knowledge of the precise amount and calorie content of the food consumed, and an analysis of the extent to which calories are not absorbed but are lost in the feces. In the free-living state, energy intake is most

commonly estimated by analysis of dietary diaries in which subjects document in detail the precise amounts of all foods and fluids consumed. The error in assessing energy (calorie) intake by this method is unlikely to be less than ±10 per cent[25] and often much greater, particularly in obese individuals in whom energy intake is likely to be substantially underestimated.[26] In practice, therefore, energy intake is rarely estimated except in carefully controlled experimental circumstances.

ENERGY EXPENDITURE

Total daily energy expenditure consists of three components: basal metabolic rate, energy expended in physical activity, and thermogenesis. In the free-living state, daily energy expenditure is difficult to measure in children. The current 'gold standard' measurement utilizes the doubly labeled water method, which is based on the measurement of carbon dioxide production over an approximate 2-week period from the difference in the elimination rates (measured in urine) of two stable non-radioactive isotopes ($^2H_2$ and ^{18}O) from the body. The method is non-invasive, has good precision (2–8 per cent)[27–30] for the measurement of total energy expenditure and is easily administered to children.[31] The disadvantage is the expense of the isotopes and the need for sophisticated mass spectrometry support. Furthermore, in a child with reduced or increased values, measurements of total daily energy expenditure do not indicate which subcomponent is abnormal (unless other components of energy expenditure are also measured), nor is it possible to evaluate abnormalities in energy balance over short-term periods, such as 24 hours. Doubly labeled water techniques have, however, demonstrated that most obese children, contrary to the findings of earlier studies, have higher total energy expenditures than lean individuals but which are normal when adjusted for body size.[26]

Basal metabolic rate

In a child, the largest component of total daily energy expenditure is that due to the basal metabolic rate. This is defined as the energy expended, shortly after waking when the subject is unstressed, in a postabsorptive (fasting) state and in a thermoneutral environment (i.e. no energy is being expended to maintain body temperature). In humans, basal metabolic rate accounts for 60–75 per cent of total daily energy expenditure[32] and is the energy expended by the body as a result of the fundamental cellular metabolic processes necessary to maintain life. The major predictors of basal metabolic rate are weight and fat-free mass.[24] Basal metabolic rate is reduced when adjusted for fat-free mass (the most metabolically active component of body composition) as children grow older and in girls compared with boys.[24,33]

Basal metabolic rate is most commonly measured by ventilated hood indirect calorimetry in which energy expenditure is estimated from measurements of oxygen consumption and carbon dioxide production. This method requires the cooperation of the child, who is required to lie still for periods of around 30 minutes, and is, therefore, difficult to measure after the neonatal period until approximately 7 years of age. When these measurements are made on a child who has been admitted to hospital fasting following waking, data are often referred to as *resting* rather than basal metabolic rate.

Physical activity

The next largest contribution to daily energy expenditure is that contributed by the effects of physical activity, mostly due to skeletal muscle activity and compensatory responses of the cardiorespiratory system. In a child, free-living physical activity levels may vary widely but account for approximately 20–30 per cent of total energy expenditure. Physical activity levels account for a lower proportion of total energy expenditure in normal pre-school children than in those who are prepubertal or adolescent.[34] Energy expended in physical activity is correlated with markers of aerobic fitness, fat-free mass and fat mass, and is greater in the spring than the autumn.[24] In the normal population, some studies have shown that reduced energy expended in physical activity may be involved in the development of obesity.[35,36] However, duration and frequency of physical activity seem more important than energy expended in activity in the regulation of energy balance.[37,38]

Free-living physical activity may be measured in children by direct observation, self reporting, heart-rate or activity monitoring. The first two of these techniques are in most circumstances impractical or inaccurate.[34] One of the more widely used methods in clinical research into factors predisposing to obesity is the measurement of heart rate continuously through the waking day. Physical activity or energy expenditure can be calculated from assumptions based on a linear relationship between heart rate and oxygen uptake. This method is relatively cheap and easy to use even in obese children[39,40] but accuracy in estimating total energy expenditure is limited to −17 to +18 per cent of values obtained by doubly labeled water.[41] This may be partly due to the effects of emotional stress, body position and other non-exercise-related influences on heart rate.[42]

Other techniques estimate physical activity using various devices to record mechanical motion. The earliest devices (pedometers) record acceleration and deceleration of movement in one direction, but fail to measure exercise intensity or the effects of cycling or increases in energy expenditure from carrying objects or walking/ running uphill.[43] In recent years, more sophisticated activity monitors, which document intensity of movement in addition to quantity, have become available.[43] Some of these measure activity in three dimensions, a particular

advantage when attempting to estimate a child's physical activity.[44]

Thermogenesis

The smallest contribution to energy expenditure (approximately 10 per cent) is that caused by thermogenesis (diet induced and cold induced). Thermogenesis is the effect on energy expenditure of a variety of stimuli, such as feeding, cold, increasing sympathetic activity due to anxiety, drugs and other unknown stimuli.[45] Thermogenesis is rarely measured and reported separately as abnormalities in this component of energy expenditure are unlikely to be a major contributing factor to the etiology of obesity.

CONSEQUENCES OF OBESITY IN CHILDHOOD AND ADOLESCENCE

Short-term consequences

The most common consequences of childhood obesity are psychosocial: anxiety, the effects of bullying, and isolation.[8] These are particularly marked in adolescence.

'Simple' obesity (due to a relatively large appetite and/or inactive lifestyle) is usually associated with an increase in growth velocity, and obese children are usually tall for age with bone age advance and earlier pubertal maturation. A number of relatively minor endocrine abnormalities are commonly associated with simple obesity (e.g. premature adrenarche, menstrual irregularity). Obesity that is endocrine in origin is much less common, and is usually associated with poor linear growth and bone age delay.

A wide range of other comorbidities exist: orthopedic, hepatic, and respiratory, most of which are common relative to non-obese children but otherwise fairly uncommon.[8] Cardiovascular risk factors are relatively common in obese children and tend to 'cluster' in the obese child.[9,46,47] Furthermore, obesity is associated with atherogenesis, even in childhood[48]. The childhood obesity epidemic in the USA was followed by an epidemic of juvenile type II diabetes and increasing presentation of adolescents with type II diabetes is likely. It is also worth noting that long-term survivors of childhood cancer have an increased risk of the 'metabolic syndrome' (a cluster of abnormalities including insulin resistance, glucose intolerance, hypertension, dyslipidemias and atherosclerotic cardiovascular disease[49]).

Longer-term consequences

PERSISTENCE OF OBESITY

While not all obese children become obese adults, childhood obesity has a strong tendency to persist into adulthood. Persistence is especially likely in older children and adolescents, where one or both parents are obese, or where obesity is more severe.[50]

PSYCHOLOGICAL

The literature on the psychological consequences of obesity in adulthood is substantial, but it suffers from a number of methodological problems and a detailed discussion is beyond the scope of this review. However, despite the methodological difficulties, a systematic review of this subject concluded that obesity that persists into adulthood is generally associated with increased risk of emotional problems, negative body image and self-perception.[51]

SOCIAL AND ECONOMIC CONSEQUENCES

Two studies, one from the USA[52] and the other from the UK,[53] have shown that obese adolescents and young adults have poorer social outcomes, corrected for IQ, (e.g. marriage; educational attainment) and economic outcomes (e.g. income) in young adulthood. These effects presumably arise because of discrimination and are more marked in women than men. One concern for long-term survivors of childhood cancer must be that these long-term social and economic effects of obesity might compound the educational deficits described in Chapter 2b.

CARDIOVASCULAR RISK FACTORS IN ADULTHOOD

There is evidence that the cardiovascular risk factors associated with obesity tend to persist into adult life. These include hypertension, adverse lipid profiles and hyperinsulinaemia.[54] In survivors of childhood cancer, the (indirect) cardiovascular effects of obesity may be exacerbated by treatment-related mechanisms, which have more direct effects on the cardiovascular system (see Chapter 4).

ADULT MORBIDITY AND MORTALITY

Obesity in childhood and adolescence increases the risk of morbidity and mortality in adult life, particularly from cardiovascular disease and type II diabetes.[55,56]

OBESITY IN PATIENTS WITH ACUTE LYMPHOBLASTIC LEUKEMIA

Prevalence

PATTERNS OF EXCESS WEIGHT GAIN AFTER DIAGNOSIS

A number of studies have reported changes in BMI standard deviation scores ('SD' or 'Z' score) or centiles following diagnosis of acute lymphoblastic leukemia (ALL). These have consistently shown weight and BMI gain in excess of population reference data but at rates that have

varied between studies.[57–71] This variation probably relates to differences in treatment protocols, definitions of excess weight gain (e.g. use of different reference data) and the relatively small sample sizes in each study (particularly given the heterogeneity of treatment within some studies). Despite the variations between studies, some patterns are clear, notably that the period of most marked excess weight gain is during therapy, particularly during the first year of therapy. Traditionally, the excess weight gain during therapy was interpreted as evidence of a medical cause of obesity, a side effect of therapy, but the actual causes are more complex and are discussed below.

There is consistent evidence of a process of excess weight gain in children with ALL that begins soon after diagnosis and is common (it occurs in most patients, including those who do not go on to become obese). Excess weight gained during therapy is usually maintained[60,61,64,65] (increases in BMI Z score are maintained relative to controls or reference populations). Some studies reported subgroups of patients in whom excess weight gain (relative to population reference data) continued after cessation of therapy,[59,64,65,67] implying an important lifestyle contribution to the development of obesity.

PREVALENCE OF OBESITY DURING THERAPY

Early reports of excess weight gain in patients with ALL[59] raised the concern that obesity was not just a 'late effect', but occurred early, before the end of therapy. A number of more recent studies have estimated obesity prevalence using the BMI centile in patients in first remission at the beginning and end of therapy and these are summarized in Table 7a.1. Prevalence estimates vary, largely as a function of the relatively small numbers and different obesity definitions. However, these studies all show that obesity is common during therapy and that many children being treated for ALL are likely to require treatment for obesity.

PREVALENCE OF OBESITY AFTER THERAPY

Table 7a.2 summarizes studies of obesity prevalence in survivors of ALL after therapy. Whereas prevalence estimates vary between studies, all of the final height studies, with one exception,[66] reported a much higher prevalence of obesity than expected and/or higher prevalence than controls, using definitions based on BMI. The only study to find no difference in obesity prevalence in long-term survivors (compared to a control group) used BMI as the definition of obesity, but did find that long-term survivors were significantly fatter than controls.[66]

An epidemic of pediatric and adult obesity occurred across the developed world in the 1980s and 1990s, but the studies summarized in Table 7a.2 confirm that obesity prevalence in long-term survivors of ALL is substantially higher than that of the general population.

Causes of obesity in ALL

ENERGY IMBALANCE

As noted above in 'Principles of energy balance', obesity is the result of chronic positive energy balance. In this

Table 7a.1 Obesity prevalence (%; defined using BMI) at diagnosis and end of therapy for acute lymphoblastic leukaemia

Study	n	Definition (BMI centile)	Prevalence (%) at diagnosis	End of therapy
Odame et al.[59]	40	>97.7th	5	43 (girls), 26 (boys)
Van Dongen-Melman et al.[60]	113	>90th	8	30
Reilly et al.[61]	98	>97.7th	2	9
Mayer et al.[62]	39	>97.7th	3	38 with cranial irradiation, 48 without

BMI, body mass index.

Table 7a.2 Obesity prevalence after therapy

Study	n	Obesity definition (centile)	Assessment period	Prevalence (%)
Schell et al.[63]	91	BMI > 24 kg/m^2	Final height	38
Odame et al.[59]	40	BMI > 97.7th	Diagnosis + 4 years	57 (girls), 21 (boys)
Van Dongen-Melman et al.[60]	113	BMI > 90th	Diagnosis + 4 years	24
Didi et al.[64]	114	BMI > 85th	Final height	46
Talvensaari et al.[49]	50	Body weight > 120% ideal	Diagnosis + 13 years	32 (vs. 10 in controls)
Birkebaeck et al.[65]	33	BMI > 90th	Final height	36
Nysom et al.[66]	95	BMI > 90th	Diagnosis + 11 years	25
Reilly et al.[61]	98	BMI > 97.7th	Diagnosis + 3 years	16
Shaw et al.[67]	33	BMI > 85th	Final height	56 (females, $n = 25$), 13 (males, $n = 8$)

BMI, body mass index.

section, the evidence for abnormalities in various components of energy balance, and the underlying mechanisms, are reviewed.

CRANIAL IRRADIATION

Cranial irradiation and/or chemotherapy directed at the central nervous system (CNS) have the potential to cause CNS (particularly hypothalamic) damage. This may promote obesity via a number of possible mechanisms: alterations in resting energy expenditure or energy expended on physical activity; growth hormone insufficiency can alter substrate oxidation and fat deposition; and hypothalamic regulation of food intake can be impaired (see Chapters 4b and 8a).

A good deal of research on the mechanisms of excess weight gain in ALL has considered the possible role of CNS damage. It is now clear that patients who have not received cranial irradiation, treated by chemotherapy only, are at increased risk of excess weight gain and obesity relative to controls.[61,62,65,70] Cranial radiotherapy/ growth hormone insufficiency is not essential to the development of obesity in ALL. For children treated on more modern protocols, which do not use cranial radiotherapy, rates and pattern of excess weight gain may be similar to those treated on older protocols with cranial radiotherapy.[61,62,70] However, there is also some evidence that risk of obesity was higher for patients treated on older protocols that used cranial irradiation.[59,71,72] Risk of growth hormone insufficiency is almost certainly higher for patients treated on protocols that used cranial radiotherapy.[72,73] In summary, CNS directed therapy probably contributes to obesity in ALL in older protocols, but is by no means the only or even the major determinant of obesity.

STEROID THERAPY

One unusual feature of ALL therapy is long-term treatment with corticosteroids. Corticosteroids could promote obesity via a range of possible mechanisms: effects on appetite/regulation of energy intake; alterations in substrate oxidation; and alterations in energy expenditure.[74] There is a widespread belief that steroid therapy is a major contributor to the development of obesity in ALL but until recently there was almost no empirical evidence of energy balance effects of corticosteroid therapy in any clinical setting. A recent study from the UK reported that energy intake in children treated for ALL during the maintenance phase of chemotherapy was significantly increased.[68] The magnitude of the increase in energy intake was substantial, around 20 per cent on average during the 5-day course of dexamethasone (6.5 mg/m^2) or prednisolone (40 mg/m^2). Even a small (1–2 per cent of energy requirement) positive energy balance can lead to obesity, if it is sustained, so an increase of this magnitude suggests that glucocorticoid therapy is an important contributor to excess weight gain in ALL. During intensification (when glucocorticoids are used for a longer period than in maintenance), the contribution to positive energy balance may be even greater.

Various attempts have been made to relate degree of weight gain to the dose or steroid used. These have been largely inconclusive, usually because of relatively small sample sizes.[60] Some studies found that dexamethasone therapy was associated with a greater magnitude of excess weight gain than prednisolone,[60,73] although others did not.[66,68]

LIFESTYLE CHANGES: PHYSICAL ACTIVITY AND INACTIVITY

The major lifestyle change, which has been shown to be common in patients treated for ALL, is reduced habitual physical activity. Patients treated for ALL are much less active than their healthy peers both during and after therapy.[75,76] The magnitude of this reduction in activity, together with other evidence that physical inactivity is an important determinant of obesity risk,[77] suggests that this behavioral change is an important contributor to the development and maintenance of obesity in ALL.

The reduction in physical activity has been demonstrated by two independent methods. Reilly et al. measured total energy expenditure by the doubly labeled water method, resting energy expenditure and energy expended on activity in 20 patients (mean age 10 years) treated for ALL between 2 and 3 years postdiagnosis.[76] Results were compared with 20 closely matched healthy controls. These patients were not obese but had shown excess weight gain. They were studied when well, living at home and attending school. Total energy expenditure was markedly reduced in the patients, by 282 kcal/day on average and this was almost entirely due to reduced energy expended on physical activity. Both total energy expenditure and energy expended on physical activity was predictive of subsequent degree of excess weight gain. Warner et al. reported differences in total energy expenditure (by heart rate monitoring), resting energy expenditure and energy expended on physical activity in 31 survivors of ALL, 21 survivors of other childhood malignancies and 32 healthy sibling controls.[75] In this study, patients with ALL were slightly older (mean 12 years old) and further from diagnosis than in the study by Reilly et al.,[76] but engagement in physical activity was also markedly reduced in the survivors of ALL. In the healthy sibling controls and controls who had survived other malignancies, mean physical activity level (the ratio total energy expenditure: resting energy expenditure) was 1.47 and 1.58, respectively. In the survivors of ALL, mean physical activity level was only 1.27, which indicates an extremely inactive lifestyle.[75] Taken together,

these studies demonstrate a substantial reduction in engagement in physical activity that begins during therapy for ALL and persists for some time after therapy. It is also worth noting that circumstances earlier in therapy (when patients are hospitalized/unwell) are even less conducive to engagement in physical activity and so physical activity levels may be even more abnormal. This, when combined with the steroid effects noted above, probably explains the observation that the rate of excess weight gain is highest in the first year of therapy.

Warner *et al.* found that abnormalities in body fatness and physical activity level were not present in the heterogenous group of children who had survived other malignancies,[75] and this is consistent with other evidence that weight gain in survivors of a variety of solid tumors was not particularly marked.[59]

The precise social or behavioral causes of reduced physical activity in children treated for ALL remain unclear, and we lack evidence on activity patterns, which might identify the precise behavioral changes that children treated for ALL undergo. It is possible to speculate that changes in parental behavior secondary to the psychosocial consequences of treatment[78] might predispose to reduced activity. Pathophysiological changes in the cardiorespiratory system, or growth hormone insufficiency, resulting from treatment of ALL,[79,80] might also contribute to reduced physical activity/reduced energy expended on physical activity in some patients, particularly those treated on older protocols. Evidence from patients treated on older protocols suggested that survivors of ALL were less physically fit than their peers[81–83] but the relevance of this to modern treatment protocols remains unclear, and reduced physical fitness *per se* need not cause reduced energy expended on physical activity. There is increasing evidence in modern children, that variations in time spent in sedentary-low intensity activities are most important to energy balance (e.g. time spent in sedentary behaviors, such as TV viewing). The role of high-intensity activities in prevention of obesity is somewhat limited, because high-intensity activity is so infrequent, and reduced physical activity in the survivors of ALL probably reflects increased time in sedentary behaviors, such as TV viewing.[77]

LIFESTYLE CHANGES: DIETARY INTAKE

There is currently only limited evidence on the dietary intakes of children treated for ALL. Available evidence indicates that gross overeating is not a feature of the development of obesity in ALL[76,84] other than during periods of steroid treatment.[68] Overeating relative to total energy expenditure must occur, by definition, for obesity to develop, but 'relative overeating' is difficult to measure given the inaccuracy and imprecision of all methods available for assessment of dietary intake.[76]

PREMATURE ADIPOSITY REBOUND

The adiposity rebound is believed to be a 'critical period' in childhood during which risk of adult obesity can be 'programmed'.[85] Indices of adiposity in healthy children, such as the BMI, increase dramatically during the first year of life, then decline to a nadir at around 4–5 years of age. The period (typically between 5 and 7 years of age) when the BMI begins to increase after its nadir has been termed the adiposity rebound. Children with early adiposity rebound are at substantially increased risk of adult obesity, with current estimates suggesting a relative risk of adult obesity of around 5 compared to children with more typical timing of adiposity rebound. This relationship is independent of other risk factors for adult obesity and independent of BMI at the time of adiposity rebound.[85] The mechanisms by which programming at the adiposity rebound occurs are unknown at present.

Peak age of diagnosis of ALL is just before the typical age at adiposity rebound and prolonged positive energy balance begins shortly after diagnosis, so it seems reasonable to expect that timing of adiposity rebound might be affected by diagnosis of ALL. Evidence of this is limited at present but one recent study found a dramatically advanced adiposity rebound in children treated for ALL.[69] In 68 patients with ALL in continuous complete remission adiposity rebound had occurred in 81 per cent by age 4, but in only 21 per cent of 889 healthy controls at the same age. Extremely early adiposity rebound (by age 3) had occurred in 43 per cent of the patients, but only 4 per cent of controls. Premature adiposity rebound is, therefore, likely to contribute to increased risk of adult obesity in children treated for ALL, at least for those who have not experienced adiposity rebound by the time of diagnosis (most patients under the age of about 5 years at diagnosis).

EVIDENCE ON OTHER POSSIBLE CAUSES

A number of other possible mechanisms might underlie the development of obesity in children treated for ALL. Many studies have tested for abnormalities in resting energy expenditure (REE). In the early stages of therapy, REE may show a short-term increase but this is probably of limited clinical significance.[86] Substrate oxidation may also be subtly altered by steroid therapy during periods of intensive treatment, but again the extent to which this might contribute to the development of obesity is unclear.[87] Most studies have compared REE of patients and healthy controls during maintenance chemotherapy or after the end of therapy, and most have found no significant differences between patients and controls.[70,84,87,88] Two studies have reported small reductions in REE relative to controls, but this abnormality in energy metabolism is probably of limited biological significance, since both demonstrated a much larger reduction in the energy

expended on physical activity in the same patients.[75,76] Diet-induced thermogenesis (DIT) is a small component of total energy expenditure (see 'Energy expenditure') that varies little between individuals. One study found that DIT was normal in children with ALL.[86]

Predictive models

A number of studies have attempted to identify risk factors for excess weight gain or obesity in patients treated for ALL. The aim of this research was to derive clinical algorithms that predict risk of obesity in individual patients. Ultimately, these might offer the prospect of modifying treatment or offering other measures that may facilitate prevention of obesity. The present review will focus on the three studies that used regression models to consider a number of potential risk factors simultaneously. Schell et al. studied patients who had reached final height treated on older protocols between 1973 and 1975 in the USA, and attempted to identify risk factors for obesity in adulthood.[63] Didi et al. studied patients treated between 1971 and 1987 in the UK, at final height.[64] Reilly et al. studied younger patients (at 3 years postdiagnosis), treated in the UK during the 1990s, and attempted to identify risk factors for excess weight gain.[61] All three studies were limited by relatively small sample sizes and by the need for caution in generalizing their findings, specifically because of changes in treatment protocols over the years.

More generally, the statistical procedures used tend to generate population-specific predictive models that should be cross-validated, in a different sample or population, before they can be considered generalizable. The studies also tended to concentrate on potential risk factors that were routinely available from patient records. It is worth noting that a number of well-established risk factors for child and adolescent obesity (such as parental obesity and socioeconomic status[89]) are not routinely recorded during ALL therapy. These risk factors might well exacerbate the existing predisposition to obesity in ALL, but evidence on this to date is limited.[60,67]

Both studies from the UK that used regression models identified risk factors, which were statistically significant, notably age at diagnosis (greater risk in younger patients) but concluded that these results would be of limited clinical value when attempting to identify high-risk subgroups of patients.[61,63] An additional concern was that, since the problem of excess weight gain and obesity in survivors of ALL is so common, an approach that targets 'high-risk' groups for treatment or prevention may be inappropriate. It may be more helpful to consider all patients as high risk of obesity and its sequelae.

One valuable outcome of these and other studies of risk factors for obesity has been to confirm or refute hypotheses in relation to causes of obesity in ALL. For example, it is now clear that gender differences in obesity risk are minor and that CNS therapy is not a common cause of obesity, in contrast to earlier evidence based on older treatment protocols.

OBESITY FOLLOWING INTRACRANIAL TUMORS

Introduction

Obesity is a well-recognized complication of tumors in the hypothalamo-pituitary region.[90,91] There are a number of mechanisms whereby such tumors result in obesity. Energy intake may be increased in excess of requirements owing to impaired satiety and hyperphagia caused by disruption of the ventromedial hypothalamic nuclei owing to direct effects of the tumor[92] or following surgical trauma.[93,94] Increased appetite may also occur following steroid therapy to prevent increased intracranial pressure. Energy expenditure may be reduced below energy intake as a consequence of hypopituitarism. This may be due to tumor-induced disruption of hypothalamo-pituitary signaling, direct tumor or surgical damage to the pituitary gland, or a result of cranial radiotherapy. Furthermore, the tumor or its treatment may result in specific neurological or behavioral effects that may reduce habitual levels of physical activity.

Tumors affecting the hypothalamus

Craniopharyngioma is the most common tumor in the hypothalamic region associated with obesity. Although craniopharyngioma like germinoma have their origins in the pituitary stalk, they often extend to involve the hypothalamus. Other tumors that may affect the hypothalamus include epithelioma, pinealoma, endothelioma, hamartoma, colloid cysts and benign tumors, epidermoids, ganglioneuroma, ependymoma and gliomas.[90] The obesity that is associated with tumors in the hypothalamic region is partly a consequence of their adverse effects on the ventromedial hypothalamus.[90] Animal studies suggest that obesity results from increased parasympathetic and decreased sympathetic activity.[95] As energy stores are increased, circulating insulin and leptin concentrations increase with developing peripheral resistance to insulin action, and central and peripheral resistance to leptin action.[96,97] In addition, hypothalamic tumors may induce obesity by injury of the paraventricular nuclei, which directly leads to hyperphagia.

Severe weight gain (see Figure 7a.1) is very common in childhood craniopharyngioma. In a large study of 63 children, 17 per cent had a history of significant weight gain

in the 3.5 years prior to the diagnosis of a craniopharyngioma. All these individuals had preoperative evidence on magnetic resonance imaging of tumor extension into the hypothalamus.[94] Following surgery, mean BMI SD score for all 63 subjects increased from 0.0 to +2.7 at 6 months and to +2.4 at 1 year. The increase in BMI was greatest in those with severe hypothalamic damage on preoperative imaging. This increase in BMI was unrelated to steroid therapy or time to start of growth hormone treatment.[94] Others have shown similar results with 52 per cent of children becoming obese following aggressive surgical intervention.[93] Therapeutic behavioral interventions to control obesity in these circumstances have had poor outcomes.[98] These observations suggest that, wherever possible, surgical intervention for craniopharyngioma should avoid further hypothalamic injury.

Steroid therapy

Children with intracranial tumors frequently receive high-dose glucocorticoid treatment either at presentation to ameliorate the symptoms of raised intracranial pressure or following surgery to limit postoperative edema. The mechanisms whereby such treatment may be associated in the short term with increasing obesity are discussed above (see earlier section on steroid therapy).

Hypopituitarism

Almost all children undergoing surgery for a craniopharyngioma develop multiple pituitary hormone deficiencies.[94] Pituitary dysfunction is also a common complication of other tumors in the hypothalamic region. Furthermore, cranial radiotherapy used to treat a variety of intracranial tumors (e.g. medulloblastoma) commonly results in hypopituitarism (see Chapter 8a).

Although the adverse effects of radiotherapy are dependent on dose, fractionation, age when irradiated, time from irradiation and site of radiotherapy, there is evidence that growth hormone is the most sensitive to these effects.[99] It is now known that irradiation of the hypothalamo-pituitary axis with fractionated doses of 30 Gy or more is associated with a 60–100 per cent risk within 2–5 years of growth hormone deficiency sufficiently severe to cause growth failure.[100–102] Growth hormone is known to have numerous metabolic effects, including stimulation of lipolysis, nitrogen retention and protein synthesis.[103–105] When growth hormone deficiency is prolonged and severe, affected individuals demonstrate a reduction in resting metabolic rate, increased relative adiposity and are at increased risk of obesity.[18,106,107] Young adults have also been shown to have reduced maximal exercise capacity.[108] Growth hormone therapy reverses these effects and, within 6 weeks, leads to increased resting metabolic rate

and fat-free mass,[31] with coincidental reductions in body fat and redistribution of fat from central abdominal to peripheral sites.[109] There is, however, no evidence that the anabolic effects of therapy and increased maximal exercise capacity result in increased physical activity.[31]

Radiotherapy-induced growth hormone deficiency may have particular adverse implications in the long term. Follow-up studies have shown that young adult survivors of childhood brain cancer who received cranial radiotherapy are at increased risk of cardiovascular disease *with* evidence of elevated systolic blood pressure, increased waist–hip ratio and adverse lipid profiles. These abnormalities were particularly pronounced in those with untreated growth hormone deficiency.[110]

Hypothyroidism may also occur following hypothalamo-pituitary irradiation. Hypothyroidism impairs both linear growth and weight gain. Because growth is more severely affected than weight gain, affected children demonstrate a relative increase in weight compared to height. However, this is rarely severe enough to cause obesity.[111]

Neurological complications and lifestyle changes

Intracranial tumors and their treatment are associated with neurological complications that may have adverse effects on motor function (see Chapter 2). Impaired motor function may also result in significantly reduced physical activity, thus predisposing the child to obesity. This finding, particularly when associated with the adverse effects of growth hormone deficiency, may result in rapid changes in body composition (see Figure 7a.2).

PREVENTION AND TREATMENT OF OBESITY IN SURVIVORS OF CHILDHOOD CANCER

To date, there is no published evidence on strategies for prevention or treatment of obesity in children with ALL, and only very limited evidence from children with other malignancies. Guidance on potentially useful strategies can be obtained from the literature on pediatric obesity prevention and treatment. Expert committee advice on the identification and management of child and adolescent obesity is widely available,[3] and a recent systematic review of the subject considered the evidence on prevention and treatment.[89] Strategies for prevention that are well established as being successful in the long term are lacking but a number of approaches to prevention are promising.

Of particular note is the paradigm shifts that have occurred, first from physical fitness to physical activity, and more recently to a focus on physical inactivity/

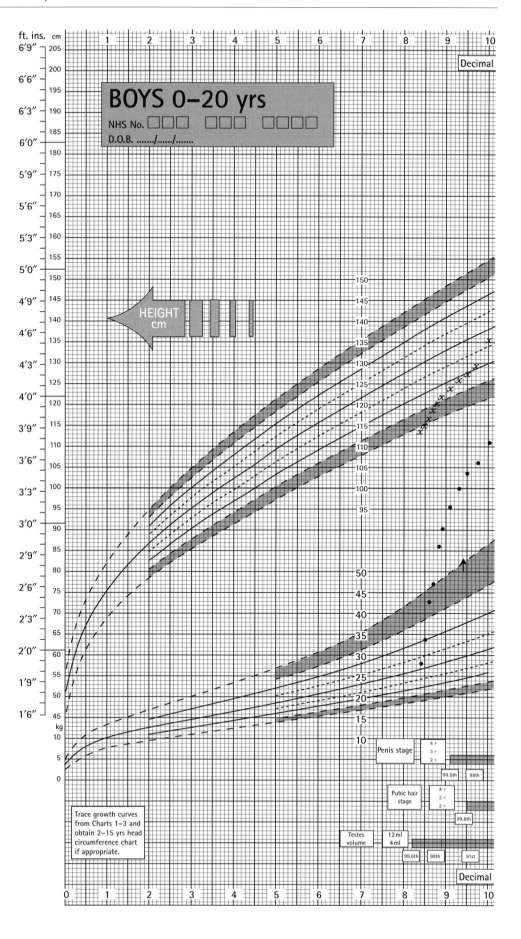

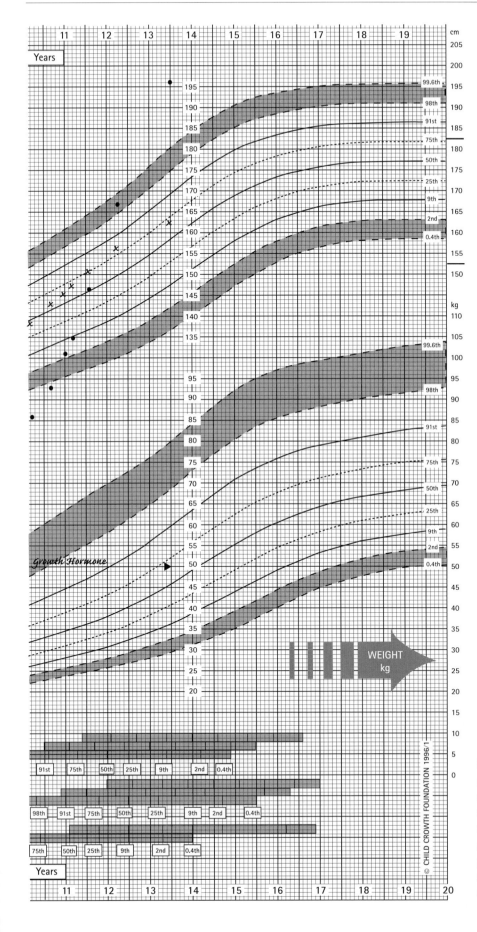

Figure 7a.1 *Severe weight gain in a child treated surgically for a craniopharyngioma. This child was treated postoperatively with thyroxine and hydrocortisone, with growth hormone added at 9.4 years old.* ✕ *, height measurements; •, weight measurements.*

Figure 7a.2 *The effect of stopping and then restarting growth hormone therapy on body composition in a patient with impaired motor function and growth hormone deficiency following treatment for an intracranial tumor.*

sedentary behaviors such as TV viewing.[77] Promotion of a reduction in sedentary behavior (e.g. TV viewing) appears to be more successful in increasing activity levels of children than the more obvious and traditional strategy of promoting an increase in structured physical activity.[3,77] Reducing behaviors such as TV viewing may also reduce the 'relative overeating', which characterizes the development of obesity in modern children. This strategy is also more likely to be practical in a clinical situation, with limited access to exercise specialists, and both safer and more likely to be tolerated by children than promotion of structured aerobic exercise. Targeting sedentary behavior using simple rules (such as limiting TV viewing and computer use to an agreed maximum of 14 hours/week), and encouraging the ability of the family to self-monitor sedentary behavior may be beneficial in both prevention and treatment of obesity. The strategy is especially relevant in ALL because it is clear that lifestyle, in particular a dramatically reduced engagement in physical activity, is central to the development and maintenance of obesity. Promotion of 'active living' by targeting sedentary behavior is also attractive because it may also have beneficial implications for the problems with bone health common in the survivors of childhood cancer (see Chapter 13).

If strategies for the prevention and treatment of obesity in children treated for cancer are adopted, it is likely that family involvement will be beneficial.[3,89] Alteration of steroid therapy with the aim of preventing obesity is unlikely, so changes in patient and family lifestyles would appear to be the only available option for preventive strategies. Finally, the issue of when to intervene to prevent obesity in children treated for cancer has not been clearly established. However, the evidence, summarized above, confirms that obesity is an early as well as a late

effect, and that its origins can lie in the excess weight gain and lifestyle changes during therapy. When taken together with the high failure rate that characterizes obesity treatment in adulthood, prevention seems the most attractive option, and it should probably start early, perhaps during treatment.

KEY POINTS

- Body mass index may be used to monitor indirectly for evolving childhood obesity.
- Dual-energy X-ray absorptiometry provides the most reliable clinical measurement of body fat.
- Obesity occurs when energy intake exceeds energy expenditure.
- Psychosocial consequences are the most common adverse effects of childhood obesity.
- Long-term survivors of childhood cancer have increased risks of 'the multimetabolic syndrome'.
- Obesity in survivors of acute lymphoblastic leukemia is due to the adverse effects of cranial radiotherapy, glucocorticoid therapy and a reduction in physical activity.
- Intracranial tumors predispose to obesity either by direct hypothalamic effects causing impaired satiety and hyperphagia, or as a consequence of hypopituitarism, steroid therapy or reductions in physical activity secondary to neurodisability.
- Severe obesity is very common in children undergoing treatment for craniopharyngioma.
- There is little evidence for effective interventions to treat childhood obesity; these should most probably be focused around persuading children to adjust their lifestyles by increasing their levels of habitual physical activity.

REFERENCES

1. Freedman DS, Srinavasan GL, Burke CL, *et al.* Relation of body fat distribution to hyperinsulinaemia in children and adolescents: Bogalusa Heart Study. *Am J Clin Nutr* 1987; **46**:403–410.
2. Freedman DS, Serdula MK, Srinavasan SR, Berenson GS. Relation of circumferences and skinfold thickness to lipid in children and adolescents: Bogalusa Heart Study. *Am J Clin Nutr* 1999; **69**:308–317.
3. Barlow S, Dietz WH. Obesity evaluation and treatment: expert committee recommendations. *Pediatrics* 1998; **102**:e29.
4. Power C, Lake J, Cole TJ. Measurement and long term health risks of child and adolescent fatness. *Int J Obes* 1997; **21**:507–526.
◆5. Cole TJ, Freeman JV, Preece MA. BMI reference curves for the UK, 1990. *Arch Dis Child* 1995; **73**:25–29.
6. CDC Growth Charts USA. http://www.cdc.gov/nchs/about/major/ nhanes/growthcharts /datafiles.htm (access verified 1.12.2001).

7. Reilly JJ, Dorosty AR, Emmett PM, ALSPAC Study Team. Identification of the obese child: adequacy of the BMI for clinical practice and epidemiology. *Int J Obes* 2000; **24**:1623–1627.

8. Dietz WH. Health consequences of obesity in youth: childhood predictors of adult disease. *Pediatrics* 1998; **101**:518–525.

9. Freedman DS, Dietz WH, Srinavasan SR, Berenson GS. The relation of overweight to cardiovascular risk factors among children and adolescents: Bogalusa Heart Study. Pediatrics 1999; **103**:1175–1182.

10. Warner JT, Cowan FJ, Dunstan FOJ, Gregory JW. Validity of BMI for assessment of adiposity in children with disease states. *Ann Hum Biol* 1997; **24**:209–215.

11. Maynard LM, Wisemandle W, Roche AF, *et al.* Childhood body composition in relation to body mass index. *Pediatrics* 2001; **107**:344–350.

12. Mazess RB, Barden HS, Bisek JP, Hanson J. Dual energy X-ray absorptiometry for total-body and regional bone-mineral and soft-tissue composition. *Am J Clin Nutr* 1990; **51**:1106–1112.

13. Ellis KJ, Shypailo RJ, Pratt JA, Pond WG. Accuracy of dual-energy X-ray absorptiometry for body-composition measurements in children. *Am J Clin Nutr* 1994; **60**:660–665.

14. Goran MI, Driscoll P, Johnson R, *et al.* Cross-calibration of body-composition techniques against dual-energy X-ray absorptiometry in young children. *Am J Clin Nutr* 1996; **63**:299–305.

15. Gutin B, Litaker M, Islam S, *et al.* Body-composition measurement in 9–11-y-old children by dual-energy X-ray absorptiometry, skinfold-thickness measurements, and bioimpedance analysis. *Am J Clin Nutr* 1996; **63**:287–292.

16. Tanner JM, Whitehouse RH. Revised standards for triceps and subscapular skinfolds in British children. *Arch Dis Child* 1975; **50**:142–145.

17. Rudolf MCJ, Sahota P, Barth JH, Walker J. Increasing prevalence of obesity in primary school children: cohort study. *Br Med J* 2001; **322**:1094–1095.

18. Tanner JM, Whitehouse RH. The effect of human growth hormone on subcutaneous fat thickness in hyposomatotrophic and panhypopituitary dwarfs. *J Endocrinol* 1967; **39**:263–275.

19. Durnin JVGA, Rahaman MM. The assessment of the amount of fat in the human body from measurements of skinfold thickness. *Br J Nutr* 1967; **21**:681–689.

20. Brook CGD. Determination of body composition of children from skinfold mesaurements. *Arch Dis Child* 1971; **46**:182–184.

21. Gregory JW, Greene SA, Scrimgeour CM, Rennie MJ. Body water measurement in growth disorders: a comparison of bioelectrical impedance and skinfold thickness techniques with isotope dilution. *Arch Dis Child* 1991; **66**:220–222.

22. Davies PSW, Gregory JW. Body water measurements in growth disorders. *Arch Dis Child* 1991; **66**:1467.

23. Goran MI, Kaskoun MC, Carpenter WH, *et al.* Estimating body composition in young children using bioelectrical resistance. *J Appl Physiol* 1993; **75**:1776–1780.

24. Goran MI, Sun M. Total energy expenditure and physical activity in prepubertal children: recent advances based on the application of the doubly labeled water method. *Am J Clin Nutr* 1998; **68**(Suppl.):944S–949S.

25. Passmore R. Energy balance in man. *Proc Nutr Soc* 1967; **26**:97–101.

•26. DeLany JP. Role of energy expenditure in the development of pediatric obesity. *Am J Clin Nutr* 1998; **68**(Suppl.):950S–955S.

27. Schoeller DA, van Santen E. Measurement of energy expenditure in humans by doubly-labeled water method. *J Appl Physiol* 1982; **53**:955–959.

28. Klein PD, James WPT, Wong WW *et al.* Calorimetric validation of the doubly-labelled water method for determination of energy expenditure in man. *Hum Nutr Clin Nutr* 1984; **38C**:95–106.

29. Prentice AM, Coward WA, Davies HL *et al.* Unexpectedly low levels of energy expenditure in healthy women. *Lancet* 1985; **i**:1419–1422.

30. Roberts SB, Coward WA, Schlingenseipen K-H, *et al.* Comparison of the doubly labeled water ($^2H_2{}^{18}O$) method with indirect calorimetry and a nutrient-balance study for simultaneous determination of energy expenditure, water intake, and metabolizable energy intake in preterm infants. *Am J Clin Nutr* 1986; **44**:315–322.

31. Gregory JW, Greene SA, Jung RT, *et al.* Changes in body composition and energy expenditure after six weeks' growth hormone treatment. *Arch Dis Child* 1991; **66**:598–602.

32. Sims EAH, Danforth E. Expenditure and storage of energy in man. *J Clin Invest* 1987; **79**:1019–1025.

33. Weinsier RL, Schutz Y, Bracco D. Reexamination of the relationship of resting metabolic rate to fat-free mass and to the metabolically active components of fat-free mass in humans. *Am J Clin Nutr* 1992; **55**:790–794.

•34. Goran MI, Treuth MS. Energy expenditure, physical activity and obesity in children. *Pediatr Clin N Am* 2001; **48**:931–953.

35. Berkowitz RI, Agras WS, Korner AF *et al.* Physical activity and adiposity: a longitudinal study from birth to childhood. *J Pediatr* 1985; **106**:734–738.

36. Eck LH, Klesges RC, Hanson CL, *et al.* Children at familial risk for obesity: an examination of dietary intake, physical activity and weight status. *Int J Obes* 1992; **16**:71–78.

37. Goran MI, Hunter G, Nagy TR, *et al.* Physical activity related energy expenditure and fat mass in young children. *Int J Obes* 1997; **21**:171–178.

38. Maffeis C, Zaffanello M, Schutz Y. Relationship between physical inactivity and adiposity in prepubertal boys. *J Pediatr* 1997; **131**:288–292.

39. Bradfield RB, Paulos J, Grossman L. Energy expenditure and heart rate of obese high school girls. *Am J Clin Nutr* 1971; **24**:1482–1488.

◆40. Armstrong N, Balding J, Gentle P, Kirby B. Patterns of physical activity among 11 to 16 year old British children. *Br Med J* 1990; **301**:203–205.

41. Livingstone MBE, Coward WA, Prentice AM, *et al.* Daily energy expenditure in free-living children: comparison of heart-rate monitoring with the doubly labeled water ($^2H_2{}^{18}O$) method. *Am J Clin Nutr* 1992; **56**:343–352.

42. Saris WHM. Habitual activity in children: methodology and findings in health and disease. *Med Sci Sports Exerc* 1986; **18**:253–263.

•43. Rowlands AV, Eston RG, Ingledew DK. Measurement of physical activity in children with particular reference to the use of heart rate and pedometry. *Sports Med* 1997; **24**:258–272.

44. Eston RG, Rowlands AV, Ingledew DK. Validity of heart rate, pedometry, and accelerometry for predicting the energy cost of children's activities. *J Appl Physiol* 1998; **84**:362–371.

45. Garrow JS. *Obesity and related diseases.* Edinburgh: Churchill Livingstone, 1988.

46. Morrison JA, Barton BA, Biro FM, Daniels SR, Sprecker DL. Overweight, fat patterning, and cardiovascular disease risk factors in black and white boys. *J Pediatr* 1999; **135**:451–457.

47. Morrison JA, Sprecker DL, Barton BA, *et al.* Overweight, fat patterning, and cardiovascular disease risk factors in black and white girls. *J Pediatr* 1999; **135**:458–464.

48. Berenson GS, Srinavasan SR, Bao W, *et al.* Association between multiple cardiovascular risk factors and atherosclerosis in children and young adults. *N Engl J Med* 1998; **338**:1650–1656.

49. Talvensaari KK, Larning M, Tapanainer P, Knip M. Long term survivors of childhood cancer have an increased risk of manifesting the metabolic syndrome. *J Clin Endorinol Metab* 1996; **81**:3051–3055.

50. Whitaker RC. Predicting obesity in young adulthood from childhood and parental obesity. *N Engl J Med* 1997; **337**:869–873.

51. *Clinical guidelines on the identification, evaluation, and treatment of overweight and obesity in adults.* Bethesda, MD: National Institutes of Health/National Heart Lung and Blood Institute, 1998.

◆52. Gortmaker SL. Social and economic consequences of overweight in adolescence and young adulthood. *N Engl J Med* 1993; **329**:1008–1012.

53. Sargent J, Blanchflower DG. Obesity and stature in adolescence and earnings in young adulthood. *Arch Pediatr Adolesc Med* 1994; **148**:681–687.

54. Must A. The disease burden associated with obesity. *JAMA* 1999; **282**:1523–1529.

55. Must A, Jacques PF, Dallali GE, *et al.* Long term morbidity and mortality of overweight adolescents: follow up of the Harvard Growth Study of 1922–1935. *N Engl J Med* 1992; **327**:1350–1355.

56. Vanhala MJ, Vanhala PT, Keinanen-Kiukaanniemi SM, *et al.* Relative weight gain and obesity as a child predict metabolic syndrome as an adult. *Int J Obes* 1999; **23**:656–659.

57. Sainsbury CP, Newcombe RG, Hughes IA. Weight gain and height velocity during prolonged first remission from acute lymphoblastic leukaemia. *Arch Dis Child* 1985; **60**:832–836.

58. Zee P, Chen CH. Prevalence of obesity in children after therapy for ALL. *Am J Pediatr Hematol Oncol* 1986; **8**:294–299.

59. Odame I, Reilly JJ, Gibson BES, Donaldson MDC. Patterns of obesity in boys and girls after treatment for ALL. *Arch Dis Child* 1994; **7**:147–149.

60. Van Dongen-Melman JEWM, Hokken-Koelaga ACS, Hahlen K, *et al.* Obesity after successful treatment of ALL in childhood. *Pediatr Res* 1995; **38**:86–90.

61. Reilly JJ, Ventham JC, Newell J, *et al.* Risk factors for excess weight gain in children treated for acute lymphoblastic leukaemia. *Int J Obes* 2000; **24**:1537–1541.

62. Mayer EI, Reuter M, Dopfer RE, Ranke MB. Energy expenditure, energy intake, and prevalence of obesity during therapy for acute lymphoblastic leukemia during childhood. *Horm Res* 2000; **53**:193–199.

63. Schell MJ, Ochs JJ, Schrock EA, Carter M. A method of predicting adult weight and obesity in long term survivors of childhood ALL. *J Clin Oncol* 1992; **10**:128–133.

◆64. Didi M, Didcock E, Davies HA, *et al.* High incidence of obesity in young adults after treatment for ALL. *J Pediatr* 1995; **127**:63–67.

65. Birkebaek NH, Clausen N. Height and weight pattern up to 20 years after treatment for acute lymphoblastic leukaemia. *Arch Dis Child* 1998; **79**:161–164.

66. Nysom K, Holm K, Michaelsen KF, *et al.* Degree of fatness after treatment for ALL in childhood. *J Clin Endocrinol Metab* 1999; **84**:4591–4596.

67. Shaw MP, Bath LE, Duff J, *et al.* Obesity in leukaemia survivors: the familial contribution. *Pediatr Hematol Oncol* 2000; **17**:231–237.

68. Reilly JJ, Brougham M, Montgomery C, *et al.* Effect of glucocorticoid therapy on energy intake in children treated for ALL. *J Clin Endocrinol Metab* 2001; **86**:3742–3745.

69. Reilly JJ, Kelly A, Ness P, *et al.* Premature adiposity rebound in children treated for acute lymphoblastic leukaemia. *J Clin Endocrinol Metab* 2001; **86**:2775–2778.

70. Reilly JJ, Blacklock CJ, Dale E, *et al.* Resting metabolic rate and obesity in childhood acute lymphoblastic leukaemia. *Int J Obes* 1996; **20**:1130–1132.

71. Groot-Loonen JJ, Otten BJ, V'ant Hof MA, *et al.* Influence of treatment modalities on body weight in ALL. *Med Pediatr Oncol* 1996; **27**:92–97.

72. Brennan BMD, Rahim A, Blum WF, *et al.* Hyperleptinaemia in young adults following cranial irradiation in childhood: growth hormone deficiency or leptin insensitivity? *Clin Endocrinol* 1999; **50**:163–169.

73. Birkebaeck NH, Fisker S, Clausen N, *et al.* Growth and endocrinological disorders up to 21 years after treatment for ALL in childhood. *Med Pediatr Oncol* 1998; **30**:351–356.

74. Tatatanni PA, Larson DE, Snitkers S, *et al.* Effects of glucocorticoids on energy metabolism and food intake in humans. *Am J Physiol* 1996; **271**:E317–325.

◆75. Warner JT, Bell W, Webb DKH, Gregory JW. Daily energy expenditure and physical activity in survivors of childhood malignancy. *Pediatr Res* 1998; **43**:607–613.

◆76. Reilly JJ, Ventham JC, Ralston JM, *et al.* Reduced energy expenditure in pre-obese children treated for acute lymphoblastic leukemia. *Pediatr Res* 1998; **44**:557–562.

77. Robinson TN. Reducing childrens' TV viewing to prevent obesity. *JAMA* 1999; **282**:1561–1567.

78. Zeltzer LK, Chen E, Weiss R. Comparison of psychologic outcome in adult survivors of childhood ALL vs. sibling controls. *J Clin Oncol* 1997; **15**:547–556.

79. Warner JT, Bell W, Webb DK, Gregory JW. Relationship between cardiopulmonary response to exercise and adiposity in survivors of childhood malignancy. *Arch Dis Child* 1997; **76**:298–303.

80. Nysom K, Holm K, Olsen JH, *et al.* Pulmonary function after treatment for ALL in childhood. *Br J Cancer* 1998; **78**:21–27.

81. Jenney MEM, Faragher EB, Morris-Jones PH, Woodcock A. Lung function and exercise capacity in survivors of childhood leukaemia. *Med Pediatr Oncol* 1995; **24**:222–230.

82. Matthys D, Verhaaren H, Beroit Y, *et al.* Gender difference in aerobic capacity in adolescents after cure from malignant disease in childhood. *Acta Paediatrica* 1993; **82**:459–462.

83. Calzolari A, Baroni C, Biondi G, *et al.* Evaluation of a group of leukaemic children towards their inclusion in physical activities. *Int J Sports Cardiol* 1985; **2**:108–115.

84. Bond SA, Han AM, Wootton SA, Kohler JA. Energy intake and basal metabolic rate during maintenance chemotherapy. *Arch Dis Child* 1992; **67**:229–232.

85. Whitaker RC, Pepe MS, Wright JA, *et al.* Early adiposity rebound and risk of adult obesity. *Pediatrics* 1998; **101**:1–6.

86. Vaisman N, Stallings VA, Chan H, *et al.* Effect of chemotherapy on energy and protein metabolism of children near the end of treatment for ALL. *Am J Clin Nutr* 1993; **57**:679–684.

87. Stallings VA, Vaisman N, Chan HSL, *et al.* Energy metabolism in children with newly diagnosed ALL. *Pediatr Res* 1989; **26**:154–157.

88. Delbecque-Boussard L, Gottrand F, Ategbo S, *et al.* Nutritional status of children with acute lymphoblastic leukaemia: a longitudinal study. *Am J Clin Nutr* 1997; **65**:95–100.

89. Reilly JJ, Wilson M, Summerbell CD, Wilson DC. Obesity diagnosis, prevention and treatment: evidence based answers to common questions. *Arch Dis Child* (in press).

90. Bray GA, Gallagher TF. Manifestations of hypothalamic obesity in man: a comprehensive investigation of eight patients and a review of the literature. *Medicine* 1975; **54**:301–330.

91. Ortiz-Suarez H, Erickson DL. Pituitary adenomas of adolescents. *J Neurosurg* 1975: **43**:437–439.

92. Reeves AG, Plum F. Hyperphagia, rage, and dementia accompanying a ventromedial hypothalamic neoplasm. *Arch Neurol* 1969; **20**:616–624.

93. Hoffman HJ, De Silva M, Humphreys RP, *et al.* Aggressive surgical management of craniopharyngiomas in children. *J Neurosurg* 1992; **76**:47–52.

◆94. De Vile CJ, Grant DB, Hayward RD, *et al.* Obesity in childhood craniopharyngioma: relation to post-operative hypothalamic damage shown by magnetic resonance imaging. *J Clin Endocrinol Metab* 1996; **81**:2734–2737.

95. Bray GA, York DA. Hypothalamic and genetic obesity in experimental animals: an autonomic and endocrine hypothesis. *Physiol Rev* 1979; **59**:719–809.

96. Smith FJ, Campfield LA. Pancreatic adaptation in VMH obesity: in vivo compensatory responses to altered neural input. *Am J Physiol* 1986; **251**:R70–76.

97. Campfield LA, Smith FJ. Overview: neurobiology of OB protein (leptin). *Proc Nutr Soc* 1998; **57**:429–440.

98. Skorzewska A, Lal S, Waserman J, Guyda H. Abnormal food-seeking behavior after surgery for craniopharyngioma. *Neuropsychobiology* 1989; **21**:17–20.

99. Shalet SM. Irradiation induced growth failure. *Clin Endocrinol Metab* 1986; **15**:591–606.

100. Brauner R, Rappaport R, Prevot C, *et al.* A prospective study of the development of growth hormone deficiency in children given cranial irradiation, and its relation to statural growth. *J Clin Endocrinol Metab* 1989; **68**:346–351.

101. Darendeliler F, Livesey EA, Hindmarsh PC, Brook CGD. Growth and growth hormone secretion in children following treatment of brain tumours with radiotherapy. *Acta Paediatr Scand* 1990; **79**:121–127.

102. Clayton PE, Shalet SM. Dose dependency of time of onset of radiation-induced growth hormone deficiency. *J Pediatr* 1991; **118**:226–228.

103. Henneman DH, Henneman PH. Effects of human growth hormone on levels of blood and urinary carbohydrate and fat metabolites in man. *J Clin Invest* 1960; **39**:1239–1245.

104. Dempsher DP, Bier DM, Tollefsen SE, *et al.* Whole body nitrogen kinetics and their relationship to growth in short children treated with recombinant human growth hormone. *Pediatr Res* 1990; **28**:394–400.

105. Zeisel HJ, Willgerodt H, Richter I, *et al.* Stimulation of nitrogen and whole-body protein metabolism in growth hormone-deficient children by recombinant human growth hormone: relationship to growth. *Horm Res* 1992; **37**(Suppl. 2):14–21.

106. Tanner JM, Whitehouse RH, Hughes PCR, Vince FP. Effect of human growth hormone treatment for 1 to 7 years on growth of 100 children, with growth hormone deficiency, low birthweight, inherited smallness, Turner's Syndrome, and other complaints. *Arch Dis Child* 1971; **46**:745–782.

107. Salomon F, Cuneo RC, Hesp R, Sonksen PH. The effects of treatment with recombinant human growth hormone on body composition and metabolism in adults with growth hormone deficiency. *N Engl J Med* 1989; **321**:1797–1803.

108. Cuneo RC, Salomon F, Wiles CM, *et al.* Growth hormone treatment in growth hormone-deficient adults. II. Effects on exercise performance. *J Appl Physiol* 1991; **70**:695–700.

♦109. Rosenbaum M, Gertner JM, Leibel RL. Effects of systemic growth hormone (GH) administration on regional adipose tissue distribution and metabolism in GH-deficient children. *J Clin Endocrinol Metab* 1989; **69**:1274–1281.

♦110. Heikens J, Ubbink MC, van der Pal HPJ, *et al.* Long term survivors of childhood brain cancer have an increased risk for cardiovascular disease. *Cancer* 2000; **88**:2116–2121.

111. Brown RS, Larsen PR. Thyroid gland development and disease in infancy and childhood. In: DeGroot L, Henneman G (eds) *Thyroid disease manager.* http://www.thyroidmanager.org, 1989.

The late effects of pediatric cancer treatment on the gastrointestinal tract

NIGEL MEADOWS

INTRODUCTION

The last three decades have been witness to great advances in the management of children with cancer. This is largely due to the combined use of different combinations of treatment. It has been estimated that 1:1000 20-year-olds is a survivor of some form of cancer.[1] The aim of treatment has now progressed from not just survival alone, but to establish normal growth and development in the long-term survivors. Many organ systems are affected initially but the potentially toxic treatment given to these children can have long lasting effects, which may declare themselves later. The average half-life of the enterocyte is 4 days. The gastrointestinal tract is a prime candidate for problems associated with the treatment of cancers in children because of its rapid turnover. This susceptibility is well known in the acute stage and is easily visible as mucositis, which may extend beyond the oral cavity. Although this is the most visible sign of gut involvement, there are many other conditions that are not so easily seen but have equally important effects. These include factors such as increased gastrointestinal permeability, mucosal damage and alteration of inflammatory response, such as cytokine release. It is these that are most likely to result in long-term complications. Nutritional status and the composition of the bowel bacterial flora may also influence outcome.

The results of gastrointestinal involvement are the onset of malnutrition and associated electrolyte disturbances. If there is pre-existing malnutrition due to the disease itself, the situation will be exacerbated. Malnutrition can contribute not only to treatment failure but also to further damage of the bowel. This can be the result of protein energy malnutrition, or the more subtle effects of trace metal and vitamin deficiencies.[2] Malnutrition will result in an increase in bowel permeability. This may potentiate the crossing of large molecules capable of inducing an allergic response into the circulation. This can provoke an enteropathy with subsequent malabsorption.[3] Increased permeability will also allow translocation of bacteria across the mucosal barrier and, in some cases, can lead to septicemia. The function of the immune system is also compromised in protein malnutrition with the main effect on the T-lymphocyte population. The net effect of this is to render the patient more susceptible to infection.

Malabsorption, particularly of fat, is often the result of a concurrent pancreatic deficiency, which improves with the improvement in nutritional status.[4]

Trace metals and vitamins are important cofactors in the defence against free-radical damage, which can cause disruption of enterocyte membranes and consequent malabsorption. Vitamin E, α-tocopherol, is the most important antioxidant in the body and is commonly deficient in situations of fat malabsorption. Zinc and copper, in the form of the enzyme superoxide dismutase, are also an essential part of the protection against free-radical attack on enterocyte membranes. All of these deficiencies will potentiate the toxic effects of oncological therapies, such as chemotherapy, radiotherapy and surgery.

While much is known about the acute effects of therapy on the gastrointestinal tract, there is a paucity of information regarding the long-term effects. This is obviously of importance if we are to consider the long-term survival of such children. This subchapter will concentrate on the late effects of chemotherapy, radiation and surgery on the gastrointestinal tract. Graft-versus-host disease will also be considered owing to the increasing number of children receiving bone marrow transplantation for malignancies such as leukemia. This is an artificial cut-off and it will be appreciated that most of the commonly used treatments will potentiate the effects of each other. It is also important when discussing the gastrointestinal tract to consider the role of infection, as the bowel contains more bacteria within the lumen than there are cells in the body.

The role of infections

During the acute treatment of malignant disease, infections are an important part of the increased, and often sudden, mortality. Infections of the gastrointestinal tract result in sudden and excessive loss of fluid and electrolytes because of the associated diarrhea.

In the chronic phase of treatment, infection is much less likely. Those patients who are maintained on long-term immunosuppressants, as, for example, following a bone marrow transplantation, may develop life-threatening infection. Because of the unusual nature of the pathogens involved, infection may not be recognized, or may be confused with chronic or late-onset graft rejection. The relative deficiency of T-cell responsiveness will not only increase susceptibility to these infections but will also impair the recovery from them. The most important of these infections are *Cryptosporidia* and cytomegalovirus.

Guerrant in 1997[5] was one of the first people to recognize the importance of cryptosporidia, a protozoan, in adult patients with AIDS. It is now appreciated that the organism is present in asymptomatic carriers and may cause diarrhea in children without immunocompromise. The protozoan produces a Th 1 response, explaining its importance following treatments such as long-term steroids and cyclosporin, which may impair such a response. Ingestion of oocytes results in infection of the enterocyte, which is induced to produce the neutrophil-recruiting cytokine interleukin-8. Further evidence for the importance of T cells in this infection is provided by work from MacDonald *et al.* in 1996, who showed that the best protection was from transfer of CD4 helper cells from immune individuals.[6] *Cryptosporidia* infections result in massive amounts of diarrhea and fluid loss, and some studies have suggested a secretory mechanism for its production, such as an enterotoxin. However, perfusion studies by Kelly *et al.* of the upper small intestine have failed to demonstrate any such increased secretion.[7]

Affected individuals have a high mortality, which is especially increased in those patients who are severely immunocompromised. The clinical features, in addition to the diarrhea, are severe abdominal pain and nausea, both of which are non-specific. The diagnosis has to be actively sought by examination of the stools using a modified Ziehl–Neelson technique[8] or electron microscopy; either will reveal the oocytes.

The treatment of infected symptomatic individuals is not very effective and, realistically, the most that can be currently achieved is the relief of symptoms. In those patients who are immunocompetent, a trial of spiramycin is indicated to achieve eradication of the organism. In those patients who are compromised, pain relief and maintenance of nutrition are important. Nutrition may need to be given as a continuous enteral feed during the initial stages of the infection, although occasionally total parenteral nutrition is required. Cholestyramine may be effective in relief of the diarrhea. The mode of action is to bind to bile salts, which act as a prosecretory agent on the colonic mucosa. Loperamide may also be helpful in controlling the amount of diarrhea, owing to its antisecretory action, and by slowing gastrointestinal motility.[9]

Another pathogen that is an important cause of diarrhea in the late stages of cancer management is cytomegalovirus (CMV). This virus may reactivate at any time and is especially important in the post-bone marrow transplant patient. This leads to a CMV viremia. The virus then invades the gastrointestinal epithelium, the result of which is a secondary vasculitis and submucosal ischemia. It may have generalized effects, including both bowel and liver involvement. As for *Cryptosporidia*, the most devastating symptom is diarrhea. Anorexia and concurrent malnutrition are also frequent but, unlike cryptosporidia infection, abdominal pain is not such a well-recognized feature. Infection arises by the reactivation of a latent infection in an immunocompromised host. The poor submucosal perfusion can lead to secondary ulceration, which may then progress to perforation. The major gastrointestinal sites of involvement are the esophagus and colon. The colonic disease results in the clinical symptoms of gastrointestinal rectal bleeding or bloody diarrhea, and tenesmus. The esophageal involvement may result in dysphagia. The predominance of colonic symptoms means that colonoscopy is probably the investigation of first choice to exclude other causes of bloody diarrhea, such as ulcerative colitis. The histological changes of intranuclear inclusion bodies are diagnostic, although unfortunately their absence does not preclude the diagnosis. [10]

Eradication as with *Cryptosporidia* is not generally effective and, in the immunocompromised patient, CMV carries a high mortality. Therapeutic agents, such as ganciclovir, intravenously for several weeks have been tried and have been effective in some centers. Unfortunately,

reactivation is well described and there is little reported long-term improvement.

LONG–TERM COMPLICATIONS ASSOCIATED WITH DRUG THERAPY

The modern treatment of cancer in children relies heavily on regimes of combinations of cytotoxic drugs. These therapeutic agents are designed to kill actively dividing cells. It should, therefore, not be surprising to find that one of the major sites of complication, as a bystander effect, is the gastrointestinal tract. The life span of an enterocyte is 4 days and, therefore, is a direct target for such therapy. The most widely used drugs fall into the categories of alkylating agents, such as nitrogen mustard, cyclophophamide, carmustine, lomustine and antimetabolites, such as methotrexate, 5-fluoruracil, cytosine arabinoside, 6-mercaptopurine, vincristine and vinblastine. All of these agents affect the bowel. The side effects vary, not only with the combination used, but also from patient to patient. It also has to be appreciated that there is a narrow therapeutic window for these agents. The effects of these regimes, particularly in the acute episode, may be potentiated by other factors, such as malnutrition, radiotherapy and infection. Nutrition is further compromised by the associated nausea and vomiting that occurs with these regimes.[11,12]

The most common effect of cytotoxic agents is a reduction of mitotic activity of the enterocyte, which can decrease as early as 2 hours following ingestion. At 21 hours, after a single bolus of methotrexate, there is little to see under the light microscope. However, using electron microscopy even at such an early stage, there is evidence of swollen mitochondria, swollen Golgi apparatus and endoplasmic reticulum. These degenerative changes rapidly lead to progressive mucosal injury, which becomes manifest as mucositis. Later effects become visible under light microscopy as partial villous atrophy and superficial erosions, with ulceration and hemorrhage throughout the intestine.[13,14] More recent experimental work using animal models has suggested that these early light microscopy changes are preceded by evidence of increased enterocyte apoptosis or early cell death. These changes again precede the crypt hyperplasia, which is a response to such an injury. These microscopic changes result in ileus or diarrhea, protein-losing enteropathy secondary to the inflammation, and profound electrolyte disturbance, such as hypokalemia. Fortunately, the regenerative changes are equally rapid and, although the inflammation may persist for 3–4 weeks, repair and regeneration start at 14 days.[15,16]

During the acute period, the net effect of these changes in the small intestinal epithelium is to produce diarrhea, which in turn leads to malabsorption. In very young infants, this may result in the passage of protein into the portal blood stream and in susceptible infants may lead to food intolerance with further damage to the mucosa from an immune response. This effect may last for several months and is important to consider in any infant with longstanding diarrhea following chemotherapy. Infection has to be excluded by stool culture and electron microscopy for viral agents, and generally a biopsy is performed to examine the mucosa. This shows partial villous atrophy with a generalized increase in inflammatory cells. The treatment is to exclude antigen by feeding with a protein hydrolysate. This may have to be given initially by continuous infusion, if the damage has been severe. Most of these infants will recover within a couple of months, when a food challenge with cows' milk protein is appropriate. The role of increased bowel permeability during chemotherapy is debated, but certainly from work in animal models, such as cats, the measurement of intestinal permeability does not seem to correlate with the degree of mucosal damage. Novel approaches to the prevention of intestinal injury during chemotherapy have been tried in animals, such as administration of glucagon-like peptide-2 to rats, and growth hormone in methotrexate infusions, but there is little evidence to recommend the routine use in children. The main treatment remains supportive only.[17,18]

Vincristine results in intestinal symptoms, of pain and distension, accompanied by diarrhea. This may occur early within 3 days of treatment and is the result of pseudo-obstruction. In this clinical situation, the bowel develops poor motility with the build-up of bacteria within the small intestine. The net effect of this is fat malabsorption owing to bile salt deconjugation, and vomiting because of the obstructive-like picture. The symptoms usually resolve within a couple of weeks, but they may be severe requiring total parenteral nutrition (TPN) to support the child's nutritional status and fluid balance.[19]

From this discussion, it can be seen that most of the problems and side effects associated with chemotherapy are acute and rarely result in long-term effects. It is in combination with infection and radiotherapy that they may produce chronic problems.

RADIATION ENTERITIS

Of all the different types of therapy available for children undergoing treatment for oncological disease, radiotherapy is the one that is most likely to result in long-term complications in the gastrointestinal tract. It is rare, however, for radiotherapy to be used in isolation, and what is really being observed is a cumulative effect of both drug regimes and radiotherapy, or in some cases the addition of surgical procedures. Radiation enteritis can be

regarded as having three main phases in which complications may occur: early; delayed, which is taken as months after treatment; and late, which may occur several years after the treatment.[20] The data on children are very limited, which is surprising in view of the long duration of follow-up of these children. Most data have come from the USA. One such study, from an oncology center in Boston, examined the outcome of 44 children undergoing abdominal radiotherapy. Two-thirds had acute symptoms, which were vomiting and diarrhea. Of this group, one-third were considered severe enough to require intravenous fluids, although the duration of the symptoms was brief, lasting days only.

Eleven per cent had symptoms within 2 months of therapy; these patients formed the delayed group. The presentation of these children was different. In addition to vomiting and diarrhea, they also had an increased incidence of signs of obstruction, such as abdominal distension and pain. It was felt by the authors that the true incidence of problems may have been higher because early deaths were not taken into consideration. All of the patients with delayed symptoms had been symptomatic in the early phase of treatment but these may have been relatively mild in some cases. This study did not take into account the late symptoms, although it can be seen that the incidence of acute complications versus delayed is much greater. In terms of the diagnoses of the patients who were obstructed, the majority had received abdominal radiotherapy for either Hodgkin's lymphoma or rhabdomyosarcoma, although other centers have highlighted the increased incidence in those children receiving radiotherapy following surgery for Wilms' tumors.[21]

The most common pathological findings in the delayed group are those of diffuse fibrosis, in addition to enteritis. While the stomach and small intestine appear to be the most sensitive to irradiation, the late effects are quite widespread from the esophagous to the rectum. The acute histopathology of the mucosa shows villous blunting, with an increased plasma cell infiltrate in the lamina propria.

Electron microscopy shows shortened microvilli, enlarged nuleoli, dilated mitochondria and endoplasmic reticulum. At 3–4 weeks there is an infiltration of neutrophils that results in the development of microabscesses. An examination of the histology of the delayed changes shows extensive fibrosis involving the full thickness of the bowel wall and vascular inclusions suggesting that this may be the causative mechanism. This argument is further strengthened by the finding that a concurrent vasculitis during radiotherapy is a further risk factor for the development of complications. The mucosal fibrosis leads to stricture formation, and resultant mucosal ulceration and malabsorption.[22,23]

The incidence of significant fibrosis is related to the dose of radiation. One study of adults reported an incidence of

5 per cent after 4000–5000 cGy, increasing to 36 per cent over 6000 cGy. The majority of strictures developed within 5 years of treatment. Further factors appear to be the number of portals used, the dose rate and the treatment duration. The most important associated risk factor was previous abdominal surgery. The most likely explanation is that, following abdominal surgery, the development of adhesions and a relative fixation of the mesentery are common. This means that the intestine is held relatively fixed in the radiation field, which increases the relative dose. Coexisting malnutrition, resulting in a thin abdominal wall, will act in a similar manner to increase the incidence of complications. Drug therapy as a risk factor has been alluded to before. The most common candidate drugs are actinomycin, doxorubicin, bleomycin and fluouracil. The mechanism by which they increase the effect of radiation is unknown.[24]

In animal studies there has been some interest in the role of nitric oxide in the development of intestinal changes associated with radiation. Rat studies have demonstrated that ionizing radiation induces nitric oxide synthetase-mediated epithelial function, even in the absence of an inflammatory response.[25] Further, animal studies have examined the role of lipid peroxidation and protection against free-radical damage. They have shown some potential protective effect by using supplements of vitamin E and selenium, but this was only protective, if the supplementation was started prior to the irradiation.[26]

Rapidly dividing cells, such as the enterocyte, require glutamine as an energy substrate. Animal studies have suggested that this may be useful in conjunction with arginine as a supplement prior to treatment. This produced an improvement in villous height but measurement of functional improvement was not included in the study design. Much further experimental work and clinical trials are needed before glutamine administration can be interpreted as giving benefit to children undergoing radiotherapy, and whether it will have any effect on the reduction of long-term complications.[27]

The symptoms of radiation in the acute phase are straightforward and will usually respond well to simple supportive therapy, such as intravenous rehydration and antiemetic treatment alone. The delayed and late complications may present more insidiously. Diarrhea is common and can be the result of a protein-losing enteropathy. The mechanism is by lymphatic obstruction in the mucosa or mesentery, leading to secondary lymphangiectasia. This results in loss of lymph with a subsequent loss of albumin and lymphocytes into the bowel lumen. Diarrhea may also be secondary to bile salt loss and fat malabsorption. The loss of bile salts may be a primary event or may in turn be secondary to degradation by increased bacteria in a blind loop of bowel. There is mounting interest in the possible role of altered bowel bacterial flora in the production of symptoms and there is some evidence to suggest that a change in the microflora

may result in changes in the small bowel motility patterns, thereby exacerbating the diarrhea. At the present time there have been no long-term trials reported looking at the use of probiotics, such as *Lactobacillus acidophilus* in the management of radiation enteritis.[28,29]

The onset of vomiting, abdominal pain and distension would indicate obstruction, and the presence of fibrous adhesion bands, or a critical stenosis. Investigation, unlike the investigation of drug-induced problems, is much more centered on defining the anatomy. In the presence of predominant diarrhea, it is still essential to exclude the presence of an infection, and the patient's stools should be examined for bacterial and viral pathogens. A plain abdominal X-ray should be obtained to exclude an obstruction. If this is partial or a blind loop is considered, then a barium meal with complete follow through should be requested to look for fixed dilated loops of bowel associated with bands of fibrous adhesions. The investigation of blind loop and lymphangiectasia will be discussed in subsequent sections.[30]

A novel approach to treatment has been to look at reversing the vasculitic changes with hyperbaric oxygen. One study evaluated 32 patients, all of whom were adults, with established radiation enteritis. A total of 53 per cent of the patients showed some improvement or cure, and 47 per cent showed no change in symptoms. In those patients with long-term complications, 66 per cent were cured and 34 per cent failed to show any improvement. An approach such as this may warrant larger scale studies.[31]

LYMPHATIC OBSTRUCTION

Lymphatic obstruction is a potential problem following radiotherapy, and is due either to lymph node enlargement at the root of the mesentery or more local blockage within the bowel wall leading to secondary lymphangiectasia. The histology of the mucosa shows a dilated central lacteal, with normal villous height and crypt depth, and no other associated signs of an enteropathy. The dilated lacteal results in losses of both albumin and lymphocytes, leading to both diarrhea and edema. There may also be an associated pleural effusion and ascites, depending on the degree of hypoalbuminemia. Investigation will show isolated lymphopaenia with low albumin and, in some cases, this may be accompanied by low immunoglobulin levels.[32]

Investigation is required to determine if there is an isolated segment or if this is due to obstruction at the route of the mesentery. Protein loss in the stool can be demonstrated by finding increased levels of α1-antitrypsin in stool collections. More exact quantification is possible using radiolabeled chromium chloride injected into the blood and, in some circumstances, this may also aid localization. An endoscopic biopsy may show dilated lacteals

but as secondary lymphangiectasia is usually patchy this may not contribute to management. Changes on barium examination are also difficult to interpret and, in our practice, we have found an abdominal computed tomography (CT) scan is able to provide the most information, especially looking for sites of obstruction. Provided there is no evidence of luminal obstruction, information may be available using the new technique of capsule radio-endoscopy. This involves swallowing a capsule with a radio transmitter. The signal is then picked up by a jacket worn by the patient. Although in its infancy, this method is available and currently undergoing trial into the indications for its use in clinical practice. It is important that investigations are undertaken of dietary treatment, as the lacteal distension and bowel thickening will not be visible.

Treatment is surgical if a mesenteric lymphatic obstruction can be demonstrated but, if a large segment of bowel mucosa is involved, dietary manipulation is indicated. Medical management is to restrict the amount of dietary fat to about 5–10 g daily in an adult. This is usually supplemented with medium-chain triglycerides as these are absorbed directly into the portal blood stream and will result in resolution of the lacteal dilatation. Some long-chain fatty acids must still be given to provide an intake of essential fatty acids and to avoid deficiency states.[33]

SURGICAL COMPLICATIONS

The majority of surgical complications of cancer treatment are either as a result of previous surgery or radiotherapy, but most commonly a combination of both. The most typical types of problem are adhesions, strictures and blind loops. Adhesions and strictures present with symptoms of obstruction and blind loops, which are often missed, present with diarrhea.

Adhesions develop commonly following abdominal surgery and, as has been discussed in previous sections, may be potentiated by both drugs and radiotherapy. The onset may be insidious with episodes of abdominal pain, accompanied by vomiting, or acutely as obstruction. The first-line investigation is a plain abdominal X-ray, which may demonstrate fixed distended loops of bowel. In the more insidious group, the partial obstruction is best defined by a barium X-ray. Treatment requires skilled clinical judgment, as repeated further surgery will result in an increased adhesion formation and a cycle of further need for surgery is created. In this situation, it is often helpful for a period of bowel rest, with nutrition given either as an enteral liquid diet or TPN. In the acute presentation, surgery is usually the treatment of choice. The prognosis in this group of patients, although not subject to much in the way of clinical studies, is probably one of repeated episodes of symptoms.

Strictures present in a similar manner with signs of acute or subacute obstruction. The patient may notice that particularly fibrous foods, such as mushrooms, which are often eaten without much chewing, are responsible for an exacerbation of pain. The investigation of first choice is a barium meal and follow through, which is able to demonstrate the degree and length of bowel involved.

The surgical technique will depend on the degree of stenosis and length of area. The most common etiology of these strictures is radiotherapy. They are frequently extensive, needing bowel resection. Lesser degrees of stricture may be approached by stricturoplasty. Because of the densely fibrotic nature of this type of stricture, they are unlikely to be amenable to newer techniques, such as balloon dilatation.

Blind loops are areas of small intestine that have bacterial proliferation. It was Gorbach in 1967 who observed that the normal bacterial flora of the small intestine were sparse colonies of Gram-positive organisms.[34] It was also noted that bacterial proliferation resulted in steatorrhea and malabsorption of vitamin B_{12}. Burke and Anderson at about the same period also observed that this was accompanied by sugar malabsorption that is not related to mucosal damage.[35] The steatorrhea is an effect of the deconjugation of bile salts as a result of bacterial degradation. The commonest form of blind loop is not in fact a true blind-ending bowel as such, but an area of bowel with poor motility, as a result of previous surgery or radiotherapy. Normal bowel motility, particularly the migrating motor complex, which is a continuous contraction from the mouth to the anus, enables the small intestine to clear bacteria.

The identification of blind loops is difficult. They may be identified by barium meal and follow through but are easily missed. The glucose malabsorption may be used as a diagnostic investigation using the glucose hydrogen breath test. This method utilizes the observation that bacteria digesting unabsorbed glucose will produce hydrogen that is absorbed and excreted in the breath. A portable analyser can be used to sample aliquots of expired air and a rise of 20 parts per million above fasting is diagnostic. This, unfortunately, confirms the presence of a blind loop, not its location. A different breath test using ^{14}C-labeled glycocholate is also available but confers little advantage. The older tests, such as measuring urinary indicans are seldom used. Treatment is initially with antibiotics, such as metronidazole orally, which will eradicate bacteria in the lumen. Surgery is indicated, if the symptoms are severe, difficult to control with recurrent antibiotics or a loop is able to be localized.[36]

An interesting but rare surgical complication has recently been reported by Kiely et al. They have identified a group of children following surgical resection of abdominal neuroblastoma with severe long-term postoperative diarrhea. They studied 77 children of whom 30 per cent had postoperative diarrhea. In 5 per cent this was severe, requiring rehydration intravenously, and in 7 per cent it was moderate. A total of 65 per cent did not respond to loperamide given to control the diarrhea. It was felt that the most likely etiology was disruption of the celiac plexus of nerves, as those children with the highest incidence and the most severe symptoms were those who had had surgery involving difficult dissection around the superior mesenteric artery. This is in accordance with an increasing body of evidence, suggesting that the interplay of the enteric nervous system in addition to a role in the control of motility may also be involved in secretion. In this situation the use of agents such as octreotide may be helpful in relieving the diarrhea.[37]

GRAFT-VERSUS-HOST DISEASE

Bone marrow transplantation has become an accepted form of treatment for many malignancies, primarily of leukemia. The complication rate is high and transplantation is available only in centers that are experienced in the acute management, and the chronic problems associated with such treatment. The primary target organs for graft-versus-host disease are skin, lymphoid tissue, liver and intestinal mucosa.[38,39]

The incidence of acute complications of the gastrointestinal tract in children is approximately 30 per cent. The presenting symptoms are usually severe abdominal pain, diarrhea, anorexia and vomiting. The manifestation of gastrointestinal involvement follows that of the skin and can involve any region of the intestine, but most commonly affects the terminal ileum and proximal colon.[40] The symptoms are, therefore, often accompanied by bleeding. Predisposing factors appear to be the use of pretransplant chemotherapy and infection. Infectious episodes following transplant appear to be particularly important and it is hypothesized that this activates the immune system, resulting in rejection. Recent evidence would suggest that acute graft-versus-host disease is more common after peripheral stem-cell transplantation than bone marrow, and is most likely to be related to the increased T-cell load associated with bone marrow transplants.[41] The first line of investigation in these patients is endoscopy and stool culture to exclude infectious gastroenteritis. If there is rectal bleeding, colonoscopy is the preferred endoscopic examination but many centers would also include an upper gastrointestinal endoscopy. The mucosal changes are non-specific, with patchy areas of erythema, and an increased friability. It is important to examine the specimens for evidence of CMV infection. The treatment is to replace the fluid and electrolytes. Antidiarrhea medication, such as codeine and loperamide, should be used

with caution, as they may precipitate an ileus, particularly in the presence of electrolyte disturbance.

Chronic graft-versus-host disease occurs between 3 and 12 months following transplantation, and is estimated to involve about 30 per cent of the long-term survivors. Unlike the acute enteritis, the onset is more insidious and may be missed in the early stages, particularly as, in one study, 25 per cent had not had any evidence of acute problems. The major site of involvement is different from the acute episode, with the esophagus being commonly involved. The presenting features are, therefore, swallowing difficulties, retrosternal pain and anorexia, and these are usually accompanied by severe weight loss.[42] As in common with most of the other gastrointestinal complications of cancer treatment, the mortality is increased with infection and the continued use of immunosuppressant therapy. In a minority of patients, there is an associated secretory diarrhea, which may be confused with the presence of infection. The cause is unknown but may respond to antisecretory agents such as octreotide.[43,44]

The primary aim of investigation is to determine the degree of esophageal involvement. A barium swallow will show evidence of narrowing or stenosis and, if coupled with video, will give information regarding esophageal motility. To obtain the maximum amount of information, particularly about the presence of esophagitis, it is best combined with upper gastrointestinal endoscopy. Macroscopically the presence of stenosis or web formation and stenosis are visible with desquamation of the proximal esophagus. The histology of the changes under light microscopy shows a significant loss of the surface epithelium, with mixed acute and chronic inflammatory infiltrates. There is also necrosis of the basal squamous cells. The accompanying submucosal fibrosis is responsible for the obstructive symptoms but this may not be easily visible at biopsy, as these are often fairly superficial when taken at the time of upper gastrointestinal endoscopy.

The management of these patients is difficult, especially if there is an associated esophageal dysmotility. Nutrition may have to be maintained by nasogastric tube or gastrostomy feeding. There is limited evidence that supplementation with nucleotides may be beneficial, although the evidence is more compelling for the acute complications. They may, however, have a role in the prevention of more chronic complications.[45,46]

CONCLUSIONS

The importance of the gastrointestinal complications of the long-term treatment of children's cancer is the interaction between nutrition and growth. It is essential that, in planning regimes, damage to the gut is minimized, and

that delayed complications are considered and diagnosed early before the effects of malnutrition intervene. It is difficult to separate the different types of therapy in terms of which has the most adverse impact. They all potentiate each other. However, it can be appreciated from the preceding discussion that radiotherapy is probably responsible for most of the long-term effects seen. It is essential, therefore, in those children who receive abdominal irradiation, that the dose is suitable to protect the intestine. The advent of endoscopic techniques has enabled the intestine to be examined in increasing detail, which aids rapid diagnosis, particularly in the acute phase. The bowel is at considerable risk of infection and, in all cases where diarrhea is the major presenting symptom, this has to be actively excluded as a first priority, especially in those patients undergoing long-term immunosuppression.

The management of long-term complications of the bowel is a multidisciplinary exercise. There should be close cooperation between not only oncologists and gastroenterologists, but the assistance of surgeons and dieticians is essential in planning treatment. The number of gastrointestinal complications appears small, but there are very few studies that address the issue. Much more work is required in this area to ensure that long-term survivors of childhood cancers reach maturity with optimal growth and nutrition.

KEY POINTS

- The exact incidence of chronic gastrointestinal complications of childhood cancer is unknown but they appear to be uncommon.
- The risks are highest with radiotherapy and surgery.
- Failure to thrive is often an early sign of problems.
- Vomiting suggests stricture formation.

REFERENCES

- 1. Schwartz C. Long-term survivors of childhood cancer: The late effects of therapy. *The Oncologist* 1999; **4**:45–54.
2. Sullivan PB, Lunn PG, Northrop-Clewes C, *et al.* Persistent diarrhoea and malnutrition – the impact of treatment on small bowel structure and permeability. *J Pediatr Gasteroenterol Nutr* 1992; **14**:208–215.
3. Walker-Smith JA. Milk intolerance in children. *Clin Allergy* 1986; **16**:183–190.
4. Boedeker EC, Latimer JS. Flora of the gut and protective function. In: Walker WA, Drurie PR, Hamilton JR, *et al.* (eds) *Pediatric gastrointestinal disease*, Vol. 1. Philadelphia: BC Decker, 1991:281–299.
5. Guerrant RL. Cryptosporidiosis: an emerging, highly infectious threat. *Emerging Infect Dis* 1997; **3**:51–57.
6. MacDonald V, Robinson HA, Kelly JP, Bancroft GJ. Immunity to Cryptosporidium muris infection in mice is expressed through gut

CD4+ intraepithelial lymphocytes. *Infect Immun* 1996; **64**:2556–2562.

7. Kelly P, Thillainayagam AV, Smithson J. Jejunal water and electrolyte transport in human cryptosporidiosis. *Dig Dis Sci* 1996; **41**:2095–2099.

8. Henriksen SA, Pohlenz JFL. Staining of cryptosporidia by a modified Ziehl–Neelsen technique. *Acta Vet Scand* 1981; **22**:594–596.

9. Farthing MJG. Parasitic and fungal infections of the digestive tract. In: Walker WA, Drurie PR, Hamilton JR, *et al.* (eds) *Pediatric gastrointestinal disease*, Vol. 1. Philadelphia: BC Decker, 1991:546–555.

10. Saavedra IM, Abi-Hanna A. Diarrheal disease in CMV infection. In: Gracey M, Walker-Smith J (eds) *Diarrheal disease*. Nestle Nutriton Workshop Series, Vol. 38, 1997:191–209.

●11. Shaw MT, Spector MI, Ladman AJ. Effects of cancer, radiotherapy, and cytotoxic drugs on intestinal structure and function. *Cancer Treat Rev* 1979; **6**:141–151.

●12. Riddell RH. The gastrointestinal tract. In: Riddell RH (ed.) *Pathology of drug induced and toxic disorders*. Edinburgh: Churchill Livingstone, 1982:515.

13. Craft AW. Methotrexate-induced malabsorption in children with acute lymphoblastic leukaemia. *Br Med J* 1977; **4**:1511–1512.

14. Smith FP. Chemotherapeutic alterations of small intestinal morphology and function: a progress report. *J Clin Gastroenterol* 1979; **1**:203–207.

15. Pinkerton CR, Cameron CH, Sloan JM, *et al.* Jejunal crypt cell abnormalities associated with methotrexate treatment in children with acute lymphoblastic leukaemia. *J Clin Pathol* 1982; **35**:1272–1277.

16. Keefe DM, Brealey J, Goland GJ, Cummins AG. Chemotherapy for cancer causes apoptosis that precedes hypoplasia in crypts of the small intestine in humans. *Gut* 2000; **47**:632–637.

17. Marks SL, Cook AK, Reader R, *et al.* Effects of glutamine supplementation of an amino acid based purified diet on intestinal mucosal integrity in cats with methotrexate induced enteritis. *Am J Vet Res* 1999; **60**:755–763.

18. Ortega M, de Segura IA, Vazquez I, *et al.* Growth hormone and nutrition as protective agents against methotrexate induced enteritis. *Revista Esp Enfermedades Digestivas* 2001; **93**:148–155.

19. Weiss H, Walker M, Wiernik P. Neurotoxicity of commonly used antineoplastic agents. *N Engl J Med* 1974; **291**:75–81.

●20. Donaldson SS. Radiation enteritis in children: a retrospective, clinicopathological correlation and dietary management. *Cancer* 1975; **35**:1167.

21. Hirsch BZ, Kleinman RE. Radiation enteritis. In: Walker WA, Drurie PR, Hamilton RJ, *et al.* (eds) *Pediatric gastrointestinal disease*, Vol. 2. Philadelphia: BC Decker, 1991:915–918.

22. Tarpilla S. Morphological and functional response of human small intestine to ionizing irradiation. *Scand J Gastroenterol Suppl* 1971; **6**:9.

23. Potish RA, Jones TK, Levitt SH. Factors predisposing to radiation-related small bowel damage. *Radiology* 1980; **135**:219.

24. Phillips T, Fu K. Quantification of combined radiation therapy and chemotherapy: effects on critical normal tissue. *Cancer* 1976; **37**:1186.

25. Freeman SL, MacNaughton WK. Ionizing radiation induces iNOS-mediated epitheleal dysfunction in the absence of an inflammatory response. *Am J Physiol Gastro Liver Physiol* 2000; **278**:G243–G250.

26. Mutlu-Turkoglu U, Erbil Y, Oztezcan S, *et al.* The effect of selenium and/or vitamin E treatments on radiation-induced intestinal injury. *Life Sci* 2000; **66**:1905–1913.

27. Ersin S, Tuncyurek P, Esassolak M, *et al.* The prophylactic and therapeutic effects of glutamine and arginine enriched diets on radiation induced enteritis in rats. *J Surg Res* 2000; **89**:121–125.

28. MacNaughton. Review article: new insights into the pathogenesis of radiation-induced intestinal dysfunction. *Aliment Pharmacol Therapeut* 2000; **14**:523–528.

29. Classen J, Belka C, Paulsen F, *et al.* Radiation-induced gastrointestinal toxicity. Pathophysiology, approaches to treatment and prophylaxis. *Strahlenther Onkol* 1998; (Suppl. 3):82–84.

30. Darsini CP, Rangabashyam OP, Vijayan J, Rangabashyam N. Management of chronic radiation enteritis our experience. *Nat Med J India* 1999; **12**:140–141.

31. Gouello JP, Bouachour G, Person B, *et al.* The role of hyperbaric oxygen in radiation-induced digestive disorders. *Presse Med* 1999; **28**:1579.

32. Waldmann TA. Protein losing enteropathy. *Gastroenterology* 1966; **50**:422–443.

33. Tift WL, Lloyd JK. Intestinal lymphangiectasia. Long-term results with an MCT diet. *Arch Dis Child* 1975; **50**:269–276.

34. Gorbach SL, Plaut AG, Nahas L. Studies of intestinal microflora. *Gastroenterology* 1967; **53**:856–859.

35. Burke V, Anderson CM. Sugar intolerance as a cause of protracted diarrhoea following surgery of the gastrointestinal tract in neonates. *Austr Paediatr J* 1966; **2**:219–220.

36. Fromm H, Hoffman AF. Breath test for altered bile-acid metabolism. *Lancet* 1971; **2**:621–622.

37. Rees H, Markley MA, Kiely EM, *et al.* Diarrhea after resection of advanced abdominal neuroblastoma: a common management problem. *Surgery* 1998; **123**:568–572.

38. Bostram B, Brunning R, McGlave P, *et al.* Factors predicting relapse following bone marrow transplantation for acute nonlymphocytic leukaemia. *Blood* 1985; **65**:1191–1196.

39. Anderson CC, Goldstone AH, Linch DC, *et al.* Autologous bone marrow transplantation for patients with acute myeloid leukaemia and acute lymphoblastic leukaemia – a comparison. *Bone Marrow Transplant* 1987; **1**:271–279.

40. Lazarus HM, Coccia PF, Herzig RH. Incidence of graft versus host disease with and without methotrexate prophylaxis in allogenic bone marrow transplant patients. *Blood* 1984; **64**:215–222.

41. Cutler C, Giri S, Jeyapalan S, *et al.* Acute and chronic graft versus host disease after allogenieic peripheral blood stem cell and bone marrow transplantation: a meta analysis. *J Clin Oncol* 2001; **19**:3685–3691.

●42. McDonald GB. Intestinal and hepatic complications of human bone marrow transplantation. *Gastroenterology* 1986; **90**:460–470.

43. Deeg HJ. Bone marrow transplantation: a review of delayed complications. *Br J Haematol* 1984; **57**:185–189.

44. Ely P, Dunitz J, Rogosheske J, *et al.* Use of somatostatin analogue, octreotide acetate, in the management of acute gastrointestinal graft versus host disease. *Am J Med* 1991; **90**:707–710.

45. Dunn SP, Kreuger IJ, Butani L, Punnett H. Late onset of severe graft versus host disease in a pediatric liver transplant recipient. *Transplantation* 2001; **71**:1483–1485.

46. Grimble GK, Westwood OM. Nucleotides as immunomodulators in clinical nutrition and metabolic care. *Curr Opin Clin Nutr Metabol Care* 2001; **4**:57–64.

7c

Hepatic complications

MELISSA M HUDSON

INTRODUCTION

Hepatic complications resulting from childhood cancer therapy are uncommon and observed primarily as acute treatment toxicities. Although radiation and specific chemotherapeutic agents have established hepatotoxicity, limited information is available about long-term outcomes related to liver injury. Moreover, the majority of studies describe hepatic complications resulting from now obsolete treatment modalities or developing in patients potentially predisposed by transfusion-acquired hepatitis. The present dearth of studies describing persistent or late-onset hepatic complications may result from the low frequency of these events in children treated with contemporary antineoplastic therapy. However, the long-term consequences of hepatic injury related to veno-occlusive disease, chronic graft-versus-host disease and transfusion-acquired hepatitis have not been established. Thus, childhood cancer survivors with asymptomatic subclinical liver injury may present later in life with clinically significant liver disease. Continued monitoring of aging childhood cancer survivors is, therefore, critical to determine these outcomes. This subchapter will review what is currently understood about hepatic complications developing after treatment of childhood cancer. Guidelines for health monitoring of predisposed childhood cancer survivors and counseling recommendations for risk reduction will also be provided.

RADIATION-INDUCED HEPATOTOXICITY

The liver is relatively resistant to radiation injury up to a dose of 3000–3500 cGy delivered using conventional fractionation.[1,2] A significant proportion of patients treated with doses exceeding 3500 cGy will develop hepatotoxicity but smaller volumes of the liver can be safely irradiated to higher doses. In a review evaluating hepatic tolerance relative to radiation dose and volume, Jirtle et al. estimated that the whole liver could tolerate doses of 2000 cGy, while one-third to one-half of the liver could be irradiated to 4000 cGy without complications.[3] The development of three-dimensional treatment planning has permitted both high-dose treatment to liver tumors with normal liver sparing and more accurate quantification of the radiation dose administered. However, longitudinal prospective studies using this technology are not available.

Several investigations have reported factors predisposing to radiation-induced hepatic injury in children with Wilms' tumor, neuroblastoma and hepatoblastoma.[4–10] The risk of radiation-induced hepatic injury increases with increasing radiation dose and volume. Younger age at treatment, prior partial hepatectomy, and concomitant use of dactinomycin and doxorubicin also predispose to greater injury.[4] The majority of patients with radiation-induced hepatotoxicity present in a subacute phase that begins 1–12 weeks after completion of radiation. Delayed and chronic toxicity following hepatic radiation have only rarely been reported.[11]

Acute radiation liver injury usually manifests several weeks after radiation and is characterized by centrolobular hemorrhage and sinusoidal congestion with adjacent minimal hepatic cellular atrophy. A subacute phase may develop after several months, eventually progressing to a chronic phase after 3–6 months. Histologic studies of acute radiation liver disease indicate a veno-occlusive process resulting from focal endothelial injury with fibrin deposition. In most cases, the liver gradually heals after

subacute radiation injury, when fibrin deposits are invaded by fibroblasts and collagen deposition occurs. With persistent chronic injury, congestion of the sinusoids resolves and fibrosis becomes the predominant histologic finding. Transforming growth factor β (TGFβ) is felt to play a role in the abnormal fibrinogenesis and resulting hepatic fibrosis.[12]

The majority of reports describing acute radiation hepatopathy in pediatric patients involve dated radiation technology and treatment approaches. Persistent or late-onset radiation hepatopathy after contemporary treatment regimens are exceedingly rare in the absence of other predisposing conditions, such as viral hepatitis. The low frequency of hepatopathy in pediatric cancer survivors treated with contemporary radiation is consistent with complete resolution of acute liver injury, although this has not been histologically confirmed in prospective studies.

CHEMOTHERAPY-INDUCED HEPATOTOXICITY

Several chemotherapeutic agents commonly used to treat pediatric malignancies produce hepatocellular toxicity (Table 7c.1).[13] Generally, most children experience complete recovery from acute hepatic injury, unless there is an underlying process like transfusion-acquired hepatitis.[14–17] The majority of reports in the literature summarize the clinical features of methotrexate-induced hepatotoxicity, while relatively few provide information about long-term liver outcomes.[18–20] Information regarding other known hepatotoxins, for example, 6-mercaptopurine and actinomycin-D, is restricted to descriptions of acute toxicity.[21–23] These limited studies suggest that the incidence of clinically significant liver disease induced by chemotherapy is low or that the latency for manifestation of liver toxicity has not been reached.

Methotrexate hepatotoxicity was first described in studies of adult patients with psoriasis.[24] Methotrexate-induced hepatic injury is typically manifest by transient elevations of serum transaminases [alanine aminotransferase (ALT) and aspartate aminotransferase (AST)], alkaline phosphatase or lactate dehydrogenase levels; biochemical changes do not correlate with the severity of hepatic disease.[25–27] The risk of methotrexate hepatotoxicity increases with duration of therapy and cumulative dose when the agent is taken continuously by mouth.[13] Daily oral methotrexate predisposes to a risk of fibrosis or cirrhosis that is more than two times the incidence observed with intermittent parenteral administration.[28,29] Early studies of the agent reported hepatic fibrosis in up to 80 per cent of children with acute lymphoblastic leukemia treated with oral low-dose methotrexate 2.5–10 mg daily over 2.5–5 years. Later investigations using intermediate-dose

Table 7c.1 *Chemotherapy with reported hepatotoxicity. (Adapted with permission from Perry, 1992.[13])*

Alkylating agents	Antibiotics
Busulfan[a][BMT]	Bleomycin
Chlorambucil	Dactinomycin[a]
Cyclophosphamide[a][BMT]	Daunorubicin
Ifosfamide	Doxorubicin
Melphalan	**Plant alkaloids**
Nitrogen mustard	Etoposide
Thiotepa	Vinblastine
Nitrosureas	Vincristine
Carmustine (BCNU)[a][BMT]	**Miscellaneous agents**
Lomustine (CCNU)[a][BMT]	L-Asparaginase
Antimetabolites	Cisplatin
Cytosine arabinoside[a]	Carboplatin[a]
5-Fluorouracil	Dacarbazine[a]
6-Mercaptopurine[a]	Procarbazine
Methotrexate	
6-Thioguanine[a]	

[a]Agents associated with veno-occlusive disease.
[a][BMT] associated with veno-occlusive disease as an agent used in transplant conditioning.

parenteral administration observed hepatic fibrosis in less than 5 per cent of cases.[26,27] In studies correlating liver function and histology, mild structural changes predominated and the incidence of portal fibrosis was low.[25–27] These findings are consistent with a clinical course in which methotrexate-induced fibrosis regresses or stabilizes after completion of therapy and is rarely associated with end-stage liver disease.[25,27,30]

HEPATIC VENO-OCCLUSIVE DISEASE

Hepatic veno-occlusive disease (VOD) is characterized by the clinical features of jaundice, right upper quadrant pain, hepatomegaly, ascites, liver dysfunction and thrombocytopenia. The clinical course of VOD may be mild and reversible or life threatening with progressive hepatic failure. VOD has been attributed to hepatic radiation as well as a variety of chemotherapeutic agents used in conventional treatment regimens for pediatric malignancies, including dactinomycin, cytosine arabinoside, dacarbazine and 6-mercaptopurine (Table 7c.1).[13] Myeloablative chemotherapy used in conditioning regimens before allogeneic or autologous bone marrow transplantation may also produce VOD. Most commonly these include cyclophosphamide, carmustine and busulfan.

Initially, pediatric investigators observed that VOD was predisposed by hepatic irradiation and exacerbated by the concomitant administration of radiosensitizing drugs, such as dactinomycin and doxorubicin.[4,7,9] Later studies indicated that treatment with dactinomycin and vincristine chemotherapy alone could produce VOD,[10,22,23]

which was observed after both pulse-intensive (60 μg/kg) and modified pulse-intensive (45 μg/kg) administration of dactinomycin. Following withdrawal of the predisposing drug(s), treatment of VOD is largely supportive. The clinical course described in most series indicates full recovery for the majority of children.[22,23] Long-term sequelae after hepatic VOD have not been studied.

GRAFT–VERSUS–HOST DISEASE

Graft-versus-host disease (GvHD) is one of the most common causes of chronic liver disease in childhood cancer survivors treated with bone marrow transplantation.[31] Approximately 80 per cent of patients with chronic GvHD have liver involvement that is characterized by pruritus, fatigue and weight loss.[32] Laboratory abnormalities include elevations of alkaline phosphatase and serum transaminases; bilirubin elevation is variable and does not correlate well with clinical outcome. Chronic GvHD may be further exacerbated by drug toxicity and chronic viral infection. Liver biopsies are usually necessary to establish the diagnosis and define the extent of liver dysfunction. Again, information about the long-term impact of chronic liver GvHD is limited, but reports documenting deaths from cirrhosis and hepatic failure suggest that chronic liver disease may predispose to early mortality.[33–35]

TRANSFUSION–ACQUIRED CHRONIC HEPATITIS

Over the last 30 years, standardization of blood bank practices related to donor screening has resulted in a dramatic decline in transfusion-acquired hepatitis. However, patients treated for childhood cancer before implementation of blood-donor screening constitute a large population at risk for transfusion-acquired hepatitis. In the USA, hepatitis B donor screening was implemented in mid-1971. From 1986 to 1990, recognition of non-A, non-B hepatitis led to the practice of excluding self-reported high-risk individuals from the donor pool and the introduction of surrogate testing of donors with ALT. Hepatitis C screening by the first-generation enzyme immunoassay (EIA) was initiated in 1990; a more sensitive, second-generation EIA became available in 1992. Blood-donor screening practices, which may vary geographically, should be considered when evaluating childhood cancer survivors with a history of transfusion. Every patient presenting with abnormal liver function should be screened for hepatitis A, B and C. Survivors transfused before implantation of EIA-II blood-donor screening in 1992 should be screened for hepatitis C regardless of liver function, as chronic infection may be present in patients with normal liver function.

Viral hepatitis B and C may complicate the treatment course of childhood cancer and result in chronic hepatic dysfunction. In most series, the majority of children are presumed to have transfusion-acquired hepatitis; however, other modes of transmission should also be considered, particularly in areas where hepatitis B and C are endemic. Of the two, hepatitis B tends to have a more aggressive acute clinical course and a lower rate of chronic infection in the range of 1–10 per cent.[36] In contrast, acute infection with hepatitis C is usually mild but chronic infection occurs in approximately 80 per cent of patients. Patients chronically infected with hepatitis B or C are predisposed to liver-related morbidity and mortality from cirrhosis, end-stage liver disease and hepatocellular carcinoma.[37] Concurrent infection with both viruses appears to accelerate the progression of liver disease.[38,39]

Early investigations correlated hepatitis B infection with chronic liver dysfunction in childhood cancer patients.[14] With identification of hepatitis C as the agent responsible for the majority of cases of non-A, non-B hepatitis, more recent studies have described the clinical course of childhood cancer patients with chronic hepatitis C infection. The risk of significant liver disease in childhood cancer survivors with chronic hepatitis C virus (HCV) infection is unknown. This cohort is unique in having acquired the infection when they were young, and receiving immunosuppressive or hepatotoxic chemotherapy. Thus, the disease course may be different in childhood cancer patients because cancer therapy may significantly alter the initial immune response to HCV or hepatotoxic antineoplastic therapy may accelerate the progression of liver disease.

In studies of adults with chronic hepatitis C, cirrhosis develops in 20 per cent an average of 20 years after diagnosis of acute infection.[40] Of these, 1–5 per cent of patients will subsequently develop hepatocellular carcinoma an average of 10 years after diagnosis of cirrhosis.[41] The natural history of infection and the role of the immune system in the progression to clinically significant liver disease are complex and poorly understood. Likewise, little is known about risk factors predisposing to progression of liver disease.

Predicting outcomes in chronically infected adult patients has been difficult because many studies do not correlate histologic findings from liver biopsies with clinical and laboratory parameters. The common clinical symptoms of chronic infection, malaise, fatigue, nausea, abdominal pain, myalgia and arthritis are not consistent with the degree of liver disease as determined by laboratory evaluations and biopsy.[42] ALT elevation has been variably correlated with histologic findings on biopsy.[40] The level of viremia, as measured by the polymerase chain reaction (PCR) appears to have the strongest relationship

to liver histology, though HCV has been detected in some patients repeatedly negative by PCR testing.[43]

The long-term sequelae of transfusion-associated hepatitis C infection acquired during childhood have not been established. Based on the hepatitis B experience, investigators speculate that age at infection and immunocompetence may be a determinant for the chronicity of infection and progression of hepatocellular damage.[44,45] To date, cohort studies of chronically infected patients suggest that fibrosis develops more slowly in patients who acquired the infection when they were 20 years or younger, but longer follow-up is required to define the true incidence of HCV-related liver disease.[45,46]

Several investigations have described preliminary outcomes in childhood cancer survivors with chronic hepatitis C infection.[38,47–53] The prevalence of hepatitis C infection in childhood cancer survivors varies geographically and ranges from 5 to almost 50 per cent. As in adult series, chronic infection is common, with PCR detection of viral RNA ranging from 70 to 100 per cent in cohorts studied.[38,48,49,53,54] Most patients are asymptomatic, but laboratory evaluations of ALT demonstrate liver dysfunction in 29–79 per cent. Biopsy documentation of liver disease has not been uniformly pursued to permit consistent correlation of clinical and laboratory features with histologic findings. Early investigations of childhood cancer survivors with chronic hepatitis C reported a mild clinical course without progression to end-stage liver disease or cirrhosis. However, recent reports of hepatocellular carcinoma in childhood cancer survivors with chronic hepatitis C confirm the suspicion that chronic infection may be associated with clinically significant liver disease.[55] More aggressive chronic infection has been observed in patients with concurrent hepatitis B infection and in bone marrow transplant recipients.[25,39,56]

SCREENING AND LONG-TERM FOLLOW-UP GUIDELINES

For the most part, screening of childhood cancer survivors at risk for late hepatic complications can be accomplished through a careful annual physical examination and minimal laboratory evaluation of liver function. Physical findings of spider angioma, palmar erythema, hepatomegaly, splenomegaly, icterus or ascites are generally limited to individuals with longstanding liver dysfunction. Patients with a history of transfusion before 1992 should be tested for hepatitis C antibody; others presenting with abnormal liver function should be screened for hepatitis A, B and C. Other laboratory screening should include serum transaminases, alkaline phosphatase and bilirubin. In patients with established chronic liver disease, for example, those with chronic hepatitis C, the albumin level and international normalized ratio (INR) provide a good indicator of liver synthetic function. Abnormalities of blood counts, such as anemia and thrombocytopenia, may be associated with complications related to portal hypertension including hypersplenism and variceal bleeding. Persistently abnormal liver function should prompt referral for liver biopsy. In patients with established cirrhosis and end-stage liver disease, esophagogastroduodenoscopy is recommended to evaluate for varices; initiation of beta blockade therapy significantly reduces the incidence of variceal bleeding.[57] Patients with cirrhosis should have periodic ultrasound scans to screen for neoplastic sequelae, such as hepatoma or hepatocellular carcinoma, which have been associated with chronic hepatitis; alpha-fetoprotein is a useful screening tumor marker for these complications.

Survivors with liver dysfunction should be counseled regarding risk reduction methods to prevent hepatic injury. Standard recommendations include abstinence from alcohol use and immunization against hepatitis A and B viruses. In patients with chronic hepatitis, precautions to reduce viral transmission to household and sexual contacts should also be reviewed. Patients with chronic hepatitis associated with liver dysfunction may benefit from antiviral therapy. Periodic monitoring by a subspecialist in gastroenterology/hepatology will facilitate access to optimal antiviral therapies, which are evolving as new agents are developed. These consultants also expedite arrangements for liver transplantation in appropriate candidates with progressive unremitting liver dysfunction.

KEY POINTS

- Hepatic complications resulting from childhood cancer therapy are uncommon and observed primarily as acute treatment toxicities. Limited information is available about long-term outcomes related to liver injury.
- The long-term consequences of hepatic injury related to veno-occlusive disease, chronic graft-versus-host disease and transfusion-acquired hepatitis have not been established.
- Viral hepatitis B and C may complicate the treatment course of childhood cancer and result in chronic hepatic dysfunction.
- Hepatitis B tends to have a more aggressive acute clinical course and a lower rate of chronic infection.
- Hepatitis C is characterized by a mild acute infection and a high rate of chronic infection.
- Chronic hepatitis B and C predispose to liver-related morbidity and mortality from cirrhosis, end-stage liver disease and hepatocellular

carcinoma. Concurrent infection with both viruses accelerates the progression of liver disease.

- Survivors with liver dysfunction should be counseled regarding risk reduction methods to prevent hepatic injury. Standard recommendations include abstinence from alcohol use and immunization against hepatitis A and B viruses.
- In patients with chronic hepatitis, precautions to reduce viral transmission to household and sexual contacts should also be reviewed.

REFERENCES

1. Ingold JA, Reed GB, Kaplan HS, Bagshaw MA. Radiation hepatitis. *Am J Roentgenol* 1965; **93**:200–208.

♦2. Emami B, Lyman J, Brown A, *et al.* Tolerance of normal tissue to therapeutic irradiation. *Int J Radiat Oncol Biol Phys* 1991; **21**:109–122.

●3. Jirtle RL, Anscher MS, Alati T. Radiation sensitivity of the liver. *Adv Radiat Biol* 1990; **14**:269–311.

4. Tefft M. Radiation related toxicities in National Wilms' Tumor Study Number 1. *Int J Radiat Oncol Biol Phys* 1977; **2**:455–463.

♦5. Tefft M, Mitus A, Das L, *et al.* Irradiation of the liver in children: review of the experience in the acute and chronic phases, and in the intact normal and partially resected. *Am J Roentgenol Rad Ther Nucl Med* 1970; **108**:365–385.

6. Tefft M, Mitus A, Jaffe. Irradiation of the liver in children: acute effects enhanced by concomitant chemotherapeutic administration. *Am J Roentgenol Rad Ther Nucl Med* 1971; **111**:165–173.

7. Kun LE, Camitta BM. Hepatopathy following irradiation and Adriamycin. *Cancer* 1978; **42**:81–84.

8. Bhanot P, Cushing B, Philippart A, *et al.* Hepatic irradiation and Adriamycin cardiotoxicity. *J Pediatr* 1979; **95**:561–563.

9. Johnson FL, Balis FM. Hepatopathy following irradiation and chemotherapy for Wilms' tumor. *Am J Pediatr Hematol Oncol* 1982; **4**:217–221.

10. Flentje M, Weirich A, Potter R, Ludwig R. Hepatotoxicity in irradiated nephroblastoma patients during postoperative treatment according to SIOP9/GPOH. *Radiother Oncol* 1994; **31**:222–228.

11. Barnard JA, Marshall GS, Neblett WW, *et al.* Noncirrhotic portal fibrosis after Wilms' tumor therapy. *Gastroenterology* 1986; **90**:1054–1056.

♦12. Lawrence TS, Robertson JM, Anscher MS, *et al.* Hepatic toxicity resulting from cancer treatment. *Int J Radiat Oncol Biol Phys* 1995; **31**:1237–1248.

●13. Perry M. Chemotherapeutic agents and hepatotoxicity. *Semin Oncol* 1992; **19**:551–565.

14. Locasciulli A, Vergani GM, Uderzo C, *et al.* Chronic liver disease in children with leukemia in long-term remission. *Cancer* 1983; **52**:1080–1087.

♦15. Weber BL, Tanyer G, Poplack DG, *et al.* Transient acute hepatotoxicity of high-dose methotrexate therapy during childhood. *Natl Cance Inst Monogr* 1987:207–212.

16. Bessho F, Kinumaki H, Yokota S, *et al.* Liver function studies in children with acute lymphocytic leukemia after cessation of therapy. *Med Pediatr Oncol* 1994; **23**:111–115.

17. Ballauff A, Krahe J, Jansen B, *et al.* [Chronic liver disease after treatment of malignancies in children]. *Klin Padiatr* 1999; **211**:49–52.

18. Lascari AD, Givler RL, Soper RT, Hill LF. Portal hypertension in a case of acute leukemia treated with antimetabolites for ten years. *N Engl J Med* 1968; **279**:303–306.

19. Ruymann FB, Mosijczuk AD, Sayers RJ. Hepatoma in a child with methotrexate-induced hepatic fibrosis. *JAMA* 1977; **238**:2631–2633.

20. Nesbit M, Krivit W, Heyn R, Sharp H. Acute and chronic effects of methotrexate on hepatic, pulmonary, and skeletal systems. *Cancer* 1976; **37**:1048–1057.

21. Einhorn M, Davidsohn I. Hepatotoxicity of mercaptopurine. *JAMA* 1964; **188**:802–806.

22. Green DM, Norkool P, Breslow NE, *et al.* Severe hepatic toxicity after treatment with vincristine and dactinomycin using single-dose or divided-dose schedules: a report from the National Wilms' Tumor Study. *J Clin Oncol* 1990; **8**:1525–1530.

23. Raine J, Bowman A, Wallendszus K, Pritchard J. Hepatopathy–thrombocytopenia syndrome – a complication of dactinomycin therapy for Wilms' tumor: a report from the United Kingdom Childrens Cancer Study Group. *J Clin Oncol* 1991; **9**:268–273.

24. Dahl MG, Gregory MM, Scheuer PJ. Methotrexate hepatotoxicity in psoriasis – comparison of different dose regimens. *Br Med J* 1972; **1**:654–656.

25. Parker D, Bate CM, Craft AW, *et al.* Liver damage in children with acute leukaemia and non-Hodgkin's lymphoma on oral maintenance chemotherapy. *Cancer Chemother Pharmacol* 1980; **4**:121–127.

26. McIntosh S, Davidson DL, O'Brien RT, Pearson HA. Methotrexate hepatotoxicity in children with leukemia. *J Pediatr* 1977; **90**:1019–1021.

27. Topley JM, Benson J, Squier MV, Chessells JM. Hepatotoxicity in the treatment of acute lymphoblastic leukemia. *Med Pediatr Oncol* 1979; **7**:393–399.

28. Colsky J, Greenspan EM, Warren TN. Hepatic fibrosis in children with acute leukemia after therapy with folic acid antagonists. *Arch Pathol Lab Med* 1955; **59**:198–206.

29. Hutter RVP, Shipkey FH, Tan CTC, *et al.* Hepatic fibrosis in children with acute leukemia: a complication of therapy. *Cancer* 1960; **13**:288–307.

30. Hersh EM, Wong VG, Henderson ES, Freireich E. Hepatotoxic effects of methotrexate. *Cancer* 1966; **19**:600–606.

31. Sullivan KM, Agura E, Anasetti C, *et al.* Chronic graft-versus-host disease and other late complications of bone marrow transplantation. *Semin Hematol* 1991; **28**:250–259.

32. Fisher VL. Long-term follow-up in hematopoietic stem-cell transplant patients. *Pediatr Transplant* 1999; **3**(Suppl. 1):122–129.

33. Knapp AB, Crawford JM, Rappeport JM, Gollan JL. Cirrhosis as a consequence of graft versus host disease. *Gastroenterology* 1987; **92**:513–519.

♦34. Socie G, Stone JV, Wingard JR, *et al.* Long-term survival and late deaths after allogeneic bone marrow transplantation. Late Effects Working Committee of the International Bone Marrow Transplant Registry. *N Engl J Med* 1999; **341**:14–21.

35. Yau JC, Zander AR, Srigley JR, *et al.* Chronic graft-versus-host disease complicated by micronodular cirrhosis and esophageal varices. *Transplantation* 1986; **41**:129–130.

36. http://www.fda.gov/cber/products/testkitshtm. 04/29/02.

●37. Seeff LB, Koff RS. Evolving concepts of the clinical and serologic consequences of hepatitis B virus infection. *Semin Liver Dis* 1986; **6**:11–22.

38. Villano SA, Vlahov D, Nelson KE, *et al.* Persistence of viremia and the importance of long-term follow-up after acute hepatitis C infection. *Hepatology* 1999; **29**:908–914.

39. Paul IM, Sanders J, Ruggiero F, *et al.* Chronic hepatitis C virus infections in leukemia survivors: prevalence, viral load, and severity of liver disease. *Blood* 1999; **93**:3672–3677.

◆40. Locasciulli A, Testa M, Valsecchi MG, *et al.* Morbidity and mortality due to liver disease in children undergoing allogeneic bone marrow transplantation: a 10-year prospective study. *Blood* 1997; **90**:3799–3805.

◆41. Shakil AO, Conry-Cantilena C, Alter HJ, *et al.* Volunteer blood donors with antibody to hepatitis C virus: clinical, biochemical, virologic, and histologic features. The Hepatitis C Study Group. *Ann Intern Med* 1995; **123**:330–337.

42. Yano M, Yatsuhashi H, Inoue O, *et al.* Epidemiology and long term prognosis of hepatitis C virus infection in Japan. *Gut* 1993; **34**:S13–16.

43. Desmet VJ, Gerber M, Hoofnagle JH, *et al.* Classification of chronic hepatitis: diagnosis, grading and staging. *Hepatology* 1994; **19**:1513–1520.

44. Haydon GH, Flegg PJ, Blair CS, *et al.* The impact of chronic hepatitis C virus infection on HIV disease and progression in intravenous drug users. *Eur J Gastroenterol Hepatol* 1998; **10**:485–489.

45. Lucidarme D, Dumas F, Arpurt J, *et al.* and a French Collaborative Study Group. Natural history of hepatitis C: age at the time of transfusion might be an important predictive factor of progression to cirrhosis. *Gastroenterology* 1997; **112**:A516.

46. Poynard T, Bedossa P, Opolon P. Natural history of liver fibrosis progression in patients with chronic hepatitis C. The OBSVIRC, METAVIR, CLINIVIR, and DOSVIRC groups. *Lancet* 1997; **349**:825–832.

47. Vogt M, Lang T, Frosner G, *et al.* Prevalence and clinical outcome of hepatitis C infection in children who underwent cardiac surgery before the implementation of blood-donor screening. *N Engl J Med* 1999; **341**:866–870.

48. Fink FM, Hocker-Schulz S, Mor W, *et al.* Association of hepatitis C virus infection with chronic liver disease in paediatric cancer patients. *Eur J Pediatr* 1993; **152**:490–492.

49. Arico M, Maggiore G, Silini E, *et al.* Hepatitis C virus infection in children treated for acute lymphoblastic leukemia. *Blood* 1994; **84**:2919–2922.

50. Locasciulli A, Testa M, Pontisso P, *et al.* Prevalence and natural history of hepatitis C infection in patients cured of childhood leukemia. *Blood* 1997; **90**:4628–4633.

51. Locasciulli A, Cavalletto D, Pontisso P, *et al.* Hepatitis C virus serum markers and liver disease in children with leukemia during and after chemotherapy. *Blood* 1993; **82**:2564–2567.

52. Neilson JR, Harrison P, Skidmore SJ, *et al.* Chronic hepatitis C in long term survivors of haematological malignancy treated in a single centre. *J Clin Pathol* 1996; **49**:230–232.

53. Cesaro S, Petris MG, Rossetti F, *et al.* Chronic hepatitis C virus infection after treatment for pediatric malignancy. *Blood* 1997; **90**:1315–1320.

54. Strickland DK, Riely CA, Patrick CC, *et al.* Hepatitis C infection among survivors of childhood cancer. *Blood* 2000; **95**:3065–3070.

55. Cesaro S, Rossetti F, De Moliner L, *et al.* Interferon for chronic hepatitis C in patients cured of malignancy. *Eur J Pediatr* 1994; **153**:659–662.

56. Strickland DK, Jenkins JJ, Hudson MM. Hepatitis C infection and hepatocellular carcinoma after treatment of childhood cancer. *J Pediatr Hematol Oncol* 2001; **23**:527–529.

57. Locasciulli A, Testa M, Pontisso P, *et al.* Hepatitis C virus genotypes and liver disease in patients undergoing allogeneic bone marrow transplantation. *Bone Marrow Transplant* 1997; **19**:237–240.

58. Bernard B, Lebrec D, Mathurin P, *et al.* Beta-adrenergic antagonists in the prevention of gastrointestinal rebleeding in patients with cirrhosis: a meta-analysis. *Hepatology* 1997; **25**:63–70.

7d

Craniofacial development, teeth and salivary glands

ANDREW L SONIS

It has long been recognized that antineoplastic therapies can adversely affect the developing dentofacial structures and oral environment. Anomalous orofacial development involving bone, soft tissues and teeth can contribute to altered function and appearance, resulting in both physical and psychosocial morbidity. Alterations in the oral environment induced by cancer therapy can also have a detrimental effect on dental health. The extent of these complications is dependent upon the age of the patient at the time of treatment and the choice of therapeutic modalities.

EFFECTS ON CRANIOFACIAL DEVELOPMENT

Hard tissue development of the facial skeleton occurs through three different processes: intramembranous bone formation, endochondral bone formation, and odontogenesis or tooth formation. Change in bone morphology or spatial relationship is accomplished by one of two processes: remodeling and translation. Remodeling occurs through apposition and resorption of bone resulting in differential changes and alterations in the size and morphology of a given bone. As a result of this phenomenon, referred to as primary translation, the relative position of the bone in space will change. Secondary translation occurs when the growth of a given bone results in the spatial positional change of an adjacent bone. The adjoining soft tissues also influence hard tissue development. Consequently, a structure directly affected by therapy may also result in anomalies of adjacent structures.[1,2]

The capacity of ionizing radiation to injure growing bone and cartilage has been known since the studies of Perth in the early 1900s.[3] However, its effect on the developing craniofacial skeleton remained largely unexplored until some 50 years later. In examining these effects it is convenient to subdivide the various areas of the facial skeleton.

Conventionally, craniofacial growth is described by each of its components, namely, the calvarium, cranial base, nasomaxillary complex, mandible and dentition. The intramembranous sutural growth system of the calvarium allows for the rapidly expanding brain of the growing child. Therefore, size of the hard tissue cranial vault is determined by the underlying neural mass, provided the sutural growth system is functional. The expanding brain exerts separating tensional forces on the sutures secondarily stimulating compensatory sutural bone growth. The calvarium, paralleling the growth of the developing brain, achieves 87 per cent of its adult size by age 2 years, 90 per cent by 5 years and 98 per cent by 15 years of age.[4] Consequently, children whose craniums are exposed to growth-inhibiting levels of radiation prior to age 5 years are at particular risk of demonstrating clinical manifestations of such an insult.

Studies of long-term survivors of acute lymphoblastic leukemia (ALL) who had received 2400 cGy of cranial irradiation found that approximately 50 per cent of patients had head circumferences below the second percentile.[5]

While the average age at diagnosis was 4.5 years, younger patients were observed to be at higher risk of microcephaly. A similar ALL study by Appleton et al. found that those patients under the age of 3 years who received 1800 cGy or 2400 cGy all demonstrated smaller head circumferences.[6] The smaller head circumference observed in these patients was likely due to endocrine and/or neurotoxicity of treatment resulting in smaller brain size, as opposed to a direct effect on the bone.[7,8] This same phenomenon likely occurs in children receiving cranial irradiation for brain tumors, where dosages are significantly higher than 2400 cGy.[9] Although growth failure as measured by height has been observed in ALL patients receiving no cranial irradiation or 1800 cGy, clinical observation would suggest little if any effect on head circumference in the patient older than 6 years.[10] Consequently, radiation levels greater than 1800 cGy in the patient under 6 years of age are likely necessary to affect calvarial development indirectly in the growing child.

Changes in the cranial base occur primarily due to endochondral growth along a series of bones interposed by cartilaginous abutments, or synchondroses. The cartilages between these bones contribute variably to cranial elongation and lateral expansion. Growth in the anteroposterior length of the cranial fossa depends on growth at the sphenofrontal, frontal-ethmoidal, spheno-ethmoidal and spheno-occipital sutures. The anterior cranial base is completely ossified by age 6 years, but the spheno-occipital synchondrosis remains active through early adolescence and is likely the major contributor to growth of the cranial base.[11,12] Anomalies of cranial base development typically result in a lack of midface development or the 'dished in' appearance characteristic of conditions, such as achondroplasia or Down syndrome.

The effects of irradiation on endochondral bone growth are well documented.[13,14] Radiation injury to the epiphysis results in arrested chrondrogenesis and a reduction in chrondroblasts. And while microscopic changes may be observed with dosages as low as 200 cGy, significant growth abnormalities typically are not observed until dosages approach or exceed 2000 cGy.[15] The threshold dose for interference with cranial base development is unclear. Sonis et al. studied a cohort of ALL survivors at least 5 years post-diagnosis[16] None of the 51 patients who received 2400 cGy cranial irradiation, including 20 under the age of 5 years at time of treatment, had deficient midfaces as measured by cephalometric analysis. In one of the first comprehensive reports of dentofacial abnormalities in long-term survivors of pediatric cancer, Jaffe et al. also reported no facial deformities in any ALL patients who received 2400 cGy or less of cranial irradiation.[17] However, included in this same report was a photograph of a 22-year-old female demonstrating an obvious midface hypoplasia. This patient had received 5040 cGy of radiotherapy for a rhabdomyosarcoma at age 11 years.

In an extremely interesting case report, Berkowitz et al. compared the effects of therapy on a child with rhabdomyosarcoma involving the left buccinator with his unaffected identical twin.[18] The patient was initially treated at age 2½ years and received 6000 cGy of radiotherapy. Dentofacial growth evaluation was performed some 6 years later. Cephalometric analysis revealed a generalized craniofacial deficiency including a significant anteroposterior hypoplasia of the midface. Kaste and Hopkins describe a patient who at age 5 years received 3500 cGy of radiotherapy for a rhabdomysarcoma of the right nasopharynx.[19] Follow-up 10 years later revealed significant maxillary hypoplasia. These reports would suggest that dosages exceeding 2400 cGy are required to affect growth of the cranial base and, although younger children are more severely affected, the window of insult likely extends throughout the adolescent growth period.

Growth in width of the maxilla occurs at the palatal suture during the first 5 years of life. Subsequent increases in the width of the anterior maxilla occur through bone deposition on the outer surfaces of the maxilla and by the more labial eruption of the permanent teeth. The developing eye also contributes to midface development. Just as the brain stimulates the calvarium to expand, so does growth of the eye provide an expanding force separating the neural and facial skeleton, particularly at the frontomaxillary and frontozygomatic sutures. In utero, the rapidly growing eye contributes significantly to widening of the fetal face. By age 2 years it obtains 50 per cent of adult size and full adult size by age 7 years.[20] However, the size of the orbital cavity is dependent upon the size of the eye. Enucleation and/or radiation therapy may inhibit the growth of the bony structure, resulting in diminished orbital growth with a subsequent effect on transverse facial development.[21] While some studies have demonstrated equally adverse effects of enucleation and irradiation on orbital development, radiotherapy to the orbit is far more detrimental to facial growth.[22,23] These same studies would suggest that young children (under 6–7 years) with retinoblastomas receiving radiotherapy in excess of 3000 cGy are at high risk of these types of craniofacial deformities. Similar findings are reported for children receiving radiotherapy for nasopharyngeal carcinoma and rhabdomyosarcoma[24] (Figure 7d.1).

Growth of the nasomaxillary complex occurs by two mechanisms. Growth of the cranial base displaces the maxilla in a downward and forward direction, while active growth of the cartilaginous nasal septum and maxillary sutures contribute more directly. The influence of the nasal septal cartilage is clearly demonstrated in the patient with bilateral cleft lip and palate, where the tip of the nose, columella, philtrum, prolabium and primary palate, free of their facial attachments, protrude conspicuously from the face. In addition, surface deposition and resorption contribute significantly to increases in the size

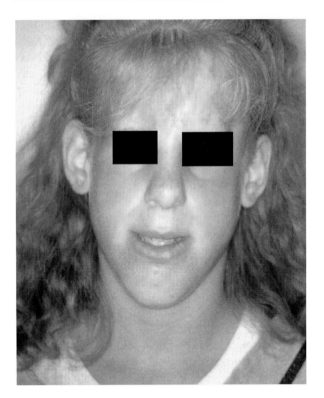

Figure 7d.1 *Effect of radiotherapy on the transverse development of facial skeleton. Patient with retinoblastoma received 4000 cGy to the right lateral field and 3600 cGy to the left field at age 3 months.*

of the nasal cavities and maxillary tuberosities. The close proximity of these structures to the cranial base make it likely that anomalies in growth in this region of the face are the result of both direct and indirect effects.

The mandible is formed from intramembranous bone; consequently the mandibular condyles are derived from secondary cartilage and, although the cartilage of the mandibular condyle appears somewhat similar to the cartilage of the epiphyseal plates, it behaves quite differently.[12] Rather than initiating and directing growth of the mandible, the condyles adapt to the forward and downward displacement of the jaw by growing upward and backward. These vertical changes provide for some of the required changes of the growing child essential for life, namely increased respiration and deglutition, as well as eruption of the teeth. Bilateral interference with this condylar growth will typically result in a small mandible, while unilateral interference will typically result in a mandibular asymmetry.[25] The mandible, unlike other parts of the facial skeleton, continues to grow throughout adolescence. The site of growth interference in the mandible has been found to be in the region of the condylar head. Animal studies demonstrate that mandibular dosages as low as 400–440 cGy may cause incomplete damage to the condylar regions. Damage may occur to growth centers, with osteocyte death, microvascular

injury, periosteal damage, aplasia and fibrous replacement of marrow spaces, in addition to a decrease in the number of cells in the immediate and hypertrophic zones of the condylar cartilage. However, there typically are no visible deficiencies of the mandible until radiation dosages are significantly greater than these levels. Studies specifically examining mandibular growth suggest irradiation must exceed 1800 cGy before there are clinically detectable effects on mandibular development. Not surprisingly, these defects are both age and dose dependent.[16]

Growth of the tooth-supporting alveolar bone is completely dependent on the presence, eruption and root length of teeth. The lack of teeth will result in the alveolus never forming, and extraction of teeth will ultimately lead to the resorption of this bone. When many teeth are missing or the length of the teeth is compromised, the vertical dimension of the face is markedly decreased, characterized by a shortened lower face and overclosure of the mandible. Consequently, while there is no evidence of a direct effect of radiation upon alveolar bone development, tooth agenesis or disturbed root development caused by radiotherapy can have an indirect effect.

Craniofacial growth is not proportional. So while calvarial growth is almost completed by age 5 years, the nasomaxillary complex, mandible and dentition continue with significant growth into adolescence, explaining the dramatic differences in facial appearance of the infant and adolescent. Most studies would suggest that after 12 years of age, radiation-induced facial growth alterations are minimal.[17,26]

Craniofacial growth may also be indirectly affected by radiotherapy, as is likely the case in patients receiving total body irradiation for bone marrow transplantation. These children experience a proportional overall decrease in length of both the maxilla and mandible, which is likely related to diminished growth hormone production, as opposed to a direct effect of the radiation upon these structures.[27,28]

DENTAL DEVELOPMENT

All teeth go through a series of developmental stages (Table 7d.1). Dental development begins approximately 28 days *in utero* with the initiation of the 20 primary teeth and is typically completed around age 18 years with completed root development of the third molars. The 20 primary teeth are ultimately replaced by corresponding permanent teeth, which arise from an epithelial structure originating from the primary tooth germ, the successional dental lamina. Those permanent teeth with no primary teeth predecessor develop directly from a dental lamina arising from the oral epithelium. An insult to either of these dental lamina typically results in lack of the corresponding tooth. Eruption of the primary dentition

Table 7d.1 *Chronology of development and eruption of teeth*

Tooth	Tooth germ completed	Calcification commences	Crown completed	Eruption in mouth	Root completed
Primary					
Incisors		3–4 months iu	2–4 months	6–8 months	1.5–2 years
Canines		5 months iu	9 months	16–20 months	2.5–3 years
1st molars	12–16 weeks iu	5 months iu	6 months	12–15 months	2–2.5 years
2nd molars		6–7 months iu	11–12 months	20–30 months	3 years
Permanent					
Central incisors	30 weeks iu	3–4 months	4–5 years	Max: 7–9 years Mand: 6–8 years	9–10 years
Lateral incisors	32 weeks iu	Max: 10–12 months Mand: 3–4 months	4–5 years	7–9 years	10–11 years
Canines	30 weeks iu	4–5 months	6–7 years	Max: 11–12 years Mand: 9–10 years	12–15 years
1st premolars	30 weeks iu	1.5–2 years	5–6 years	10–12 years	12–14 years
2nd premolars	31 weeks iu	2–2.5 years	6–7 years	10–12 years	12–14 years
1st molars	24 weeks iu	Birth	3–5 years	6–7 years	9–10 years
2nd molars	6 months	2.5–3 years	7–8 years	12–13 years	14–16 years
3rd molars	6 years	7–10 years	12–16 years	17–21 years	18–25 years

iu, *in utero.*

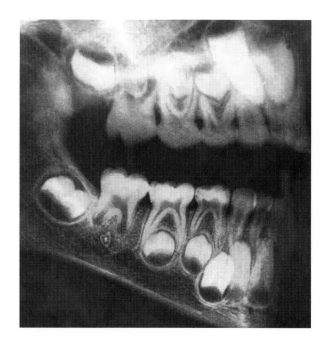

Figure 7d.2 *Radiograph of a 6-year-old, demonstrating relationship of developing permanent teeth to overlying primary teeth.*

begins on average at 7 months of age and is completed at about 29 months. Dental eruption is then quiescent for nearly 4 years. At the age of 6 years, the jaws contain more teeth than at any other time. Twenty-four teeth are jammed between the orbits and the nasal cavity, while another 24 fill the body of the mandible (Figure 7d.2). Between 6 and 8 years of age, all eight primary incisors are lost and 12 permanent teeth erupt, the permanent incisors and the first permanent molars. After this extreme level of activity, there is a quiet period relative to eruption until around 10½ years of age, although much activity is occurring in the way of root development of the remaining permanent teeth. During the next 18 months the remaining 12 primary teeth are lost and 16 permanent teeth erupt.

Individual tooth development proceeds through several characteristic stages; initiation, proliferation, histodifferentiation, morphodifferentiation, apposition, mineralization and maturation. Initiation is characterized by a proliferation of the basal cell layer of the oral epithelium and its ingrowth into the underlying mesochyme. During the proliferation stage, individual tooth formation proceeds through increased mitotic activity leading to histodifferentiation, the stage when ameloblasts and odontoblasts develop, the precursors to enamel and dentin, respectively. Histodifferentiation marks the end of the proliferation stage as these cells lose the ability to multiply. Disturbances in initiation and proliferation typically result in failure of tooth development, while insults during histodifferentiation result in abnormal structure of dentin and/or enamel. The basic form of each tooth is determined during morphodifferentiation. Recombinant studies in the 1970s and 1980s demonstrated that interactions between epithelial and mesechymal cells regulate both morphogenesis of the tooth and the differentiation of the dental cells.[29] Aberrations in morphodifferentiation will result in abnormal shapes and sizes of teeth. Appositional growth is the result of a layer-like deposition of an extracellular organic matrix. This

matrix, produced by the ameloblasts and odontoblasts, is deposited according to a definite pattern and rate.

Mineralization of the enamel requires a properly mineralized dentin matrix. Consequently, altered dentinogenesis will result in abnormal enamel mineralization. Normal mineralization occurs when inorganic calcium salts precipitate within the deposited organic matrix. The process begins with the precipitation of a small nidus about which further precipitation occurs. The original nidus increases in size by the addition of concentric laminations. There is eventual approximation and fusion of these individual calcospherites into a homogeneously mineralized layer. If the calcification process is disturbed, there is lack of fusion of the calcospherites. These deficiencies are not readily identified in the enamel, but in the dentin are microscopically evident and referred to as interglobular dentin. Interference in this stage will result in hypomineralization, which may make the tooth less resistant to dental caries.

Root development begins following the completion of crown morphogenesis and coronal dentin and enamel matrix formation. Its normal development is dependent upon a bilaminar epithelial structure referred to as Hertwig's root sheath. This sheath continues to exist as long as the root continues to elongate. Consequently, an insult capable of arresting root sheath development may result in a total lack of root structure or a shortened blunted root depending on the stage of root development. Although root development may play a significant role in the eruption of the dentition, not infrequently rootless teeth are observed to erupt normally.

EFFECTS OF RADIATION ON DENTAL DEVELOPMENT

While animal models have demonstrated minimal doses required to cause localized dental defects to be in the range of 200 cGy, most but not all human studies suggest a minimal dose of around 400 cGy. Fromm *et al.* found that any developing tooth within a radiation-treated field receiving greater that 400 cGy showed some developmental abnormalities but even levels below this may be detrimental to the developing dentition.[26] Indeed, one of the earliest case reports was of a 5-month-old with a congenital nevus of the lip and adjacent cheek treated with a single superficial dose of 400 cGy of radiation with an estimated bone dose of 200 cGy.[30] The result was enamel hypoplasia of the maxillary primary incisors and permanent central incisors. Consequently, developing teeth lying outside a field may still receive toxic levels of radiation as a result of scatter.

Dental defects secondary to radiotherapy have been widely documented and include tooth dwarfism, root underdevelopment (blunting and tapering), incomplete

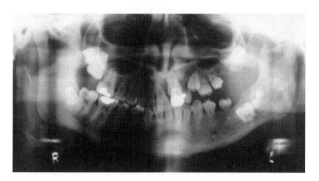

Figure 7d.3 *Panoramic radiograph of a 20-year-old patient treated with 5600 cGy radiation at age 5 years for rhabdomyosarcoma. Note atypical root morphology, rootless teeth and arrested tooth eruption.*

calcification, premature apical closure, delayed or arrested root development, agenesis and lack of eruption.[16,17,26,31–41] Odontogenic cell sensitivity depends upon their position in the cell cycle and their mitotic activity at the time of treatment. Odontoblasts are most susceptible to low-dose radiation just prior to their initiation of dentin matrix formation, likely because these presecretory odontoblasts are rapidly proliferating.[42] Following radiation exposure, odontoblastic mitotic activity ceases. Osteodentin produced by odontoblast-like cells is deposited between the arrested odontoblasts and the pulp, interfering with the normal interaction of dentin with enamel. The result is defective enamel.

It was thought that 1000 cGy was sufficient to damage mature ameloblasts permanently and 3000 cGy to arrest tooth development. However, more recent data suggest that, when combined with chemotherapy, significantly lower doses can result in these same defects. When dosages of 1000–1800 cGy of radiation are administered late in dental development, apical root distortion may occur. Larger doses at earlier stages of dental development may result in complete clinical agenesis and apices of irradiated developing teeth tend to close earlier than normal, resulting in shortened roots with atypical morphology (Figure 7d.3).

DENTOFACIAL COMPLICATIONS OF CHEMOTHERAPY

The adverse effects of chemotherapy on the developing dentofacial structures are limited to the direct effects on the developing dentition and the indirect effects on the oral environment, central nervous system and endocrine system. Although animal and human studies have demonstrated toxic effects of chemotherapeutic agents on bone formation, it has not been shown to affect facial growth directly in humans.[43,44]

Animal studies have shown that the chemotherapeutic agents colchicine, vincristine, cyclophosphamide, Adriamycin, methotrexate and Daunorubinocin can all directly affect dental development. Jaffe *et al.* were among the first to report the adverse effects of chemotherapy upon the developing dentition.[45–49] Five of 23 patients who received chemotherapy only demonstrated significant defects in their enamel described as acquired amelogenesis imperfecta, microdontia of the premolars and a tendency of thinning of the roots with enlarged pulp chambers.[17] In a study of ALL patients who received chemotherapy exclusively, Rosenberg observed similar findings related to root development. Three-quarters of the children who received treatment between the ages of 4 and 10 years demonstrated developmental root anomalies.[50]

EFFECTS OF CANCER TREATMENT ON DENTAL DISEASE

The two most prevalent dental diseases afflicting man are dental caries and periodontal disease. Dental caries is an infectious multifactorial disease, resulting in the destruction of teeth through acid demineralization. The onset of this disease requires the interaction of three principal factors: the host (teeth and saliva), the microflora (primarily mutans streptococcus), and the substrate or diet. Periodontal disease encompasses a group of diseases that affect the supporting tissues of the dentition, namely, the gingiva and underlying bone. Like dental caries, these diseases are typically multifactorial, involving the host (teeth, saliva, systemic factors) and the microflora. Gingivitis, the most common form of the disease observed in children, is a bacterial-mediated inflammation of the gingiva. The initial manifestations of this disease typically occur via bacterial colonization of the tooth surface (plaque) resulting in a gingival inflammation. Consequently, those factors that increase an individual's susceptibility to dental caries may also have the same effect on periodontal disease. Cancer therapy can affect all of these factors either directly or indirectly.

Clinical manifestations of dental caries occur when cariogenic bacteria colonize the tooth surface and are exposed to a fermentable carbohydrate. The bacteria then produce lactic acid, which demineralizes the tooth subsurface, ultimately resulting in cavitation.

The previously discussed consequences of both chemotherapy and radiotherapy on dental development, specifically as it relates to enamel, may increase the susceptibility of a tooth to bacterial colonization. The roughened surface of malformed enamel promotes increased bacterial plaque colonization and thinner enamel likely makes the tooth less resistant to the acid produced by this plaque.

This increased susceptibility to plaque accumulation may also be a cofactor in the development of a unique periodontal condition in patients receiving cyclosporin A.[51–53] Gingival hyperplasia is reported to occur in 25–80 per cent of solid-organ transplant patients receiving cyclosporin A.[51] However, the prevalence of gingival hyperplasia in bone marrow transplant recipients receiving cyclosporin A is likely much lower, although not well documented.[54] This gingival overgrowth is thought to be the result of fibroblast proliferation. Several fibroblast subpopulations are sensitive responders to this cyclosporin A, resulting in a stimulation of increased collagen synthesis.[55] Patients with significant plaque accumulation have been observed to have much higher levels of gingival hyperplasia. This response is apparently dose dependent.[52,53,56,57]

Saliva, which plays an extremely important role in protecting the dentition, is also affected by therapy. Salivary protection for the dentition occurs through four mechanisms. First, saliva aids in buffering the acidic pH generated by dental plaque. Second, the mechanical washing of the tooth surface decreases bacterial colonies and helps to remove retained foodstuffs. Third, saliva contains several antimicrobial factors that protect oral mucosal and hard surfaces. Fourth, it serves as a vehicle for calcium phosphate and fluoride, and thereby aids in controlling demineralization, while contributing to remineralization.[58]

Obviously, even in the normal individual, this protective function of saliva can be overwhelmed by bacterial action resulting in dental caries. However, when salivary function is severely compromised, dental caries susceptibility increases dramatically. Bleomycin, busulfan and doxorubicin have all been found to contribute to xerostomia.[59] However, chemotherapeutic induced xerostomia tends to be limited to treatment periods and not long term. Although quantitative decreases in salivary flow rates have been reported in children receiving total body irradiation (TBI) at levels of around 1000 cGy, it is unclear whether these changes impact oral health.[60] Typically, salivary flow rates begin to decline 5–10 days into preconditioning with TBI for bone marrow transplantation (BMT) to levels approximately 50 per cent of normal and continue to decrease to 25 per cent of normal until about 2–3 months post-transplant. Salivary secretion rates then tend to increase slowly over the next 3 years until they reach approximately 75 per cent of pretreatment values. Chemotherapy-conditioned BMT patients experience similar changes in salivary function up to 1 year following transplant, just not to the same magnitude as those patients receiving TBI. After 4 years, their salivary secretion rates are indistinguishable from healthy children. Although these salivary changes are inversely related to increases observed in caries-associated bacteria, most studies show actual decay rates are no different than those observed in normal controls.

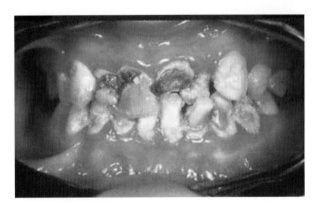

Figure 7d.4 *Example of severe radiation caries.*

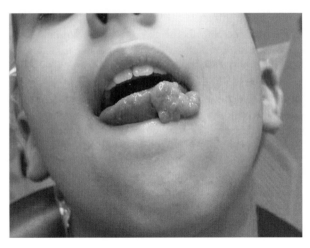

Figure 7d.5 *Exophytic soft tissue lesions of BMT patient with CGvHD receiving cyclosporin A.*

Children receiving high-dose irradiation (4000–6000 cGy) apparently are at greater risk of dental caries secondary to salivary dysfunction. Fromm *et al.* found that 6 of 15 patients receiving 4000–6000 cGy of head and neck irradiation developed radiation caries.[26] Typically, patients whose salivary glands are exposed to this level of radiation demonstrate markedly reduced salivary flow, resulting in an increased risk of an atypical pattern of dental decay. Radiation caries is characterized by decay involving the neck or cervical portion of the tooth. Over the course of several months, it progesses rapidly inward to the dentin and cementum, to the point where the entire crown of the tooth may be undermined (Figure 7d.4). Prevention of this severe form of dental caries is aimed at making the teeth more acid resistant with topical fluorides, decreasing the bacterial burden with chlorhexidene rinses and increasing salivary flow via pilocarpine.[61–64]

Another often unrecognized contributing factor to caries development is the long-term administration of sucrose-containing medications.[65–68] Many commonly prescribed pediatric oral medications are sweetened with sucrose to improve their flavor and, therefore, compliance. However, children who are exposed to these medications are at significantly higher risk of developing dental caries.[69]

ORAL COMPLICATIONS OF CHRONIC GRAFT–VERSUS–HOST DISEASE (CGVHD)

Decreased salivary function with subjective complaints of xerostomia is a common finding in patients with chronic graft-versus-host disease.[70,71] The extent of their diminished salivary function is not nearly as severe or apparently as devastating to the dentition as those patients receiving high-dose radiotherapy. The salivary function of these patients responds well to pilocarpine administration.

Allogeneic BMT patients with CGvHD receiving cyclosporin A may also be at risk of developing non-gingival soft tissue growths (Figure 7d.5).[72,73] These lesions are similar to pyogenic granulomas that grow rapidly over several months. They are composed of fibrous and granulation tissue with acute and chronic inflammation. It has been suggested that the gingival hyperplasia frequently associated with cyclosporin A likely plays a role in the development of these lesions. These lesions may spontaneously exfoliate, although more often are surgically excised. Pediatric patients with CGvHD disease frequently display the same oral changes observed in adult patients, including mucosal lichenoid changes, erythema, atrophy, mucoceles and ulceration. The prevalence of oral involvement in children with CGvHD ranges from 80 to 100 per cent.[71,74]

RECOMMENDATIONS FOR DENTAL CARE OF LONG–TERM SURVIVORS OF PEDIATRIC CANCER

Those patients who suffer some of the dentofacial effects of cancer therapy may have some unique dental care requirements. Lifelong aggressive prevention programs aimed at minimizing the risk of dental disease are certainly indicated for all these patients. In addition, the restoration of function and esthetics through dental implants, orthodontic therapy, and plastic and maxillofacial surgery is now a viable option for many of these patients.[75–83]

KEY POINTS

- Both chemotherapy and radiotherapy can have significant effects on the developing dental and facial structures.

- Radiation effects on the facial skeleton are typically more severe in children below the age of 5 years at the time of their therapy and receiving radiation levels at or above 2400 cGy.
- Developing teeth exposed to radiation levels as low as 400 cGy may demonstrate significant defects. These include enamel hypoplasia, tooth dwarfism, root defects, incomplete calcification, agenesis and lack of eruption.
- Chemotherapeutic agents given during dental development can result in significant anomalies of the dentition. These defects include enamel hypoplasias, tooth dwarfism and root anomalies.
- Children receiving cancer therapy may be at greater risk of dental disease owing to the adverse effects of therapy on the dental structures and salivary glands. Additionally, sucrose-containing medications may also contribute to increased risk of dental caries.

REFERENCES

1. Enlow D, *Facial growth*, 3rd edn. Philadelphia: WB Saunders, 1990.
2. Guyuron B, Dagys AP, Munro IR, *et al.* Effect of irradiation on facial growth: a 7- to 25-year follow-up. *Ann Plastic Surg* 1983. **11**:423–427.
3. Perthes G. Uber den Einfluss der Rontgensteahlen auf epitheliale gewehe insbesondere auf carcinom. *Arch Klin Chir* 1903; **71**:955.
4. Graber T. *Orthodontics*, 3rd edn. Philadelphia: WB Saunders, 1972.
5. Waber DP, Urion DK, Tarbell NJ, *et al.* Late effects of central nervous system treatment of acute lymphoblastic leukemia in childhood are sex-dependent. *Dev Med Child Neurol* 1990. **32**:238–248.
6. Appleton RE, Farrell K, Zaide J, *et al.* Decline in head growth and cognitive impairment in survivors of acute lymphoblastic leukaemia. *Arch Dis Child* 1990; **65**:530–534.
7. Shalet SM, Whitehead E, Chapman AJ, *et al.* The effects of growth hormone therapy in children with radiation-induced growth hormone deficiency. *Acta Paediatr Scand* 1981; **70**:81–86.
8. Gleeson HK, Shalet SM. Endocrine complications of neoplastic diseases in children and adolescents. *Curr Opin Pediatr* 2001; **13**:346–351.
9. Habrand JL, De Crevoisier R. Radiation therapy in the management of childhood brain tumors. *Childs Nervous System* 2001; **17**:121–133.
10. Sklar C, Mertens A, Walter A, *et al.* Final height after treatment for childhood acute lymphoblastic leukemia: comparison of no cranial irradiation with 1800 and 2400 centigrays of cranial irradiation. *J Pediatr* 1993; **123**:59–64.
11. Sarnat BG. Craniofacial change and non-change after experimental surgery in young and adult animals. *Angle Orthodontist* 1988; **58**:321–342.
12. Koski K. Cranial growth centers: facts of fallacies? *Am J Orthodont* 1968; **54**:566–583.
13. Goldwein JW. Effects of radiation therapy on skeletal growth in childhood. *Clin Orthopaed Related Res* 1991; **262**:101–107.
14. Probert JC, Parker BR. The effects of radiation therapy on bone growth. *Radiology* 1975; **114**:155–162.
15. Neuhauser EDB, Berman Z, Cohen J. Irradiation effects of roentgen therapy on the growing spine. *Radiology* 1952; **59**:637–650.
◆16. Sonis AL, Tarbell N, Valachovic RW, *et al.* Dentofacial development in long-term survivors of acute lymphoblastic leukemia. A comparison of three treatment modalities. *Cancer* 1990; **66**:2645–2652.
17. Jaffe N, Toth BB, Hoar RE, *et al.* Dental and maxillofacial abnormalities in long-term survivors of childhood cancer: effects of treatment with chemotherapy and radiation to the head and neck. *Pediatrics* 1984; **73**:816–823.
18. Berkowitz RJ, Neuman P, Spalding P, *et al.* Developmental orofacial deficits associated with multimodal cancer therapy: case report. *Pediatr Dentistry* 1989; **11**:227–231.
19. Kaste SC, Hopkins KP. Micrognathia after radiation therapy for childhood facial tumors. Report of two cases with long-term follow-up. *Oral Surg Oral Med Oral Pathol* 1994; **77**:95–99.
20. Sperber G. *Craniofacial embryology*, 4th edn. D. DD. Boston: Wright, 1989:246.
21. Kennedy R. Growth retardation and volume determinations of the anopthalmic orbit. *Am J Opthalmol* 1973: **76**:294–302.
22. Doline S, Needleman HL, Petersen RA, *et al.* The effect of radiotherapy in the treatment of retinoblastoma upon the developing dentition. *J Pediatr Ophthalmol Strabismus* 1980; **17**:109–113.
23. Mohr C, Fritze H, Messmer E, *et al.* [The question of midface growth inhibition following retinoblastoma treatment in early childhood]. *Deutsche Zeitschrift Mund Kiefer Gesichts-Chir* 1990; **14**:391–394.
◆24. Denys D, Kaste SC, Kun LE, *et al.* The effects of radiation on craniofacial skeletal growth: a quantitative study. *Int J Pediatr Otorhinolaryngol* 1998; **45**:7–13.
25. Nwoku AL, Koch H. Effect of radiation injury on the growing face. *J Maxillofac Surg* 1975; **3**:28–34.
26. Fromm M, Littman P, Raney RB, *et al.* Late effects after treatment of twenty children with soft tissue sarcomas of the head and neck. Experience at a single institution with a review of the literature. *Cancer* 1986; **57**:2070–2076.
27. Dahllof G, Forsberg CM, Ringden O, *et al.* Facial growth and morphology in long-term survivors after bone marrow transplantation. *Eur J Orthodont* 1989; **11**:332–340.
28. Brauner R, Adan L, Souberbielle JC, *et al.* Contribution of growth hormone deficiency to the growth failure that follows bone marrow transplantation. *J Pediatr* 1997; **130**:785–792.
29. Kollar EJ, B.G. Tissue interactions in embryonic mouse tooth germs: II. The inductive role of the dental papilla. *J Embryon Expression Morphogen* 1970; **24**:173–186.
30. Weyman J. The effect of irradiation on developing teeth. *Oral Surg Oral Med Oral Pathol* 1968; **25**:623–629.
31. Alpaslan G, Alpaslan C, Gogen H, *et al.* Disturbances in oral and dental structures in patients with pediatric lymphoma after chemotherapy: a preliminary report. *Oral Surg Oral Med Pathol Oral Radiol Endodont* 1999; **87**:317–321.
◆32. Dahllof G, Barr M, Bolme P, *et al.* Disturbances in dental development after total body irradiation in bone marrow transplant recipients. *Oral Surg Oral Med Oral Pathol* 1988. **65**:41–44.
33. Dury DC, Roberts MW, Miser JS, *et al.* Dental root agenesis secondary to irradiation therapy in a case of rhabdomyosarcoma of the middle ear. *Oral Surg Oral Med Oral Pathol* 1984; **57**:595–599.
34. Fronman S, Ratzkowski E. Two cases of radiation damage to the growing dentition and their supporting structures in children. *Dent Practitioner Dent Rec* 1966; **16**:344–348.

35. Guggenheimer J, Fischer WG, Pechersky JL. Anticipation of dental anomalies induced by radiation therapy. *Radiology* 1975; **117**:405–406.

36. Kaste SC, Hopkins KP, Jones D, *et al.* Dental abnormalities in children treated for acute lymphoblastic leukemia. *Leukemia* 1997; **11**:792–796.

37. Katalin G, Mihaly O, Arpad C. [Dental complications of radiotherapy of tumors of the nasal cavity in childhood]. *Fogorvosi Szemle* 1995; **88**:387–391.

38. Koppang HS. [Dental damage after radiotherapy for malignant lesions in the head and neck region]. *Norske Tannlaegeforenings Tidende* 1975; **85**:159–165.

39. Majorana A, Gastaldi G, Angiola C, *et al.* [Dental anomalies in pediatric patients undergoing radiotherapy: a preliminary study of a population of 15 subjects]. *Minerva Stomatologica* 1994; **43**:65–69.

40. Nasman M, Bjork O, Soderhall S, *et al.* Disturbances in the oral cavity in pediatric long-term survivors after different forms of antineoplastic therapy. *Pediatr Dentistry* 1994; **16**:217–223.

41. Sian JS. The effects of radiation on the teeth: patient management. *Dental Update* 1987; **14**:442–443.

42. Pajari U, Lahtela P, Lanning M, *et al.* Effect of anti-neoplastic therapy on dental maturity and tooth development. *J Pedodontics* 1988; **12**:266–274.

43. Friedlaender GE, Tross RB, Doganis AC, *et al.* Effects of chemotherapeutic agents on bone. I. Short-term methotrexate and doxorubicin (adriamycin) treatment in a rat model. *J Bone Joint Surg Am Vol* 1984; **66**:602–607.

44. Glasser DB. The effect of chemotherapy on growth in the skeletally immature individual. *Clin Orthopaed Related Res* 1991; **262**:93–100.

45. Reade PC, Roberts ML. Some long-term effects of cyclophosphamide on the growth of rat incisor teeth. *Arch Oral Biol* 1978; **23**:1001–1005.

46. McKee MD, Warshawsky H. Modification of the enamel maturation pattern by vinblastine as revealed by glyoxal bis(2-hydroxyanil) staining and 45calcium radioautography. *Histochemistry* 1986; **86**:141–145.

47. Moe H. On the effect of vinblastine on ameloblasts of rat incisors *in vivo*. 3. Acute and protracted effect on differentiating ameloblasts. A light microscopic study. *Acta Pathol Microbiol Scand Sect A Pathol* 1977; **85**:330–334.

48. Moe H, Mikkelsen H. On the effect of vinblastine on ameloblasts of rat incisors *in vivo*. 2. Protracted effect on secretory ameloblasts. A light microscopical study. *Acta Pathol Microbiol Scand Sect A Pathol* 1977; **85**:319–329.

49. Moe H, Mikkelsen H. Light microscopical and ultrastructural observations on the effect of vinblastine on ameloblasts of rat incisors *in vivo*. I. Short-term effect on secretory ameloblasts. *Acta Pathol Microbiol Scand Sect A Pathol* 1977; **85A**:73–88.

50. Rosenberg SW, Kolodney H, Wong GY, *et al.* Altered dental root development in long-term survivors of pediatric acute lymphoblastic leukemia. A review of 17 cases. *Cancer* 1987; **59**:1640–1648.

51. Boltchi FE. Cyclosporine A-induced gingival overgrowth: a comprehensive review. *Quintessence Int* 1999; **30**:775–783.

52. Somacarrera ML, Hernandez G, Acero J, *et al.* Factors related to the incidence and severity of cyclosporin-induced gingival overgrowth in transplant patients. A longitudinal study. *J Periodontol* 1994; **65**:671–675.

53. Thomas DW, Newcombe RG, Osborne GR. Risk factors in the development of cyclosporine-induced gingival overgrowth. *Transplantation* 2000; **69**:522–526.

54. Beveridge T. Cyclosporin A: an evaluation of clinical results. *Transplant Proc* 1983; **15**:433–436.

55. James JA. Gingival fibroblast response to cyclosporin A and transforming growth factor beta 1. *J Periodont Res* 1998; **33**:40–48.

56. Fu E, Nieh S, Chang HL, *et al.* Dose-dependent gingival overgrowth induced by cyclosporin in rats. *J Periodontol* 1995; **66**:594–598.

57. Karpinia KA. Factors affecting cyclosporine-induced gingival overgrowth in pediatric renal transplant recipients. *Pediatr Dentistry* 1996; **18**:450–455.

58. Newburn E. *Cariology*, 3rd edn. Chicago: Quintessence, 1989.

59. Schubert MM, a.I., K.T., Iatrogenic causes of salivary gland dysfunction. *J Dent Res* 1987; **66**:680–688.

◆60. Dahllof G, Bagesund M, Ringden O. Impact of conditioning regimens on salivary function, caries-associated microorganisms and dental caries in children after bone marrow transplantation. A 4-year longitudinal study. *Bone Marrow Transplantation* 1997; **20**:479–483.

61. Deutsch M. The use of pilocarpine hydrochloride to prevent xerostomia in a child treated with high dose radiotherapy for nasopharynx carcinoma. *Oral Oncol* 1998; **34**:381–382.

62. Dreizen S, Brown LR, Daly TE, *et al.* Prevention of xerostomia-related dental caries in irradiated cancer patients. *J Dent Res* 1977; **56**:99–104.

63. Hamlar DD, Schuller DE, Gahbauer RA, *et al.* Determination of the efficacy of topical oral pilocarpine for postirradiation xerostomia in patients with head and neck carcinoma. *Laryngoscope* 1996; **106**:972–976.

64. Papas AS, Joshi A, MacDonald SL, *et al.* Caries prevalence in xerostomic individuals. *J Can Dent Assoc J Assoc Dent Can* 1993; **59**:171–174, 177–179.

65. Babington MA. Cariogenic medications. *Pediatr Nurs* 1982; **8**:165–171.

66. Feigal RJ. Dental caries potential of liquid medications. *Pediatrics* 1981; **68**:416–419.

67. Feigal RJ. The cariogenic potential of liquid medications: a concern for the handicapped patient. *Special Care Dentistry* 1982; **2**:20–24.

68. Feigal RJ. Dental caries related to liquid medication intake in young cardiac patients. *J Dentistry Children* 1984; **51**:360–362.

69. Maguire A, Rugg-Gunn AJ, Butler TJ. Dental health of children taking antimicrobial and non-antimicrobial liquid oral medication long-term. *Caries Res* 1996; **30**:16–21.

70. Nagler RM, Nagler A. Major salivary gland involvement in graft-versus-host disease: considerations related to pathogenesis, the role of cytokines and therapy. *Cytokines Cell Molec Ther* 1999; **5**:227–232.

71. Nicolatou-Galitis O, Kitra V, Van Vliet-Constantinidou C, *et al.* The oral manifestations of chronic graft-versus-host disease (cGVHD) in paediatric allogeneic bone marrow transplant recipients. *J Oral Pathol Med* 2001; **30**:148–153.

72. Lee L, Miller PA, Maxymiw WG, *et al.* Intraoral pyogenic granuloma after allogeneic bone marrow transplant. Report of three cases. *Oral Surg Oral Med Oral Pathol* 1994; **78**:607–610.

73. Woo SB, Lee SJ, Schubert MM. Graft-vs.-host disease. *Crit Rev Oral Biol Med* 1997; **8**:201–216.

74. Dahllof G, Heimdahl A, Modeer T, *et al.* Oral mucous membrane lesions in children treated with bone marrow transplantation. *Scand J Dent Res* 1989; **97**:268–277.

75. Arcuri MR, Fridrich KL, Funk GF, *et al.* Titanium osseointegrated implants combined with hyperbaric oxygen therapy in previously irradiated mandibles. *J Prosthet Dent* 1997; **77**:177–183.

76. Jacobsson M, Tjellstrom A, Thomsen P, *et al.* Integration of titanium implants in irradiated bone. Histologic and clinical study. *Ann Otol Rhinol Laryngol* 1988; **97**(4 Pt 1):337–340.

77. Leake DL, Habal MB. Reconstitution of craniofacial osseous contour deformities, sequelae of trauma and post resection for

tumors, with an alloplastic-autogenous graft. *J Trauma Injury Infect Crit Care* 1977; **17**:299–303.

78. Dahllof G, Jonsson A, Ulmner M, *et al.* Orthodontic treatment in long-term survivors after pediatric bone marrow transplantation. *Am J Orthodont Dentofacial Orthoped* 2001; **120**:459–465.

79. Stevens MC, Mahler H, Parkes S. The health status of adult survivors of cancer in childhood. *Eur J Cancer* 1998; **34**:694–698.

80. Buchbinder D, Urken ML, Vickery C, *et al.* Functional mandibular reconstruction of patients with oral cancer. *Oral Surg Oral Med Oral Pathol* 1989; **68**:499–503; discussion 503–504.

81. Makkonen TA, Kiminki A, Makkonen TK, *et al.* Dental extractions in relation to radiation therapy of 224 patients. *Int J Oral Maxillofac Surg* 1987; **16**:56–64.

82. Maxymiw WG, Wood RE, Liu FF. Postradiation dental extractions without hyperbaric oxygen. *Oral Surg Oral Med Oral Pathol* 1991; **72**:270–274.

83. Newman GV, Newman RA. A longitudinal study of the effects of surgery, radiation, growth hormone, and orthodontic therapy on the craniofacial skeleton of a patient evidencing hypopituitarism and a Class II malocclusion: report of a case. *Am J Orthodont Dentofacial Orthoped* 1994; **106**:571–582.

8

Endocrine and fertility effects

8a

Growth and neuroendocrine consequences

KEN H DARZY, HELENA K GLEESON AND STEPHEN M SHALET

INTRODUCTION

While cure of childhood cancer is now a realistic target, the consequences of cancer treatment still pose major concerns for the surviving child and all those involved in their subsequent care. Amongst the complications of cancer therapy, endocrine abnormalities are the most common and inflict a negative impact on growth, body image, sexual function and quality of life.

The spectrum of endocrine complications includes gonadal damage, thyroid disorders and dysfunction of the hypothalamic – pituitary (h-p) axis.

Neuroendocrine abnormalities may follow external radiotherapy for a variety of tumors when the h-p axis falls within the fields of radiation. Deficiency of one or more anterior pituitary hormones has been described following therapeutic cranial irradiation for primary brain tumors, tumors involving the h-p axis, nasopharyngeal tumors, tumors of the base of the skull and solid tumors of the face and neck, as well as following prophylactic cranial irradiation in childhood acute lymphoblastic leukemia (ALL) and total body irradiation (TBI) prior to bone marrow transplant (BMT).

In this subchapter we consider the pathogenesis, presentation and clinical management of the neuroendocrine abnormalities that occur secondary to radiation therapy with particular emphasis on the impact of growth hormone (GH) deficiency on growth, and the benefits of GH treatment both in childhood and adulthood.

RADIOBIOLOGY

The radiobiological impact of a radiation schedule depends on the total dose, fraction size, number of fractions and the duration.

Studies have consistently shown a strong correlation between the total radiation dose and the development of pituitary hormone deficits.[1–6] Thus, after lower radiation doses, isolated GH deficiency ensues, while higher doses may produce panhypopituitarism. Radiation schedules used in children with ALL or brain tumors (18–50 Gy with a fraction size of 1.8–2.5 Gy/day) usually cause isolated growth hormone deficiency. More intensive irradiation schedules used, in particular, for those with nasopharyngeal carcinoma, deliver a higher dose of radiation ($\geq$60 Gy), and lead to early and multiple pituitary hormone deficits.[7,8] Furthermore, the same total dose given in fewer fractions over a shorter time period is likely to cause a greater incidence of pituitary hormone deficiency than if the schedule is spread over a longer time interval with a greater number of fractions.[9]

More recently, the degree of anterior pituitary hormone deficit following radiation exposure has been correlated with the biological effective dose (BED) of the radiation affecting the h-p axis. The formula used to calculate the BED incorporates total dose, fraction size and tissue (h-p axis) response to radiation.[10] The calculation of BED provides a useful method of comparing radiation schedules and predicting the development of radiation-induced GH deficiency.[10]

Age of the patient at the time of radiotherapy may be an additional factor that determines the extent of radiation damage sustained by the h-p axis for a given BED and consequently the severity of the neuroendocrine abnormalities. Some data suggest that children are more sensitive than adults and that older children are less vulnerable than younger children to the risk of developing GH deficiency following radiation to the h-p axis.[1]

The damaging effects of radiation on h-p function are also increased when the h-p axis is already affected by another pathology. A radiation dose of 35–42.5 Gy to the h-p axis caused isolated GH deficiency in the majority of children treated for non-pituitary brain tumors,[6,11] whereas a similar dose in adult patients irradiated for pituitary adenomas led to multiple pituitary hormone deficits in more than 80 per cent within a similar time scale after radiotherapy.[12]

PATHOPHYSIOLOGY, SITE AND NATURE OF RADIATION DAMAGE

There is evidence that the hypothalamus is more radiosensitive than the pituitary and is damaged by lower doses of cranial radiation. For instance, after lower doses of cranial irradiation (<50 Gy) and after TBI,[13–19] the primary site of radiation damage is hypothalamic and is usually associated with isolated GH deficiency, whereas higher doses, as used in the treatment of nasopharyngeal carcinomas[5,7,18–20] or tumors of the base of the skull,[21] may produce direct anterior pituitary damage, which contributes to early and multiple pituitary hormone deficiencies.

Patients with pituitary adenomas treated by the implantation of yttrium-90 into the pituitary gland, with radiation doses of 500–1500 Gy to the pituitary, had a combined incidence of thyroid-stimulating hormone (TSH) and adrenocorticotrophin (ACTH) deficiency of 39 per cent at 14 years[22] compared with an incidence of over 90 per cent at 10 years among patients who underwent external irradiation with doses ranging from 37.5 to 42.5 Gy.[12] The most likely explanation for the difference in the incidence of hypopituitarism after the two types of irradiation is that the fields for external irradiation included the hypothalamus, which was relatively unaffected by yttrium-90 treatment.

The pattern of neuroendocrine disturbances following cranial irradiation provides further evidence that the hypothalamus is the primary site for radiation-induced damage. Many studies in patients who received cranial irradiation demonstrate:

- an increased basal serum prolactin concentration, which is rarely observed after interstitial radiotherapy with yittrium-90 implants;
- delayed luteinizing hormone/follicle-stimulating hormone (LH/FSH) release following stimulation with an intravenous bolus of gonadotrophin-releasing hormone (GnRH) in patients with gonadotrophin deficiency and delayed rise and/or delayed decline in the TSH response to intravenous thyrotrophin-releasing hormone (TRH) stimulation in patients with TSH deficiency (hypothalamic hypothyroidism);
- impaired peak GH responses to stimuli that act through hypothalamic pathways, e.g. insulin-induced hypoglycemia and intravenous arginine infusion in the presence of intact pituitary (somatotroph) responsiveness to a bolus of exogenous growth hormone-releasing hormone (GHRH); and reduced spontaneous (physiological) GH secretion despite normal serum GH responses to pharmacological stimuli (GH neurosecretory dysfunction).

These are the characteristic abnormalities in anterior pituitary hormone secretion in patients with pathologically documented hypothalamic disease.

Hypothalamic-pituitary dysfunction secondary to radiation is also time dependent.[5,12] There is an increase in the frequency and severity of hormonal deficits with a longer time interval after radiotherapy irrespective of whether the latter is administered for pituitary tumor or non-pituitary pathology (Figures 8a.1 and 8a.2). The progressive nature of the hormonal deficits following radiation damage to the h-p axis can be attributed to the delayed effects of radiotherapy on the axis or the development of secondary pituitary atrophy consequent upon lack of hypothalamic releasing/trophic factors.[3,23,24] Achermann et al.[25] demonstrated that long-term survivors who received cranial irradiation had impaired GH pulse generation, and secretion in response to continuous GHRH and intermittent somatostatin (SS) infusion in comparison with normal controls, suggesting that GH secretory dysfunction does not simply reflect reduced GHRH and SS secretion, and that trophic effects or pituitary damage may be important over time. In a study by the authors involving 49 cranially irradiated adult survivors, the time dependency of pituitary (somatotroph) dysfunction was supported by the finding of a strong and significant negative correlation between the peak GH response to the combined GHRH plus arginine stimulation test and the time interval after irradiation.[26] Similarly,

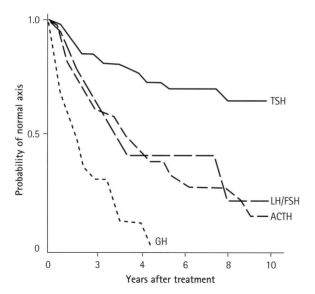

Figure 8a.1 *Life-table analysis indicating probabilities of initially normal hypothalamic-pituitary-target gland axes remaining normal after radiotherapy. ACTH, adrenocorticotrophin; FSH, follicle-stimulating hormone; GH, growth hormone; LH, luteinizing hormone; TSH, thyroid-stimulating hormone. (Reproduced from Littley MD, Shalet SM, Beardwell CG, et al. Hypopituitarism following external radiotherapy for pituitary tumors in adults. Q J Med 1989; 70:145–160 with permission.)*

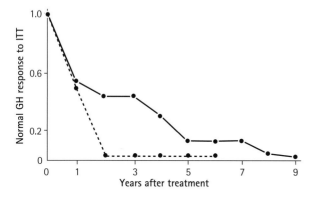

Figure 8a.2 *The incidence of growth hormone (GH) deficiency in children receiving 27–32 Gy -·--·- or ≥ —·— 35 Gy of cranial irradiation for a brain tumor in relation to time from irradiation. ITT, insulin tolerance test. (Adapted from Clayton PE, Shalet SM. Dose dependency of time of onset of radiation-induced growth hormone deficiency. J Pediatr 1991;118:226–228 with permission.)*

the observation of attenuated pituitary responses to GnRH or TRH stimulation is also compatible with progressive pituitary failure.

The pathophysiology of radiation-induced damage remains poorly understood: does it reflect vascular damage or direct neuronal damage? Studies of regional cerebral blood flow by Chieng and colleagues[27] using ^{99m}Tc-hexamethyl propyleneamine oxime (HMPAO) in 34 patients with nasopharyngeal cancer before irradiation, at 6 months, 1 year and more than 5 years after irradiation showed that regional hypothalamic blood flow was reduced after cranial irradiation, but there was no significant difference in the hypothalamic/occipital blood flow ratio between 6 months and 5 years after irradiation. These observations were in stark contrast to the progressive endocrine dysfunction with time in these patients. These results suggest that direct injury to the hypothalamic neurons, rather than reduced cerebral blood flow, is the major cause of progressive hypothalamic-pituitary dysfunction after fractionated cranial irradiation.

The remarkable difference in the incidence of anterior pituitary hormone deficiencies, with secretion of GH being most frequently affected, suggests that selective hypothalamic neuronal and pituitary cell damage by direct radiation occurs. In this context, differential radiosensitivity of hypothalamic-pituitary function has been proposed and clinical observations reveal that the GH axis is the most radiosensitive followed by the gonadotrophin, ACTH and TSH axes. In an experimental study by Robinson et al.,[28] differential radiosensitivity of hypothalamic-pituitary function was clearly demonstrated in the young adult rat. In this experiment, irradiation induced time- and dose-dependent changes in pituitary hormone contents. GH and prolactin (PRL) were most sensitive and decreased by more than 90 per cent after irradiation. TSH contents were unaffected 8 weeks after the lowest dose of irradiation but were reduced at 14 and 20 weeks. LH and ACTH were the slowest to be affected and then only at the higher doses of radiation. Further evidence for direct neuronal damage came from the observations of Hochberg et al.[29] who studied rat pituitary cell survival and growth hormone secretion after *in vitro* irradiation of pituitary cell culture. Their data reveal the marked sensitivity of the somatotrophs to single doses of radiation as low as 300 cGy, and the remarkable resistance of the gonadotrophin- and TSH-secreting cells to doses as high as 1000 cGy. The findings of both studies are consistent with most of the clinical observations in human.

Neuropharmacology has provided an additional tool to explore the pathophysiology of radiation injury. The observations of Jorgensen and colleagues[30] also suggest that radiation-induced hypothalamic dysfunction may be secondary to radiation damage of the suprahypothalamic neurotransmitter pathways. In their study, they explored the neurotransmitter control of GH secretion in children after radiotherapy by using neurotransmitter-excitatory substances to study the GH secretory response in 17 children who had received 12–60 Gy to the cranium and 40 short children with normal endocrine function. Their

study was based on the principle that neurotransmitter stimuli provoke GH secretion by inducing changes in hypothalamic GHRH and/or somatostatin release, and patients who respond to one or more of these stimuli must have intact hypothalamic responsiveness. The irradiated children had decreased mean GH secretion in response to insulin-induced hypoglycemia and arginine infusion, and decreased mean 24-hour GH concentrations, compared to the control group. In contrast, the two groups had similar GH secretory responses to stimulation with exogenous GHRH and suppression with somatostatin infusion, indicating that the irradiated pituitary responsiveness was relatively preserved. Assessment of neurotransmitter pathways in the irradiated children revealed significantly lower mean peak GH concentrations in response to five of the six substances tested compared to control children: α-adrenergic stimulation (clonidine), β-adrenergic blockade (propranalol), cholinergic stimulation, dopaminergic stimulation (L-dopa) and gamma-aminobutyric acid (GABA)-ergic stimulation (valproic acid). Results of serotonergic stimulation (L-tryptophan) were not statistically significant. However, eight of the GH-deficient irradiated patients were able to respond normally to one or more neurotransmitter stimuli, suggesting that their impaired GH secretion is not related to defects in GHRH or somatostatin production, but rather to defects in neurotransmitter input from suprahypothalamic pathways.

Further insight into the impact of cranial irradiation on neuroregulatory control of GH secretion was provided by the work of Ogilvy-Stuart and coworkers.[31] Their investigation was based on manipulating cholinergic tone in young adults rendered GH-deficient in childhood after cranial irradiation; this approach is based on the established contribution of cholinergic input in modifying somatostatin tone and thereby GH secretion.

One of ten controls and four of eight irradiated subjects with documented GH deficiency had a peak GH level to GHRH analogue of less than 20 mU/l. After pretreatment with pyridostigmine (acetylcholinesterase inhibitor), all subjects except one irradiated subject had a peak GH level of greater than 20 mU/l. Pretreatment with pyridostigmine and pirenzepine (cholinergic antagonist) significantly modified the GH response to GHRH analogue within both groups. Pretreatment with pyridostigmine significantly enhanced the GH response to GHRH analogue compared with GHRH analogue alone, and pretreatment with pirenzepine significantly attenuated the response to GHRH analogue. The data may be interpreted in several ways, but suggest that cranial irradiation reduces but does not abolish somatostatin tone and also reduces endogenous GHRH secretion. Although somatostatin tone is reduced, it can be increased by cholinergic manipulation and, therefore, is not irreversibly fixed. This has possible implications if GHRH analogues are used to treat patients with radiation-induced GH deficiency.[32]

Further studies in animals and human are needed to achieve better understanding of the exact mechanisms underlying radiation-induced h-p dysfunction; these may provide the opportunity subsequently to test novel interventions in patients with these abnormalities, which might minimize the development or degree of associated neuroendocrine injury.

GROWTH HORMONE DEFICIENCY

Growth hormone deficiency is usually the first and is frequently the only manifestation of neuroendocrine injury following cranial irradiation. The severity and speed of onset of radiation-induced GH deficiency is dose dependent and the incidence increases with time-elapsed after irradiation.

Current evidence suggests that nearly 100 per cent of children treated with radiation doses in excess of 30 Gy will have blunted GH responses to insulin tolerance test (ITT), whilst 35 per cent of those receiving less than 30 Gy still show a normal peak GH response to the ITT between 2 and 5 years after radiotherapy[3] (Figure 8a.2). Low-dose cranial irradiation (18–24 Gy) as used prophylactically in ALL often leads to isolated GH deficiency.[9,16,33–35] Isolated GH deficiency has also been noted following total radiation doses as low as 10 Gy as used in TBI.[35,36] Prospective studies also suggest that impaired GH responses to provocative tests can occur as early as 3 months and certainly in the first 12 months postirradiation for brain tumors.[6,11] In a study by Chen et al., GH responses to ITT dropped substantially 1 month after high-dose radiation therapy (>60 Gy) for nasopharyngeal carcinoma with very little further decrease by 18 months.[8]

Clinical studies of GH secretion after cranial irradiation in humans support the experimental animal data by showing that the h-p axis of the young is more radiosensitive than that of older children or adults. For instance, in a study of children and adults undergoing TBI, after a mean time of 2.8 years following TBI (1000–1320 cGy in 5–6 fractions over 3 days), all 18 adults showed a normal GH response to an ITT,[37] whilst after a mean time of 2.4 years after a similar TBI schedule (1100–1520 cGy in 3–8 fractions over 2–5 days), 15 out of 29 children showed subnormal GH responses to an ITT.[36] In three of the 15 children, previous cranial irradiation might have explained the GH deficiency, but no irradiation other than TBI had been administered to the remaining 12 children. In addition, younger children receiving prophylactic cranial irradiation for ALL are more susceptible to radiation-induced GH deficiency than older children.[38] Similarly, Samaan et al., in their study of 166 patients, who had received high-dose irradiation for tumors of the head and neck, showed that children younger than 15 years of

age had a higher incidence of GH deficiency soon after radiotherapy than older patients.[39]

Radiation-induced growth hormone neurosecretory dysfunction

Radiation-induced growth hormone neurosecretory dysfunction (GHNSD) is well-described following radiation injury of the h-p axis.[14,24,40] It is classically characterized by diminished spontaneous (physiological) GH secretion in the presence of preserved peak GH responses to provocative tests.[41] Under normal circumstances, GH is secreted in an intermittent pulsatile pattern with the most profound secretory bursts occurring during sleep. Spontaneous GH secretion is determined by the number of the pulses, pulse amplitude and the total 24-hour integrated GH concentration derived from sampling every 20 minutes over a 24-hour period.

Thus, the frequency of radiation-induced GH deficiency reported can be influenced by the type of investigation used to assess GH secretion, i.e. physiological versus pharmacological tests. Most prospective studies have concentrated on provocative tests and, therefore, the exact prevalence of radiation-induced GH deficiency may well be underestimated. For example, Albertsson-Wikland et al. showed that spontaneous GH secretion was severely disturbed in all children more than 2 years after they had received cranial irradiation (>40 Gy) for brain tumors.[42] This is in contrast to the lower incidence of GH deficiency with the same radiation schedules and time scale reported in other studies that relied on stimulation tests.

Radiation-induced GHNSD appears to be dose dependent and is usually encountered in children treated for ALL who have received a radiation dose in the range of 18–24 Gy.[40] Eventually, higher radiation doses (>27 Gy) affect both spontaneous and stimulated GH secretion fairly equally.[43]

Reduced spontaneous GH secretion has been described in both prepubertal and pubertal girls following cranial irradiation for ALL (24 Gy) with a failure of the expected increase in GH secretion at puberty,[44] associated with an attenuated pubertal growth.[45] In an attempt to minimize neuropsychological disturbance and abnormalities in GH secretion, the dose of prophylactic cranial irradiation was reduced to 18 Gy after 1981 without any change in prognosis. The effect of this lower dose on GH secretion is, however, disputed. Crowne et al. showed a reduction in spontaneous GH secretion only during puberty with, in addition, a disturbance in the periodicity of GH secretion,[46] whereas Lannering et al. showed a reduction in spontaneous GH secretion prepubertally and during puberty, but with normal periodicity throughout.[47] Stubberfield et al. showed greater reduction in spontaneous GH secretion in children who had

received 24 Gy as compared to those who had received 18 Gy;[48] however, growth rates in both groups did not differ for the first 5 years after diagnosis but there was a greater impact of 24 Gy on long-term growth.[48]

There are no longitudinal studies involving regular assessment of spontaneous GH secretion and, hence, the natural history of GH deficiency following cranial irradiation or TBI remains unknown. However, with physiological tests most studies showed a higher prevalence of GH deficiency in the early years after irradiation and a progressive increase in the frequency of GH deficiency as assessed by pharmacological tests. This suggests that the discrepancy between stimulated and spontaneous GH secretion tends to disappear with time after radiotherapy and it is likely that patients who develop impaired GH responses to provocative tests late after irradiation may have had GHNSD at an earlier stage. Further studies are needed to define the exact incidence of radiation-induced GHNSD in children and the factors that influence its transformation into classical GH deficiency with time or its 'persistence' into adult life.

Diagnosis of radiation-induced GH deficiency

AUXOLOGICAL

Growth in children is a sensitive marker of GH status. Thus, in the absence of other etiologies for growth retardation, the presence of significant growth deviation over a 1-year period, that is, growth velocity below the 25th centile or a drop in height of $\geqslant 1$ standard deviation (SD), is highly suggestive of clinically significant GH deficiency, particularly in the appropriate clinical context, i.e. previous irradiation.

Growth monitoring is an essential part of the follow-up of all children who have received cranial irradiation as part of their cancer treatment. Accurate measurement of the standing and sitting height should be recorded every 3–6 months. The sitting height is obtained by direct measurement using a sitting height stadiometer and provides invaluable information in patients who have received spinal irradiation or TBI. The impact of spinal irradiation on spinal growth is such that, in children who received craniospinal irradiation, greater auxological emphasis must be placed on the leg length changes rather than total height.

BIOCHEMICAL

The biochemical diagnosis of GH deficiency classically relies on the demonstration of attenuated GH responses to pharmacological stimuli. Standard provocative tests may be misleading, however, in these patients because false-negative results are not unusual, particularly after low-dose cranial irradiation. Although, measurement of

GROWTH AND CANCER TREATMENT

Growth impairment is frequently seen following successful cancer treatment in children. In many patients, this results in reduced statural growth and final height. Although radiation-induced GH deficiency is a common cause of growth impairment in cancer survivors, a variety of other factors could also contribute, including the disease process itself, decreased nutritional intake, psychosocial dysfunction, chemotherapy, steroid therapy, spinal irradiation, hypothyroidism, hypogonadism, precocious puberty and the non-endocrine complications of various treatment modalities.

GROWTH IN CHILDREN TREATED FOR ALL

Many controversies and, therefore, confusion have been generated over the growth patterns of children treated for ALL. A major reason for the difficulty in interpretation of data is that most studies have analyzed growth in children treated with both prophylactic cranial irradiation and combination chemotherapy (CT) schedules. Thus, disentangling the adverse contribution of these two major therapeutic modalities on growth has proved difficult. However, some conclusions acceptable to most investigators can be drawn.

Early growth deceleration with bone age retardation during treatment for ALL is well recognized and is mainly attributed to the adverse effects of chemotherapy on growth. Schriock et al. showed that the mean decrease in height standard deviation score (SDS) at the end of chemotherapy in 70 out of 115 patients (90 per cent) was -0.74 ± 0.53 and -0.91 ± 0.47 in patients who received prophylactic cranial or craniospinal irradiation, respectively.[96] The greatest drop in height SDS occurs in the first year of chemotherapy[97] and is most marked in the very young children (<4 years).[96,97] Unlike final height, early growth impairment is unrelated to the radiation schedule used for prophylaxis[98] and occurs to the same extent in those who did not receive prophylactic cranial radiation.[99,100]

On completion of chemotherapy, 70 per cent of patients will show a variable degree of catch-up growth, if the chemotherapy was not intensive and prolonged.[2] Catch-up growth occurs in the irradiated and non-irradiated patients[99] and is associated with a progression in bone age maturation.[101] It lasts at least 1 year and, in some patients, can result in a return of height SDS to baseline values,[96,102] usually within 2–3 years. Catch-up growth tends to be complete in the non-irradiated patients but suboptimal in the irradiated patients.[100]

Other factors contributing to growth impairment in these early stages may include malnutrition, recurrent infection, sickness and the disease itself. It is difficult to quantify the role of GH deficiency at this stage. GH secretion, assessed longitudinally during the first 24 months of treatment for ALL, was suppressed completely during dexamethasone treatment.[103]

Before 1981 most children with ALL received a cranial irradiation dose of 24–25 Gy. Although studies of growth for the first few years after irradiation suggested that any impact on growth was minor, final height data show unequivocally that height loss from the time of primary therapy is significant with between 31 and 48 per cent of children losing 10 cm or more of height.[104] Contributing factors include evolving radiation-induced GH deficiency, precocious puberty and possibly spinal irradiation. Kirk et al. demonstrated a final height of 1.37 SD below the population mean in 71 per cent of survivors 6 years after therapy that involved cranial irradiation with 24 Gy.[34] GH deficiency was documented in most patients either pharmacologically or physiologically. Schriock et al. showed that 74 per cent and 37 per cent will achieve a final height that is >1 SD or 2 SD below population mean, respectively.[96] Similarly, Robison et al. found a threefold excess in the proportion of males and a 4.2-fold excess in the proportion of females below the fifth percentile.[105] The height distributions observed for patients treated with craniospinal radiation only or cranial radiation plus intrathecal methotrexate were not different, although both deviated significantly from expected.[105]

As the lower cranial irradiation dose of 18 Gy was only introduced in the 1980, less final height data are available in children receiving this dose of irradiation. Nonetheless, Davies et al. showed that significant loss of standing height occurred in both 18-Gy as well as the 24-Gy cohorts of children, and although the height loss was greater in the higher dose group, this difference was not significant.[104] Indeed, with time it may be that the difference between the 18-Gy and 24-Gy groups is shown to be even less than in this study,[104] as the median age at diagnosis for the 24-Gy group (4.2 years girls, 4.9 years boys) was significantly younger than for the 18-Gy group (7.3 years girls, 9.4 years boys), allowing them more time for height loss. In contrast, Sklar et al. showed a significant difference in height loss in patients treated with 24 Gy compared to 18 Gy with a change in height SDS between diagnosis and achievement of final height of -1.38 ± 0.16 and -0.65 ± 0.15, respectively.[106] In both these studies, no spinal irradiation was given.[104,106]

Chemotherapy may also play a role in growth impairment. The discrepancy in height loss between two groups of children who received similar cranial irradiation schedules but CT of varying intensity provided indirect evidence for the effect of CT.[34,97] There is also in vitro evidence from rat liver perfusion experiments that GH-stimulated production of IGF-1 is inhibited by 6-mercaptopurine[107] and chronic administration of 6-mercaptopurine has been

age had a higher incidence of GH deficiency soon after radiotherapy than older patients.[39]

Radiation-induced growth hormone neurosecretory dysfunction

Radiation-induced growth hormone neurosecretory dysfunction (GHNSD) is well-described following radiation injury of the h-p axis.[14,24,40] It is classically characterized by diminished spontaneous (physiological) GH secretion in the presence of preserved peak GH responses to provocative tests.[41] Under normal circumstances, GH is secreted in an intermittent pulsatile pattern with the most profound secretory bursts occurring during sleep. Spontaneous GH secretion is determined by the number of the pulses, pulse amplitude and the total 24-hour integrated GH concentration derived from sampling every 20 minutes over a 24-hour period.

Thus, the frequency of radiation-induced GH deficiency reported can be influenced by the type of investigation used to assess GH secretion, i.e. physiological versus pharmacological tests. Most prospective studies have concentrated on provocative tests and, therefore, the exact prevalence of radiation-induced GH deficiency may well be underestimated. For example, Albertsson-Wikland et al. showed that spontaneous GH secretion was severely disturbed in all children more than 2 years after they had received cranial irradiation (>40 Gy) for brain tumors.[42] This is in contrast to the lower incidence of GH deficiency with the same radiation schedules and time scale reported in other studies that relied on stimulation tests.

Radiation-induced GHNSD appears to be dose dependent and is usually encountered in children treated for ALL who have received a radiation dose in the range of 18–24 Gy.[40] Eventually, higher radiation doses (>27 Gy) affect both spontaneous and stimulated GH secretion fairly equally.[43]

Reduced spontaneous GH secretion has been described in both prepubertal and pubertal girls following cranial irradiation for ALL (24 Gy) with a failure of the expected increase in GH secretion at puberty,[44] associated with an attenuated pubertal growth.[45] In an attempt to minimize neuropsychological disturbance and abnormalities in GH secretion, the dose of prophylactic cranial irradiation was reduced to 18 Gy after 1981 without any change in prognosis. The effect of this lower dose on GH secretion is, however, disputed. Crowne et al. showed a reduction in spontaneous GH secretion only during puberty with, in addition, a disturbance in the periodicity of GH secretion,[46] whereas Lannering et al. showed a reduction in spontaneous GH secretion prepubertally and during puberty, but with normal periodicity throughout.[47] Stubberfield et al. showed greater reduction in spontaneous GH secretion in children who had

received 24 Gy as compared to those who had received 18 Gy;[48] however, growth rates in both groups did not differ for the first 5 years after diagnosis but there was a greater impact of 24 Gy on long-term growth.[48]

There are no longitudinal studies involving regular assessment of spontaneous GH secretion and, hence, the natural history of GH deficiency following cranial irradiation or TBI remains unknown. However, with physiological tests most studies showed a higher prevalence of GH deficiency in the early years after irradiation and a progressive increase in the frequency of GH deficiency as assessed by pharmacological tests. This suggests that the discrepancy between stimulated and spontaneous GH secretion tends to disappear with time after radiotherapy and it is likely that patients who develop impaired GH responses to provocative tests late after irradiation may have had GHNSD at an earlier stage. Further studies are needed to define the exact incidence of radiation-induced GHNSD in children and the factors that influence its transformation into classical GH deficiency with time or its 'persistence' into adult life.

Diagnosis of radiation-induced GH deficiency

AUXOLOGICAL

Growth in children is a sensitive marker of GH status. Thus, in the absence of other etiologies for growth retardation, the presence of significant growth deviation over a 1-year period, that is, growth velocity below the 25th centile or a drop in height of ≥ 1 standard deviation (SD), is highly suggestive of clinically significant GH deficiency, particularly in the appropriate clinical context, i.e. previous irradiation.

Growth monitoring is an essential part of the follow-up of all children who have received cranial irradiation as part of their cancer treatment. Accurate measurement of the standing and sitting height should be recorded every 3–6 months. The sitting height is obtained by direct measurement using a sitting height stadiometer and provides invaluable information in patients who have received spinal irradiation or TBI. The impact of spinal irradiation on spinal growth is such that, in children who received craniospinal irradiation, greater auxological emphasis must be placed on the leg length changes rather than total height.

BIOCHEMICAL

The biochemical diagnosis of GH deficiency classically relies on the demonstration of attenuated GH responses to pharmacological stimuli. Standard provocative tests may be misleading, however, in these patients because false-negative results are not unusual, particularly after low-dose cranial irradiation. Although, measurement of

spontaneous GH secretion over 24 hours appears to be the most sensitive means of determining GH status in the irradiated patients, it is very time consuming and is only available in research centers. A practical approach would, therefore, involve performing pharmacological tests using stimuli that work through hypothalamic pathways. Two provocative tests are usually needed to make the diagnosis of isolated GH deficiency with certainty.[49]

Amongst all provocative tests, the insulin tolerance test is the 'gold standard' for assessment of GH deficiency.[50,51] Insulin-induced hypoglycemia stimulates GH secretion through hypothalamic pathways and there is overwhelming evidence that the ITT is the most sensitive test to identify radiation damage,[52,53] and that impaired GH responses to the ITT may occur in association with normal GH responses to arginine infusion following low-dose cranial irradiation.[53]

The cut-off peak GH threshold used to define GH status following various stimuli is arbitrarily defined.[50,54] In children, the peak GH response to the ITT below which a child is considered to be suffering from GH deficiency has been gradually increased and, currently, most pediatric endocrinologists would consider GH replacement therapy, in the appropriate clinical context, if that child failed to achieve a peak GH response above 20 mU/l (7 μg/l).[51,54]

A reduction in the GH-dependent markers, insulin-like growth factor 1 (IGF-1) and IGF binding protein 3 (IGFBP-3) is consistent with GH deficiency. However, reduced IGF-1 and IGFBP-3 are not specific for GH deficiency, and may occur in children with malnutrition, hypothyroidism, renal failure, liver disease or diabetes mellitus.[54] In addition, normal age and puberty-corrected IGF-1 and/or IGFBP-3 levels are frequently seen in patients with documented radiation-induced GH deficiency defined by physiological and/or pharmacological tests.[55-60] Thus, it had been thought that neither of these markers can be used as a reliable index of the development of radiation-induced GH deficiency.[54] In contrast to these conclusions, in a recent study by Adan et al., 95 per cent of cancer survivors with severe GH deficiency were shown to have an IGF-1 standard deviation score of less than −2.[61] It is to be noted, however, that most of the studied patients were adults with longstanding severe GH deficiency, which might explain the higher prevalence of abnormally low IGF-I levels in their cohort.[61]

ABNORMALITIES OF GONADOTROPHIN SECRETION

Gonadotrophin deficiency

Gonadotrophin deficiency is infrequent when the radiation dose to the h-p axis is less than 40 Gy.[62,63] However, the incidence is remarkably increased in an irradiated pituitary tumor cohort. Littley et al. demonstrated that 5 years after irradiation of tumors involving the pituitary or anatomically related structures, the incidence of LH/FSH deficiency in patients with initially normal gonadotrophin secretion who received 20 Gy delivered in eight fractions over 11 days was 33 per cent.[4] However, 66 per cent of patients with previously normal gonadotrophin secretion developed LH/FSH deficiency 5 years after receiving 35–40 Gy delivered in 15 fractions over 21 days.

There is a progressive increase in the incidence of gonadotrophin deficiency following cranial irradiation for non-pituitary brain tumors, or tumors of the neck and face as the radiation dose received by the h-p axis exceeds 50 Gy. Rappaport et al. reported that 14 out of 45 children studied following high-dose cranial irradiation for head and neck tumors showed evidence of partial or severe gonadotrophin deficiency.[64] The prevalence of gonadotrophin deficiency also increases with time postirradiation, a cumulative incidence of 20–50 per cent has been reported in patients followed long term, making it the second most common anterior pituitary hormone deficit in many series.[2,5,7,64] In addition, Lam et al. demonstrated a progressive decrease in stimulated but not the basal LH level 1, 2, 3, 4 and 5 years after irradiation, whereas basal and stimulated FSH level increased after irradiation and were significantly higher than pretreatment values at 1 year.[5] After the first year, there was a tendency for both basal and stimulated FSH levels to fall with increasing time since radiotherapy. Mean integrated FSH responses to GnRH stimulation at 3, 4 and 5 years were significantly lower than the mean value at 1 year. The authors suggested that the fall in serum LH but rise in serum FSH in the first year following radiation is due to a radiation-induced decrease in the pulse frequency of hypothalamic GnRH secretion.[5] The progressive decrease in secretion of both LH and FSH after the first year is in keeping with a progressive reduction in hypothalamic GnRH pulse amplitude.[5]

Gonadotrophin deficiency provides a spectrum of severity from subtle (subclinical) abnormalities in secretion detected only by GnRH testing to severe impairment associated with diminished circulating sex hormone levels. Although abnormalities in LH/FSH secretion can be demonstrated on dynamic testing, sometimes as early as 1 month following high-dose irradiation,[8] clinically significant LH/FSH deficiency is usually a long-term complication.[5] Basal LH/FSH levels are usually normal or low normal with diminished sex hormone concentrations, and GnRH testing reveals a delayed peak gonadotrophin response and/or a delayed decline indicating hypothalamic damage; a blunted response indicating pituitary damage or a mixed pattern of responses indicates possible damage at both sites. Repeated intermittent infusion of GnRH may restore pituitary responsiveness and, therefore, differentiate

between primary and secondary pituitary atrophy[65] and, with prolonged treatment, there is the potential for restoring gonadal function and fertility.[66]

Precocious or early puberty

The effect of cerebral irradiation on the hypothalamic–pituitary–gonadal axis (HPGA) appears to be dose dependent. Radiation doses in excess of 50 Gy may render a child gondotrophin deficient,[64] whereas lesser doses of irradiation may, paradoxically, cause premature activation of the axis resulting in early or precocious puberty.[67–72] The mechanism for early puberty following irradiation is thought to be due to the disinhibition of cortical influences on the hypothalamus.

Low-dose cranial irradiation employed in central nervous system (CNS) prophylaxis for ALL is associated with a higher incidence of early or precocious puberty, which predominantly affects girls.[69] The frequency of male ALL survivors with documented early or precocious puberty is no greater than seen in a normal population.[69,70] This sexual dichotomy has been attributed to fundamental differences in the interaction between the higher centers in the CNS and hypothalamic function. It has been postulated that the CNS restraint on the onset of puberty is more readily disrupted in girls than in boys by any insult, including irradiation.

At higher radiation doses employed in the treatment of brain tumors (25–50 Gy) early puberty is not restricted to girls. Ogilvy-Stuart *et al.* demonstrated that in 46 GH-deficient children previously irradiated for brain tumors (25–47.5 Gy) the onset of puberty occurred at an early age in both sexes, and there was a significant linear association between age at irradiation and age at onset of puberty[71] (Figure 8a.3). Thus, the mean chronological age at the onset of puberty was 8.5 years in girls and 9.2 years in boys plus 0.29 year for every year of age at the time of irradiation; for example, the estimated age at onset of puberty in a boy irradiated at 2 years of age would be 9.79 years and that for a boy irradiated at 9 years of age would be 11.82 years. In the context of GH deficiency, which is usually associated with a delay in the onset of puberty, this is abnormal. In a more recent study, Lannering *et al.* also showed that boys who received high doses of irradiation for brain tumors entered puberty at a median age of 10.5 years compared to an average age for Swedish boys of 12.4 years;[72] again emphasizing the disappearance of sexual dichotomy with higher radiation doses.

The mechanism for early puberty after irradiation is likely to be related to disinhibition of cortical influences on the hypothalamus. Puberty then proceeds through the increased frequency and amplitude of GnRH pulsatile secretion by the hypothalamus. The clinical observations in humans of radiation dose dependency of

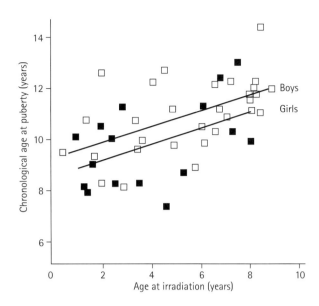

Figure 8a.3 *Estimated and fitted chronological ages at the onset of puberty for age at irradiation.* ■, *girls;* □, *boys. (Reproduced from Ogilvy-Stuart AL, Clayton PE, Shalet SM. Cranial irradiation and early puberty. J Clin Endocrinol Metab 1994; **78**:1282–1286 with permission of the copyright holder, The Endocrine Society.)*

abnormalities in gonadotrophin secretion have been recently confirmed in an animal model. Roth *et al.* selectively irradiated the h-p region of infantile or juvenile female rats with a single dose of 4, 5, 6, 9 or 2 × 9 Gy.[73] High radiation doses (9 Gy or more) caused retardation of sexual maturation, lower gonadotrophin levels and growth retardation associated with GH deficiency, whereas low radiation doses (5 or 6 Gy) led to accelerated onset of puberty as well as elevated LH and estradiol levels in 20 per cent of infantile rats, but not the older (juvenile) rats suggesting, in addition, age dependency for the premature activation of the hypothalamic GnRH-pulse generator. The authors also showed that, in animals irradiated with 5 Gy, the release rates of the inhibitory neurotransmitter GABA from hypothalamic explants were significantly lower and the GnRH expression in the hypothalamic preoptic area was significantly higher than in controls.[74] They postulated that radiation-induced precocious puberty might be caused by damage to inhibitory GABAergic neurons leading to disinhibition and premature activation of GnRH neurons. A single whole-brain dose of 10 Gy in rats has been shown to be biologically equivalent to a dose of 24 Gy in human given in 12–14 fractions.[75]

The outcome of precocious puberty is usually worse in irradiated children as GH deficiency is almost always present leading to attenuation of the pubertal growth spurt, resulting in a further loss of growth potential. Furthermore, the window of opportunity offered by GH replacement is reduced in the GH-deficient child

GROWTH AND CANCER TREATMENT

Growth impairment is frequently seen following successful cancer treatment in children. In many patients, this results in reduced statural growth and final height. Although radiation-induced GH deficiency is a common cause of growth impairment in cancer survivors, a variety of other factors could also contribute, including the disease process itself, decreased nutritional intake, psychosocial dysfunction, chemotherapy, steroid therapy, spinal irradiation, hypothyroidism, hypogonadism, precocious puberty and the non-endocrine complications of various treatment modalities.

GROWTH IN CHILDREN TREATED FOR ALL

Many controversies and, therefore, confusion have been generated over the growth patterns of children treated for ALL. A major reason for the difficulty in interpretation of data is that most studies have analyzed growth in children treated with both prophylactic cranial irradiation and combination chemotherapy (CT) schedules. Thus, disentangling the adverse contribution of these two major therapeutic modalities on growth has proved difficult. However, some conclusions acceptable to most investigators can be drawn.

Early growth deceleration with bone age retardation during treatment for ALL is well recognized and is mainly attributed to the adverse effects of chemotherapy on growth. Schriock et al. showed that the mean decrease in height standard deviation score (SDS) at the end of chemotherapy in 70 out of 115 patients (90 per cent) was -0.74 ± 0.53 and -0.91 ± 0.47 in patients who received prophylactic cranial or craniospinal irradiation, respectively.[96] The greatest drop in height SDS occurs in the first year of chemotherapy[97] and is most marked in the very young children (<4 years).[96,97] Unlike final height, early growth impairment is unrelated to the radiation schedule used for prophylaxis[98] and occurs to the same extent in those who did not receive prophylactic cranial radiation.[99,100]

On completion of chemotherapy, 70 per cent of patients will show a variable degree of catch-up growth, if the chemotherapy was not intensive and prolonged.[2] Catch-up growth occurs in the irradiated and non-irradiated patients[99] and is associated with a progression in bone age maturation.[101] It lasts at least 1 year and, in some patients, can result in a return of height SDS to baseline values,[96,102] usually within 2–3 years. Catch-up growth tends to be complete in the non-irradiated patients but suboptimal in the irradiated patients.[100]

Other factors contributing to growth impairment in these early stages may include malnutrition, recurrent infection, sickness and the disease itself. It is difficult to quantify the role of GH deficiency at this stage. GH secretion, assessed longitudinally during the first 24 months of treatment for ALL, was suppressed completely during dexamethasone treatment.[103]

Before 1981 most children with ALL received a cranial irradiation dose of 24–25 Gy. Although studies of growth for the first few years after irradiation suggested that any impact on growth was minor, final height data show unequivocally that height loss from the time of primary therapy is significant with between 31 and 48 per cent of children losing 10 cm or more of height.[104] Contributing factors include evolving radiation-induced GH deficiency, precocious puberty and possibly spinal irradiation. Kirk et al. demonstrated a final height of 1.37 SD below the population mean in 71 per cent of survivors 6 years after therapy that involved cranial irradiation with 24 Gy.[34] GH deficiency was documented in most patients either pharmacologically or physiologically. Schriock et al. showed that 74 per cent and 37 per cent will achieve a final height that is >1 SD or 2 SD below population mean, respectively.[96] Similarly, Robison et al. found a threefold excess in the proportion of males and a 4.2-fold excess in the proportion of females below the fifth percentile.[105] The height distributions observed for patients treated with craniospinal radiation only or cranial radiation plus intrathecal methotrexate were not different, although both deviated significantly from expected.[105]

As the lower cranial irradiation dose of 18 Gy was only introduced in the 1980, less final height data are available in children receiving this dose of irradiation. Nonetheless, Davies et al. showed that significant loss of standing height occurred in both 18-Gy as well as the 24-Gy cohorts of children, and although the height loss was greater in the higher dose group, this difference was not significant.[104] Indeed, with time it may be that the difference between the 18-Gy and 24-Gy groups is shown to be even less than in this study,[104] as the median age at diagnosis for the 24-Gy group (4.2 years girls, 4.9 years boys) was significantly younger than for the 18-Gy group (7.3 years girls, 9.4 years boys), allowing them more time for height loss. In contrast, Sklar et al. showed a significant difference in height loss in patients treated with 24 Gy compared to 18 Gy with a change in height SDS between diagnosis and achievement of final height of -1.38 ± 0.16 and -0.65 ± 0.15, respectively.[106] In both these studies, no spinal irradiation was given.[104,106]

Chemotherapy may also play a role in growth impairment. The discrepancy in height loss between two groups of children who received similar cranial irradiation schedules but CT of varying intensity provided indirect evidence for the effect of CT.[34,97] There is also in vitro evidence from rat liver perfusion experiments that GH-stimulated production of IGF-1 is inhibited by 6-mercaptopurine[107] and chronic administration of 6-mercaptopurine has been

shown experimentally to impair the growth of animals.[108] There may also be a direct effect of CT on the epiphyses. This has been demonstrated in growth plate specimens from children with osteosarcoma[109] and also by studying the impact of CT on short-term leg growth by performing knemometry on unirradiated children during the first 6 months of combination CT for ALL. The median leg length velocity was at its lowest at the end of the intensification block of CT, but markers of GH status remained within 2 SD of the mean, suggesting that the mechanism of growth failure at this time was related to the impact of CT on the growth plate.[110,111] CT-induced GH deficiency appears to be a real entity,[112] which needed to be excluded in the knemometry studies; however, there are no detailed studies of GH status in children who received CT alone for ALL. Furthermore, in a large USA final-height study, Sklar et al. showed that there was significant but modest height loss in children who received CT alone for ALL (height SD -0.49 ± 0.14), the height loss was appreciably less than in those who also received cranial irradiation (height SD -1.38 after 24-Gy irradiation).[106] If the CT was capable of causing sustained severe GH deficiency, one would have anticipated much greater height loss in the CT-only cohort. In addition, other workers[99,113,114] have not found a significant height reduction 5 years from diagnosis or at final height in children treated with CT alone. Thus, the variation in reported results almost certainly reflects differences in the intensity and duration of CT schedules.

The use of short-term growth data in the irradiated patient to predict the final height outcome can be misleading. Some children may have a 'normal' growth pattern initially; however, their growth curve may deteriorate in subsequent years. It is possible that the detrimental effects of prophylactic cranial irradiation in some patients may become apparent only several years after therapy and usually around the time of puberty or shortly before. This could be explained on the basis of late occurrence of GH deficiency and/or precocious puberty or that the h-p axis is not damaged to the extent that will impair the production of GH prepubertally and hence growth, but will fail to cope with the increased demands for GH during puberty resulting in an obvious growth deceleration.[115]

Spinal irradiation is a documented cause of impaired spinal growth,[116] which in severe cases can lead to skeletal disproportion and short stature.[117] It is likely that this effect is dose related but very few studies exist with growth data that allow one to analyze this relationship. The work of Robison et al. suggests that the dose of spinal irradiation received during craniospinal irradiation (24 Gy; fraction size 120–200 cGy) alone was insufficient to impair spinal growth.[105] Unfortunately, in this study no measurements of sitting height were available.

A major surprise in the final height data reported by Davies et al. was significant disproportion with relatively short spine in patients treated with either 18 or 24 Gy of cranial irradiation but no spinal irradiation.[104] A total of 81 per cent of those children in whom sitting height data were available had relatively shorter backs than legs and in nearly quarter of the children the disproportion was of a marked degree (greater than 2 SD difference between leg length and sitting height). After mathematical correction for sitting height loss, there was no longer a significant reduction in standing height SD score at final height in all except the 24 Gy group of girls. These data suggest that, at least in some children, much if not all of the height loss seen is due to a reduction in sitting height. The explanation for the disproportion is not yet resolved, but the timing of pubertal onset does not explain the observation, as the latter is not systematically delayed in either sex. Possible hypotheses include an effect of CT on the epiphysial growth plate of the spine or, alternatively, GH insufficiency confined primarily to the pubertal phase of growth during which spinal growth normally exceeds leg length growth.

It is now accepted that cranial irradiation with 18–25 Gy is capable of inducing GH deficiency during childhood. The major problems have been, however, to determine the exact contribution of the GH deficiency to the adverse growth pattern, how to diagnose the GH deficiency and to establish if such children benefit from GH replacement therapy. Patients with pharmacologically documented GH deficiency have the worst final height prognosis,[118,119] with a loss in height SDS as high as 1.7 ± 0.2 compared to 0.9 ± 0.2 in children with a normal peak GH response to stimulation. Furthermore, in a recent study of GH status and final height in adult survivors of childhood ALL, Brennan et al. showed that the worst final height outcome with a median loss in height of -2.1 SD was seen in patients with severe GH deficiency, suggesting that much of the height loss could have been prevented by GH replacement therapy.[35]

GROWTH IN CHILDREN AFTER BMT

Bone marrow transplantation preparative regimens are designed to suppress the immune system and to eradicate the underlying hematological disorder or malignancy. Commonly used regimens have included high-dose cyclophosphamide (CY) given alone or in combination with TBI or total lymphoid irradiation; more recently, the combination of high-dose busulphan (BU) with CY has been used. The number of children with leukemia receiving BMT is increasing and, in particular, approximately 20 per cent of children with acute myeloid leukemia will receive a BMT. The post-BMT growth of these children may be adversely affected; potential mechanisms include the direct impact of CT and/or radiotherapy on the skeleton, graft-versus-host disease (GvHD), radiation-induced

GH deficiency and hypothyroidism. The situation is complicated further in that many of these children will have received cranial irradiation and/or CT before undergoing BMT. Thus, the reported post-BMT growth pattern varies considerably; poor growth being observed during the first year after TBI in those who had received previous cranial irradiation but significantly later in those undergoing TBI alone.[120] The medium-term growth data are more contentious: Giorgiani et al. found that growth rates did not differ between these latter two cohorts of children 3 years post-BMT.[120] In contrast, in a study containing less detailed information on the evolution of the growth pattern but data more in line with expectations, Huma et al. reported significantly greater loss in height SD 4 years after BMT in those children who had received previous cranial irradiation in addition to TBI as compared with those who underwent TBI alone.[121]

Thus, therapy, such as cranial irradiation, administered well before the BMT and TBI, may profoundly influence the evolution and severity of the adverse growth pattern witnessed after BMT.

CT–preparative regimens

Children treated for aplastic anemia appear to grow normally after high-dose CY alone[122,123] but, if they received a combination of high-dose Cy and lymphoid irradiation (7.5-Gy single-dose irradiation), the standing height SD was significantly reduced 3 years after transplantation as compared with the pretransplant height.[124] TBI, however, appears to have a much more profound adverse impact on growth.[78,124–127]

The impact of combination of Bu/CY on growth is contentious. Wingard et al. found no difference between the impairment of growth rates over the first 2 post-transplant years in patients treated with BU/CY and those treated with CY/TBI.[128] Sanders reported similar findings[129] and Manenti et al. described reduced growth velocity in children aged between 10 and 12 years following a BMT for thalassemia major with a BU/CY preparative regimen.[130] The latter situation must be complicated by the potential contribution of iron overload-induced gonadotrophin deficiency and pubertal delay. Sanders et al., however, also reported a significant incidence of GH deficiency in children transplanted for leukemia following BU/CY alone.[129]

In contrast to the above reports, Liesner et al.[131] and Giorgiani et al.[120] did not find any significant growth impairment in 31 children (combined series) for up to 4 years after BU/CY and a BMT; interestingly, however, two individual children did grow poorly and showed subnormal GH responses to two provocative stimuli 2 years after BMT.[120]

At this time we can draw no firm conclusions about the impact of BU/CY on growth. Minimal final height data are available, and substantial biochemical evidence to either confirm or refute the existence of CT-induced GH deficiency is not available, although the growth data of Liesner et al.[131] and Giorgiani et al.[120] suggest that if BU/CY-induced GH deficiency exists, it is very uncommon. On the other hand, there is suggestive evidence that intensive pre-BMT CT may adversely influence growth; in a 6-year follow-up of 32 transplanted long-term survivors of childhood cancer, Willi et al. observed that the 11 patients with neuroblastoma continued to grow poorly, whereas a comparison group of 21 patients treated for leukemia has essentially normal growth 2 years after the procedure.[132] The major therapeutic differences between the two groups included the doses of local radiotherapy, and type and number of cytotoxic drugs used. In comparison with the relatively mild growth-inhibiting effects of the CT regimen for leukemia, the very intensive CT-preparative regimen used in patients with neuroblastoma had significant adverse effects on growth.[132]

Skeletal dysplasia

Several reports have intimated that radiation-induced skeletal dysplasia induces poor growth, if the TBI is administered in a single rather than multiple fractions.[126,127] Curiously, Brauner et al. described a marked difference in the growth outcome in children receiving a single TBI dose of 8 Gy rather than 10 Gy, suggesting a critical threshold;[127] alternatively, the variation in post-BMT growth between their two groups of children might be explained by differences in underlying pathologies and pre-BMT treatment schedules.[127] Furthermore, in the latter study,[127] only four children received 8-Gy single-dose TBI with follow-up for 5 years. More recently, Clement-De Boers et al. have reported final height data, which indicate that substantial height is lost (approximately 2 SD for boys and 1 SD for girls) following 7–8-Gy single-dose TBI and that much of this height loss is late, taking place during puberty.[123]

The proposal that fractionation of the TBI schedule may be a significant factor in the adverse growth outcome has been supported by Huma et al. in a study of children who received hyperfractionated TBI;[121] those children who received hyperfractionated TBI alone showed a decrease in standing height from -0.11 to -0.73 over the first 4 post-BMT years, which the authors interpreted as a smaller decrease in SD than might have been anticipated following conventional-schedule TBI.[121] Unfortunately, follow-up was only for 4 years and no comparative group receiving a conventional TBI schedule was available for study.

In complete contrast, Sanders observed that the type of TBI administered (single or fractionated) had no major effect on growth velocity![129] Sanders reported growth data in 112 girls (30 received 10-Gy single-dose

TBI and 82 received 12–15.57-Gy single dose TBI) and 154 boys (48 received 10 Gy single-dose TBI and 106 received fractionated-dose TBI).[129] Despite these apparently very large numbers, detailed longitudinal growth data are not available in these populations of children. In support of the observations of Sanders, Brauner et al. showed that the growth rate rapidly decreased during the 3 years after TBI only in those patients given the 10-Gy TBI as a single exposure but not in children given 12 Gy in six fractions.[127] If, however, follow-up was extended for a longer period of time, the same group showed that the effects of a single 10-Gy dose and a 12-Gy fractionated dose on growth are similar 5 years after BMT.[133]

In addition to the significant reduction in standing height SD after TBI, altered body proportions with a relatively short spine have been described.[126] This disproportion has been seen as early as 1 year after TBI for ALL, irrespective of the schedule of irradiation, single or fractionated; caution is necessary, however, before incriminating the TBI, as significant disproportion at final height has been observed in children treated for ALL by combination CT and cranial irradiation only,[104] with protocols identical to those of the pretransplant children with ALL studied by Thomas et al.[126]

Graft-versus-host disease

Graft-versus-host disease complicating BMT may be associated with considerable impairment of growth.[126] The acute growth suppressive effects of glucocorticoids would explain the deceleration of linear growth in most chronic GvHD patients. In some patients, however, once chronic GvHD is controlled, growth rates may return to normal and catch-up growth may be seen.[129] Other children fail to achieve catch-up growth after completion of treatment and equally decreased growth rates of the patients with chronic GvHD who did not receive treatment suggest that factors other than steroids contributed to their decreased growth,[78] i.e. the disease process itself.

Growth hormone status

There are now abundant studies which have shown a significant incidence of GH deficiency (20–70 per cent) following TBI and high-dose CT.[36,120,133–138] The majority of these studies have reported impaired GH responses to provocative stimuli, although a few groups have described reduced spontaneous GH secretion.[136,138]

Initially, there was some dispute about the impact of fractionation of the TBI schedule on GH status, the suggestion being that fractionation might reduce the risk of GH deficiency.[127] Subsequently, however, Thomas et al. and Brauner et al. could find no evidence that fractionation was beneficial in this regard.[133,139] Furthermore,

there is no evidence that hyperfractionation of the TBI schedules preserves GH status, as Huma et al. reported GH deficiency in three of five children growing poorly after hyperfractionated TBI alone for a BMT without any history of previous cranial irradiation.[121]

There is also a clearer picture with regard to the radiation threshold dose required to induce GH deficiency. On the basis of GH provocative tests and IGF-1 estimations, Clement-De Boers et al. found no evidence of GH deficiency in eight children growing poorly after a single TBI dose of 7–8 Gy,[123] whereas a single TBI dose of 10 Gy or fractionated doses of 12 Gy clearly do induce GH deficiency.[36,133] These conclusions should be treated with caution, however, as Clement-De Boers et al. did not carry out repeated GH provocative testing over time.[123] Therefore, the possibility remains that a TBI dose of 7–8 Gy may induce GH deficiency but not until many years have elapsed.

GROWTH IN CHILDREN TREATED FOR BRAIN TUMORS

Growth impairment during the first year of treatment for brain tumors is well described.[43,140,141] Shalet et al. showed that children whose GH secretion to pharmacological stimuli was adequate over the first year of treatment grew just as poorly as those who developed GH deficiency.[140] Therefore, growth deceleration in the first year does not appear to be related to the development of GH deficiency.

Unlike the situation in leukemia patients, growth deceleration in children with brain tumors during the first year of treatment is not usually followed up by catch-up growth. In contrast, growth impairment may continue progressively and become clinically obvious after the second or third year of starting treatment. This can be attributed to the quick evolution of GH deficiency in view of the higher cranial radiation doses and the effects of spinal irradiation on spinal growth. Albertsson-Wikland et al. found severely disturbed spontaneous 24-hour GH secretion in all children who showed growth deviation of more than 1 SD 2 years after radiotherapy (≥40 Gy).[42] In their study, prepubertal children aged between 3 and 8 years at irradiation were at particular risk of having both impaired growth and GH secretion. In this study, however, the contribution of spinal irradiation was not examined and growth impairment was presumed to reflect impaired GH secretion only. In a later study, Brauner et al. examined the impact of spinal irradiation on growth.[43] At the 2-year follow-up, children treated by cranial and spinal irradiation had a mean height of 1.46 ± 0.40 SD below the normal mean, while children given only cranial irradiation (with a similar dose) had a mean height SDS of -0.15 ± 0.18 ($p < 0.02$). Therefore, the loss in total height following craniospinal

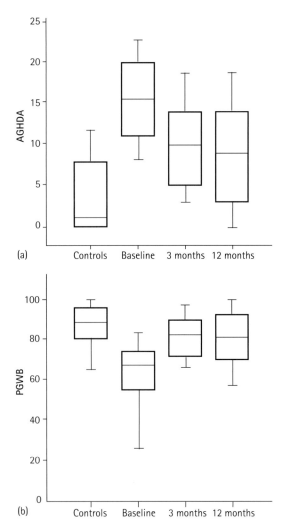

(a)

(b)

Figure 8a.6 *Box and whisker plots, representing quality of life as represented by (a) the Adult Growth-Hormone Deficiency Assessment (AGHDA; range 0–25; high values represent greater morbidity) and (b) the Psychological General Well-Being Index (PGWB; range 0–110; low values represent greater morbidity) in growth hormone (GH)-deficient survivors of childhood cancer during 12 months GH treatment and in healthy control subjects. The lower boundary of the box indicates the 25th percentile, a line within the box marks the median and the upper boundary of the box indicates the 75th percentile. Error bars above and below the box indicate the 90th and 10th percentiles. (Reproduced from Murray RD, Darzy KH, Gleeson HK, et al. GH-deficient survivors of childhood cancer: GH replacement during adult life.* J Clin Endocrinol Metab *2002; 87:129–135 with permission of the copyright holder, The Endocrine Society.)*

KEY POINTS

- Isolated GH deficiency is the most common manifestation of radiation damage to the h-p axis and can occur with low radiation doses.

- Gonadotrophin, TSH and ACTH deficiency and hyperprolactinemia can occur with radiation doses in excess of 40 Gy.
- Precocious or early puberty mostly affects young girls with low radiation doses (<24 Gy) and both sexes equally with higher doses (24–50 Gy).
- Growth impairment and a final height that is well below the target height range are common in cancer survivors, owing to GH deficiency, precocious puberty and spinal irradiation.
- GH therapy can improve final height by preventing further height loss.
- Final height depends on prepubertal height gain and is optimized by GH replacement.
- Precocious puberty reduces the time available for GH therapy to induce height gain.
- GnRH analogue therapy in addition to GH replacement can delay puberty and maximize height gain.
- GH therapy is safe and does not lead to an increased risk of tumor recurrence or *de novo* malignancies.
- Endocrine deficits are persistent and long-term follow up is needed.
- GH replacement therapy in the adult GH deficient survivors of childhood cancer treatment can improve quality of life.

REFERENCES

◆1. Shalet SM, Beardwell CG, Pearson D, *et al.* The effect of varying doses of cerebral irradiation on growth hormone production in childhood. *Clin Endocrinol Oxf* 1976; **5**:287–290.

◆2. Constine LS, Woolf PD, Cann D, *et al.* Hypothalamic-pituitary dysfunction after radiation for brain tumors. *N Engl J Med* 1993; **328**:87–94.

◆3. Clayton PE, Shalet SM. Dose dependency of time of onset of radiation-induced growth hormone deficiency. *J Pediatr* 1991; **118**:226–228.

◆4. Littley MD, Shalet SM, Beardwell CG, *et al.* Radiation-induced hypopituitarism is dose-dependent. *Clin Endocrinol Oxf* 1989; **31**:363–373.

◆5. Lam KS, Tse VK, Wang C, *et al.* Effects of cranial irradiation on hypothalamic-pituitary function – a 5-year longitudinal study in patients with nasopharyngeal carcinoma. *Q J Med* 1991; **78**(286):165–176.

◆6. Duffner PK, Cohen ME, Voorhess ML, *et al.* Long-term effects of cranial irradiation on endocrine function in children with brain tumors. A prospective study. *Cancer* 1985; **56**:2189–2193.

◆7. Samaan NA, Vieto R, Schultz PN, *et al.* Hypothalamic, pituitary and thyroid dysfunction after radiotherapy to the head and neck. *Int J Radiat Oncol Biol Phys* 1982; **8**:1857–1867.

◆8. Chen MS, Lin FJ, Huang MJ, *et al.* Prospective hormone study of hypothalamic-pituitary function in patients with nasopharyngeal

TBI and 82 received 12–15.57-Gy single dose TBI) and 154 boys (48 received 10 Gy single-dose TBI and 106 received fractionated-dose TBI).[129] Despite these apparently very large numbers, detailed longitudinal growth data are not available in these populations of children. In support of the observations of Sanders, Brauner et al. showed that the growth rate rapidly decreased during the 3 years after TBI only in those patients given the 10-Gy TBI as a single exposure but not in children given 12 Gy in six fractions.[127] If, however, follow-up was extended for a longer period of time, the same group showed that the effects of a single 10-Gy dose and a 12-Gy fractionated dose on growth are similar 5 years after BMT.[133]

In addition to the significant reduction in standing height SD after TBI, altered body proportions with a relatively short spine have been described.[126] This disproportion has been seen as early as 1 year after TBI for ALL, irrespective of the schedule of irradiation, single or fractionated; caution is necessary, however, before incriminating the TBI, as significant disproportion at final height has been observed in children treated for ALL by combination CT and cranial irradiation only,[104] with protocols identical to those of the pretransplant children with ALL studied by Thomas et al.[126]

Graft-versus-host disease

Graft-versus-host disease complicating BMT may be associated with considerable impairment of growth.[126] The acute growth suppressive effects of glucocorticoids would explain the deceleration of linear growth in most chronic GvHD patients. In some patients, however, once chronic GvHD is controlled, growth rates may return to normal and catch-up growth may be seen.[129] Other children fail to achieve catch-up growth after completion of treatment and equally decreased growth rates of the patients with chronic GvHD who did not receive treatment suggest that factors other than steroids contributed to their decreased growth,[78] i.e. the disease process itself.

Growth hormone status

There are now abundant studies which have shown a significant incidence of GH deficiency (20–70 per cent) following TBI and high-dose CT.[36,120,133–138] The majority of these studies have reported impaired GH responses to provocative stimuli, although a few groups have described reduced spontaneous GH secretion.[136,138]

Initially, there was some dispute about the impact of fractionation of the TBI schedule on GH status, the suggestion being that fractionation might reduce the risk of GH deficiency.[127] Subsequently, however, Thomas et al. and Brauner et al. could find no evidence that fractionation was beneficial in this regard.[133,139] Furthermore,

there is no evidence that hyperfractionation of the TBI schedules preserves GH status, as Huma et al. reported GH deficiency in three of five children growing poorly after hyperfractionated TBI alone for a BMT without any history of previous cranial irradiation.[121]

There is also a clearer picture with regard to the radiation threshold dose required to induce GH deficiency. On the basis of GH provocative tests and IGF-1 estimations, Clement-De Boers et al. found no evidence of GH deficiency in eight children growing poorly after a single TBI dose of 7–8 Gy,[123] whereas a single TBI dose of 10 Gy or fractionated doses of 12 Gy clearly do induce GH deficiency.[36,133] These conclusions should be treated with caution, however, as Clement-De Boers et al. did not carry out repeated GH provocative testing over time.[123] Therefore, the possibility remains that a TBI dose of 7–8 Gy may induce GH deficiency but not until many years have elapsed.

GROWTH IN CHILDREN TREATED FOR BRAIN TUMORS

Growth impairment during the first year of treatment for brain tumors is well described.[43,140,141] Shalet et al. showed that children whose GH secretion to pharmacological stimuli was adequate over the first year of treatment grew just as poorly as those who developed GH deficiency.[140] Therefore, growth deceleration in the first year does not appear to be related to the development of GH deficiency.

Unlike the situation in leukemia patients, growth deceleration in children with brain tumors during the first year of treatment is not usually followed up by catch-up growth. In contrast, growth impairment may continue progressively and become clinically obvious after the second or third year of starting treatment. This can be attributed to the quick evolution of GH deficiency in view of the higher cranial radiation doses and the effects of spinal irradiation on spinal growth. Albertsson-Wikland et al. found severely disturbed spontaneous 24-hour GH secretion in all children who showed growth deviation of more than 1 SD 2 years after radiotherapy ($\geqslant$40 Gy).[42] In their study, prepubertal children aged between 3 and 8 years at irradiation were at particular risk of having both impaired growth and GH secretion. In this study, however, the contribution of spinal irradiation was not examined and growth impairment was presumed to reflect impaired GH secretion only. In a later study, Brauner et al. examined the impact of spinal irradiation on growth.[43] At the 2-year follow-up, children treated by cranial and spinal irradiation had a mean height of 1.46 $\pm$ 0.40 SD below the normal mean, while children given only cranial irradiation (with a similar dose) had a mean height SDS of -0.15 ± 0.18 ($p < 0.02$). Therefore, the loss in total height following craniospinal

irradiation was, in fact, related to lack of spinal growth. Similar findings were reported a year later by Darendeliler et al.[142] The detailed auxological data over the first 3 years clearly illustrated that sitting height reduction was the major contributing factor to the observed reduction in standing height in patients who received craniospinal irradiation. Later on GH deficiency becomes a significant adverse factor in the growth of irradiated children.[143–149]

The need for spinal irradiation, to prevent spinal relapse, is inevitable in the treatment of brain tumors that exfoliate cells into the cerebrospinal fluid such as medulloblastoma and ependymoma. The impact of direct radiation-damage of the spine is considerable in terms of height loss and disproportionate growth; the latter is reflected by decreased upper-to-lower segment ratios.[150] Shalet et al. studied the final standing and sitting height in adult survivors who had received craniospinal irradiation in comparison with those who had received cranial irradiation only.[151] The median standing height SDS in the first group was −2.37 compared to −1.14 in the second group and, in both groups, both height parameters were significantly correlated with age at irradiation. The latter reflects the fact that the younger the age at which GH deficiency or other adverse factors affecting growth occur then the greater the loss in growth potential. The eventual loss in height due to impaired spinal growth was estimated to be 9 cm, if irradiation was given at 1 year, 7 cm if given at 5 years, and 5.5 cm if given at 10 years.[151]

It has been shown that growth in the first 4 years after treatment with craniospinal irradiation is more profoundly affected in children who have received adjuvant chemotherapy than in those receiving craniospinal irradiation alone, suggesting a synergistic effect on growth retardation when both treatment modalities are combined.[152] More recently, Ogilvy-Stuart and Shalet studied in detail the effects of chemotherapy on final height and found that the detrimental effect of chemotherapy on growth could be as profound as the spinal effect of craniospinal irradiation, and the effect of these two therapies was additive, causing the most severe growth restriction when used in combination.[76] In addition, the degree of height loss was related to the age at irradiation, with the most profound effect on final height occurring in children who were youngest at irradiation (Figure 8a.4). The study also revealed that the use of chemotherapy did not exacerbate skeletal disproportion.[76]

RESPONSE TO GROWTH HORMONE THERAPY

In patients with documented radiation-induced GH deficiency, GH replacement increases growth velocity in the first 3 years of treatment compared with pretreatment

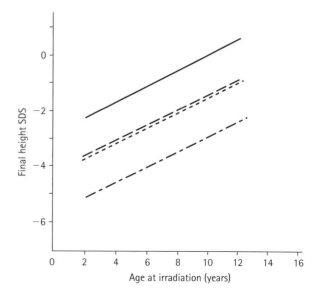

Figure 8a.4 *Parallel linear regression of final height standard deviation score (SDS) on age at irradiation, according to the four treatment groups. Cranial irradiation alone (___), cranial irradiation + chemotherapy alone (_ _ _), craniospinal irradiation alone (____), craniospinal irradiation + chemotherapy (_ . _). (Reproduced from Ogilvy-Stuart AL, Shalet SM. Growth and puberty after growth hormone treatment after irradiation for brain tumors.* Arch Dis Child *1995; 73:141–146 with permission.)*

growth velocity.[120,142,144–148,153–155] However, long-term studies are the most critical and, ideally, these should include an analysis of the final height, and gain or loss in stature (standard deviation score) from initiation of GH therapy until the end of growth in children with radiation-induced GH deficiency, contrasted with the growth pattern in those who did not receive GH therapy.

A few studies have shown that short-term growth responses to GH therapy in cranially irradiated GH deficient patients are comparable in magnitude to those in patients with idiopathic GH deficiency. Continuation of GH therapy until completion of growth, however, failed to produce catch-up growth in the irradiated patients.[147,148,154] Nevertheless, GH therapy in those patients maintained their initial height centile to adulthood, while those who did not receive treatment showed further deterioration in their height centiles with a tendency for extreme short stature.[148,154] Thus, it appears that the role of GH therapy in the irradiated patients is to prevent further loss in stature, rather than induce catch-up growth, which is normally the expected outcome in patients with idiopathic or classical GH deficiency, in whom the change in height SDS to completion of growth may exceed 2 SD compared with a change of less than 0.3 in the irradiated patient.

There are a number of factors that may contribute to the suboptimal growth response, including spinal irradiation, precocious or early puberty, and delayed initiation and inadequacy of GH therapy.

The growth promoting effect of GH therapy on the non-irradiated spine normally matches that observed in the legs and, therefore, GH therapy does not lead to disproportionate final stature in patients with classical GH deficiency.[156] Radiation injury of the spine results in impaired spinal growth resistant to GH therapy.[148,154] Thus, although GH therapy prevents further height loss, it does so at the expense of exaggerating skeletal disproportion (Figure 8a.5), which already exists in the majority of these patients.

GROWTH HORMONE THERAPY AND FINAL HEIGHT OUTCOME

Acute lymphoblastic leukemia

There are very few data on the impact of GH therapy in children with radiation-induced GH deficiency following

the treatment of leukemia. Didi *et al.* reported a mean final height of 159.8 ± 8.5 cm, which was significantly less than the mean midparental height of 165 ± 5.2 cm, but 9 of the 15 children achieved their target height.[157] Adan *et al.* reported similar findings in 17 boys of normal pubertal age who received GH replacement therapy for GH deficiency following 24-Gy cranial irradiation for ALL.[118] In their study, the mean height loss was 1.7 SD in the untreated cohort with subnormal GH status ($n = 15$) compared with 0.6 SD in those who received GH replacement ($n = 17$).

Bone marrow transplant

The literature contains no data on pubertal growth or final height achieved in response to GH replacement in children with TBI-induced GH deficiency. The majority of the therapeutic results are short-term, usually 1 year,

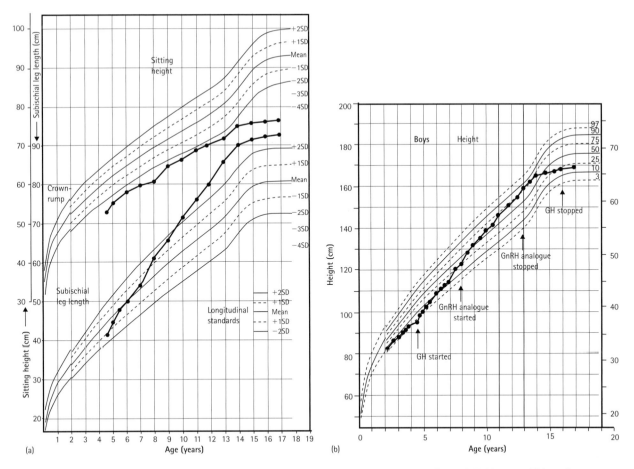

Figure 8a.5 *Severe skeletal disproportion in a patient who received craniospinal irradiation for medulloblastoma. This patient received growth hormone (GH) replacement between age 4 and 16 years, and gonadotrophin-releasing hormone (GnRH) analogue treatment between age 8 and 13 years. Note the excellent growth response in the legs compared to that achieved in the spine (a). Using combined therapy, it was possible to achieve the target height in this patient (b) by extending the period of prepubertal height gain, but at the expense of exaggerating his skeletal disproportion.*

with occasional studies extended to 3 years.[135] There is a general agreement that there is a significant improvement in height velocity over the first year of GH treatment compared with the pretreatment velocity, with responses that range between a modest improvement in growth velocity[133,135,137] and frank catch-up growth.[120,121,136]

Brain tumors

Patients treated for brain tumors have the worst final height prognosis, presumably related to the effects of spinal irradiation, and the earlier onset and more severe degree of GH deficiency. Analysis of final height data from different series showed that the vast majority of such patients do not achieve an adult height above the 50th centile and more than half of them will be below the third centile, despite GH therapy[76,154] (Figure 8a.4).

The disappointing final height results in many series can be attributed, in part, to the delayed initiation of GH therapy and the inadequacy of GH schedules in the early studies.

To date, almost all final height data are derived from observational studies comparing patients' groups who were treated with GH therapy to those who did not. Optimally, prospective, randomized, placebo-controlled trials using various GH therapy schedules in radiation-induced GH deficiency are required to define the exact response to treatment and to explore the optimum GH schedule. Such trials, however, are extremely difficult to carry out for a variety of reasons; they require international coordination and standardization of methods used to diagnose GH deficiency between centers. Most importantly, such trials would be unethical, as many children would have to remain in the untreated arm while growing poorly with biochemical evidence of GH deficiency.

Indications, timing, and safety of GH therapy

There remains an obvious concern about the oncogenic potential of GH replacement in patients treated for a childhood malignancy. Current data from single-center and large multicenter surveillance studies do not suggest either an increase in the risk of brain tumor recurrence or an increase in the incidence of de novo malignancies during GH replacement initiated 2 years or more after the primary treatment.[158–165] Surveillance programs also failed to demonstrate any increase in the risk of leukemia relapse in those treated in first remission.[161,162,164,166] However, substantial data do not exist to determine whether GH replacement might adversely influence the prognosis of the child with a previous history of relapse.[167]

The chance of a brain tumor recurrence is greatest in the first 2 years following the completion of the primary treatment. Consequently, GH therapy is not offered within this time period, as it may be associated with a number of tumor recurrences and deaths. Therefore, despite a lack of proof of a causal relationship, many families and doctors would associate GH therapy with tumor recurrence. A reasonable approach, therefore, at 2 years (a time point that is negotiable with the pediatric oncologist) after primary treatment would be to consider for GH therapy all children with brain tumors treated by standard radiation schedules, including a dose to the hypothalamic-pituitary axis in excess of 30 Gy. By this time they would no longer be receiving cytotoxic chemotherapy, the risk of tumor recurrence is low and it is established that most, if not all, will be GH-deficient. In certain centers, GH therapy would be offered routinely at 2 years without recourse to GH tests or evidence of impaired growth. Alternatively, others would consider GH therapy when GH deficiency is established biochemically irrespective of growth rate. These approaches assume, given the epidemiological evidence, that it is highly likely that growth will soon decline in those patients or that an 'apparently' normal growth rate is perhaps subnormal. A more selective approach, however, is still adopted by some endocrinologists who would insist on biochemical evidence of GH deficiency and a subnormal growth rate before initiating GH treatment.

Where the natural history of radiation-induced GH deficiency is less predictable or less well known, for example, after a radiation dose of 20–30 Gy, standard provocative tests of GH release are performed at 2 years and, if the results are abnormal, the children receive GH therapy, again independent of the growth rate. If GH status appears to be normal and the growth rate is appropriate for pubertal status, then growth is observed closely and the GH stimulation tests are repeated annually. However, if the growth rate is subnormal in the presence of normal GH responses to pharmacological stimuli, then GH neurosecretory dysfunction may be a possible explanation. Alternative approaches to this situation would be either an appraisal of physiological GH secretion, such as a 24-hour profile, or an empirical trial of GH therapy. In practice, 24-hour GH profiles are reserved for research studies and not clinical management.

These guidelines assume that, in craniospinal-irradiated children, growth is assessed by leg-length velocity, and that other endocrine and non-endocrine causes of poor growth have been excluded or treated. In the clinic, the timing of the introduction of GH therapy is matched with the special circumstances, age, pubertal status and needs of an individual child. Early treatment is particularly suitable for the craniospinally irradiated young child of short parents.

MANAGEMENT OF GH DEFICIENCY DURING PUBERTY – THE ROLE OF GnRH ANALOGUE THERAPY

Normal pubertal growth and development requires intact gonadotrophic and somatotrophic axes. Puberty is normally associated with about a twofold increase in daily GH production. It is unclear whether this rise represents an epiphenomenon or a real physiological requirement. Children with GH deficiency enter puberty late and fail to achieve a satisfactory pubertal growth spurt. Therefore, it has been advocated, previously, that the GH dose should be increased during puberty to aid this growth spurt and mimic normal physiology. However, there is no convincing evidence of additional benefit from using higher GH doses.[168] The lack of further height gain may be attributed to accelerated skeletal maturation and shortened duration of puberty as a consequence of higher GH doses.[168] This is particularly pertinent in cranially irradiated patients, in whom increasing the dose of GH during puberty may be counterproductive because these patients are already prone to accelerated skeletal maturation and attenuated duration of puberty.[170]

An alternative strategy would be the addition of GnRH analogue therapy to GH therapy to halt pubertal progression and delay epiphyseal closure in order to extend the window of opportunity for GH to promote linear growth. This approach is particularly appealing in patients with early or precocious puberty and GH deficiency.

Results of this strategy in the non-irradiated patient are promising.[171–173] Proven benefit of the combined GH and GnRH analogue therapy in the irradiated patients is not yet established. No prospective randomized controlled trial of GnRH analogue plus GH versus GH alone has been carried out in children with radiation-induced GH deficiency and early puberty. Limited observations exist that indicate a better final height outcome for those receiving GnRH analogue plus GH replacement with the additional suggestion that the gain in statural height is primarily a consequence of better spinal growth in those receiving cranial irradiation only.[174] In contrast, height gain in craniospinally irradiated patients is mostly in the legs and, thus, skeletal disproportion, which is already present in most of these patients, is exacerbated (Figure 8a.5).

THE ADULT SURVIVOR

Radiation-induced pituitary hormone deficiencies are irreversible and persist into adult life. Therefore, continued surveillance and management of hormone replacement therapy is required into adult life, and it is imperative

Table 8a.1 *Features of adult growth hormone deficiency*

Low bone mineral density and increased fracture risk

Abnormal body composition:
Increased fat mass with abdominal preponderance
Increased waist/hip ratio
Reduced lean body mass
Reduced muscle bulk
Decreased extracellular water

Metabolic abnormalities:
Abnormal lipid profile
Glucose intolerance
Insulin resistance
Impaired fibrinolysis

Reduced muscle strength and exercise performance

Impaired cardiac function and structure

Premature atherosclerosis

Impaired quality of life and psychological well-being – in particular, reduced energy

that irradiated patients are not lost to follow-up in the transition from pediatric to adult clinics.

Growth hormone deficiency is common in long-term survivors of childhood malignancy. The clinical features of adult GH deficiency syndrome have been described over the last 13 years[175,176] (Table 8a.1) and the benefits of GH replacement therapy in GH-deficient adults proven in double-blind placebo-controlled trials. These include improvement in quality of life and psychological well-being, body composition (increased lean mass and decreased fat mass), lipid profile and other cardiovascular risk factors, and bone mineral density.[176] Currently, in the UK impaired quality of life remains the major indication for a trial of GH replacement in adults.[177,178]

Young adult survivors show an increased prevalence of obesity,[179,180] reduced bone mineral density[181] and adverse lipid profile[182] and impaired quality of life.[183] Many of these abnormalities resemble those associated with the adult GH deficiency syndrome. However, the relative contribution of GH deficiency toward these abnormalities is difficult to disentangle from the direct effects of the primary pathology, irradiation, chemotherapy, high-dose corticosteroids, insufficient exercise and excessive caloric intake. In a recent study, Murray *et al.* analyzed the effects of physiological GH replacement therapy for 12–18 months in GH-deficient adult survivors.[184] Significant improvement in quality of life was observed, but improvements in body composition, the abnormal lipid profile and bone mineral density were minor, suggesting that GH deficiency is not the only etiological factor in the pathogenesis of these abnormalities (Figure 8a.6).

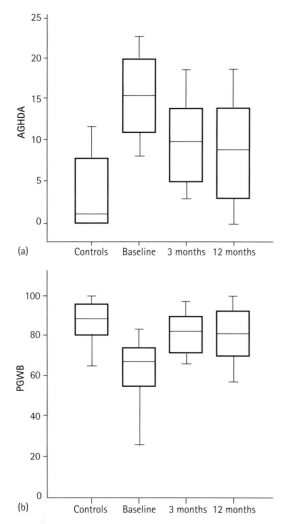

(a)

(b)

Figure 8a.6 *Box and whisker plots, representing quality of life as represented by (a) the Adult Growth-Hormone Deficiency Assessment (AGHDA; range 0–25; high values represent greater morbidity) and (b) the Psychological General Well-Being Index (PGWB; range 0–110; low values represent greater morbidity) in growth hormone (GH)-deficient survivors of childhood cancer during 12 months GH treatment and in healthy control subjects. The lower boundary of the box indicates the 25th percentile, a line within the box marks the median and the upper boundary of the box indicates the 75th percentile. Error bars above and below the box indicate the 90th and 10th percentiles. (Reproduced from Murray RD, Darzy KH, Gleeson HK, et al. GH-deficient survivors of childhood cancer: GH replacement during adult life.* J Clin Endocrinol Metab *2002; 87:129–135 with permission of the copyright holder, The Endocrine Society.)*

KEY POINTS

- Isolated GH deficiency is the most common manifestation of radiation damage to the h-p axis and can occur with low radiation doses.

- Gonadotrophin, TSH and ACTH deficiency and hyperprolactinemia can occur with radiation doses in excess of 40 Gy.
- Precocious or early puberty mostly affects young girls with low radiation doses (<24 Gy) and both sexes equally with higher doses (24–50 Gy).
- Growth impairment and a final height that is well below the target height range are common in cancer survivors, owing to GH deficiency, precocious puberty and spinal irradiation.
- GH therapy can improve final height by preventing further height loss.
- Final height depends on prepubertal height gain and is optimized by GH replacement.
- Precocious puberty reduces the time available for GH therapy to induce height gain.
- GnRH analogue therapy in addition to GH replacement can delay puberty and maximize height gain.
- GH therapy is safe and does not lead to an increased risk of tumor recurrence or *de novo* malignancies.
- Endocrine deficits are persistent and long-term follow up is needed.
- GH replacement therapy in the adult GH deficient survivors of childhood cancer treatment can improve quality of life.

REFERENCES

◆1. Shalet SM, Beardwell CG, Pearson D, *et al.* The effect of varying doses of cerebral irradiation on growth hormone production in childhood. *Clin Endocrinol Oxf* 1976; **5**:287–290.
◆2. Constine LS, Woolf PD, Cann D, *et al.* Hypothalamic-pituitary dysfunction after radiation for brain tumors. *N Engl J Med* 1993; **328**:87–94.
◆3. Clayton PE, Shalet SM. Dose dependency of time of onset of radiation-induced growth hormone deficiency. *J Pediatr* 1991; **118**:226–228.
◆4. Littley MD, Shalet SM, Beardwell CG, *et al.* Radiation-induced hypopituitarism is dose-dependent. *Clin Endocrinol Oxf* 1989; **31**:363–373.
◆5. Lam KS, Tse VK, Wang C, *et al.* Effects of cranial irradiation on hypothalamic-pituitary function – a 5-year longitudinal study in patients with nasopharyngeal carcinoma. *Q J Med* 1991; **78**(286):165–176.
◆6. Duffner PK, Cohen ME, Voorhess ML, *et al.* Long-term effects of cranial irradiation on endocrine function in children with brain tumors. A prospective study. *Cancer* 1985; **56**:2189–2193.
◆7. Samaan NA, Vieto R, Schultz PN, *et al.* Hypothalamic, pituitary and thyroid dysfunction after radiotherapy to the head and neck. *Int J Radiat Oncol Biol Phys* 1982; **8**:1857–1867.
◆8. Chen MS, Lin FJ, Huang MJ, *et al.* Prospective hormone study of hypothalamic-pituitary function in patients with nasopharyngeal

carcinoma after high dose irradiation. *Jpn J Clin Oncol* 1989; **19**:265–270.

◆9. Shalet SM, Price DA, Beardwell CG, *et al.* Normal growth despite abnormalities of growth hormone secretion in children treated for acute leukemia. *J Pediatr* 1979; **94**:719–722.

◆10. Schmiegelow M, Lassen S, Poulsen HS, *et al.* Cranial radiotherapy of childhood brain tumours: growth hormone deficiency and its relation to the biological effective dose of irradiation in a large population based study. *Clin Endocrinol* 2000; **53**:191–197.

◆11. Shalet SM, Beardwell CG, Morris-Jones PH, *et al.* Pituitary function after treatment of intracranial tumours in children. *Lancet* 1975; **2**(7925):104–107.

◆12. Littley MD, Shalet SM, Beardwell CG, *et al.* Hypopituitarism following external radiotherapy for pituitary tumours in adults. *Q J Med* 1989; **70**(262):145–160.

◆13. Ahmed SR, Shalet SM, Beardwell CG. The effects of cranial irradiation on growth hormone secretion. *Acta Paediatr Scand* 1986; **75**:255–260.

◆14. Chrousos GP, Poplack D, Brown T, *et al.* Effects of cranial radiation on hypothalamic-adenohypophyseal function: abnormal growth hormone secretory dynamics. *J Clin Endocrinol Metab* 1982; **54**:1135–1139.

◆15. Lannering B, Albertsson-Wikland K. Growth hormone release in children after cranial irradiation. *Horm Res* 1987; **27**:13–22.

◆16. Costin G. Effects of low-dose cranial radiation on growth hormone secretory dynamics and hypothalamic–pituitary function. *Am J Dis Child* 1988; **142**:847–852.

◆17. Ryalls M, Spoudeas HA, Hindmarsh PC, *et al.* Short-term endocrine consequences of total body irradiation and bone marrow transplantation in children treated for leukemia. *J Endocrinol* 1993; **136**:331–338.

◆18. Samaan NA, Bakdash MM, Caderao JB, *et al.* Hypopituitarism after external irradiation. Evidence for both hypothalamic and pituitary origin. *Ann Intern Med* 1975; **83**:771–777.

◆19. Blacklay A, Grossman A, Ross RJ, *et al.* Cranial irradiation for cerebral and nasopharyngeal tumours in children: evidence for the production of a hypothalamic defect in growth hormone release. *J Endocrinol* 1986; **108**:25–29.

◆20. Lam KS, Wang C, Yeung RT, *et al.* Hypothalamic hypopituitarism following cranial irradiation for nasopharyngeal carcinoma. *Clin Endocrinol (Oxf)* 1986; **24**:643–651.

◆21. Pai HH, Thornton A, Katznelson L, *et al.* Hypothalamic/pituitary function following high-dose conformal radiotherapy to the base of skull: demonstration of a dose–effect relationship using dose–volume histogram analysis. *J Radiat Oncol Biol Phys* 2001; **49**:1079–1092.

◆22. Jadresic A, Jimenez LE, Joplin GF. Long-term effect of 90Y pituitary implantation in acromegaly. *Acta Endocrinol* 1987; **115**:301–306.

◆23. Schmiegelow M, Lassen S, Poulsen HS, *et al.* Growth hormone response to a growth hormone-releasing hormone stimulation test in a population-based study following cranial irradiation of childhood brain tumors. *Horm Res* 2000; **54**:53–59.

◆24. Spoudeas HA, Hindmarsh PC, Matthews DR, *et al.* Evolution of growth hormone neurosecretory disturbance after cranial irradiation for childhood brain tumours: a prospective study. *J Endocrinol* 1996; **150**:329–342.

◆25. Achermann JC, Hindmarsh PC, Robinson IC, *et al.* The relative roles of continuous growth hormone-releasing hormone (GHRH(1-29)NH2) and intermittent somatostatin(1-14)(SS) in growth hormone (GH) pulse generation: studies in normal and post cranial irradiated individuals. *Clin Endocrinol (Oxf)* 1999; **51**:575–585.

◆26. Dorzy KH, Aimaretti G, Wieringa G, *et al.* The usefulnes of the combined growth hormone (GH)-releasing hormone and arginine stimulation test in the diagnosis of radiation-induced GH deficiency is dependent on the post-irradiation time interval. *J Clin Endocrinol Metab* 2003; **88**:95–102.

◆27. Chieng PU, Huang TS, Chang CC, *et al.* Reduced hypothalamic blood flow after radiation treatment of nasopharyngeal cancer: SPECT studies in 34 patients. *AJNR Am J Neuroradiol* 1991; **12**:661–665.

◆28. Robinson IC, Fairhall KM, Hendry JH, *et al.* Differential radiosensitivity of hypothalamo-pituitary function in the young adult rat. *J Endocrinol* 2001; **169**:519–526.

◆29. Hochberg Z, Kuten A, Hertz P, *et al.* The effect of single-dose radiation on cell survival and growth hormone secretion by rat anterior pituitary cells. *Radiat Res* 1983; **94**:508–512.

◆30. Jorgensen EV, Schwartz ID, Hvizdala E, *et al.* Neurotransmitter control of growth hormone secretion in children after cranial radiation therapy. *J Pediatr Endocrinol* 1993; **6**:131–142.

◆31. Ogilvy-Stuart AL, Wallace WH, Shalet SM. Radiation and neuroregulatory control of growth hormone secretion. *Clin Endocrinol (Oxf)* 1994; **41**:163–168.

◆32. Ogilvy-Stuart AL, Stirling HF, Kelnar CJ, *et al.* Treatment of radiation-induced growth hormone deficiency with growth hormone-releasing hormone. *Clin Endocrinol (Oxf)* 1997; **46**:571–578.

◆33. Shalet SM, Beardwell CG, Jones PH, *et al.* Growth hormone deficiency after treatment of acute leukaemia in children. *Arch Dis Child* 1976; **51**:489–493.

◆34. Kirk JA, Raghupathy P, Stevens MM, *et al.* Growth failure and growth-hormone deficiency after treatment for acute lymphoblastic leukaemia. *Lancet* 1987; **1**(8526):190–193.

◆35. Brennan BM, Rahim A, Mackie EM, *et al.* Growth hormone status in adults treated for acute lymphoblastic leukaemia in childhood. *Clin Endocrinol (Oxf)* 1998; **48**:777–783.

◆36. Ogilvy-Stuart AL, Clark DJ, Wallace WH, *et al.* Endocrine deficit after fractionated total body irradiation. *Arch Dis Child* 1992; **67**:1107–1110.

◆37. Littley MD, Shalet SM, Morgenstern GR, *et al.* Endocrine and reproductive dysfunction following fractionated total body irradiation in adults. *Q J Med* 1991; **78**(287):265–274.

◆38. Brauner R, Czernichow P, Rappaport R. Greater susceptibility to hypothalamopituitary irradiation in younger children with acute lymphoblastic leukemia. *J Pediatr* 1986; **108**:332.

◆39. Samaan NA, Schultz PN, Yang KP, *et al.* Endocrine complications after radiotherapy for tumors of the head and neck. *J Lab Clin Med* 1987; **109**:364–372.

◆40. Blatt J, Bercu BB, Gillin JC, *et al.* Reduced pulsatile growth hormone secretion in children after therapy for acute lymphoblastic leukemia. *J Pediatr* 1984; **104**:182–186.

◆41. Bercu BB, Diamond FB Jr. Growth hormone neurosecretory dysfunction. *Clin Endocrinol Metab* 1986; **15**:537–590.

◆42. Albertsson-Wikland K, Lannering B, Marky I, *et al.* A longitudinal study on growth and spontaneous growth hormone (GH) secretion in children with irradiated brain tumors. *Acta Paediatr Scand* 1987; **76**:966–973.

◆43. Brauner R, Rappaport R, Prevot C, *et al.* A prospective study of the development of growth hormone deficiency in children given cranial irradiation, and its relation to statural growth. *J Clin Endocrinol Metab* 1989; **68**:346–351.

◆44. Moell C, Garwicz S, Westgren U, *et al.* Suppressed spontaneous secretion of growth hormone in girls after treatment for acute lymphoblastic leukaemia. *Arch Dis Child* 1989; **64**:252–258.

◆45. Moell C, Garwicz S, Westgren U, *et al.* Disturbed pubertal growth in girls treated for acute lymphoblastic leukemia. *Pediatr Hematol Oncol* 1987; **4**:1–5.

◆46. Crowne EC, Moore C, Wallace WH, et al. A novel variant of growth hormone (GH) insufficiency following low dose cranial irradiation. Clin Endocrinol (Oxf) 1992; 36:59–68.

◆47. Lannering B, Rosberg S, Marky I, et al. Reduced growth hormone secretion with maintained periodicity following cranial irradiation in children with acute lymphoblastic leukaemia. Clin Endocrinol (Oxf) 1995; 42:153–159.

◆48. Stubberfield TG, Byrne GC, Jones TW. Growth and growth hormone secretion after treatment for acute lymphoblastic leukemia in childhood. 18-Gy versus 24-Gy cranial irradiation. J Pediatr Hematol Oncol 1995; 17:167–171.

◆49. Shalet SM, Brennan BM. Growth and growth hormone status following treatment for childhood leukaemia. Horm Res 1998; 50:1–10.

◆50. Hoffman DM, O'Sullivan AJ, Baxter RC, et al. Diagnosis of growth-hormone deficiency in adults. Lancet 1994; 343(8905):1064–1068.

◆51. Growth Hormone Research Society. Consensus guidelines for the diagnosis and treatment of adults with growth hormone deficiency: summary statement of the Growth Hormone Research Society Workshop on Adult Growth Hormone Deficiency. J Clin Endocrinol Metab 1998; 83:379–381.

◆52. Lissett CA, Saleem S, Rahim A, et al. The impact of irradiation on growth hormone responsiveness to provocative agents is stimulus dependent: results in 161 individuals with radiation damage to the somatotropic axis. Clin Endocrinol Metab 2001; 86:663–668.

◆53. Dickinson WP, Berry DH, Dickinson L, et al. Differential effects of cranial radiation on growth hormone response to arginine and insulin infusion. J Pediatr 1978; 92:754–757.

◆54. Shalet SM, Toogood AA, Rahim A, et al. The diagnosis of growth hormone deficiency in children and adults. Endocrine Rev 1998; 19:203–223.

◆55. Tillmann V, Buckler JM, Kibirige MS, et al. Biochemical tests in the diagnosis of childhood growth hormone deficiency. J Clin Endocrinol Metab 1997; 82:531–535.

◆56. Sklar C, Sarafoglou K, Whittam E. Efficacy of insulin-like growth factor binding protein 3 in predicting the growth hormone response to provocative testing in children treated with cranial irradiation. Acta Endocrinol 1993; 129:511–515.

◆57. Nivot S, Benelli C, Clot JP, et al. Nonparallel changes of growth hormone (GH) and insulin-like growth factor-I, insulin-like growth factor binding protein-3, and GH-binding protein, after craniospinal irradiation and chemotherapy. J Clin Endocrinol Metab 1994; 78:597–601.

◆58. Tillmann V, Shalet SM, Price DA, et al. Serum insulin-like growth factor-I, IGF binding protein-3 and IGFBP-3 protease activity after cranial irradiation. Horm Res 1998; 50:71–77.

◆59. Achermann JC, Hindmarsh PC, Brook CG. The relationship between the growth hormone and insulin-like growth factor axis in long-term survivors of childhood brain tumours. Clin Endocrinol Oxf 1998; 49:639–645.

◆60. Cicognani A, Cacciari E, Pession A, et al. Insulin-like growth factor-I (IGF-I) and IGF-binding protein-3 (IGFBP-3) concentrations compared to stimulated growth hormone (GH) in the evaluation of children treated for malignancy. J Pediatr Endocrinol Metab 1999; 12:629–638.

◆61. Adan L, Trivin C, Sainte-Rose C, et al. GH deficiency caused by cranial irradiation during childhood: factors and markers in young adults. J Clin Endocrinol Metab 2001; 86:5245–5251.

◆62. Pasqualini T, Escobar ME, Domene H, et al. Evaluation of gonadal function following long-term treatment for acute lymphoblastic leukemia in girls. Am J Pediatr Hematol Oncol 1987; 9:15–22.

◆63. Sanders JE, Buckner CD, Leonard JM, et al. Late effects on gonadal function of cyclophosphamide, total-body irradiation, and marrow transplantation. Transplantation 1983; 36:252–255.

◆64. Rappaport R, Brauner R, Czernichow P, et al. Effect of hypothalamic and pituitary irradiation on pubertal development in children with cranial tumors. J Clin Endocrinol Metab 1982; 54:1164–1168.

◆65. Yoshimoto Y, Moridera K, Imura H. Restoration of normal pituitary gonadotropin reserve by administration of luteinizing-hormone-releasing hormone in patients with hypogonadotropic hypogonadism. N Engl J Med 1975; 292:242–245.

◆66. Hall JE, Martin KA, Whitney HA, et al. Potential for fertility with replacement of hypothalamic gonadotropin-releasing hormone in long term female survivors of cranial tumors. J Clin Endocrinol Metab 1994; 79:1166–1172.

◆67. Brauner R, Czernichow P, Rappaport R. Precocious puberty after hypothalamic and pituitary irradiation in young children. N Engl J Med 1984; 311:920.

◆68. Brauner R, Rappaport R. Precocious puberty secondary to cranial irradiation for tumors distant from the hypothalamo-pituitary area. Horm Res 1985; 22(1–2):78–82.

◆69. Leiper AD, Stanhope R, Kitching P, et al. Precocious and premature puberty associated with treatment of acute lymphoblastic leukaemia. Arch Dis Child 1987; 62:1107–1112.

◆70. Quigley C, Cowell C, Jimenez M, et al. Normal or early development of puberty despite gonadal damage in children treated for acute lymphoblastic leukemia. N Engl J Med 1989; 321:143–151.

◆71. Ogilvy-Stuart AL, Clayton PE, Shalet SM. Cranial irradiation and early puberty. J Clin Endocrinol Metab 1994; 78:1282–1286.

◆72. Lannering B, Jansson C, Rosberg S, et al. Increased LH and FSH secretion after cranial irradiation in boys. Med Pediatr Oncol 1997; 29:280–287.

◆73. Roth C, Schmidberger H, Schaper O, et al. Cranial irradiation of female rats causes dose-dependent and age-dependent activation or inhibition of pubertal development. Pediatr Res 2000; 47:586–591.

◆74. Roth C, Lakomek M, Schmidberger H, et al. Cranial irradiation induces premature activation of the gonadotropin-releasing-hormone. Klin Padiatr 2001; 213:239–243.

◆75. Schunior A, Zengel AE, Mullenix PJ, et al. An animal model to study toxicity of central nervous system therapy for childhood acute lymphoblastic leukemia: effects on growth and craniofacial proportion. Cancer Res 1990; 50:6455–6460.

◆76. Ogilvy-Stuart AL, Shalet SM. Growth and puberty after growth hormone treatment after irradiation for brain tumours. Arch Dis Child 1995; 73:141–146.

◆77. Livesey EA, Hindmarsh PC, Brook CG, et al. Endocrine disorders following treatment of childhood brain tumours. Br J Cancer 1990; 61:622–625.

◆78. Sanders JE, Pritchard S, Mahoney P, et al. Growth and development following marrow transplantation for leukemia. Blood 1986; 68:1129–1135.

◆79. Shankar RR, Jakacki RI, Haider A, et al. Testing the hypothalamic-pituitary-adrenal axis in survivors of childhood brain and skull-based tumors. J Clin Endocrinol Metab 1997; 82:1995–1998.

◆80. Rose SR, Lustig RH, Burstein S, et al. Diagnosis of ACTH deficiency. Comparison of overnight metyrapone test to either low-dose or high-dose ACTH test. Horm Res 1999; 52:73–79.

◆81. Tsatsoulis A, Shalet SM, Harrison J, et al. Adrenocorticotrophin (ACTH) deficiency undetected by standard dynamic tests of the hypothalamic-pituitary-adrenal axis. Clin Endocrinol (Oxf) 1988; 28:225–232.

◆82. Crowne EC, Wallace WH, Gibson S, et al. Adrenocorticotrophin and cortisol secretion in children after low dose cranial irradiation. Clin Endocrinol (Oxf) 1993; 39:297–305.

•83. Oberfield SE, Sklar C, Allen J, et al. Thyroid and gonadal function and growth of long-term survivors of medulloblastoma/PNET.

In: Green DM, D'Angio GJ (eds) *Late effects of treatment for childhood cancer.* New York: Wiley-Liss, 1992:55–62.

◆84. Mohn A, Chiarelli F, Di Marzio A, *et al.* Thyroid function in children treated for acute lymphoblastic leukemia. *J Endocrinol Invest* 1997; **20**:215–219.

◆85. Lando A, Holm K, Nysom K, *et al.* Thyroid function in survivors of childhood acute lymphoblastic leukaemia: the significance of prophylactic cranial irradiation. *Clin Endocrinol (Oxf)* 2001; **55**:21–25.

◆86. Voorhess ML, Brecher ML, Glicksman AS, *et al.* Hypothalamic-pituitary function of children with acute lymphocytic leukemia after three forms of central nervous system prophylaxis. A retrospective study. *Cancer* 1986; **57**:1287–1291.

◆87. Shalet SM, Beardwell CG, Twomey JA, *et al.* Endocrine function following the treatment of acute leukemia in childhood. *J Pediatr* 1977; **90**:920–923.

◆88. Carter EP, Leiper AD, Chessells JM, *et al.* Thyroid function in children after treatment for acute lymphoblastic leukaemia. *Arch Dis Child* 1989; **64**:631.

◆89. Robison LL, Nesbit ME, Sather HN, *et al.* Thyroid abnormalities in long-term survivors of childhood acute lymphoblastic leukemia. *Pediatr Res* 1985; **19**:266A.

◆90. Caron PJ, Nieman LK, Rose SR, *et al.* Deficient nocturnal surge of thyrotropin in central hypothyroidism. *J Clin Endocrinol Metab* 1986; **62**:960–964.

◆91. Trejbal D, Sulla I, Trejbalova L, *et al.* Central hypothyroidism – various types of TSH responses to TRH stimulation. *Endocr Regul* 1994; **28**:35–40.

◆92. Rose SR, Lustig RH, Pitukcheewanont P, *et al.* Diagnosis of hidden central hypothyroidism in survivors of child-hood cancer. *J Clin Endocrinol Metab* 1999; **84**:4472–4479.

◆93. Lee KO, Macjida T, Beck-Peccoz P. Central hypothalamic hypothyroidism with thyrotropin of decreased biological activity: a delayed consequence of cranial irradiation. *American Endocrinology Society* 73rd Annual Meeting, 1991:Abstract 420.

◆94. Lee KO, Persani L, Tan M, *et al.* Thyrotropin with decreased biological activity, a delayed consequence of cranial irradiation for nasopharyngeal carcinoma. *J Endocrinol Invest* 1995; **18**:800–805.

◆95. Jyotsna VP, Singh SK, Chaturvedi R, *et al.* Cranial irradiation – an unusual cause for diabetes insipidus. *J Assoc Physicians India* 2000; **48**:1107–1108.

◆96. Schriock EA, Schell MJ, Carter M, *et al.* Abnormal growth patterns and adult short stature in 115 long-term survivors of childhood leukemia. *J Clin Oncol* 1991; **9**:400–405.

◆97. Clayton PE, Shalet SM, Morris-Jones PH, *et al.* Growth in children treated for acute lymphoblastic leukaemia. *Lancet* 1988; **1**(8583):460–462.

◆98. Starceski PJ, Lee PA, Blatt J, *et al.* Comparable effects of 1800- and 2400-rad (18- and 24-Gy) cranial irradiation on height and weight in children treated for acute lymphocytic leukemia. *Am J Dis Child* 1987; **141**:550–552.

◆99. Hokken-Koelega AC, van Doorn JW, Hahlen K, *et al.* Long-term effects of treatment for acute lymphoblastic leukemia with and without cranial irradiation on growth and puberty: a comparative study. *Pediatr Res* 1993; **33**:577–582.

◆100. Moell C, Garwicz S, Marky I, *et al.* Growth in children treated for acute lymphoblastic leukemia with and without prophylactic cranial irradiation. *Acta Paediatr Scand* 1988; **77**:688–692.

◆101. Tamminga RY, Zweens M, Kamps W, *et al.* Longitudinal study of bone age in acute lymphoblastic leukaemia. *Med Pediatr Oncol* 1993; **21**:14–18.

◆102. Berglund G, Karlberg J, Marky I, *et al.* A longitudinal study of growth in children with acute lymphoblastic leukemia. *Acta Paediatr Scand* 1985; **74**:530–533.

◆103. Marky I, Mellander L, Lannering B, *et al.* A longitudinal study of growth and growth hormone secretion in children during treatment for acute lymphoblastic leukemia. *Med Pediatr Oncol* 1991; **19**:258–264.

◆104. Davies HA, Didcock E, Didi M, *et al.* Disproportionate short stature after cranial irradiation and combination chemotherapy for leukaemia. *Arch Dis Child* 1994; **70**:472–475.

◆105. Robison LL, Nesbit ME, Jr., Sather HN, *et al.* Height of children successfully treated for acute lymphoblastic leukemia: a report from the Late Effects Study Committee of Childrens Cancer Study Group. *Med Pediatr Oncol* 1985; **13**:14–21.

◆106. Sklar C, Mertens A, Walter A, *et al.* Final height after treatment for childhood acute lymphoblastic leukaemia: comparison of no cranial irradiation with 1800 and 2400 centigrays of cranial irradiation. *J Pediatr* 1993; **123**:59–64.

◆107. Price DA, Morris MJ, Rosewell KV, *et al.* The effects on anti-leukemic drugs on somatomedin production and cartilage responsiveness to somatomedin in vitro. *Pediatr Res* 1981; **15**:1553 (Abstract).

◆108. Green DM, Williams PD, Simpson L, *et al.* Evaluation of the chronic hepatic toxicity of 6-mercaptopurine in the wistar rat. *Oncology* 1983; **40**:138–142.

◆109. Bar-On E, Beckwith JB, Odom LF, *et al.* Effect of chemotherapy on human growth plate. *J Pediatr Orthop* 1993; **13**:220–224.

◆110. Ahmed SF, Wallace WH, Kelnar CJ. An anthropometric study of children during intensive chemotherapy for acute lymphoblastic leukaemia. *Horm Res* 1997; **48**:178–183.

◆111. Crofton PM, Ahmed SF, Wade JC, *et al.* Growth markers during intensive chemotherapy in children with acute lymphoblastic leukemia. *Horm Res* 1997; **48**(Suppl 2):62.

◆112. Romain J, Villaizan CJ, Garcia-Foncillas J, *et al.* Chemotherapy-induced growth hormone deficiency in children with cancer. *Med Pediatr Oncol* 1995; **25**:90–95.

◆113. Katz JA, Pollock BH, Jacaruso D, *et al.* Final attained height in patients successfully treated for childhood acute lymphoblastic leukemia. *J Pediatr* 1993; **123**:546–552.

◆114. Holm K, Nysom K, Hertz H, *et al.* Normal final height after treatment for acute lymphoblastic leukemia without irradiation. *Acta Paediatr* 1994; **83**:1287–1290.

◆115. Moell C, Marky I, Hovi L, *et al.* Cerebral irradiation causes blunted pubertal growth in girls treated for acute leukemia. *Med Pediatr Oncol* 1994; **22**:375–359.

◆116. Clayton PE, Shalet SM. The evolution of spinal growth after irradiation. *Clin Oncol (R Coll Radiol)* 1991; **3**:220–222.

◆117. Probert JC, Parker BR, Kaplan HS. Growth retardation in children after megavoltage irradiation of the spine. *Cancer* 1973; **32**:634–639.

◆118. Adan L, Souberbielle JC, Blanche S, *et al.* Adult height after cranial irradiation with 24 Gy: factors and markers of height loss. *Acta Paediatr* 1996; **85**:1096–1101.

◆119. Melin AE, Adan L, Leverger G, *et al.* Growth hormone secretion, puberty and adult height after cranial irradiation with 18 Gy for leukaemia. *Eur J Pediatr* 1998; **157**:703–707.

◆120. Giorgiani G, Bozzola M, Locatelli F, *et al.* Role of busulfan and total body irradiation on growth of prepubertal children receiving bone marrow transplantation and results of treatment with recombinant human growth hormone. *Blood* 1995; **86**:825–831.

◆121. Huma Z, Boulad F, Black P, *et al.* Growth in children after bone marrow transplantation for acute leukemia. *Blood* 1995; **86**:819–824.

◆122. Sullivan KM, Deeg HJ, Sanders JE, *et al.* Late complications after marrow transplantation. *Semin Hematol* 1984; **21**:53–63.

◆123. Clement-De Boers A, Oostdijk W, Van Weel-Sipman MH, *et al.* Final height and hormonal function after bone marrow transplantation in children. *J Pediatr* 1996; **129**:544–550.

◆124. Bushhouse S, Ramsay NK, Pescovitz OH, *et al.* Growth in children following irradiation for bone marrow transplantation. *Am J Pediatr Hematol Oncol* 1989; **11**:134–140.

◆125. Leiper AD, Stanhope R, Lau T, *et al.* The effect of total body irradiation and bone marrow transplantation during childhood and adolescence on growth and endocrine function. *Br J Haematol* 1987; **67**:419–426.

◆126. Thomas BC, Stanhope R, Plowman PN, *et al.* Growth following single fraction and fractionated total body irradiation for bone marrow transplantation. *Eur J Pediatr* 1993; **152**:888–892.

◆127. Brauner R, Fontoura M, Zucker JM, *et al.* Growth and growth hormone secretion after bone marrow transplantation. *Arch Dis Child* 1993; **68**:458–463.

◆128. Wingard JR, Plotnick LP, Freemer CS, *et al.* Growth in children after bone marrow transplantation: busulfan plus cyclophosphamide versus cyclophosphamide plus total body irradiation. *Blood* 1992; **79**:1068–1073.

◆129. Sanders JE. Growth and development after bone marrow trasnplantation. In: Forman SJ, Blume KG, Thomas ED (eds) *Bone marrow transplantation.* London: Blackwell, 1994:527–537.

◆130. Manenti F, Galimberti M, Lucarelli G. Growth and endocrine function after bone marrow transplantation for thalassemia. In: Buckner CD, Gale RP, Lucarelli G (eds) *Advances and controversies in thalassemia therapy: bone marrow transplantation and other approaches.* New York: Liss, 1989:273–280.

◆131. Liesner RJ, Leiper AD, Hann IM, *et al.* Late effects of intensive treatment for acute myeloid leukemia and myelodysplasia in childhood. *J Clin Oncol* 1994; **12**:916–924.

◆132. Willi SM, Cooke K, Goldwein J, *et al.* Growth in children after bone marrow transplantation for advanced neuroblastoma compared with growth after transplantation for leukemia or aplastic anemia. *J Pediatr* 1992; **120**:726–732.

◆133. Brauner R, Adan L, Souberbielle JC, *et al.* Contribution of growth hormone deficiency to the growth failure that follows bone marrow transplantation. *J Pediatr* 1997; **130**:785–792.

◆134. Sanders JE, Buckner CD, Sullivan KM, *et al.* Growth and development in children after bone marrow transplantation. *Horm Res* 1988; **30**:92–97.

◆135. Papadimitriou A, Urena M, Hamill G, *et al.* Growth hormone treatment of growth failure secondary to total body irradiation and bone marrow transplantation. *Arch Dis Child* 1991; **66**:689–692.

◆136. Borgstrom B, Bolme P. Growth and growth hormone in children after bone marrow transplantation. *Horm Res* 1988; **30**(2–3):98–100.

◆137. Olshan JS, Willi SM, Gruccio D, *et al.* Growth hormone function and treatment following bone marrow transplant for neuroblastoma. *Bone Marrow Transplant* 1993; **12**:381–385.

◆138. Hovi L, Saarinen UM, Siimes MA. Growth failure in children after total body irradiation preparative for bone marrow transplantation. *Bone Marrow Transplant* 1991; **8**(Suppl. 1):10–13.

◆139. Thomas BC, Stanhope R, Plowman PN, *et al.* Endocrine function following single fraction and fractionated total body irradiation for bone marrow transplantation in childhood. *Acta Endocrinol* 1993; **128**:508–512.

◆140. Shalet SM, Beardwell CG, Aarons BM, *et al.* Growth impairment in children treated for brain tumours. *Arch Dis Child* 1978; **53**:491–494.

◆141. Brown IH, Lee TJ, Eden OB, *et al.* Growth and endocrine function after treatment for medulloblastoma. *Arch Dis Child* 1983; **58**:722–727.

◆142. Darendeliler F, Livesey EA, Hindmarsh PC, *et al.* Growth and growth hormone secretion in children following treatment of brain tumours with radiotherapy. *Acta Paediatr Scand* 1990; **79**:950–956.

◆143. Clarson CL, Del Maestro RF. Growth failure after treatment of pediatric brain tumors. *Pediatrics* 1999; **103**:E37.

◆144. Shalet SM, Whitehead E, Chapman AJ, *et al.* The effects of growth hormone therapy in children with radiation-induced growth hormone deficiency. *Acta Paediatr Scand* 1981; **70**: 81–86.

◆145. Lannering B, Marky I, Mellander L, *et al.* Growth hormone secretion and response to growth hormone therapy after treatment for brain tumour. *Acta Paediatr Scand Suppl* 1988; **343**:146–151.

◆146. Ilveskoski I, Saarinen UM, Wiklund T, *et al.* Growth impairment and growth hormone therapy in children treated for malignant brain tumours. *Eur J Pediatr* 1997; **156**:764–769.

◆147. Clayton PE, Shalet SM, Price DA. Growth response to growth hormone therapy following cranial irradiation. *Eur J Pediatr* 1988; **147**:593–596.

◆148. Clayton PE, Shalet SM, Price DA. Growth response to growth hormone therapy following craniospinal irradiation. *Eur J Pediatr* 1988; **47**:597–601.

◆149. Lannering B, Marky I, Mellander L, *et al.* Growth hormone secretion and response to growth hormone therapy after treatment for brain tumour. *Acta Paediatr Scand Suppl* 1988; **343**:146–151.

◆150. Oberfield SE, Allen JC, Pollack J, *et al.* Long-term endocrine sequelae after treatment of medulloblastoma: prospective study of growth and thyroid function. *J Pediatr* 1986; **108**:219–223.

◆151. Shalet SM, Gibson B, Swindell R, *et al.* Effect of spinal irradiation on growth. *Arch Dis Child* 1987; **62**:461–464.

◆152. Olshan JS, Gubernick J, Packer RJ, *et al.* The effects of adjuvant chemotherapy on growth in children with medulloblastoma. *Cancer* 1992; **70**:2013–2017.

◆153. Romshe CA, Zipf WB, Miser A, *et al.* Evaluation of growth hormone release and human growth hormone treatment in children with cranial irradiation-associated short stature. *J Pediatr* 1984; **104**:177–181.

◆154. Sulmont V, Brauner R, Fontoura M, *et al.* Response to growth hormone treatment and final height after cranial or craniospinal irradiation. *Acta Paediatr Scand* 1990; **79**:542–549.

◆155. Vassilopoulou S, Klein MJ, Moore BD 3rd, *et al.* Efficacy of growth hormone replacement therapy in children with organic growth hormone deficiency after cranial irradiation. *Horm Res* 1995; **43**:188–193.

◆156. Bundak R, Hindmarsh PC, Brook CG. Body segments and growth hormone. *Arch Dis Child* 1988; **63**:839–840.

◆157. Didi M, Brennan BMD, Shalet SM. Growth hormone replacement in children treated for leukemia in childhood. *Horm Res* 1997; **48**(Suppl. 2):65.

◆158. Clayton PE, Shalet SM, Gattamaneni HR, *et al.* Does growth hormone cause relapse of brain tumours? *Lancet* 1987; **1**(8535):711–713.

●159. Clayton PE, Cowell CT. Safety issues in children and adolescents during growth hormone therapy – a review. *Growth Horm IGF Res* 2000; **10**:306–317.

◆160. Swerdlow AJ, Reddingius RE, Higgins CD, *et al.* Growth hormone treatment of children with brain tumors and risk of tumor recurrence. *J Clin Endocrinol Metab* 2000; **85**:4444–4449.

◆161. Ogilvy-Stuart AL, Ryder WD, Gattamaneni HR, *et al.* Growth hormone and tumour recurrence. *Br Med J* 1992; **304**(6842):1601–1605.

◆162. Wilton P, on behalf of the International Board of the Kabi Pharmacia International Growth Study. Safety of growth hormone (GH) – value of a large data base. *Clin Pediatr Endocrinol* 1994; **3**(Suppl. 5):61–71.

●163. Shalet SM. Growth hormone (GH) replacement therapy: cancer in children receiving GH. *Growth Horm IGF Res* 2000; **10**(Suppl. A):S49.

◆164. Maneatis T, Baptista J, Connelly K, *et al*. Growth hormone safety update from the National Cooperative Growth Study. *J Pediatr Endocrinol Metab* 2000; **13**(Suppl. 2):1035–1044.

●165. Shalet SM, Brennan BM, Reddingius RE. Growth hormone therapy and malignancy. *Horm Res* 1997; **48**(Suppl. 4):29–32.

◆166. Taha DR, Bastian W, Castells S. Growth hormone replacement therapy in children with leukemia in remission. *Clin Pediatr* 2001; **40**:441–445.

◆167. Leiper A. Growth hormone deficiency in children treated for leukemia. *Acta Paediatr Scand* 1995; **84**(Suppl. 411):41–44.

●168. Drake WM, Howell SJ, Monson JP, *et al*. Optimizing gh therapy in adults and children. *Endocr Rev* 2001; **22**:425–450.

◆169. Darendeliler F, Hindmarsh PC, Preece MA, *et al*. Growth hormone increases rate of pubertal maturation. *Acta Endocrinol* 1990; **122**:414–416.

◆170. Stanhope R, Uruena M, Hindmarsh P *et al*. Management of growth hormone deficiency through puberty. *Acta Pediatr Scand Suppl* 1991; **372**:47–52.

◆171. Cassorla F, Mericq V, Eggers M, *et al*. Effects of luteinizing hormone-releasing hormone analog-induced pubertal delay in growth hormone (GH)-deficient children treated with GH: preliminary results. *J Clin Endocrinol Metab* 1997; **82**:3989–3992.

◆172. Cara JF, Kreiter ML, Rosenfield RL. Height prognosis of children with true precocious puberty and growth hormone deficiency: effect of combination therapy with gonadotropin releasing hormone agonist and growth hormone. *J Pediatr* 1992; **120**:709–715.

◆173. Mericq MV, Eggers M, Avila A, *et al*. Near final height in pubertal growth hormone (GH)-deficient patients treated with GH alone or in combination with luteinizing hormone-releasing hormone analog: results of a prospective, randomized trial. *J Clin Endocrinol Metab* 2000; **85**:569–573.

◆174. Adan L, Sainte-Rose C, Souberbielle JC, *et al*. Adult height after growth hormone (GH) treatment for GH deficiency due to cranial irradiation. *Med Pediatr Oncol* 2000; **34**:14–19.

●175. de Boer H, Blok GJ, Van der Veen EA. Clinical aspects of growth hormone deficiency in adults. *Endocr Rev* 1995; **16**:63–86.

●176. Carroll PV, Christ ER, Bengtsson BA, *et al*. Growth hormone deficiency in adulthood and the effects of growth hormone replacement: a review. Growth Hormone Research Society Scientific Committee. *J Clin Endocrinol Metab* 1998; **83**:382–395.

●177. Bengtsson BA, Johannsson G, Shalet SM, *et al*. Therapeutic controversy. Treatment of growth hormone deficiency in adults. *J Clin Endocrinol Metab* 2000; **85**:933–942.

◆178. Murray RD, Skillicorn CJ, Howell SJ, *et al*. Dose titration and patient selection increases the efficacy of GH replacement in severely GH deficient adults. *Clin Endocrinol* 1999; **50**:749–757.

◆179. Didi M, Didcock E, Davies HA, *et al*. High incidence of obesity in young adults after treatment of acute lymphoblastic leukemia in childhood. *J Pediatr* 1995; **127**:63–67.

◆180. Sklar CA, Mertens AC, Walter A, *et al*. Changes in body mass index and prevalence of overweight in survivors of childhood acute lymphoblastic leukemia: role of cranial irradiation. *Med Pediatr Oncol* 2000; **35**:91–95.

◆181. Brennan BM, Rahim A, Adams JA, *et al*. Reduced bone mineral density in young adults following cure of acute lymphoblastic leukaemia in childhood. *Br J Cancer* 1999; **79**(11–12):1859–1863.

◆182. Talvensaari KK, Lanning M, Tapanainen P, *et al*. Long-term survivors of childhood cancer have an increased risk of manifesting the metabolic syndrome. *J Clin Endocrinol Metab* 1996; **81**:3051–3055.

◆183. Herold AH, Roetzheim RG. Cancer survivors. *Prim Care* 1992; **19**:779–791.

◆184. Murray RD, Darzy KH, Gleeson HK, *et al*. GH-deficient survivors of childhood cancer: GH replacement during adult life. *J Clin Endocrinol Metab* 2002; **87**:129–135.

8b

Disturbance of the hypothalamic–pituitary thyroid axis

HELEN A SPOUDEAS

INTRODUCTION

Late treatment effects on the pituitary–thyroid axis have been overshadowed by direct effects of irradiation on the thyroid gland itself, namely, the induction of hypothyroidism and thyroid tumors. The latter literature has benefited from the unfortunate 'natural' experiments in atomic bomb or radiation fall-out victims as well as the outcomes after mantle irradiation therapy used to cure Hodgkin's disease. What is harder to disentangle is the possible cranial irradiation effect on pituitary thyrotrophin (TSH) secretion, particularly when direct or scattered thyroid irradiation may have been coadministered in the treatment plan (e.g. craniospinal or total body irradiation, or a posterior fossa beam), or where brain tumor studies have included central (e.g. optic or suprasellar) tumors whose proximity, mass effect or surgery may also influence pituitary hormone secretion.

As physiological hormone secretion has been increasingly studied, it has become evident that the difficulties in accurately assessing damage to the endocrine system are compounded by the limitations of standard pharmacological stimulation tests, the mainstay of endocrine assessment. Subtle neurosecretory dysregulation may be manifest in physiological profiles before frank thyroid dysfunction and clinical symptoms. It is possible such disturbances and their evolutionary profile may help to define the etiopathology and spectrum of thyroid disturbances after cancer therapy just as they have for the growth hormone (GH) axis (see Chapter 8a). For this reason, it is important to understand and explore the parallel hypothalamic neuroregulatory control mechanisms between the pituitary hormones, TSH and GH, as well as the better recognized late thyroid gland dysfunction.

COMMON HYPOTHALAMIC NEUROREGULATORY MECHANISMS INFLUENCING PITUITARY THYROTROPHIN AND GROWTH HORMONE RELEASE

Growth hormone secretion

A compelling body of evidence in animals[1,2] and humans[3] suggest that the secretion of GH from the anterior pituitary is under the control of two interacting and opposing neurohumoral hypothalamic factors – one stimulatory, growth hormone-releasing hormone (GHRH), and the other inhibitory, somatostatin (SS) – each in turn under the control of the central nervous system (CNS). The human somatotrope is increasingly able to respond to this regulatory control from the ninth but particularly after the 13th week of fetal life.[4]

Thyrotrophin secretion

Thyroid-stimulating hormone (TSH) secretion, like that of GH, is pulsatile[5] but, unlike GH, these small pulses occur upon a background of tonic secretion.[6] The relative contributions of stimulatory hypothalamic thyrotrophin-releasing hormone (TRH) and inhibitory somatostatin in the regulation of these pulses, is unclear. While SS has been shown to inhibit TSH secretion[7] in a dose-dependent manner, this is more obvious in the experimental situation after TRH stimulation.[8] SS does not apparently alter the already suppressed daytime TSH levels,[9] although it does inhibit the physiological nocturnal rise in TSH, without ablating inherent pulsatility or changing plasma thyroxine (T4) or tri-iodothyronine (T3).[5,8,9]

There is evidence to suggest that physiological decreases in inhibitory SS tone modulate the nocturnal circadian rise in both pituitary TSH[9,10] and GH secretion,[11] GH being more and TSH less differentially sensitive to inhibition by SS.[7] This explains why pharmacological suppression of inhibitory SS tone does not alter daytime basal or stimulated TSH concentrations, although GH levels are significantly increased.[12]

At birth, TSH levels are high as a result of amplified basal and pulsatile release, and fall dramatically within a few days.[13] Michaud and colleagues demonstrated a subsequent prepubertal age-dependent increase in children between 7.5 and 9.5 years, and decreased levels at puberty.[14] Several studies document a sleep-independent nocturnal increase in frequency and amplitude of TSH secretion in children[15] and adults.[5,10] Although the latter is susceptible to inhibition by both SS and dopamine, the continued TSH pulsatility suggests an important regulatory predominance of TRH.[5]

Thus, pituitary TSH secretion is importantly regulated by the interplay of hypothalamic factors TRH and SS and thyroid hormone feedback, the latter probably acting through a somatostatinergic mechanism.[16] Dopamine has an additional inhibitory influence (see below)[5,10] but TRH is most likely the predominant regulatory factor.[5,12]

Somatostatin

The predominant human variety is SS(1–14); other forms and related peptides have common effects on target tissues, but demonstrate differences in potency and neuromodulation,[4] suggesting different receptors mediate their actions. SS is extensively distributed within the nervous system, the gut and both endocrine and exocrine glands, and it has diverse tissue-specific effects. Somatostatinergic neurons in the hypothalamus mainly originate in the anterior and medial divisions of the paraventricular nucleus, and terminate in the median eminence, the source of the hypophyseal-portal microvasculature.[17]

Somatostatin exerts its biological effects by binding to a family of at least two, probably five, high-affinity, tissue-specific G-coupled receptors[18] with differing affinities for native SS and its analogues, explaining the diversity of function of this hormone. Possible postreceptor mechanisms include coupling with a single but multi-potent calcium-dependent inhibitory pathway, which negatively influences at least three signal transduction systems.[18–20] Unlike GHRH, SS has no trophic effect on GH synthesis and does not inhibit GHRH-induced GH gene transcription.[20]

Dopamine

The hypothalamic factor, dopamine, also controls two pituitary hormones, thyrotrophin and prolactin (PRL) secretion, possibly through somatostatinergic mechanisms. TRH stimulates both TSH and PRL release,[5,8] but through different hormone-specific and calcium-dependent mechanisms, which require both intracellular calcium mobilization and extracellular calcium influx for TSH release, but only the former for PRL release.[21]

Prolactin secretion is tonically inhibited by dopamine[22] and the disruption of this latter hypothalamic hormone has been postulated as the reason behind postirradiation elevations in PRL noted after brain tumor therapy.[23–25] D-2 receptor agonists (bromocriptine and dopamine) inhibit PRL and TSH secretion, while D-2 antagonists (metoclopramide) promote PRL release.[5,10] Dopamine, like SS, also inhibits basal and stimulated TSH release[5,10] and further inhibits TSH subunit gene expression.[26] However, its role in the control of TSH secretion or its circadian modulation is unclear; most reports have concluded it is a minor player to TRH and SS in this respect.[5,9,10] These discrepancies may in part result from the overriding physiological inhibitory feedback effects of T3 and T4.

Thyroxine and growth hormone

Thyroid hormones influence GH secretion, mainly at hypothalamic but also at pituitary level, and, like cortisol, are necessary for GH gene transcription.[27] Hypothyroid animals exhibit both increased SS and decreased GHRH hypothalamic content, decreased pituitary GH content and increased GHRH mRNA, reversible with thyroid hormone.[28] It is uncertain whether these changes result from direct hypothalamic effects or from effective reductions in circulating GH. In hypothyroid patients, the low spontaneous and stimulated GH secretion observed can be reversed by thyroxine administration and augmented by pharmacological suppression of inhibitory SS tone, although less so than in healthy volunteers.[29]

Table 8b.1 *Likely endocrine deficit according to cranial irradiation dose (brain tumors distant from pituitary area)*

Dose	Endocrinopathy
>55–70 Gy	Hyperprolactinaemia, Panhypopituitarism
30–55 Gy	GH insufficiency, Evolving Endocrinopathy, ?Loss of nocturnal TSH surge
18–24 Gy	GH neurosecretory disturbance, Pubertal GH insufficiency, Early puberty, Adult GH Deficiency
10–15 Gy	GH neurosecretory disturbance, Adult GH Deficiency

RADIOBIOLOGY AND THE CNS

Radiation sensitivity

The radiosensitivity of a tissue is directly proportional to its mitotic activity and inversely proportional to its differentiation. Thus, highly active tissues like skin and bone marrow are 'radiosensitive', whereas the specialized mature and quiescent cells of the brain or bone are 'radioresistant'.[30] Nevertheless, if a quiescent cell is stimulated to divide, the radiation dose required to cause chromosome damage, mitotic delay and inhibition of DNA synthesis is similar in all tissues. Thus, all organ systems in the body will be damaged by irradiation, although the late effects on slowly or non-proliferating cell populations, such as the CNS, may not be immediately apparent.

Radiation-induced mammalian cell death has two components. Radiosensitive tissues are susceptible to 'single-hit' non-reparable injury quantified by a high α coefficient. Slowly proliferating neural tissue is more susceptible to 'multihit' injury, either the accumulation of sublethal injuries, the sum of which is lethal, and/or the progressive destruction of the cell's ability to repair itself. The latter both result in cell depletion quantified by a high β coefficient.[31,32] Since β is proportional to the square of the dose, fractionation effectively reduces 'multihit' mechanisms and enhances the therapeutic ratio (between late effects and tumor control). Dose fractions larger than 2 Gy (not in general use in children) increase the injury relatively more to late (neural) than early responding (or tumor) tissues, while smaller fractions over the same treatment duration (hyperfractionation) may be further beneficial in reducing late toxicity, provided sufficient time (ideally >6 hours) is allowed between fractions for tissue repair.[31]

With conventional external-beam radiotherapy, late neuroendocrine toxicity depends on the volume of the brain irradiated, the fraction size, the interfraction interval, the age of the child and the total dose delivered. Irradiation scatter is greater for ^{60}Co sources than linear accelerators, which tend to have a more penetrating beam, but since the irradiation field for most childhood brain tumors

(infratentorial) is so close to the pituitary margins (demarcated by the posterior clinoids), this is generally academic in terms of pituitary dose (at least 40–45 Gy). The highest estimated hypothalamic–pituitary doses (up to 70 Gy) occur after treatment for nasopharyngeal tumors[24] (accounting for the high incidence of hypothalamo-pituitary deficits in these cases), while yttrium-90 implants and the newer stereotactic irradiation techniques, although more focused, have a very limited application in childhood malignancy.

Chemotherapy, radiation and additive toxicity

A radiosensitizing effect of certain drugs is often postulated, but this would mean a change in cellular dose–survival characteristics (α and β), which is not often confirmed. Increased tumor or normal tissue responses to the concomitant administration of drugs and radiation usually represent additive effects. This may have significant implications in terms of long-term effects in late-responding tissues, since cumulative toxicity is not reduced by regeneration between the two modalities of treatment. A few studies have now documented additive morbidity after such combination therapies compared with either regimen independently, not only on peripheral target glands, such as the thyroid,[33,34] gonad[35,36] and skeleton,[37] but also centrally on hormonal secretion where the blood–brain barrier has been disrupted.[38] The recent strategy of 'holding' chemotherapy and delaying potentially curative cranial irradiation to avoid neurotoxicity in the youngest children with brain tumors, may yet result in additive injury evident only in the longer term.

IRRADIATION-INDUCED HYPOTHALAMIC–PITUITARY–THYROID AXIS DISTURBANCE

Thyrotrophin deficiency as part of an evolving panhypopituitarism

It has long been recognized that hypopituitarism may result after surgery or external radiotherapy directed at tumors lying within or close to the hypothalamic–pituitary axis (HPA) but there remained the possibility that this was due to compression effects from the underlying disease itself. However, reports of insidious hypopituitarism occurring in adults several years after irradiation for nasopharyngeal carcinoma, and in children after irradiation for orbital and middle ear tumors, where estimated total doses to the HPA were often greatly in excess of 50 Gy,[23] suggested a causative role for radiotherapy. This was supported by longitudinal studies demonstrating

suppressive effects on spontaneous GH secretion in leukemic children undergoing irradiation therapy[39] and on spontaneous and insulin-induced GH release within 1 year of 24 Gy and 40 Gy fractionated cranial irradiation doses given to rhesus monkeys.[40] These studies did not comment upon anterior pituitary deficits other than GH insufficiency.

Cranial irradiation and neuraxial prophylaxis remain the only proven curative therapy in malignant brain tumors of childhood, with 5-year survival rates at 60–70 per cent[41,42] This is at the expense, however, of significant late neural[42,43] and endocrine toxicity[25,44,45] largely attributed to a dose-dependent effect of cranial irradiation[43,46–48] causing neurotoxicity and an evolving hierarchical loss of all postoperatively intact anterior pituitary hormones with time, GH being the most and TSH the least sensitive hormone.[44,46,47] The contribution of chemotherapy, tumor- or surgically-induced late damage has not been considered significant and is more difficult to study.

The anterior pituitary deficits seen in adults irradiated postoperatively for pituitary tumors have been attributed entirely to irradiation[41,44] but few patients (18–21 per cent of 165 patients) in these studies had entirely intact pituitary function before irradiation. Only 23 of 124 (18.5 per cent) had normal GH, 34 of 165 (21 per cent) had normal gonadotrophins [luteinizing hormone (LH) and follicle-stimulating hormone (FSH)], while more (57 per cent and 80 per cent, respectively) had normal adreno-corticotrophin (ACTH) and TSH secretion. The prevalence of dysfunction with time was calculated annually for each individual hormone – rather than exclusively for those with entirely intact HPA function – to a median follow-up of just 5 years[44] (Figure 8b.1a). The older patients (mean age 48 years) and the natural decline in GH secretion with age[49] may have influenced the diagnostic criteria for GH deficiency in this cohort. Lower 'cut-offs' have since been recommended for adults[50] (Toogood *et al.* 1999) than for children or adolescents.[51]

With the exception perhaps of GH, where the few longitudinal studies of stimulated[38,52] and spontaneous 24-hour GH secretion[38] suggest subtle and persisting postoperative neuroregulatory disturbances compounded by irradiation, chemotherapy and time,[38,53] the independent neurotoxic effect of cranial irradiation, as distinct from any tumor, surgical or other treatment effect, remains unclear. Long-term cohort studies in treated children, confirm the high incidence and permanence of GH deficiency after cranial irradiation (>85 per cent) for posterior fossa tumors distant from the central area[38,45,53,54] but the prevalence of endocrinopathies other than GH deficiency after a similar surveillance time was very much less (2–6 per cent, 9.6 years after estimated pituitary doses of 40–50 Gy).[45,54] The 10 per cent and 5 per cent reported prevalence of respective ACTH and TSH insufficiency in our own recently reported longitudinal cohort[55] is very much less

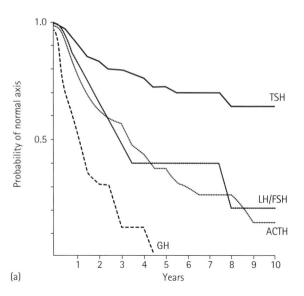

(a)

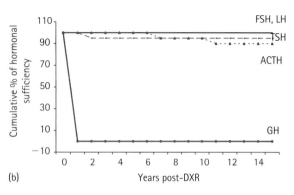

(b)

Figure 8b.1 *(a) 10-year life-table analysis, in 37 of 165 adults with intrasellar or anatomically adjacent tumors, and normal postoperative hypothalamo-pituitary function, indicating the likelihood of an evolving endocrinopathy after 37.5–42.5 Gy pituitary irradiation in 15 fractions over 20–22 days. Growth hormone (GH) is most sensitive, all adults being GH deficient within 5 years, while adrenocorticotrophin (ACTH) and gonadotrophins [luteinizing hormone (LH) and follicle-stimulating hormone (FSH)] are increasingly affected over time (80 per cent at 10 years). Thyrotrophin (TSH) is most resistant. (Redrawn from Littley* et al, 1989.[44]*) (b) Probability of an evolving endocrinopathy occurring during a 6.8–21.4-year (median 11.0 years) follow up period, after a median estimated hypothalamo-pituitary irradiation dose (DXR) of at least 40 Gy in 1.8 Gy fractions, in 16 young adult survivors of resected posterior fossa brain tumors tested twice at the onset of growth failure and at completion of growth, who were otherwise asymptomatic. Duration of follow-up was greater than 8 years in 13 patients, 12 years in seven patients and 16 years in one patient. (Redrawn from Spoudeas* et al. 2003[55] *with permission of the copyright holder, Medical and Pediatric Oncology.) GH deficiency was present in all patients tested at first assessment and was permanent. ACTH (10 per cent) and TSH (5 per cent) deficiencies were comparatively rare and there was no case of gonadotrophin deficiency or hyperprolactinemia over the duration of follow-up.*

than the 80 per cent and 57 per cent reported prevalence in the adult pituitary series[44,46] (Figure 8b.1b). Even after the highest pituitary irradiation doses of 50–70 Gy or more given for nasopharyngeal tumors, Constine *et al.* reported just 20 per cent prevalence of ACTH insufficiency and 22–65 per cent TSH insufficiency, manifest as low free T3 or T4 levels, respectively.[24]

Another explanation for our discrepant results[55] compared with those of Littley *et al.*[44] is the potentially greater biological effectivity of the same total dose if larger fractions (>2 Gy) are used,[32,56] thus causing earlier evidence of damage in the adult study. However, the young brain is known to be particularly vulnerable to irradiation-induced neural toxicity[43] despite the standard use of smaller (1.6–1.8 Gy) fraction sizes. Thus, although some evolving evidence of a wider endocrinopathy might have been expected, this was not observed even in those children followed the longest (up to 21 years),[55] and this observation has been recently confirmed in a larger cross-sectional mixed cohort of pediatric and adult tumors displaced from the central axis (S. Shalet, personal communication). A study of adult patients irradiated for prolactinomas also used smaller fraction sizes (45 Gy in 25, 1.9 Gy fractions over 35 days) to a similar total dose, and similarly failed to detect any ACTH or TSH deficiency.[57]

Pituitary irradiation experiments in rats have also failed to confirm significant ACTH or gonadotropin insufficiency, whereas TSH secretion – relatively preserved following surgical cure of GH-secreting[58] or non-functioning adenomas[59] – is paradoxically affected early, soon after GH and prolactin.[60] In the adult surgical series,[58,59] postoperative pituitary recovery occurs in exactly the reverse order of loss described by Littley *et al.*[44] after surgery and subsequent irradiation (per cent sufficiency: TSH, 57 per cent; ACTH, 38 per cent; LH and FSH, 32 per cent; and GH, 15 per cent). This is very different from the situation observed after pituitary irradiation administered in the *absence* of a coexisting pituitary lesion and pituitary surgery, whether in children[45,54] or experimentally in rats.[60] Thus, it remains unclear whether pituitary irradiation, at least in conventionally fractionated doses totaling about 40 Gy, has any direct neurotoxic effect on TSH secretion as tested by TRH stimulation tests, but overt manifestation of this consequence (like ACTH deficiency) seems rare if the tumor itself is displaced from the central axis, even though the pituitary itself may fall within the high-dose irradiation field. This does not preclude more subtle neurosecretory abnormalities in TSH secretion, as in GH secretion, whose clinical significance is as yet uncertain (see later section on nature and site of neuroendocrine deficits).

The pituitary hormonal disturbance witnessed after irradiation alone echoes its common developmental signaling cascade, exemplified by mutations in the *pit-1* (GH, PRL and TSH deficiency), *Prop-1* and *LHX3* (additionally encompassing LH and FSH deficiency) transcription factor genes, while *HESX1* homeobox gene mutations additionally cause ACTH and invariable GH deficiency.[61] Thus, is pituitary irradiation *per se* the predominant cause of the high prevalence of ACTH insufficiency (80 per cent) reported in the pituitary tumor series by Littley *et al.*[44] or might an alternative explanation exist in the form of a developmental or surgical insult? Surgery is considered a specific and discrete pituitary insult. Pituitary recovery may follow relief of pituitary-portal compression.[58,59,62] Slowly replicating neural cells may not at first demonstrate damage, but eventually cell replication failure results over time and loss of pituitary function becomes apparent. The resulting endocrinopathy may thus be due as much to delayed evidence of earlier tumor- or surgery-induced neuronal injury as to subsequent superimposed irradiation.

Nature and site of the postirradiation neuroendocrine defect

Determining the etiology of any tumor- or treatment-related neurotoxicity carries implications for future therapies aimed at reducing morbidity without compromising a 70 per cent survival.[41,42] Whether postirradiation endocrinopathy be neural or vascular, hypothalamic or pituitary in origin is still debated. The few studies on hypothalamic[63] and hypophyseal-portal blood flow[64] do not suggest this is particularly compromised. The hypothalamus or its portal connections are deemed more radiosensitive than the pituitary, particularly after doses >50 Gy,[23] but diabetes insipidus, a typical hypothalamic disorder that may long predate the radiographic appearance of a suprasellar germinoma by some 20 years,[65] has, as yet, not been reported after high-dose irradiation for non-central tumors.[24]

Selective damage to hypothalamic control centers is suggested by discordant suppression of insulin-mediated and spontaneous GH release, with preservation of GH responses to other centrally acting agents in irradiated monkeys[40] and children with leukemia[66] or brain tumors.[67] Pituitary hormone responses to their respective hypothalamic releasing hormone stimuli, may be delayed[23,46] or preserved[68] in the face of absent or attenuated responses to insulin – hypoglycemia.

Elevations in prolactin have been deemed evidence of hypothalamic damage to inhibitory dopaminergic neurons,[23,24] but these vary in severity and permanence.[46] They are more likely after high-dose radiotherapy for nasopharyngeal carcinoma[23,24] or pituitary-related tumors, particularly those causing acromegaly, and rare after treatment for extrasellar tumors in childhood.[24,69,70] Effects of previous pituitary surgery and residual tumor tissue, which may contain lactogenic as well as somatogenic activity, thus confuse the picture. We documented longitudinal

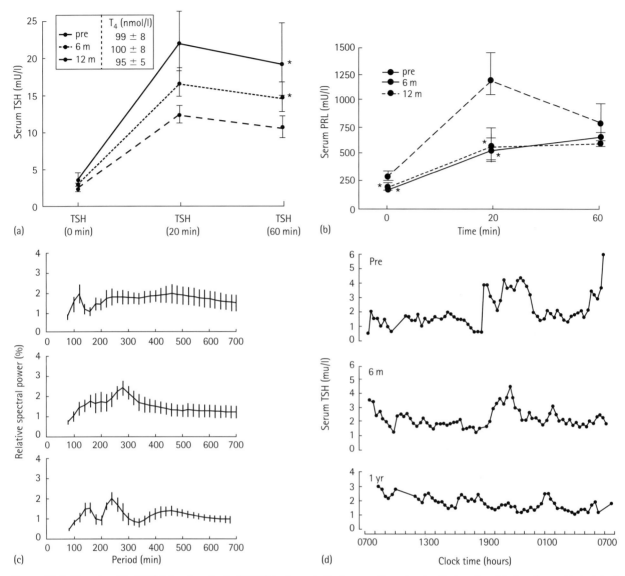

Figure 8b.2 *Thyrotrophin (TSH) (a) and prolactin (PRL) (b) release to their respective releasing factor stimuli before (pre; wide hatched lines), 6 (6 m; dotted lines) and 12 months (12 m; solid lines) in seven prepubertal children with resected posterior fossa tumors tested longitudinally after craniospinal irradiation (without chemotherapy). Note the rise (within normal values) in basal and stimulated TSH levels, and the fall in basal and stimulated PRL with time from irradiation.* indicates significance of difference from pre-irradiation values. (c) Periodicity (shown as relative spectral power) of TSH secretion before (upper panel), 6 months (middle panel) and 12 months (lower panel) after craniospinal irradiation (without chemotherapy) in seven prepubertal children with resected posterior fossa tumors. Note the slowing of the periodicity after radiotherapy. (d) Loss of TSH nocturnal surge in a representative, prepubertal individual followed longitudinally before (upper panel), 6 (middle panel) and 12 months (lower panel) after craniospinal irradiation for a posterior fossa tumor. Group data in the seven individuals followed longitudinally confirmed this was the result of an increase in 12-hour daytime (nadir) secretion, without a corresponding increase in the nocturnal mean peak secretion and is separate from recognized primary thyroid gland toxicity from the exit dose of the spinal irradiation beam. (Redrawn from Spoudeas, 1995, MD thesis.[70])*

decreases in basal and stimulated prolactin, with *increases* in stimulated TSH within the normal range 6 and 12 months after craniospinal irradiation for posterior fossa tumors (median estimated pituitary dose 45 Gy), suggesting intact dopamine secretion (Figure 8b.2a and b).[70] Nevertheless, we did note a decreased 24-hour TSH periodicity (Figure 8a.2c) and a suppression of the expected nocturnal TSH surge (Figure 8b.2d).[15] The latter is considered a good test of intact hypothalamic function,[15] suggesting that these subtle and early neuroregulatory disturbances may indicate postsurgical or irradiation-induced hypothalamic deficits in TRH and somatostatin release,[69,70] which requires further study. This 'hidden' central hypothyroidism (i.e. normal free T4 but loss of

normal TSH secretory dynamic) has also been noted by another group studying cranially irradiated childhood brain tumor survivors, whose tumor position and histological categories were mixed and included some central optic tumors.[71] The clinical ramifications of these perturbations remain to be evaluated, although a trial of thyroxine supplementation may require consideration and prove symptomatically beneficial.

These inferred hypothalamic TRH and SS secretion disturbances echo those described in the GH neuroregulatory pathway. Preserved GH responses to hypothalamic releasing hormone (GHRH), in the presence of suboptimal responses to other GH provocation tests,[68,72] suggest a primary hypothalamic GHRH deficiency but, since the GHRH doses used were supraphysiological,[73] direct pituitary damage could also be a contributory factor. Somatotroph responses to physiological GHRH doses are preserved 1 year after neurosurgery and radiation for non-central tumors,[69,70] but these are suppressed in long-term survivors of the same.[53] The majority of such late survivors retain much attenuated GH neuroregulatory responses to modulations of SS tone and GHRH,[53,74] often with disordered pulsatility and an elevated baseline,[38,53] suggestive of SS dysfunction as in animals after SS-immunoneutralization.[75]

There are potential implications of differentiating between hypothalamic and pituitary disease, and target gland dysfunction. Intermittent pulsatile subcutaneous gonadotrophin-releasing hormone (GnRH) therapy can successfully induce puberty in both sexes, and fertility in hypogonadotropic females treated for pituitary tumors.[76] Continuous subcutaneous GHRH therapy, for periods up to 1 year, promotes growth in GH-deficient children with a presumed hypothalamic etiology after irradiation therapy for brain tumors.[77] This latter response depends on the integrity of hypothalamic SS secretion and is generally less than that seen with GH alone. Significant pituitary and/or target gland dysfunction would further limit such therapeutic potential. Direct target gland damage carries independent risks of long-term mitogenicity, particularly in the thyroid. If it becomes possible to site the damage accurately, pre-irradiation endocrine strategies for protecting specific areas might be attempted.[78,79]

DIRECT AND INDIRECT RADIATION TO THE THYROID GLAND CAUSING THYROID DYSFUNCTION (HYPOTHYROIDISM, HYPERTHYROIDISM, THYROID TUMORS)

Radiation damage to the thyroid gland commonly includes hypothyroidism and thyroid tumors, with the additional possibility of hyperthyroidism and autoimmunity.

Hypothyroidism

The possible coexistence of secondary (or even tertiary) central hypothyroidism with primary hypothyroidism (recently termed 'mixed' hypothyroidism by Rose[80]) caused by cranial irradiation coadministered with that to the spine (e.g. in children with posterior fossa brain tumors) as detailed in the section above, confounds data on prevalence as well as the permanence of the dysfunction. In the majority of cases, the hypothyroidism is compensated by increased pituitary thyrotrophin concentration and thus not obviously manifest. It is dose- and time-dependent, and has been documented after fractionated doses to the thyroid area in excess of 25 Gy.[23,81] However, longer periods of follow-up in children treated in the past with low-dose cranial irradiation for non-malignant conditions, such as tinea capitis, suggest that even these low doses cause dysfunction manifest only with longer follow-up time. Although some reports have suggested an increased incidence in the younger age group,[81] this has not been confirmed by other studies.[82] Nevertheless, the irradiation risk to the thyroid may be age- as well as dose-dependent, and may be additionally influenced by the iodine status.

HODGKIN'S DISEASE

After mantle irradiation doses of 36–44 Gy in 1.5–2 Gy fractions for Hodgkin's disease in those under 16 years, prevalence rates, notably in the first 2 years, vary between 37 per cent and 88 per cent[82,83] with 25–53 per cent being compensated and 0–58 per cent overt. The use of a posterior spinal and laryngeal block at 30 Gy and 20 Gy, respectively, did not reduce the overall incidence of hypothyroidism (57 per cent) but this was overt in fewer cases (5 per cent) at a median follow-up of 65 months.[84] Although the occasional case of transient hyperthyroidism has been reported after adjuvant 'MOPP' chemotherapy,[82] an increased risk of thyroid dysfunction after chemotherapy alone has not been conclusively proven. However, one series did document primary thyroid dysfunction in 24 of 54 adults who did not receive radiotherapy.[85]

In recent years, chemotherapy has increasingly replaced neck irradiation as first-line therapy for Hodgkin's disease. In the shorter follow-up (median 6 years, range 1–20) available in these patient cohorts, the absence of hypothyroidism in those treated without radiation (COPP/ABVD) is confirmed, while in each of the two groups receiving either combined modality therapy or supradiaphragmatic irradiation alone, 34 per cent were affected.[86] In a series of 47 patients, Shafford et al. noted ultrasonically identifiable abnormalities in all irradiated thyroid glands, not readily identifiable by either clinical examination (6 per cent abnormal) or thyroid function tests (64 per cent abnormal).[87] The clinical significance of this ultrasonic abnormality remains unclear. However, the finding that the

duration of TSH hypersecretion was directly correlated with the development of focal abnormalities under surveillance underlines the recognized importance of early and annual TSH measurements (these 64 per cent occurred within 4 years) with suppression of any elevated TSH by thyroxine replacement therapy, as has been recommended in this situation.

The largest study, undertaken in 1791 young adult survivors of Hodgkin's disease in the USA, is the childhood cancer survivor cohort questionnaire study. This confirms a cumulative reported incidence of 28 per cent but an actuarial risk of 50 per cent in those receiving >45 Gy after 20 years.[88] Differences in duration and frequency of surveillance, and criteria for diagnosis and treatment (e.g. compensated vs. frank) as well as the method of ascertainment (self-reporting questionnaire vs. clinical documentation) may partially account for the differences in prevalence between the reports above.

BRAIN TUMORS

Compensated, or less commonly, frank hypothyroidism has been documented in 30–40 per cent of children treated with craniospinal irradiation for brain tumors without chemotherapy, (fractionated spinal doses 30–35 Gy), the majority occurring within 4 years. Two groups have confirmed that adjuvant chemotherapy increases this risk,[33,34] and it is noteworthy that, in our own longitudinal series of patients with posterior fossa tumors treated more recently and without chemotherapy, primary thyroid gland dysfunction was uncommon (2 out of 16 cases) at a median follow-up of 11 years.[55] Whether hyperfractionating the spinal dose further reduces the prevalence of hypothyroidism will be prospectively studied and compared to standard schedules in the forthcoming European Primitive Neuroectodermal Tumour (PNET) studies starting in 2003. This study will, for the first time, collect prospective data on hormonal function, but the spinal irradiation doses will be lower than before (24 Gy) and both arms will have identical and significant chemotherapeutic components, which will additionally influence outcome.

TOTAL BODY IRRADIATION, TOTAL LYMPHOID IRRADIATION AND CONDITIONING CHEMOTHERAPY PRIOR TO TRANSPLANTATION

A similar percentage develop thyroid dysfunction after total body irradiation (TBI),[89,90] usually compensated at first, progressing to overt hypothyroidism 5–10 years later. After 7.5–10 Gy single-fraction TBI, 28 per cent and 13 per cent developed compensated and overt hypothyroidism, respectively. After 12–15.75 Gy fractionated TBI, these figures were decreased to 12 per cent and 3 per cent, respectively, although the latter group were followed for only half the number of years.[90,91] These figures have proved overestimates, since one-third of those with compensated thyroid dysfunction recovered at a median of 60 months and there were no overt cases.[92] Although the same study documented a higher incidence of thyroid dysfunction after total lymphoid irradiation (TLI) for aplastic anemia, these patients were followed for longer. While chemotherapy may be additive to irradiation effects, its independent role in the pathogenesis of thyroid dysfunction is less obvious, since it was not observed in a large series of 105 children transplanted for thalassemia, and only 1 of 50 transplanted for aplastic anemia with conditioning chemotherapy but not TBI.[89,91]

Hyperthyroidism and hyperparathyroidism

This is much less prevalent than hypothyroidism but has been reported to occur more frequently in certain subsets of individuals treated for malignancy. In a large cross-sectional study of childhood cancer survivors, Sklar et al. reported an eightfold increased risk of hyperthyroidism after thyroid irradiation doses >35 Gy for Hodgkin's disease,[88] but this has not been consistently reported in longitudinal surveillance studies of a much smaller number of long term survivors.[87] The same group[88] have also reported hyperthyroidism after allogeneic bone marrow/stem cell transplant and hypothesize that this is most likely due to the adoptive transfer of abnormal clones of T or B cells from donor to recipient, in common with the documented increased prevalence of other autoimmune disease. Those exposed to ionizing irradiation are also at risk of primary hyperparathyroidism, which is dose dependent, and greater if exposure occurs at a young age.[93]

Autoimmunity

Autoimmune thyroiditis, with or without thyroid insufficiency, has been observed in populations after environmental exposure to radioisotopes of iodine and in the survivors of atomic bomb explosions. Since 1990, an increased prevalence of circulating thyroid antibodies not associated with significant thyroid dysfunction has also been noted in normal children exposed to radiation after the Chernobyl nuclear accident. It is likely that clinical thyroid autoimmune disease will become evident with prolonged surveillance.[94]

Etiology and management of elevated thyrotrophin levels

Elevations in TSH after spinal irradiation and TBI have been thought to reflect primary thyroid gland damage resulting from direct or scattered irradiation from the exit dose of the posterior spinal beam. Because of the recognized carcinogenic potential of megavoltage irradiation and prolonged TSH stimulation,[87,95,96] annual thyroid

palpation – with further ultrasound and needle biopsy evaluation of any nodules – and thyroid function tests (fT4 and TSH) have always been advised, with institution of thyroxine replacement when TSH is elevated on two occasions. However, increasing attention is being focused on the possibility of thyroid recovery now documented to occur after mantle irradiation,[82] spinal irradiation doses used in the neuraxial prophylaxis of children with brain tumors[34] and after TBI.[92] There remains the possibility that elevations in TSH may be a manifestation of higher irradiation damage to hypothalamic centers,[69,70] although, in the presence of a normal thyroid gland, an increase in thyroxine levels should also follow.

Thyroid (and parathyroid) tumors

Thyroid tumors are rare, accounting for less than 1 per cent of all tumors. Nevertheless, registries from Europe[97–99] and America[100] confirm their background incidence is increasing and speculation as to the reasons for this include radiation exposure (particularly causing papillary thyroid carcinomas) together with better diagnostic facilities and screening of thyroid disease. Using data from children born between 1930 and 1950 in Connecticut and Rochester, respectively, thyroid tumors have been documented to occur in the irradiated thyroid gland after irradiation doses as low as 0.3 Gy used in childhood for the treatment of benign head and neck conditions, for example, tinea capitis or a purportedly enlarged thymus gland.[100,101] The dose–response relationship was essentially linear with an estimated relative risk of 10 at 1 Gy,[101] peaking at about 25–29 years[93] and still elevated 40–45 years after irradiation, although declining with time. Those youngest at irradiation, women, and those with delayed menarche or first childbirth were at increased risk.[93,101] This statistic has been confirmed in a more recent pooled analysis of seven studies.[102] These tumors may take many years to become manifest but higher doses to the neck (>25 Gy) used for the treatment of Hodgkin's disease cause tumors more quickly.[23,81,103] Greater than 50-fold increased risks were observed for tumors of the thyroid among children treated before the age of 10,[103] and a recent report suggests that growth hormone replacement therapy may increase this risk.[104] Parathyroid adenomas are also reportedly increased by an estimated excess relative risk of 0.8 per Gray in a recent study of adults irradiated at a mean age of 49 years,[105] to palliate arthritic or spondylitic pain. Up to 30 per cent of adults presenting with primary hyperparathyroidism have been exposed to ionizing irradiation during childhood or early adult age.[106] Although these results reflect the late effects of largely outdated therapeutic modalities, they nevertheless underscore the importance of lifelong surveillance of these patients treated as children (see Rubino[107] for review).

Radiation exposure might partly explain the increased incidence of papillary thyroid cancer noted in adult tumor registries in recent decades.[98,99] However, ^{131}I treatment used in diagnostic tests and delivering an equivalent median dose of 1 Gy to the thyroid, did not increase the tumor risk [relative risk 0.86; 95 per cent confidence interval (95% CI) 0.14, 5.13] in 789 exposed subjects as compared with 1118 unexposed after 16 500 and 21 000 person-years, respectively, at a mean 20-year follow-up.[108] A similar reassuring absence of risk after ^{131}I treatment has been noted by another group.[109] Their slight excess of risk (standard incidence ratio 1.35; 95% CI 1.05–1.71) appeared related to the underlying thyroid condition rather than radiation dose exposure and was 2–10 times lower than that predicted from A-bomb survivors' data, further suggesting a benefit for fractionation of the same total dose.

The recent radioactive fall-out from the accident at Chernobyl further exemplifies the enormous risk of thyroid tumors after radiation, particularly in the youngest members of a population[94,107] and those where the diet is rich in iodine.[110] Radioactivity predisposes to papillary (solid and follicular variants) thyroid tumors, less influenced by gender, more aggressive at presentation and more frequently associated with autoimmunity. The increasing incidence of differentiated malignant papillary thyroid cancer noted amongst French adults (>15 years age) since the 1970s predates the Chernobyl accident and cannot be explained by it,[99] but these figures do not exclude the possibility that such changes may develop after a long latency, in those exposed as children in 1986. These tumors have also been noted in the childhood populations of the former USSR (i.e. where the radioactive fall-out was greatest) particularly in those aged under 5 years, and anecdotaly 15–20 years after spinal irradiation in childhood (<7 years age) for spinal tumors (50 Gy), spinal neuraxial prophylaxis for medulloblastoma (30 Gy) and TBI (12 Gy) (authors' own experience). In such cases, and because of the potential for malignant conversion, a total thyroidectomy is recommended, even if needle aspiration histology is 'benign'. Gene mutations involving the RET proto-oncogene and, less frequently, TRK have been shown to be causative events specific for papillary cancer, and RET activation was found in nearly 70 per cent of the patients who developed papillary thyroid carcinomas following the Chernobyl accident.[94]

SUMMARY

The distinction between late neural toxicity due to tumor/disease or surgery, and that due to irradiation therapy is important. Current management of children with posterior fossa tumors is based on the assumption

that virtually all neurotoxicity is irradiation induced.[42] That assumption might be challenged on the neuro-endocrine hypothalamic–pituitary evidence outlined above. Although the effects of radiotherapy and of chemotherapy are undoubtedly relevant to the adverse neuropsychological outcomes of children treated for medulloblastomas, and attempts to reduce therapeutic intensity are increasingly being made,[42,48] these treatments may arguably be no more important as determinants of functional outcome than the tumor itself, perioperative morbidity and psychosocial adversity, the 'dose' and timing of which are more difficult to measure. The apparent cognitive advantage of children treated with lower doses of cranial irradiation, perhaps at the expense of long-term cure, has only been documented in cross-sectional studies of an incomplete, and possibly self-selecting, sample of treated children whose follow-up was short. The longitudinal data in these studies do not confirm the benefit of reduced dose irradiation.[43,48] Cross-sectional rather than longitudinal assessments, differences in treatment techniques, follow-up times, tumor position, patient age and methods used to test cognition or hypothalamic–pituitary–adrenal axis integrity, may have contributed to these discrepancies.

Consistent longitudinal surveillance in multicenter studies is now necessary to accrue sufficient patient numbers to address these discrepancies in intention to treat analyses; this initial dialogue has successfully commenced in the most recent SIOP 1V (PNET) trial currently being submitted for multicenter European approval, where randomization between a hyperfractionated and standard irradiation arm will allow comparison of growth, thyroid and gonadal status between treatment groups. It is imperative that prospective surveillance continues in the long term to at least 20 years of age.

Although many survivors of childhood Hodgkin's disease have received therapy that is now outdated, the undoubted risk of thyroid autoimmune disease, and subsequent thyroid and parathyroid tumors occurring after a long latency period in those receiving direct or scattered irradiation to the thyroid gland, particularly in childhood, means that lifelong endocrine surveillance in conjunction with an adult physician, is necessary for all Hodgkin's survivors treated with mantle or neck irradiation, and all those receiving spinal or total body irradiation.

KEY POINTS

- Hypothyroidism and, less commonly hyperthyroidism and hyperparathyroidism, occurs after cancer therapy and may well be related to irradiation-induced (e.g. radiation fall-out experiments) or passively transferred (stem cell transfer) autoimmunity as well as direct glandular destruction.
- The high prevalence (30–50 per cent) of primary hypothyroidism (frank or compensated) after direct or scattered thyroid irradiation in doses >10 Gy deserves annual or 2-yearly screening and early treatment to suppress thyrotrophin (TSH) drive and tumorigenesis. Adjuvant chemotherapy increases the risk but its independent toxicity remains unclear.
- Mild or coexisting central hypothyroidism (due to neurosecretory disturbance) may be difficult to detect without detailed endocrine evaluation and its clinical import needs further scrutiny. Nevertheless, it should be considered in those with low normal fT4 and detectable TSH just within the normal range who complain of fatigue, weight gain or poor growth after cranial irradiation, and who may benefit from a trial of thyroxine replacement therapy.
- Radioidine [131]I (diagnostic or therapeutic) equivalent to 1 Gy, does not appear to increase late tumor risk.
- Thyroid irradiation doses as low as <0.1 Gy administered for benign head and neck disease significantly increase thyroid (and probably parathyroid) tumor risk (between 3 and 50 times) in a dose-dependent fashion, greatest in the first 20–30 years.
- The relationship between dose- and tumor risk is linear between 0.3 and 8–10 Gy but plateaus at higher doses (>20 Gy), although still significantly elevated even at 40 years.
- Risk factors for tumorigenesis in the irradiated gland are female sex, young age, thyroid dose and duration of TSH elevation. In part, data may be confounded by increased autoimmunity, estrogen or contraceptive use, and parity in females, factors also identified as independent risks in cross-sectional studies.
- Tumors are usually papillary in nature and have a good long-term prognosis, if effectively treated (total thyroidectomy). RET proto-oncogenes and/or autoimmunity may be implicated in the above. Total or subtotal thyroidectomy and ablative ^{131}I for those proving malignant in a recognized center of expertise are recommended.
- The specificity and sensitivity of ultrasound surveillance scans needs to be clearly ascertained, but serial thyroid function tests and annual thyroid palpation are important screens to evaluate the need for further ultrasonic scanning in high-risk groups for many years of follow-up.

REFERENCES

1. Tannenbaum GS, Ling N. The interrelationship of growth hormone-releasing factor and somatostatin in the generation of the ultradian rhythm of growth hormone secretion. *Endocrinology* 1984; **115**:1952–1957.
2. Frohman LA, Downs TR, Clarke IJ, Thomas GB. Measurement of growth hormone-releasing hormone and somatostatin in hypothalamic-portal plasma of unanaesthetized sheep. *J Clin Invest* 1990; **86**:17–24.
3. Hindmarsh PC, Brain CE, Robinson ICAF, *et al.* The interaction of growth hormone releasing hormone and somatostatin in the generation of a GH pulse in man. *Clin Endocrinol (Oxf)* 1991; **35**:353–360.
4. Goodyer CG, Branchaud CL, Lefebvre Y. Effects of growth hormone (GH)-releasing factor and somatostatin on GH secretion from early to midgestation human fetal pituitaries. *J Clin Endocrinol Metab* 1993; **76**:1259–1264.
♦5. Brabant G, Prank K, Hoang-Vu C, *et al.* Hypothalamic regulation of pulsatile thyrotropin secretion. *J Clin Endocrinol Metab* 1991; **72**:145–150.
6. Veldhuis JD, Iranmanesh A, Johnson ML, Lizarralde G. Twenty-four-hour rhythms in plasma concentrations of adenohypophyseal hormones are generated by distinct amplitude and/or frequency modulation of underlying pituitary secretory bursts. *J Clin Endocrinol Metab* 1990; **71**:1616–1623.
7. Williams TC, Kelijman M, Crelin WC, *et al.* Differential effects of somatostatin (SRIH) and a SRIH analog, SMS 201-995, on the secretion of growth hormone and thyroid-stimulating hormone in man. *J Clin Endocrinol Metab* 1988; **66**:39–45.
8. Siler TM, Yen SSC, Vale W, Guillemin R. Inhibition by somatostatin on the release of TSH induced in man by thyrotropin-releasing factor. *J Clin Endocrinol Metab* 1974; **38**:742–745.
9. Weeke J, Christensen SE, Hansen AP, *et al.* Somatostatin and the 24h levels of serum TSH, T_3, T_4 and reverse T_3 in normals, diabetics and patients treated for myxoedema. *Acta Endocrinol* 1980; **94**:30–37.
10. Rossmanith WG, Mortola JF, Laughlin GA, Yen SSC. Dopaminergic control of circadian and pulsatile pituitary thyrotropin release in women. *J Clin Endocrinol Metab* 1988; **67**:560–564.
11. Ghigo E, Imperiale E, Mazza E, *et al.* Cholinergic enhancement by pyridostigmine potentiates spontaneous diurnal but not nocturnal growth hormone secretion in short children. *Neuroendocrinology* 1989; **49**:134–137.
♦12. Spoudeas HA, Matthews DR, Brook CGD, Hindmarsh PC. The effect of changing somatostatin (SS) tone on the pituitary growth hormone (GH) and thyroid stimulating hormone (TSH) response to their respective releasing factor stimuli. *J Clin Endocrinol Metab* 1992; **75**:453–458.
13. De Zegher F, Vanhole C, Van den Berghe G. Properties of thyroid-stimulating hormone and cortisol secretion by the human newborn on the day of birth. *J Clin Endocrinol Metab* 1994; **79**:576–581.
14. Michaud P, Foradori A, Rodriguez-Portales JA, *et al.* A prepubertal surge of thyrotropin precedes an increase in thyroxine and 3,5,3-triiodothyronine in normal children. *J Clin Endocrinol Metab* 1991; **72**:976–981.
♦15. Rose SR, Manasco PK, Pearce S, Nisula BC. Hypothyroidism and deficiency of the nocturnal thyrotropin surge in children with hypothalamo-pituitary disorders. *J Clin Endocrinol Metab* 1990; **70**:1750–1755.
16. Berelowitz M, Maeda K, Harris S, Frohman LA. The effect of alterations in the pituitary–thyroid axis on hypothalamic content and in vitro release of somatostatin-like immunoreactivity. *Endocrinology* 1980; **107**:24–29.
17. Reichlin S. Somatostatin. *N Engl J Med* 1983; **309**:1495–1501.
18. Goodyer CG, Branchaud CL, Lefevre Y. In vitro modulation of growth hormone (GH) secretion from early to midgestation human fetal pituitaries by GH-releasing factor and somatostatin: role of G_S-adenylate cyclase-G_i complex and Ca5 channels. *J Clin Endocrinol Metab* 1993; **76**:1265–1270.
19. Bilezikjian L, Vale W. Stimulation of adenosine 3'5'-monophosphate production by growth hormone-releasing hormone and its inhibition by somatostatin in anterior pituitary cells in vitro. *Endocrinology* 1983; **113**:1726–1731.
20. Barinaga M, Bilezikjian LM, Vale WW, *et al.* Independent effects of growth hormone releasing factor on growth hormone release and gene transcription. *Nature* 1985; **314**:279–281.
21. Geras E, Rebecchi MJ, Gershengorn MC. Evidence that stimulation of thyrotropin and prolactin secretion by thyrotropin-releasing hormone occur via different calcium-mediated mechanisms: studies with verapamil. *Endocrinology* 1982; **110**:901–907.
22. Molitch ME. Pathologic hyperprolactinaemia. In: Veldhuis JD (ed.) *Neuroendocrinology 1. Endocrinology and Metabolism Clinics of North America.* Philadelphia: WB Saunders, 1992:877–901.
23. Samaan NA, Vieto R, Schultz PN, *et al.* Hypothalamic, pituitary and thyroid dysfunction after radiotherapy to the head and neck. *Int J Radiat Oncol Biol Phys* 1982; **8**:1857–1867.
♦24. Constine LS, Woolf PD, Cann D, *et al.* Hypothalamic–pituitary dysfunction after radiation for brain tumors. *N Engl J Med* 1993; **328**:87–94.
25. Lissett CA, Shalet SM. Management of pituitary tumours. *Horm Res* 2000; **53**(Suppl. 3):65–70.
26. Shupnik MA, Greenspan SL, Ridgeway C. Transcriptional regulation of thyrotropin subunit genes by TRH and dopamine in pituitary cell cultures. *J Biol Chem* 1986; **261**:12675–12679.
27. Martinoli MG, Pelletier G. Thyroid and glucocorticoid hormone regulation of rat pituitary growth hormone messenger ribonucleic acid as revealed by in situ hybridization. *Endocrinology* 1989; **125**:1246–1252.
28. Katakami H, Downs TR, Frohman LA. Decreased hypothalamic growth hormone-releasing hormone content and pituitary responsiveness in hypothyroidism. *J Clin Invest* 1986; **77**:1704–1711.
29. Williams T, Maxon H, Thorner MO. Blunted growth hormone (GH) response to GH-releasing hormone in hypothyroidism resolves in the euthyroid state. *J Clin Endocrinol Metab* 1985; **61**:454–456.
30. Coggle JE. The effect of radiation at the tissue level. *Biological effects of radiation.* London: Taylor and Francis, 1983:89–109.
31. Withers HR. Biology of radiation oncology. In: Tobias JS, Thomas PRM (eds) *Current radiation oncology.* Vol. 1. London: Edward Arnold, 1994:5–23.
32. Hopewell JW. Radiation injury to the central nervous system. *Med Pediatr Oncol* 1998; (Suppl.1):1–9.
♦33. Livesey EA, Brook CGD. Thyroid dysfunction after radiotherapy and chemotherapy of brain tumours. *Arch Dis Child* 1989; **64**:593–595.
34. Ogilvy-Stuart AL, Shalet SM, Gattameni HR. Thyroid function after treatment of brain tumors in children. *J Pediatr* 1991; **119**:733–737.
35. Livesey EA, Brook CGD. Gonadal dysfunction after treatment of intracranial tumours. *Arch Dis Child* 1988; **63**:495–500.
36. Byrne J, Mulvihill JJ, Myers MH, *et al.* Effects of treatment on fertility in long-term survivors of childhood or adolescent cancer. *N Engl J Med* 1987; **317**:1315–1321.

◆37. Olshan JS, Gubernick J, Packer RJ, *et al.* The effects of adjuvant chemotherapy on growth in children with medulloblastoma. *Cancer* 1992; **70**:2013–2017.

38. Spoudeas HA, Hindmarsh PC, Matthews DR, Brook CGD. Evolution of growth hormone neurosecretory disturbance after cranial irradiation for childhood brain tumours: a prospective study. *J Endocrinol* 1996; **150**:329–342.

39. Dacou-Voutetakis C, Xypolyta A, Haidas S, *et al.* Irradiation of the head. Immediate effect on growth hormone secretion in children. *J Clin Endocrinol Metab* 1977; **44**:791–794.

40. Chrousos GP, Poplack D, Brown T, *et al.* Effects of cranial radiation on hypothalamic–adenohypophyseal function: abnormal growth hormone secretory dynamics. *J Clin Endocrinol Metab* 1982; **54**:1135–1139.

41. Bailey CC, Gnekow A, Wellek S, *et al.* Prospective randomised trial of chemotherapy given before radiotherapy in childhood medulloblastoma. International Society of Paediatric Oncology (SIOP) and the (German) Society of Paediatric Oncology (GPO): SIOP II. *Med Pediatr Oncol* 1995; **25**:166–178.

42. Packer RJ, Goldwein J, Nicholson HS, *et al.* Treatment of children with medulloblastomas with reduced-dose craniospinal radiation therapy and adjuvant chemotherapy: A Children's Cancer Group Study. *J Clin Oncol* 1999; **17**:2127–2136.

◆43. Mulhern RK, Kepner JL, Thomas PR, *et al.* Neuropsychologic functioning of survivors of childhood medulloblastoma randomized to receive conventional or reduced-dose craniospinal irradiation; a pediatric oncology group study. *J Clin Oncol* 1998; **16**:1723–1728.

◆44. Littley MD, Shalet SM, Beardwell CG, *et al.* Hypopituitarism following external radiotherapy for pituitary tumours in adults. *Q J Med* 1989; **262**:145–160.

45. Livesey EA, Hindmarsh PC, Brook CG, *et al.* Endocrine disorders following treatment of childhood brain tumours. *Br J Cancer* 1990; **61**:622–625.

◆46. Littley MD, Shalet SM, Beardwell CG, *et al.* Radiation induced hypopituitarism is dose dependent. *Clin Endocrinol* 1989; **31**:363–373.

47. Clayton PE, Shalet SM. Dose dependency of time of onset of radiation-induced growth hormone deficiency. *J Pediatr* 1991; **118**:226–228.

48. Ris MD, Packer R, Goldwein J, *et al.* Intellectual outcome after reduced-dose radiation therapy plus adjuvant chemotherapy for medulloblastoma: a children's cancer study group study. *J Clin Oncol* 2001; **19**:3470–3476.

49. Iranmanesh A, Lizarralde G, Veldhuis JD. Age and relative adiposity are specific negative determinants of the frequency and amplitude of GH secretory bursts and the half-life of endogenous GH in healthy men. *J Clin Endocrinol Metab* 1991; **73**:1081–1086.

50. Toogood AA, Shalet SM. Growth hormone replacement therapy in the elderly with hypothalamic-pituitary disease: a dose-finding study. *J Clin Endocrinol Metab* 1999; **84**:131–136.

51. Dattani MT, Pringle PJ, Hindmarsh PC, Brook CGD. What is a normal stimulated growth hormone concentration? *J Endocrinol* 1992; **133**:447–450.

52. Nivot S, Benelli C, Clot JP, *et al.* Nonparallel changes of growth hormone (GH) and insulin-like growth factor-1, insulin-like growth factor binding protein-3, and GH-binding protein, after craniospinal irradiation and chemotherapy. *J Clin Endocrinol Metab* 1994; **78**:597–601.

53. Achermann JC, Hindmarsh PC, Brook CGD. The relationship between the growth hormone and insulin-like growth factor axis in long-term survivors of childhood brain tumours. *Clin Endocrinol (Oxf)* 1998; **49**:639–645.

54. Shalet SM, Beardwell CG, MacFarlane IA, *et al.* Endocrine morbidity in adults treated with cerebral irradiation for brain tumours during childhood. *Acta Endocrinol* 1977; **84**:673–680.

◆55. Spoudeas HA, Charmandari E, Brook CGD. Hypothalamo-pituitary-adrenal axis integrity after cranial irradiation for childhood posterior fossa tumours. *Med Ped Oncol* 2003; **40**:224–229.

◆56. Schmiegelow M, Lassen S, Poulsen HS, *et al.* Cranial radiotherapy of childhood brain tumours: growth hormone deficiency and its relation to the biological effective dose of irradiation in a large population based study. *Clin Endocrinol (Oxf)* 2000; **53**:191–197.

57. Grossman A, Cohen BL, Charlesworth M, *et al.* Treatment of prolactinomas with megavoltage radiotherapy. *Br Med J (Clin Res Ed)* 1984; **288**:1105–1109.

58. Sheaves R, Jenkins P, Blackburn P, *et al.* Outcome of transsphenoidal surgery for acromegaly using strict criteria for surgical cure. *Clin Endocrinol (Oxf)* 1996; **45**:407–413.

59. Arafah BM, Kailini SH, Neckl KE, *et al.* Immediate recovery of pituitary function after transphenoidal resection of pituitary macroadenomas. *J Clin Endocrinol Metab* 1994; **79**:348–354.

60. Shalet SM, Fairhall KM, Sparks E, *et al.* Radiosensitivity of hypothalamo-pituitary (HP) function in the rat is time and dose dependent. *Horm Res* 1999; **51**(Suppl. 2): P103.

61. Dattani MT, Robinson IC. The molecular basis for developmental disorders of the pituitary gland in man. *Clin Genet* 2000; **57**:337–346.

62. Ahmed S, Elsheikh M, Stratton IM, *et al.* Outcome of transphenoidal surgery for acromegaly and its relationship to surgical experience. *Clin Endocrinol (Oxf)* 1999; **50**:561–567.

63. Chieng PU, Huang TS, Chang CC, *et al.* Reduced hypothalamic blood flow after radiation treatment of nasopharyngeal cancer: SPECT studies in 34 patients. *Am J Nuclear Radiol* 1991; **12**:661–665.

64. Achermann J. The pathophysiology of post-irradiation growth hormone insufficiency. MD thesis, University of London, 1997.

65. Charmandari E, Brook CGD. 20 years of experience in idiopathic central diabetes insipidus. *Lancet* 1999; **353**:2212–2213.

66. Dickinson WP, Berry DH, Dickinson L, *et al.* Differential effects of cranial irradiation on growth hormone responses to arginine and insulin infusion. *J Pediatr* 1978; **92**:754–757.

67. Jorgensen EV, Schwartz ID, Hvizdala E, *et al.* Neurotransmitter control of growth hormone secretion in children after cranial radiation therapy. *J Pediatr Endocrinol* 1993; **6**:131–142.

68. Grossman A, Lytras N, Savage MO, *et al.* Growth hormone releasing factor: comparison of two analogues and demonstration of hypothalamic defect in growth hormone release after radiotherapy. *Br Med J* 1984; **288**:1785–1787.

69. Spoudeas HA, Hindmarsh PC, Brook CGD. Hypothalamic dysregulation after craniospinal irradiation for childhood cerebellar tumours. *Acta Paediatr Suppl* 1995; **411**:101 (abstract).

●70. Spoudeas HA. The evolution of growth hormone neurosecretory disturbance during high dose cranial irradiation and chemotherapy for childhood brain tumours. MD thesis, University of London, 1995.

◆71. Rose SR, Lustig RH, Pitukcheewanont P, *et al.* Diagnosis of central hidden hypothyroidism in survivors of childhood cancer. *J Clin Endocrinol Metab* 1999; **84**:4472–4479.

72. Lustig RH, Schriock EA, Kaplan SL, Grumbach MM. Effect of growth hormone-releasing factor on growth hormone release in children with radiation-induced growth hormone deficiency. *Pediatrics* 1985; **76**:274–279.

73. Spoudeas HA, Winrow AP, Hindmarsh PC, Brook CGD. Low dose growth hormone-releasing hormone tests: a dose response study. *Eur J Endocrinol* 1994; **131**:238–245.

74. Ogilvy-Stuart AL, Wallace WHB, Shalet SM. Radiation and neuroregulatory control of growth hormone secretion. *Clin Endocrinol (Oxf)* 1994; **41**:163–168.

75. Plotsky PM, Vale W. Patterns of growth hormone-releasing factor and somatostatin secretion into the hypophysial-portal circulation of the rat. *Science* 1985; **230**:461–463.

76. Hall JE, Martin KA, Whitney HA, *et al.* Potential for fertility with replacement of hypothalamic gonadotropin-releasing hormone in long term female survivors of cranial tumours. *J Clin Endocrinol Metab* 1994; **79**:1166–1172.

77. Ogilvy-Stuart AL, Stirling HF, Kelnar CJH, *et al.* Treatment of radiation-induced growth hormone deficiency with growth hormone-releasing hormone. *Clin Endocrinol* 1997; **46**:571–578.

78. Masala A, Faedda R, Alagna S, *et al*. Use of testosterone to prevent cyclophosphamide-induced azoospermia. *Ann Intern Med* 1997; **126**:292–295.

79. Chiarenza A, Lempereur L, Palmucci T, *et al.* Responsiveness of irradiated rat anterior pituitary cells to hypothalamic releasing hormones is restored by treatment with growth hormone. *Neuro-endocrinol* 2000; **72**:392–399.

•80. Rose SR. Cranial irradiation and central hypothyroidism trends. *Endocrinol Metab* 2001; **12**:97–104.

81. Shalet SM, Rosenstock JD, Beardwell CG, *et al.* Thyroid dysfunction following external irradiation to the neck for Hodgkin's disease in childhood. *Clin Radiol* 1977; **28**:511–515.

82. Devney RB, Sklar CA, Nesbit ME, *et al.* Serial thyroid function measurements in children with Hodgkin disease. *J Pediatr* 1984; **105**:223–227.

83. Green DEM, Brecher ML, Yakar D, *et al.* Thyroid function in pediatric patients after neck irradiation for Hodgkin disease. *Med Pediatr Oncol* 1980; **8**:127–136.

♦84. Mauch PM, Weinstein H, Botnick L, *et al.* An evaluation of long-term survival and treatment complications in children with Hodgkin's disease. *Cancer* 1983: **51**:925–932.

85. Sutcliffe SB, Chapman R, Wrigley PFM. Cyclical combination chemotherapy and thyroid function in patients with advanced Hodgkin's disease. *Med Pediatr Oncol* 1981; **9**:439–448.

86. Bethge W, Guggenberger D, Bamberg M, *et al.* Thyroid toxicity of treatment for Hodgkin's disease. *Ann Haematol* 2000; **79**:114–118.

87. Shafford EA, Kingston JE, Healy JC, *et al.* Thyroid nodular disease after radiotherapy to the neck for childhood Hodgkin's disease. *Br J Cancer* 1999; **80**:808–814.

♦88. Sklar C, Whitton J, Mertens A, *et al.* Abnormalities of the thyroid in survivors of Hodgkin's disease: data from the Childhood Cancer Survivor Study. *J Clin Endocrinol Metab* 2000; **85**:3227–3232.

89. Sklar CA, Kim TH, Ramsey NK, *et al.* Thyroid dysfunction among long term survivors of bone marrow transplantation. *Am J Med* 1982; **73**:688–694.

90. Sanders JE, Pritchard S, Mahoney P, *et al.* Growth and development following marrow transplantation for leukaemia. *Blood* 1986; **68**:1129–1135.

91. Sanders JE. The impact of marrow transplant preparative regimens on subsequent growth and development. *Semin Haematol* 1991; **28**:244–249.

♦92. Katsanis E, Shapiro RS, Robison LL, *et al.* Thyroid dysfunction following bone marrow transplantation: long term follow-up of 80 pediatric patients *Bone Marrow Transplant* 1990; **5**:335–340.

93. Schneider AB, Ron E, Lubin J, *et al.* Dose–response relationships for radiation-induced thyroid cancer and thyroid nodules: evidence for the prolonged effects of radiation on the thyroid. *J Clin Endocrinol Metab* 1993; **77**:362–369.

94. Pacini F, Vorontsova T, Molinaro E, *et al.* Thyroid consequences of the Chernobyl nuclear accident. *Acta Paediatr Suppl* 1999; **88**:23–27.

95. Modan B, Baidaty D, Mart H, *et al.* Radiation-induced head and neck tumors. *Lancet* 1974; **i**:277–279.

96. Refetoff S, Harrison J, Karanfilski BT, *et al.* Continuing occurrence of thyroid carcinoma after irradiation to the neck in infancy and childhood. *N Engl J Med* 1975; **292**:171–175.

97. Dos Santos I, Swerdlow A. Thyroid cancer epidemiology in England and Wales; time trends and geographical distribution. *Br J Cancer* 1993; **67**:330–340.

98. Pettersson B, Adami H, Wilander E, Coleman M. Trends in thyroid cancer incidence in Sweden, 1958–1981, by histopathologic type. *Int J Cancer* 1991; **48**:28–33.

99. Colonna M, Grosclaude P, Remontet L, *et al.* Incidence of thyroid cancer in adults recorded by French cancer registries (1978–1997). *Eur J Cancer* 2002; **38**:1762–1768.

100. Zheng T, Holford T, Chen Y, *et al.* Time trend and age-period-cohort effect on incidence of thyroid cancer in Connecticut, 1935–1992. *Int J Cancer* 1996; **67**:504–509.

101. Shore RE, Hildreth N, Dvoretsky P, *et al.* Thyroid cancer among persons given X-ray treatment in infancy for an enlarged thymus gland. *Am J Epidemiol* 1993; **137**:1068–1080.

♦102. Ron E, Lubin JH, Shore RE, *et al.* Thyroid cancer after exposure to external irradiation: a pooled analysis of seven studies. *Radiat Res* 1995; **141**:259–277.

103. Metayer C, Lynch CF, Clarke EA, *et al.* Second cancers among long-term survivors of Hodgkin's disease diagnosed in childhood and adolescence. *J Clin Oncol* 2000; **18**:2435–2443.

104. Sklar C, Mertens AC, Mitby P, *et al.* Risk of disease recurrence and second neoplasms in survivors of childhood cancer treated with growth hormone: a report from the Childhood Cancer Survivor Study. *J Clin Endocrinol Metab* 2002; **87**:3136–3141.

105. Rasmussen T, Damber L, Johansson L, *et al.* Increased incidence of parathyroid adenomas following X-ray treatment of benign disease in the cervical spine in adult patients. *Clin Endocrinol* 2002; **57**:731–734.

106. Tezelman S, Rodriguez JM, Shen W, *et al.* Primary hyperparathyroidism in patients who have received radiation therapy and in patients who have not received radiation therapy. *J Am Coll. Surg* 1995; **180**:81–87.

•107. Rubino C, Cailleux AF, De Vathaire F, Schlumberger M. Thyroid cancer after radiation exposure. *Eur J Cancer* 2002; **35**:645–647.

108. Hahn K, Schnell-Inderst P, Grosche B, Holn LE. Thyroid cancer after diagnostic administration of Iodine-131 in childhood. *Radiat Res* 2001; **156**:61–70.

109. Hall P, Mattson A, Boice JD Jr. Thyroid cancer after diagnostic administration of iodine-131. *Radiat Res* 1996; **145**: 86–92.

110. Memon A, Varghese A, Suresh A. Benign thyroid disease and dietary factors in thyroid cancer : a case-control study in Kuwait. *Br J Cancer* 2002; **86**:1745–1750.

Ovarian and uterine function and reproductive potential

HILARY OD CRITCHLEY, ANGELA B THOMSON AND W HAMISH B WALLACE

INTRODUCTION

The survival rate for children with cancer has dramatically increased over the past three decades, as many pediatric cancers are now treatable with multiagent chemotherapy in combination with radiotherapy and surgery.[1-3] It has been estimated that 1 in 1000 young adults are current survivors of childhood cancer and the expected 5-year survival rate following cytotoxic treatment, with or without surgery, is at least 70 per cent or higher.[4] Inevitably, some of these young survivors of childhood cancer face a future with specific problems as a consequence of their treatment.[5] The challenge for children's cancer specialists today is to maintain the current dramatic improvement in survival rates and to minimize the late effects of modern treatment regimens. The reproductive system is a vulnerable site for late effects of anticancer treatment and fertile potential is of particular concern to the young survivors of reproductive age.[6,7]

Infertility is well documented in survivors of childhood cancer. In the female, chemotherapy and radiotherapy may damage the ovary and hasten oocyte depletion, resulting in loss of hormone production, truncated fecundity and a premature menopause.[6,7] In addition, natural pubertal progression, fertility and a successful pregnancy outcome require a normally functioning hypothalamic–pituitary–ovarian-uterine axis. Thus,

adverse effects of radiotherapy or chemotherapy may be mediated through the hypothalamic–pituitary–ovarian axis,[8] the ovary[8,9] or the uterus.[10,11] The large 'Five Center Study' commissioned by the National Cancer Institute in North America, followed survivors between 1945 and 1975, and demonstrated an adjusted relative fertility in survivors of 0.85 (95 per cent confidence interval

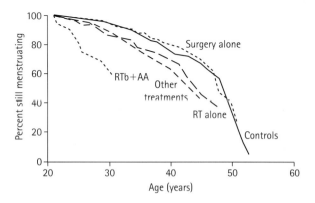

Figure 8c.1 *Menopause in childhood cancer survivors and controls expressed as the proportion of women still menstruating. Survivors' disease diagnosed between the ages of 13 and 19 years. RTb + AA, radiation below the diaphragm plus alkylating agents; RT, radiotherapy alone. (Reproduced with permission from Byrne et al. 1992.[12])*

0.78–0.92) compared with that of their siblings. The Five Center Study demonstrated that premature menopause was more commonly experienced in those patients who had been treated with infradiaphragmatic irradiation and alkylating agents, with an average age of menopause of 31 years. The risk of premature ovarian failure was greater with increasing age at the time of treatment[12,13] (Figure 8c.1).

Management of children with cancer requires an understanding of the gonadotoxic effects of therapy, counseling and, where possible, efforts made to preserve fertility. In addition, long-term follow-up of the survivors is essential to monitor for premature ovarian failure, adverse pregnancy outcome and the health of the offspring. An awareness of the impact of cancer treatment on reproductive potential has stimulated pursuit of strategies to preserve fertility. Advances in assisted reproduction techniques have focused attention on preserving gonadal tissue for future use.[14–19] Cryopreservation of immature ovarian tissue is the most promising option, with restoration of natural fertility and preservation of hormone production following autotransplantation, or maturation of oocytes *in vitro* in combination with assisted reproduction.[14,15] Many scientific, ethical and legal issues remain to be addressed before techniques to preserve fertility are available.[20] In this subchapter we consider the impact of radiotherapy and chemotherapy treatment for childhood cancer on female reproductive function, strategies for preservation of fertile potential and implications for the health of the offspring.

INVESTIGATION OF OVARIAN FUNCTION

The human ovary is endowed with a fixed pool of primordial follicles, maximal at about 5 months of age and with approximately two million oocytes present at birth. Follicle depletion, as a result of atresia and recruitment towards ovulation, leads to premature exhaustion of the follicle pool and menopause at a median age of 51 years. The fertile 'window' in females is characterized by roughly 400 monthly ovulations of a mature oocyte.[21,22] Ovarian failure and a premature menopause will arise from any cytotoxic insult, which either depletes the oocyte pool or hastens its decline.[12] Although the exact mechanisms of cytotoxic damage are uncertain, both chemotherapy and radiotherapy may inflict such an insult. If the child is peripubertal at the time of treatment, there may be arrest of pubertal development with subsequent primary amenorrhea. In postpubertal females, ovarian failure will manifest as secondary amenorrhea, often with symptoms of estrogen deficiency. Biochemically, ovarian failure is detected as elevated gonadotrophins and undetectable estradiol. It must be

remembered that follicle-stimulating hormone (FSH) levels often fluctuate and FSH testing may need repeating. Prediction of a premature menopause is difficult, although early follicular phase assay of FSH, estradiol and inhibin B, and ovarian ultrasound are potential tools to assess ovarian reserve. Elevated early follicular phase FSH with preservation of estradiol production is characteristic of the perimenopause, the length of which may vary.[23,24] Ovarian failure will require estrogen replacement for pubertal induction and cyclical hormone replacement to relieve the symptoms of estrogen deficiency (vaginal dryness, hot flushes and irritability), provide cardiovascular protection and optimize bone density.[25] While normal progression through puberty, and the onset of menarche and continuation of regular menstrual cycles are reassuring, it is not predictive of a normal reproductive life span. Quantifying the magnitude of the insult and predicting the onset of ovarian failure has become a realistic possibility following radiotherapy,[26] but remains difficult to assess following chemotherapy. In a small number of cases, recovery of menstruation is seen suggesting that additional mechanisms to cytotoxic follicle death may be involved. These women may still progress to a premature menopause and all patients will require long-term follow-up.

EFFECTS OF CANCER TREATMENT ON SUBSEQUENT OVARIAN FUNCTION

Radiation-induced ovarian damage

Although used sparingly because of damage to growing tissues, radiotherapy is administered to obtain local disease control and to consolidate remission. Total body, craniospinal, abdominal or pelvic irradiation may cause ovarian and uterine dysfunction (Table 8c.1). The degree of impairment is related to the radiation dose, fractionation schedule and age at time of treatment.[9,11,26–36]

Table 8c.1 *Radiotherapy-induced damage to the reproductive tract*

Site	Effect
Cranial/total body irradiation	Hypogonadotrophic hypogonadism
Total body irradiation/ abdomen/pelvic	Ovarian failure ($LD_{50} < 2$ Gy)
	Older women >6 Gy Younger women >20 Gy
	Uterine damage Decreased volume Decreased elasticity

The number of primordial follicles present at the time of treatment and the dose of radiotherapy will determine the fertile 'window', and dictate the age at menopause. A number of mathematical models have been proposed to explain the complex process of natural follicle decline based on a series of data describing the number of follicles present at different ages in humans.[22,26,35,36] For any given age, the size of the follicle pool can be estimated based upon a complex mathematical model of decline. In order to predict the age of menopause in patients following radiotherapy, the extent of the radiation-induced damage to the follicle pool can be determined. We have previously estimated the dose of radiation required to destroy 50 per cent of the oocytes (LD_{50}) to be less than 4 Gy, based upon an exponential model of oocyte decay.[27] The mathematical model used to calculate this value is now believed to be an oversimplification and current thinking is that follicle decay represents an instantaneous rate of temporal change based upon the remaining population pool, expressed mathematically as a differential equation.[22,37,38] Furthermore, we determined the LD_{50} to be 4 Gy from our original cohort of women, who were treated with 30 Gy at a median age (range) of 4 (1.3–13.1) years and in whom ovarian failure was detected at 12.7 (9.7–15.9) years. Given the high doses of irradiation administered, it is likely that ovarian failure would have occurred earlier but was unable to be detected clinically. This would have led to an overestimate of the calculated LD_{50}.

In a second study, ovarian function was assessed in eight patients who had received total body irradiation (TBI; 14.4 Gy) at age 11.5 (4.9–15.1) years. Ovarian failure was defined as failure to undergo or complete pubertal development or the onset of secondary amenorrhea in conjunction with persistently elevated gonadotrophin [FSH and luteinizing hormone (LH) > 32 IU/l] and low estradiol levels (<40 pmol/l). Six of the eight subjects at age 13.15 (12.5–16) years had ovarian failure.[32] Based on this new data, where diagnosis of ovarian failure was more likely to reflect the true age of onset of ovarian failure, and a revised mathematical model of natural oocyte decline, we were able to determine the surviving fraction of oocytes following irradiation and estimate the LD_{50} of the human oocyte to be less than 2 Gy.[76] This explains sterilization with total depletion of primordial follicle reserve following high doses of radiotherapy and premature ovarian failure following with lower doses that cause only partial depletion of the primordial follicle pool. Using this model, it is possible to predict the likely age of premature ovarian failure following a given dose of radiation at any age. This will enable us to counsel patients more appropriately with regard to reproductive function and, where possible, take measures to preserve fertility.

Total body irradiation, either alone or in combination with chemotherapy, is used as conditioning for bone marrow transplantation and may cause infertility.[11,30–32]

In a long-term follow-up of 708 women, median age (range) 3 (1–17) years, post bone marrow transplantation, 532 had received TBI (10–15.75 Gy, single exposure or fractionated) and cyclophosphamide (200 mg/kg) and 176 were treated with cyclophosphamide (200 mg/kg) alone or with busulphan (16 mg/kg), as conditioning therapy. Ovarian failure was observed in 90 per cent of patients following TBI and 68 per cent following chemotherapy only. Among an additional 82 patients treated prepubertally with the same regimens, ovarian failure was reported in 72 per cent.[30]

Bath et al. studied the impact of TBI on ovarian function in childhood and adolescence. Ovarian function was assessed in eight patients who had received TBI (14.4 Gy) at age 11.5 (4.9–15.1) years. Six of the eight girls, at age 13.15 (12.5–16) years, had ovarian failure. Biochemical evidence of incipient ovarian failure was observed in two girls treated prepubertally, with clinically apparent preservation of ovarian function.[11]

Matsumoto et al. studied ovarian function in 18 girls who had undergone bone marrow transplantation at age 8.5 (4.5–15.3) years, before the onset of menarche, for a variety of hematological malignant (n = 14) and non-malignant conditions (n = 4).[32] Conditioning therapy involved a variety of chemotherapy agents and fractionated TBI, 8–12 Gy and 6–8 Gy for malignant and non-malignant diseases, respectively. Twelve patients achieved menarche at a median age of 12.8 (10.8–14) years. Age at transplant was significantly younger in girls who achieved menarche than in those who developed primary amenorrhea [mean (SD), 7.2 (0.5) vs. 11.1 (1.7)]. The younger patients had a larger oocyte pool at the time of treatment and may have a shortened window of opportunity for fertility before developing a premature menopause. Furthermore, in five of the remaining six patients, gonadotrophin levels were elevated despite the onset of menses. This may reflect impending premature ovarian failure and truncated fecundity.

Abdominal and pelvic irradiation may be used in the treatment of a variety of malignancies including Wilms' tumor, pelvic rhabdomyosarcoma and Ewing's sarcoma of the pelvis or spine, with the dose and volume dependent upon the diagnosis and tumor size. Ovarian function was reviewed sequentially in 53 females treated between 1942–1985 with surgery and external abdominal radiotherapy for an intra-abdominal tumor. Ovarian failure was observed in 97 per cent (37 of 38) of females following whole abdominal irradiation in childhood (20–30 Gy). Of the 37 women, primary amenorrhea was reported in 71 per cent and a premature menopause (median age 23.5 years) in the remainder.[9] Of the 15 patients who received flank irradiation (20–30 Gy), median age at assessment 15.2 years, ovarian function was normal in all but one in whom pubertal failure had occurred. In one patient who required sex steroid replacement therapy to

achieve normal secondary sexual characteristics for pubertal failure following abdominal radiotherapy, there was evidence of recovery of ovarian function with conception reported at age 22.7 years. In total, there were four documented conceptions, all patients had received whole abdominal irradiation (20–26.5 Gy), but all had mid-trimester miscarriages and subsequently underwent a premature menopause. Poor uterine function may have contributed to the failure to sustain pregnancy. It is well recognized that the prevalence of ovarian failure following whole abdominal radiotherapy has been unacceptably high, with the majority of patients failing to complete pubertal development without hormone replacement therapy. The introduction of flank irradiation from 1972 has resulted in significantly less pubertal failure but the onset of a premature menopause may occur with time.

A permanent menopause may be induced in women over 40 years following gonadal radiotherapy treatment with 6 Gy, while significantly higher doses are required to completely destroy the oocyte pool and induce ovarian failure in younger women and children.[33] This reflects the smaller follicle reserve in older patients and hence increased susceptibility to smaller doses of irradiation.

In a retrospective study of medical records of 830 long-term female survivors of childhood cancer, Chiarelli *et al.* evaluated the risk of premature menopause and infertility following abdominal–pelvic radiation and/or alkylating agent-based chemotherapy compared with those patients treated with non-sterilizing surgery alone.[34] The results demonstrated that the risk of premature ovarian failure increased significantly with increasing dose of abdominal irradiation. The relative risk with doses <20 Gy was 1.02, increasing to 1.37 with irradiation of 20–35 Gy, and a relative risk of 3.27 with doses >35 Gy. The percentage of women with premature ovarian failure was 22 per cent and 32 per cent following radiation doses of 20–35 Gy and >35 Gy, respectively.

Cranial or craniospinal radiotherapy may be used in the treatment of some brain tumors and acute lymphoblastic leukemia with central nervous system (CNS) involvement. Scatter irradiation from craniospinal radiotherapy may directly affect ovarian function. Cranial irradiation may indirectly impair ovarian function by causing hypogonadotrophic hypogonadism. Gonadotrophins were elevated in 7 of 11 (64 per cent) females who had received cranial irradiation (mean dose 32 Gy) for brain tumors.[39]

Hypothalamic–pituitary function shows progressive compromise following high-dose cranial irradiation (>30 Gy) and the risk of gonadotrophin deficiency is 60 per cent by 4 years out from treatment.[40] Low-dose CNS-directed radiotherapy in the treatment of acute lymphoblastic leukemia (ALL) has been associated with subtle perturbations in growth hormone secretion but there are a few reports assessing the impact on the secretion of other pituitary hormones in adulthood.[41–43] In a study on reproductive function following treatment for childhood ALL, women who had received prophylactic CNS radiation had a significantly lower first birth rate than those without irradiation, indicating that doses of 18–24 Gy to the brain may be a possible risk factor.[44] The late effects of hypothalamic–pituitary–ovarian dysfunction are often subtle and may be progressive with time. Bath *et al.* report decreased LH production, reduced LH surge and short luteal phases in a group of women treated with low-dose cranial irradiation (18–24 Gy) as CNS-directed therapy for ALL.[45] Short luteal phases have been associated with reduced fertility and early miscarriage.[46] Data such as these reiterate the requirement for detailed follow-up of these patients if immediate and longer term effects on reproductive potential are to be established. A history of regular menstruation does not necessarily reflect normal hypothalamic and pituitary function. If a patient does experience hypogonadotrophic hypogonadism following cranial radiotherapy, ovulatory cycles may be achieved through the use of pulsatile gonadotrophin therapy. For women exposed to low-dose cranial irradiation, regular menses does not ensure normal hypothalamic–pituitary function, and early referral and detailed endocrine assessment is necessary, if these women present with infertility.

CHEMOTHERAPY–INDUCED OVARIAN DAMAGE

The effects on gonadal function of combination cytotoxic chemotherapy depend upon the type and total dose of drugs administered. The ovary is chemosensitive. There are few data available on threshold doses for ovarian dysfunction. The risk of gonadal damage with evolving chemotherapeutic regimens requires to be evaluated as an ongoing exercise. The age of the patient at the time of anticancer treatment plays a major role, with progressively smaller doses being required to produce ovarian failure with increasing age.[47–50] Chemotherapeutic agents known to be gonadotoxic are listed in Table 8c.2.

It is clear from the data available to date that, in children who received combination chemotherapy for ALL, a premature loss of ovarian function was uncommon.[51–53] Wallace and colleagues studied 40 female survivors of treatment for ALL.[28] Every girl achieved adult pubertal development and 37 described regular menstruation. There were 14 live births recorded in nine of the long-term survivors. Exposure to more intensive chemotherapeutic regimens for ALL may be associated with a greater risk of premature menopause.

The early reports also indicate that ovarian function is maintained after chemotherapeutic treatment of Hodgkin's disease in childhood.[54] In a recent study on

Table 8c.2 *Chemotherapeutic agents known to be gonadotoxic*

Alkylating agents
  Cyclophosphamide
  Ifosfamide
  Nitrosoureas, e.g. carmustine, lomustine
  Chlorambucil
  Melphalan
  Busulphan
Vinca–alkaloids
  Vinblastine
Antimetabolites
  Cytarabine
Platinum agents
  Cis-platinum
Others
  Procarbazine

gonadal function after chemotherapy alone for childhood Hodgkin's disease in 32 female survivors at a median age of 13.0 (9–15.2) years treated with ChlVPP (chlorambucil, vinblastine, procarbazine, prednisolone) and no radiotherapy below the diaphragm, 17 (53 per cent) of the girls had raised gonadotrophin levels, ten of whom had symptomatic ovarian failure and six received hormone replacement therapy (HRT). Nine women had 11 successful pregnancies, two of whom had previously had symptoms of ovarian failure with one requiring HRT.[55] Only the long-term follow-up of such patients will establish whether there is a potential for recovery of ovarian function or alternatively a risk of progression to premature ovarian failure.

Alkylating agents form an integral part of many treatment protocols and have long been recognized to impair gonadal function. One of the most widely studied of such agents is cyclophosphamide, which is frequently used in the treatment of many childhood malignancies. High-dose cyclophosphamide may be used as conditioning therapy before bone marrow transplantation either alone, where recovery is more likely, or in combination with other chemotherapeutic agents or total body irradiation. Ovarian function, as defined by spontaneous menstruation and normal hormone profile without hormone supplement, was assessed in 176 females following high-dose cyclophosphamide with or without high-dose busulphan and bone marrow transplantation (aged 13–58 years at transplant).[56] Of the 103 women receiving cyclophosphamide alone (200 mg/kg) ovarian function was preserved in 56 (54 per cent). The addition of busulphan (16 mg/kg) was associated with a higher prevalence of patients with ovarian dysfunction, with recovery observed in only 1 of 73 females.[29]

It is essential that there is comprehensive follow-up of the gonadal function of cancer survivors who have been exposed to the newer multiagent chemotherapeutic protocols.

INVESTIGATION OF UTERINE FUNCTION

Normal uterine shape, length and volume for prepuberty, peripuberty and postpuberty are well documented.[57] Ultrasound scanning is a reliable non-invasive technique for assessing uterine size and shape, blood supply and endometrial thickness. Uterine artery blood flow may be assessed by Doppler scanning and resistance to flow expressed as the pulsatility index. Endometrial biopsy enables assessment of endometrial function using histological and immunocytochemical techniques.[58]

EFFECTS OF CANCER TREATMENT ON UTERINE DEVELOPMENT AND FUNCTION

It is well established that uterine development and function may be compromised following radiotherapy involving the pelvis, regardless of the age at time of treatment. At the time of onset of normal puberty, there is an increase in the dimensions of the uterus and also endometrial thickness. Furthermore, there is a shape change from a tubular to a more pear-shaped organ.[59] It is, therefore, not surprising that irradiation therapies carry a significant risk of impaired uterine development, if delivered prepuberty.

The extent of the damage to the developing uterus is related to the site of radiation, total dose of radiation administered and fractionation schedule employed. Both high-dose abdominal irradiation (20–30 Gy) and the lower doses employed in TBI (14.4 Gy) may cause uterine dysfunction. Uterine physical characteristics including uterine length and blood flow, and endometrial thickness, were assessed in ten women, median age (range), 24 (15–31) years, with premature menopause secondary to whole abdominal radiotherapy (20–30 Gy) for childhood cancer. When compared to a group of 22 women, 31 (23–37) years with premature menopause who had not been exposed to cancer therapy, there was significant reduction in uterine length and uterine blood flow. Furthermore, the cancer survivors did not show any increase in endometrial thickness in response to exogenous physiologic sex steroid replacement therapy.[10,60] These observations were consistent with the view that high-dose abdominal irradiation may have long-term effects on the uterine vasculature and development of the uterus.

There is evidence that young women treated with TBI demonstrate evidence of impaired uterine growth and blood flow.[61] A small but important study by Holm and colleagues evaluated uterine function in 12 women, 4 and 10.9 years after TBI and marrow transplantation for childhood leukemia and lymphoma. Of the 12 subjects, three experienced a spontaneous puberty, eight required sex steroid replacement because of premature ovarian

failure and one described symptoms of estrogen deficiency. The median uterine and ovarian volumes were significantly reduced compared to normal controls, and uterine blood flow was impaired in survivors of childhood cancer. In the women using sex steroid replacement, the average uterine volume was reduced to 40 per cent that of the normal adult size. It would appear that, although the prescribed dose of sex steroid replacement therapy suppressed symptoms of estrogen deficiency and was sufficient to result in uterine withdrawal bleeding, the dose was unable to generate normal uterine growth and development.

A successful pregnancy will require a fully functional hypothalamic–pituitary–ovarian axis, and a uterine cavity that is not only receptive to implantation but that is able to accommodate normal growth of the developing infant to term.[62,63] Pregnancy outcome may be adversely affected by reduced uterine elasticity and fibrosis; effects secondary to abdominal irradiation and possible damage to the uterine vasculature. To date, there are only a few case series of childhood cancer survivors that have addressed issues of subsequent fertility and the health of offspring among survivors. Late effects of impaired uterine development may be associated with an increased risk of early pregnancy loss, premature labor and infants born with low birthweight.[27,30,53] Green and colleagues reported an excess risk of low birthweight infants (<2500 g) born to mothers who had received abdominal irradiation for childhood Wilms' tumor. The most recent data on survivors of Wilms' tumor continue to expose an increased risk of fetal malposition, preterm labor and low birthweight infants.[64]

Similar adverse pregnancy outcomes have been reported in women who have been exposed to TBI. In 1996, Sanders et al. evaluated the medical records of 1326 postpubertal and 196 prepubertal patients who had received high-dose chemotherapy alone or with TBI and bone marrow transplantation for either a hematological malignancy or aplastic anemia. They reported an increased risk of early pregnancy loss, preterm labor and delivery of a low or very low birthweight infant among those girls who had received TBI. There was no increased risk of congenital abnormality in the infants born. However, the authors were careful to draw attention to the fact that the potential adverse events of parental exposure to high-dose alkylating agents with or without TBI on the offspring born to women who had received a bone marrow transplant would require a longer and additional follow up.[30]

Successful pregnancies with ovum donation have been reported in women with ovarian failure secondary to exposure to TBI during childhood. Larson et al. reported the case histories of three women, who had been exposed to TBI and marrow transplantation during childhood with subsequent development of a premature menopause

during adolescence.[65] The woman with normal uterine volume (41.8 ml) delivered a healthy infant at 37 weeks gestation and had received anticancer treatment postpuberty. A second patient whose uterine volume was severely diminished (9.4 ml) miscarried in the second trimester. The third patient had not conceived at the time of publication. Observations such as these inevitably raise concerns about the uterine factor and, if conception occurs in such patients, then the pregnancy is high risk, and patients must be duly counseled about the complications of early pregnancy loss and preterm birth.

It is unknown whether the normally recommended doses and routes of administration of estrogen replacement are sufficiently adequate to facilitate uterine growth during adolescence in those young women who have been exposed to radiotherapy regimens in childhood. Bath et al. assessed both ovarian and uterine characteristics following TBI in long-term survivors of childhood cancer.[11] Pelvic ultrasound was employed to evaluate uterine size, uterine blood flow and endometrial thickness in response to exogenous sex steroid therapy in those participants with ovarian failure, and in endogenous sex steroid production in women with preservation of spontaneous ovarian activity. The physiological sex steroid replacement regimen was administered for 3 months and has previously been demonstrated to simulate endogenous estrogen and progesterone profiles of the normal ovarian cycle.[60] Baseline assessment of uterine volume (conducted 4 weeks after cessation of standard sex steroid replacement) demonstrated significant reduction in uterine volume and undetectable uterine blood flow in women with ovarian failure in comparison to those treated with chemotherapy or cranial irradiation, or a control group of healthy young women with regular menses. Re-evaluation after 3 months of physiological concentrations of sex steroid replacement therapy was associated with a significant increase in uterine volume from a median (range) 6.5 (1.7–12.7) ml at baseline to 16.5 (8.3–27.4) ml (Figure 8c.2; data derived from Bath et al.). Patients treated prepubertally demonstrated a far smaller increase in uterine volume and there was a significant correlation between uterine volume measured during the third cycle of physiological sex steroid replacement and age at irradiation ($p < 0.05$; Figure 8c.3). Improvements were also demonstrated in other uterine parameters, including an increase in endometrial thickness and uterine artery blood flow. Subsequent immunohistochemical studies of endometrial tissue from patients with ovarian failure provide evidence of a functional endometrial response to sex steroid replacement by the demonstration of expression of sex steroid (estrogen and progesterone) receptors.[66] These data support the tenet that a physiological sex steroid replacement regimen has the potential to improve uterine characteristics. It is clear that the most appropriate dose, delivery route and regimen for hormone replacement

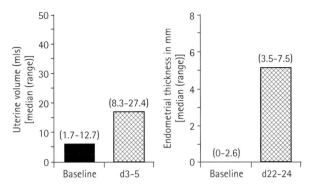

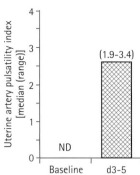

Figure 8c.2 *Physiological sex steroid replacement therapy, after 3 months administration, increased uterine volume and endometrial thickness and re-established uterine artery blood flow in subjects with premature ovarian failure as a consequence of treatment with total body irradiation for leukemia. Data derived from Bath et al. (1999).[11]*

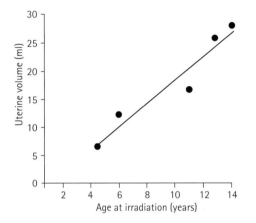

Figure 8c.3 *Demonstration of the correlation between uterine volume in the third month of physiological sex steroid replacement (n = 4) or spontaneous ovarian failure (n = 1) and the age at which irradiation was administered. (Reprinted from Bath et al., 1999[11] with permission from Elsevier Science.)*

among cancer survivors remains unknown. Ideally, a hormone replacement regimen should aim also to optimize cardiovascular and skeletal health as well as to achieve an optimal uterine response.

Chemotherapy does not appear to have any significant lasting adverse effect on uterine function. Successful pregnancy, with no increased risk of miscarriage, and healthy offspring are reported following treatment with multiagent chemotherapy regimens.[67,68]

PRESERVING FERTILITY POTENTIAL

Chemotherapy and radiotherapy may hasten oocyte depletion, with truncated fecundity and premature menopause. Consequently, efforts to develop techniques to preserve fertile potential in young cancer patients are being pursued. A number of strategies to protect the ovaries and preserve fertility during cancer therapy have been attempted with limited success. Limitation of radiation dose to the ovary is sometimes practiced in adult women but in children is technically difficult. In young

sexually mature females with partners, collection of mature oocytes for storage or fertilization and subsequent embryo cryopreservation is possible. For prepubertal girls, and the majority of young women, preservation of fertility remains experimental, and harvesting and storage of gonadal tissue before commencing cancer therapy is the most promising option.

Established practices

If a young woman is postpubertal, superovulation and mature oocyte collection is an option. The drawback of this approach is that the process of superovulation may be long,[69] at a time when the need to commence treatment is urgent and the numbers of mature oocytes available for collection is small. A further difficulty with this approach is that oocytes often fail to survive the freezing process and the live birth rate following ovum freezing is extremely low – less than 1 in every 100 oocytes collected.[70] Success rates following embryo freezing and storage (frozen embryo replacement) are higher, with reported success rates in the order of 15 per cent per cycle.[71] For women who have experienced a premature menopause as a late effect of treatment for childhood cancer, pregnancy may be achieved by ovum donation and *in-vitro* fertilization (IVF). Reported success rates for IVF with ovum donation and a normal uterus are as high as 50 per cent per cycle.[72] Chemotherapy has not resulted in an increased risk of miscarriage, an observation that may be utilized as a surrogate measure for possible lethal mutations induced by anticancer treatment.[73]

There are reports of the outcome of physically removing/shielding the ovaries from the field of planned irradiation. The technique of laparoscopic ovarian transposition (oophoropexy, moving the ovaries to the paracolic gutters) has been documented to retain ovarian function in women scheduled to receive pelvic irradiation.[74] Heterotopic ovarian autotransplantation involves grafting the ovary to a distant site in the body and anastomosing the vascular supply.[75,76] These techniques, however, do not overcome potential damage to the uterus that remains within the field of radiation insult. Another

option for postpubertal women is suppression of the hypothalamic–pituitary–ovarian axis with gonadotrophin-releasing hormone (GnRH) analogues. Unfortunately, there is little evidence that this approach achieves significant gonad protection and the decline in primordial follicle loss is not halted. There is some limited experience with the use of GnRH antagonists in ovulation induction/IVF prior to anticancer therapy in postpubertal women.[77] The conventional approaches involve GnRH agonists and treatment duration may be 20–30 days. This time interval may be reduced (median duration 12 days; range 8–13 days) with a GnRH antagonist. Moreover, stimulation of gonadotrophin secretion is avoided.

Experimental strategies

Inevitably, it is not easy to predict the risk of ovarian damage before cancer therapy. It is, therefore, not surprising that there is increasing interest in research on the potential options available to prevent or minimize the effects of chemotherapy and radiation treatment on gonadal reproductive function.[73]

One approach to preserving fertile potential was based on the original idea that the prepubertal ovary is quiescent and, therefore, protected from the cytotoxic effects of chemotherapy and radiotherapy that destroy rapidly dividing cells. It was hypothesized that suppression of hypothalamic–pituitary–gonadal axis by administration of the gonadotrophin-releasing hormone analogues (GnRH-a) would render the ovary less susceptible. A number of studies have demonstrated that GnRH-a inhibit chemotherapy-induced ovarian follicular depletion in rodents.[78] Progesterone or GnRH agonists were shown to maintain fertility and fecundity rates comparable to those of untreated control animals.[79]

While it has since become clear that the prepubertal ovary is vulnerable to the deleterious effects of cytotoxic therapy, the mechanisms by which such hormonal manipulation may offer protection of ovarian function are unclear. It is likely that the relative 'resistance' of the prepubertal ovary to cytotoxic therapy reflects the larger number of follicles present at the time of treatment rather than the avoidance of damage. In rodents, gonadotrophin analogues prevent follicular growth and mitosis by blocking gonadotrophin induction. Although the exact mechanism is uncertain, it may involve direct suppression of GnRH receptors in the ovary, with subsequent inhibition of recruitment of small follicles into the proliferating pool as well as atresia of the already developed follicles. However, there remains uncertainty about applicability in the human, particularly as the human ovary has significantly fewer numbers of GnRH receptors in the ovary. Using a primate model, Ataya *et al.* demonstrated that GnRH-a cotreatment protected the

rhesus monkey from cyclophosphamide-induced ovarian damage by significantly reducing follicular decline compared with cyclophosphamide alone, from 65 per cent to 29 per cent.[80,81] These findings are supported by clinical studies, which demonstrated that cotreatment of GnRH-a with chemotherapy resulted in premature ovarian failure (POF) in one out of 44 (2.3 per cent) compared with 26 out of 45 (58 per cent) in the group treated with chemotherapy (with or without mantle field irradiation) only.[82,83] In another study, Blumenfeld and coworkers were able to study the protective effects of GnRH agonists in patients undergoing cytotoxic alkylating agent-based treatment for systemic lupus erythematosus. Ovarian function was preserved in all eight women receiving GnRH agonists in conjunction with chlorambucil or cyclophosphamide, in contrast to five of the nine (56 per cent) of patients treated with chemotherapy only.[84] Adjuvant treatment with GnRH-a to limit the gonadal toxic effects of otherwise successful treatment regimens is potentially attractive. However, this must be viewed with some caution as, although GnRH-a provided some protection against cyclophosphamide, no advantage was conferred against irradiation or high-dose chemotherapy in the case of conditioning therapy for bone marrow transplantation, where ovarian failure was unpreventable irrespective of hormone suppression.[85] In the case of radiation, this may be explained in part by the different mechanism of gonadal damage induced by radiotherapy, namely, the destruction of primordial follicles, which are not under the influence of gonadotrophins.[86] The judicious use of GnRH-a may play a role in the appropriate patient group, such as young women and children subjected to alkylating agent-based chemotherapy for Hodgkin's disease.

Recently, attention has focused on the mechanisms involved in primordial follicle loss. Follicle death involves the process of apoptosis, and studies in mice have explored whether or not this process may be interrupted.[87] In these studies, the gene encoding acid sphingomyelinase was disrupted. The apoptotic depletion of primordial fetal oocytes was prevented and increased numbers of primordial follicles were present in the mice at birth. Furthermore, these oocytes appeared to be resistant to chemotherapy-induced apoptosis *in vitro* and radiation-induced apoptosis *in vivo*. Observations such as these have raised interesting possibilities for future research approaches to preserve fertility potential by preventing primordial follicle depletion during radiotherapy or chemotherapy.

There is a particular practical and ethical challenge to develop therapeutic strategies for the preservation of fertility in prepubertal girls. In this context, much attention has focused on the cryopreservation of primordial follicles. This approach was first explored some 50 years ago, when autografts of mouse ovarian tissue were demonstrated to

survive freezing and thawing.[88] Subsequently, Parrot demonstrated that normal offspring might be obtained from mice with orthotic ovarian grafts that had been frozen and stored.[89] The reproductive life span of these female mice was, however, limited. The last 10 years has seen a resurgence of interest in this approach to fertility preservation. The technique has been demonstrated to be successful in sheep. In these experiments, ovarian cortical strips were frozen and reimplanted after oophorectomy. Estrous cycles returned in the animals, although circulating gonadotrophin concentrations remained higher than in the precastrate range.[16,90] Unexpectedly, one of the sheep conceived and a healthy live lamb was born. Primordial follicles were detected in all grafts at post mortem some 9 months following reimplantation.

Since the mid-1990s, ovarian cortical tissue has been collected and stored for young girls and women before treatment for cancer. Usually the tissue is collected laparoscopically under general anesthetic. Cortical strips are taken with biopsy forceps from one ovary, or an entire ovary is removed and subsequently cortical strips are taken for storage. The ovarian cortical tissue is then stored in a cryoprotectant and frozen at −196°C in liquid nitrogen.[91] Several thorough reviews have recently appeared on this topic addressing the practical issues of ovarian strip cryopreservation.[92] Most importantly, standards for best practice in cryopreservation of gonadal tissue, including the criteria for providing a service, patient identification and selection, standard operating procedures and aspects of storage have been published by a working party under the auspices of the Royal College of Obstetricians and Gynaecologists.[93]

It has been demonstrated that human primordial follicles survive cryopreservation and return of ovarian endocrine activity achieved with reimplantation.[94] More recently, it has been demonstrated that orthotopic reimplantation of frozen/thawed ovarian cortical strips is a tolerable technique for the restoration of ovarian function.[95] Heterotopic transplantation of ovarian cortical strips has also recently been demonstrated as a potential method of preserving fertility if the anticancer treatment only involved pelvic irradiation.[96] The likelihood of success of this technique when the patient has additionally been administered gonadotoxic chemotherapy is still very uncertain. To date, no successful pregnancy has been reported as a consequence of replacement of frozen cortical tissue into a cancer survivor (or indeed any other women for whom there existed an appropriate indication).

The functional life span of ovarian cortical strips will be related to the number of primordial follicles that survive the reimplantation process and this is estimated to be in the order of 70 per cent.[14,97] The in vitro maturation of human primordial follicles into mature oocytes is not currently a therapeutic option for women, although it is a topical area of current research. Thus far, pregnancy after in vitro maturation of oocytes from preantral follicles has only been successful in the mouse.[98]

Attention has also been paid to the concern about the potential risk of transmission of the original disease, since the gonads are known sanctuary sites for malignant cells, particularly for hematological malignancies.[85] This risk has been demonstrated to exist in lymphoma SCID mouse models.[99] The risk of transplanting tumor cells might be avoided by maturing ovarian follicles in vitro and thereafter employing assisted reproductive techniques.[100] Recently Kim et al. addressed the safety issue in women by xenografting ovarian tissue from women with lymphoma to immunodeficient mice.[101] Ovarian tissue was collected by laparoscopic ovarian biopsy or unilateral oophorectomy from 18 patients (all postpubertal) who desired fertility preservation by low-temperature tissue banking prior to potentially sterilizing first- or second-line anticancer treatment for lymphoma. No animal (SCID mice) xenografted with human ovarian tissue from 13 women with Hodgkin's lymphoma developed signs of disease. Further, there was no microscopic evidence of residual disease in ovarian tissue prior to grafting nor in other tissues examined. Reassuring data were also derived from the women with non-Hodgkin's lymphoma. By contrast, a group of control mice grafted with human lymph node tissue from a subject with follicular lymphoma all developed B-cell lymphoma of human origin. This single small study indicates that there is some hope that ovarian tissue from lymphoma patients might be safely autotransplanted once anticancer therapy is concluded. Of course, further detailed studies are required on this important aspect of managing future fertility potential.

There are reassuring reports that the incidence of congenital abnormality and childhood malignancies are not increased in the offspring born to long-term childhood cancer survivors.[102–104] There are, however, no data concerning the outcomes in offspring born to cancer survivors as a result of assisted reproductive technologies. In the latter situation, the normal process of conception and natural selection have been bypassed. Concerns have also been raised about risk of transmission of viral diseases and contamination of storage facilities.

ETHICAL AND LEGAL ISSUES

The cryopreservation and subsequent use of prepubertal ovarian tissue presents a number of practical and ethical problems that must be addressed before embarking on any clinical program.[105,106] Consideration must be given to issues of safety relating to the harvesting of the tissue, subsequent use and possible implications for the progeny. When considering preservation of fertility in children

and young women with cancer, it is imperative that oncologists are not only aware of the advances in assisted reproduction and the options available to the young girl, but also understand the inherent legal and ethical issues surrounding such a delicate area. Inevitably, this will require multidisciplinary collaboration between oncologists and specialists in assisted reproduction, who together can help the child and their family make an informed decision about fertility preservation.

The options available for preserving fertility in females have been outlined above. While it is possible that a minority of young sexually mature girls may be able to undergo oocyte collection, for the large majority of patients the only potential option will be to harvest ovarian tissue. It is this latter option that raises many difficult issues. Germ-cell harvesting is not yet standard practice in the management of females with cancer and must be considered entirely experimental. To justify such procedures ethically and legally, consent must be obtained; however, the issue of consent itself presents many dilemmas when considering children with cancer. By definition, for consent to be valid, it must be given voluntarily by a competent and informed person. In order to fulfill these criteria, we expect the consenting person to understand complex concepts of research, which we ourselves are only just beginning to understand. Furthermore, we are asking them to make such a decision when issues relating to safety are uncertain and options for future use of the tissue remain experimental. The removal of ovarian tissue is an invasive procedure that carries an element of risk, a risk that is augmented in individuals whose health is already compromised by their disease. The subsequent reimplantation of stored tissue may carry as yet unquantified risk with the potential of reactivating disease in individuals in remission.

Given our current lack of knowledge surrounding the issues of safety and future use, it is questionable whether even competent individuals can give fully informed consent. Reiteration of the experimental nature of these procedures is necessary. Time to address some of these difficulties is restricted by the need to commence cancer therapy. Some of these practical difficulties may be alleviated if obtaining consent is considered as a continuum, which can be divided into two stages, with part one involving harvesting and cryopreservation of the tissue, and part two involving subsequent use of the tissue. The latter clearly would require separate consent. Issues relating to the use of the tissue in the event of the death of the patient should also be discussed. In addition, consideration of fertility preservation is a quality of life issue at a time of intense stress for young patients and their families. Nevertheless, in our experience, open discussion is embraced and often potentially therapeutic for the vulnerable family facing treatment for cancer. Discussion of fertility issues at the time of diagnosis provides the family with the reassurance that they can look forward to long-term survival for their child, and a future when these issues will become important.

The concept of obtaining informed consent for germ-cell harvest, storage and future use in children and their families requires further consideration of the legal framework, which defines who is eligible to give the consent, and the complex legal issues controlling harvesting and storage of reproductive tissue. In the UK, consent for procedures in children, minors, is generally obtained by proxy. However, in exceptional circumstances, minors may be deemed competent by their doctor to give valid consent. The area of assisted reproduction in the UK, is under the jurisdiction of the Human Fertilisation and Embryology Authority (HFEA),[107] which dictates that consent for storage of gametes and embryos is given by the person providing the material and cannot by given by proxy, and must be stored on licensed premises. The HFEA define a gamete as a 'reproductive cell, such as an ovum or spermatozoa, which has a haploid set of chromosomes and which is capable of taking part in fertilization with another of the opposite sex to form a zygote'.[108]

For the minority of females mature enough to be considered for oocyte preservation, the 'minor' would be able to provide consent if deemed Gillick competent.[109] In the case of germ-cell harvesting, where immature gametes would be collected, there are no laws defining storage criteria, thus the tissue could be harvested from the girls with parental consent. The HFEA framework governing the field of assisted reproduction was not designed with children in mind, and is currently undergoing a reappraisal to amend its framework to ensure children are offered the same opportunity and protection as adults.

CONCLUSIONS

As treatment for childhood cancer has become increasingly successful, adverse effects on female reproductive function are assuming greater importance. It is incumbent upon oncologists that appropriate counseling of patients at risk of impaired ovarian function and infertility forms part of their routine care. Preservation of fertility before treatment must be considered in all young patients at high risk of infertility; however, options for preservation of fertile potential are limited and largely experimental. Limitation of radiation exposure by ovarian transposition should be practiced where possible. Harvesting ovarian tissue and cryopreservation of cortical slices are practiced in a number of centers, although these procedures remain experimental and future utilization of stored tissue is uncertain. Ultimately, autografting and restoration of natural fertility is the aim of cryopreservation of ovarian

tissue but techniques need to be developed to ensure malignant cells are not transferred in the tissue. Isolation of follicles and *in vitro* maturation for assisted reproduction is an alternative option, which will eliminate any risk of transmission of malignant cells. Even where harvesting of ovarian tissue and subsequent maturation of oocytes, whether *in vivo* or *in vitro*, uterine function will play an important role in determining the success of any pregnancy.

Harvesting ovarian tissue is already practiced in some centers and is likely to become standard practice in the management of females at risk of infertility secondary to treatment for childhood cancer. Greater awareness amongst the professional bodies involved in caring for the child has fuelled the development of a comprehensive ethically and legally acceptable strategy for the practice and research related to preserving fertile potential in children and adolescents treated for cancer.

ACKNOWLEDGEMENTS

We thank Ted Pinner and Eleanor Meikle for assistance with the illustrations, and Natasha Mallion for her secretarial help.

KEY POINTS

- Whole abdominal irradiation (20–30 Gy) is associated with mid-trimester pregnancy loss. Flank radiation (as part of treatment for Wilms' tumor) and total body irradiation (14 Gy) is associated with increased risk of miscarriage, preterm labor and delivery of low birthweight infants.
- The effects on gonadal function of combination cytotoxic chemotherapy depend upon the type and total dose of drugs administered.
- It is essential that the uterine factor is recognized, as there may be associated problems in pregnancy.
- Prediction of a premature menopause is difficult, although early follicular-phase assay of follicle-stimulating hormone, estradiol and inhibin B, and ovarian ultrasound are potential tools to assess ovarian reserve.
- Ovarian failure will require estrogen replacement for pubertal induction and cyclical hormone replacement to relieve the symptoms of estrogen deficiency (vaginal dryness, hot flushes and irritability), provide cardiovascular protection and optimize bone density.
- It is essential that there is comprehensive follow-up of the gonadal function of cancer survivors

who have been exposed to the newer multiagent chemotherapeutic protocols.
- High-dose cranial irradiation (>30 Gy) may result in a compromise of hypothalamic and pituitary function.
- The cryopreservation and subsequent use of prepubertal ovarian tissue presents a number of practical and ethical problems that must be addressed before embarking on any clinical programme.
- Options for fertility preservation are limited and, in children, still remain experimental. Assisted reproductive technologies have focused efforts on the preservation of ovarian tissue for future use.

REFERENCES

1. Capocaccia R, Gatta G, Magnani C, *et al.* Childhood cancer survival in Europe 1978–1992: the EUROCARE Study. *Eur J Cancer* 2001; **37**:671–816.
2. Stiller CA. Aetiology and epidemiology. In: Pinkerton CR, Plowman PN (eds) *Paediatric oncology: clinical practice and controversies,* 2nd edn. London: Chapman and Hall Medical, 1997:3–21.
3. Wallace WHB. Growth and endocrine function following the treatment of childhood malignant disease. In: Pinkerton CR, Plowman PN (eds) *Paediatric oncology: clinical practice and controversies,* 2nd edn. London: Chapman and Hall Medical, 1997:706–31.
4. Bleyer WA. The impact of childhood cancer on the United States and the world. *Cancer* 1990; **40**:355–367.
5. Wallace WHB, Blacklay A, Eiser C, *et al.* Developing strategies for long term follow up of survivors of childhood cancer. *Br Med J* 2001; **323**:271–274.
6. Meirow D. Reproduction post chemotherapy in young cancer patients. *Mol Cell Endocrinol* 2000; **169**:123–131.
♦7. Thomson AB, Critchley HOD, Kelnar CJH, Wallace WHB. Late reproductive sequelae following treatment of childhood cancer and options for fertility preservation. Bailliere's Best Practice and Research. *Clin Endocrinol Metabol* 2002; **16**:311–334.
8. Bath LE, Anderson RA, Critchley HOD, Kelnar CJK, Wallace WHB. Hypothalamic–pituitary–ovarian dysfunction after prepubertal chemotherapy and cranial irradiation for acute leukaemia. *Hum Reprod* 2001; **16**:1838–1844.
9. Wallace WHB, Shalet SM, Crowne EC, *et al.* Ovarian failure following abdominal irradiation in childhood: natural history and prognosis. *Clin Oncol* 1989; **1**:75–79.
10. Critchley HOD, Wallace WHB, Shalet SM, *et al.* Abdominal irradiation in childhood; the potential for pregnancy. *Br J Obstet Gynaecol* 1992; **99**:392–394.
♦11. Bath LE, Critchley HOD, Chambers SE, *et al.* Ovarian and uterine characteristics after total body irradiation in childhood and adolescence: response to sex steroid replacement. *Br J Obstet Gynaecol* 1999; **106**:1265–1272.
♦12. Byrne J, Fears TR, Gail MH, *et al.* Early menopause in long term survivors of cancer during adolescence. *Am J Obstet Gynecol* 1992; **166**:788–793.
●13. Byrne J. Infertility and premature menopause in childhood cancer survivors. *Med Pediatr Oncol* 1999; **33**:24–28.

14. Oktay K, Nugent D, Newton H, *et al*. Isolation and characterization of primordial follicles from fresh and cryopreserved human ovarian tissue. *Fertil Steril* 1997; **67**:481–486.

15. Oktay K, Karlikaya GG, Aydin BA. Ovarian cryopreservation and transplantation: basic aspects. *Mol Cell Enodcrinol* 2000; **169**:105–108.

◆16. Gosden RG, Baird DT, Wade JC, Webb R. Restoration of fertility to oopherectomized sheep by ovarian autografts stored at −196°C. *Hum Reprod* 1994; **9**:597–603.

17. Gosden RG. Restitution of fertility in sterilised mice by transferring primordial ovarian follicles. *Hum Reprod* 1990; **5**:117–122.

18. Carroll J, Gosden RG. Transplantation of frozen-thawed mouse primordial follicles. *Hum Reprod* 1993; **8**:1163–1167.

19. Guanasena KT, Villines PM, Crister ES, Crister JK. Live births with autologous transplant of cryopreserved mouse ovaries. *Hum Reprod* 1997; **12**:101–116.

●20. Wallace WHB, Walker DA. Conference consensus statement: ethical and research dilemmas for fertility preservation in children treated for cancer. *Hum Fertil* 2001; **4**:69–76.

21. Block E. Quantitative morphological investigations of the follicular system in women. Variations at different ages. *Acta Anat* 1952; **14**:108–123.

22. Faddy MJ, Gosden RG, Gougeon A, *et al*. Accelerated disappearance of ovarian follicles in mid-life; implications for forecasting menopause. *Hum Reprod* 1992; **7**:1342–1346.

23. Sherman BM, West JH, Korenman SG. The menopausal transition: analysis of LH, FSH, estradiol, and progesterone concentrations during menstrual cycles of older women. *J Clin Endocrinol Metab* 1976; **42**:629–636.

24. Ahmed Eddiary NA, Lenton EA, Cooke ID. Hypothalamic–pituitary ageing: progressive increase in FSH and LH concentrations throughout the reproductive life in regularly menstruating women. *Clin Endocrinol* 1994; **41**:199–206.

25. Chapman AM, Marrett LD, Darlington G. Cytotoxic-induced ovarian failure in Hodgkin's disease. I. Hormone function. *JAMA* 1979; **242**:1877–1881.

◆26. Wallace WHB, Thomson AB, Kelsey TW. The radiosensitivity of the human oocyte. *Hum Reprod* 2003; **18**:117–121.

27. Wallace WH, Shalet SM, Hendry JH, *et al*. Ovarian failure following abdominal irradiation in childhood: the radiosensitivity of the human oocyte. *Br J Radiol* 1989; **62**:995–998.

28. Wallace WHB, Shalet SM, Tetlow LJ, Morris-Jones PH. Ovarian function following the treatment of childhood acute lymphoblastic leukaemia. *Medn Pediatr Oncol* 1993; **21**:333–339.

29. Sanders JE. The impact of marrow transplant preparation regimens on subsequent growth and development. *Semin Hematol* 1991; **28**:244–249.

◆30. Sanders JE, Hawley J, Levy W, *et al*. Pregnancies following high-dose cyclophosphamide with or without high-dose busulfan or total-body irradiation and bone marrow transplantation. *Blood* 1996; **87**:3045–3052.

31. Thibaud E, Rodriguez-Macias K, Trivin C, *et al*. Ovarian function after bone marrow transplantation. *Bone Marrow Transplant* 1998; **21**:287–290.

32. Matsumoto M, Shinohara O, Ishiguro H, *et al*. Ovarian function after bone marrow transplantation performed before menarche. *Arch Dis Child* 1999; **80**:452–454.

33. Lushbaugh CC, Casarett GW. The effects of gonadal irradiation in clinical radiation in therapy; a review. *Cancer* 1976; **37**:1111–1125.

34. Chiarelli AM, Marrett LD, Darlington G. Early menopause and infertility in females after treatment for childhood cancer diagnosed in 1964–1988 in Ontario, Canada. *Am J Epidemiol* 1999; **150**:245–254.

35. Block E. A quantitative morphological investigations of the follicular system in newborn female infants. *Acta Anat* 1953; **17**:201–206.

36. Richardson SJ, Senikas V, Nelson JF. Follicular depletion during the menopausal transition: evidence for accelerated loss and ultimate exhaustion. *J Clin Endocrinol Metab* 1987; **65**:1231–1237.

37. Faddy MJ, Gosden, RG. A model conforming the decline in follicle numbers to the age of menopause in women. *Hum Reprod* 1996; **11**:1484–1486.

38. Faddy MJ, Gosden RG, Edwards R. Ovarian follicle dynamics in mice: a comparative study of three inbred strains and an f1 hybrid. *J Endocrinol* 1983; **96**:23–33.

39. Livesey EA, Brook CGD. Gonadal dysfunction after treatment of intracranial tumours. *Arch Dis Child* 1988; **63**:495–500.

40. Littley MD, Shalet M, Beardwell CG, *et al*. Hypopituitarism following external radiotherapy for pituitary tumours in adults. *Q J Med* 1989; **70**:145–160.

41. Crowne EC, Moore C, Wallace WH, *et al*. A novel variant of growth hormone insufficiency following low dose cranial irradiation. *Clin Endocrinol* 1992; **36**:59–68.

42. Brennan BM, Rahim A, Mackie EM, *et al*. Growth hormone status in adults treated for acute lymphoblastic leukaemia in childhood. *Clin Endocrinol* 1998; **48**:777–783.

43. Birkebaek NH, Kisker S, Clausen N, *et al*. Growth and endocrinological disorders up to 21 years after treatment for acute lymphoblastic leukaemia in childhood. *Med Pediatr Oncol* 1998; **30**:351–356.

44. Nygaard R, Clausen N, Simes MA, *et al*. Reproduction following treatment for childhood leukaemia: a population based prospective cohort study of fertility and offspring. *Med Pediatr Oncol* 1991; **19**:459–466.

45. Bath LE, Anderson RA, Critchley HOD, *et al*. Hypothalamic–pituitary–ovarian dysfunction after prepubertal chemotherapy and cranial irradiation for acute leukaemia. *Hum Reprod* 2001; **16**:1838–1844.

46. Soules MR, McLachlan RI, Ek M, *et al*. Luteal phase deficiency: characterisation of reproductive hormones over the menstrual cycle. *J Clin Endocrinol Metab* 1989; **69**:804–812.

47. Whitehead E, Shalet SM, Blackledge G, *et al*. The effect of combination chemotherapy on ovarian function in women treated for Hodgkin's disease. *Cancer* 1983; **52**:988–993.

48. Clark ST, Radford JA, Crowther D, *et al*. Cytotoxic induced ovarian failure in women treated for Hodgkin's disease: a comparative study of MVPP and a seven-drug hybrid regimen. *J Clin Oncol* 1985; **13**:134–139.

49. Waxman JH, Terry YA, Wrigley PFM, *et al*. Gonadal function in Hodgkin's disease: long-term follow-up of chemotherapy. *Br Med J* 1982; **285**:1612–1613.

50. Chapman RM, Sutcliffe SB, Malpas JS. Cytotoxic-induced ovarian failure in women treated with MOPP chemotherapy for Hodgkin's disease. *Am J Med* 1981; **71**:552–556.

51. Siris ES, Leventhal BG, Vaitukaitis JL. Effects of childhood leukaemia and chemotherapy on puberty and reproductive function in girls. *N Eng J Med* 1976; **294**:1143–1146.

52. Pasqualini T, Escobar ME, Domene H, *et al*. Evaluation of gonadal function following long-term treatment for acute lymphoblastic leukaemia in girls. *Am J Pediatr Hematol Oncol* 1987; **9**: 15–22.

53. Green DM, Hall B, Zevon A. Pregnancy outcome after treatment for acute lymphoblastic leukaemia during childhood or adolescence. *Cancer* 1989; **64**:235–244.

54. Bramswig JH, Heiermann E, Heimes U, *et al*. Ovarian function in 63 girls treated for Hodgkin's disease according to the West German DAL-HD-78 and DAL-HD-82 therapy study. *Med Pediatr Oncol* 1989; **17**:344.

55. Mackie EJ, Radford M, Shalet SM. Gonadal function following chemotherapy for childhood Hodgkin's disease. *Med Pediatr Oncol* 1996; **27**:74–78.

56. Sanders JE, Buckner CD, Amos D *et al.* Ovarian failure following marrow transplantation for aplastic anaemia or leukaemia. *J Clin Oncol* 1988; **6**:813–818.

57. Holm K, Laurensen EM, Brocks, Muller J. Pubertal maturation of the internal genitalia: an ultrasound evaluation of 166 healthy girls. *Ultrasound Obstet Gynecol* 1995; **6**:175–181.

58. Critchley HOD, Wang H, Kelly RW, *et al.* Progestin receptor isoforms and prostaglandin dehydrogenase in the endometrium of women using a levonorgestrel-releasing intrauterine system. *Hum Reprod* 1998; **13**:1210–1217.

59. Bridges NA, Cooke A, Healy MJ, *et al.* Growth of the uterus. *Arch Dis Child* 1996; **75**:330–331.

60. Critchley HOD, Buckley CH, Anderson DC. Experience with a 'physiological' steroid replacement regimen for the establishment of a receptive endometrium in women with premature ovarian failure. *Br J Obstet Gynecol* 1990; **97**:804–810.

61. Holm K, Nysom K, Brocks V, *et al.* Ultrasound B-mode changes in the uterus and ovaries and Doppler changes in the uterus after total body irradiation and allogenic bone marrow transplantation in childhood. *Bone Marrow Transplant* 1999; **23**:259–263.

62. Smith RA, Hawkins MM. Pregnancies after childhood cancer. *Br J Obstet Gynecol* 1989; **96**:378–380.

63. Li FP, Gimbere K, Gelber RD, *et al.* Outcome of pregnancy in survivors of Wilms' tumour. *JAMA* 1987; **257**:216–219.

64. Green DM. Preserving fertility in children treated for cancer. *Br Med J* 2001; **323**:1201 (editorial).

65. Larsen EC, Loft A, Holm K, *et al.* Oocyte donation in women cured of cancer with bone marrow transplantation including total body irradiation in adolescence. *Hum Reprod* 2000; **15**: 1505–1508.

66. Critchley HOD, Bath LE, Wallace WHB. Radiation damage to the uterus – review of effects of treatment of childhood cancer. *Hum Fertil* 2002; **5**:61–66.

67. Nicholson HS, Byrne J. Fertility and pregnancy after treatment for cancer during childhood or adolescence. *Cancer* 1993; **71**:3392–3399.

68. Salooja N, Szydlo RM, Socie G, *et al.* Pregnancy outcomes after peripheral blood or bone marrow transplantation: a retrospective survey. *Lancet* 2001; **358**:271–276.

69. Filicori M, Cognigni GE, Arnone R, *et al.* Role of different GnRH agonist regimens in pituitary suppression and the outcome of controlled ovarian hyperstimulation. *Hum Reprod* 1996; **11**:123–132.

70. Salha O, Picton H, Balen A, Rutherford A. Human oocyte cryopreservation. *Hosp Med* 2001; **62**:18–24.

71. Human Fertilisation and Embryology Authority. *9th Annual Report and Accounts.* 2000. www.hfea.gov.uk.

72. Soderstrom-Antilla V. Pregnancy and child outcome after oocyte donation. *Hum Reprod Update* 2001; **7**:28–32.

♦73. Green DM, Whitton JA, Stovall M, *et al.* Pregnancy outcome of female survivors of childhood cancer: a report from the Childhood Cancer Survivor Study. *Am J Obstet Gynecol* 2002; **187**:1070–1080.

74. Clough KB, Goffinet F, Labib A, *et al.* Laparascopic unilateral ovarian transposition prior to irradiation. *Cancer* 1996; **77**:2638–2645.

75. Leporrier M, von Theobold P, Roffe J-L, Muller G. A new technique to protect ovarian function in young women undergoing pelvic irradiation. Heterotopic ovarian autotransplantation. *Cancer* 1987; **60**:2201–2204.

76. Thomas PRM, Winstanly D, Peckham MJ, *et al.* Reproductive and endocrine function in patients with Hodgkin's disease: effects of oopheropexy and irradiation. *Br J Cancer* 1976; **33**:226–231.

77. Anderson RAA, Kinniburgh D, Baird DT. Preliminary experience of the use of a gonadotrophin-releasing hormone antagonist in ovulation induction/in-vitro fertilization prior to cancer treatment. *Hum Reprod* 1999; **14**:2665–2668.

78. Ataya K, Ramahi-Ataya A. Reproductive performance of female rats treated with cyclophosphamide and/or LHRH agonist. *Reprod Toxicol* 1993; **7**: 229–235.

79. Montz FJ, Wolff AJ, Gambone JC. Gonadal protection and fecundity rates in cyclophosphamide-treated rats. *Cancer Res* 1991; **51**:2124–2126.

80. Ataya K, Rao LV, Lawrence E, Kimmel R. Luteinizing hormone-releasing hormone agonist inhibits cyclophosphamide-induced ovarian follicle depletion in rhesus monkeys. *Biol Reprod* 1995; **52**:365–372.

81. Ataya K, Pydyn E, Ramahi-Ataya A, Orton CG. Is radiation-induced ovarian failure in rhesus monkeys preventable by leuteinizing hormone-releasing hormone agonist? Preliminary observations. *J Clin Oncol Endocrinol Metab* 1995; **80**:790–795.

82. Blumenfeld Z, Avivi I, Linn S, *et al.* Prevention of irreversible chemotherapy-induced ovarian damage in young women with lymphoma by a gonadotrophin-releasing hormone agonist in parallel to chemotherapy. *Hum Reprod* 1996; **11**:1620–1626.

83. Blumenfeld Z. Ovarian rescue/protection from chemotherapeutic agents (1). *J Soc Gynecol Invest* 2001; **8**:S60–S64.

84. Blumenfeld Z, Shapiro D, Shteinberg M, *et al.* Preservation of fertility and ovarian function and minimizing gonadotoxicity in young women with systemic lupus erythematosus treated by chemotherapy. *Lupus* 2000; **9**:401–405.

85. Meirow D. Ovarian injury and modern options to preserve fertility in female cancer patients treated with high-dose radio-chemotherapy for haemato-oncological neoplasias and other cancers. *Leuk Lymphoma* 1999; **33**:65–76.

86. Gosden RG, Wade JC, Fraser HM, *et al.* Impact of congenital and experimental hypogonadism on the radiation sensitivity of the mouse ovary. *Hum Reprod* 1997; **12**:2483–2488.

87. Morita Y, Perez GI, Paris F, *et al.* Oocyte apoptosis is suppressed by disruption of the acid sphingomyelinase gene or by sphingosine-1-phosphate therapy. *Nature Med* 2000; **6**: 1109–1114.

88. Parkes AS, Smith AU. Regeneration of rat ovarian tissue grafted after exposure to low temperatures. *Proc Roy Soc* 1952; **140**:455–467.

89. Parrot DM. The fertility of mice with orthotopic grafts derived from frozen tissue. *J Reprod Fertil* 1960; **1**:230–241.

90. Baird DT, Webb R, Campbell BK, *et al.* Long-term ovarian function in sheep after ovariectomy and transplantation of autografts stored at −196°C. *Endocrinology* 1999; **140**:462–471.

91. Newton H, Aubard Y, Rutherford A, *et al.* Low temperature storage and grafting of human ovarian tissue. *Hum Reprod* 1996; **11**:1487–1491.

92. Gosden RG, Rutherford AJ, Norfolk DR. Ovarian banking for cancer patients transmission of malignant cells in ovarian grafts. *Hum Reprod* 1997; **12**:403.

●93. Royal College of Obstetricians and Gynaecologists. *Storage of ovarian and prepubertal testicular tissue: report of a working party.* London: Royal College of Obstetricians and Gynaecologists, 2000.

94. Oktay K, Newton H, Gosden RG. Transplantation of cryopreserved human ovarian tissue results in follicle growth initiation in SCID mice. *Fertil Steril* 2000; **73**:599–603.

95. Radford JA, Leibermann BA, Brison DR, *et al.* Orthotopic reimplantation of cryopreserved ovarian cortical strips after high-dose chemotherapy for Hodgkin's lymphoma. *Lancet* 2001; **357**:1172–1175.

96. Oktay K, Economos K, Kan M, *et al.* Endocrine function and oocyte retrieval after autologous transplantation of ovarian cortical strips to the forearm. *JAMA* 2001; **286**:1490–1493.

97. Oktay K, Karlikaya G. Ovarian function after transplantation of frozen, banked, autologous ovarian tissue. *N Engl J Med* 2000; **342**:1919.

98. Eppig JJ, O'Brien M. Development in vitro of mouse oocytes from primordial follicles. *Biol Reprod* 1996; **54**:197–207.

99. Shaw JM, Bowles J, Koopman P, *et al.* Fresh and cryopreserved ovarian tissue samples from donors with lymphoma transmit the cancer to graft recipients. *Hum Reprod* 1996; **11**:1668–1673.

100. Gosden RG, Rutherford AJ, Norfolk DR. Ovarian banking for cancer patients – transmission of malignant cells in ovarian grafts. *Hum Reprod* 1997; **12**:403.

101. Kim SS, Gosden RG, Radford JA, *et al.* A model to test the safety of human ovarian tissue transplantation after cryopreservation: xenografts of ovarian tissue from cancer patients into NOD/LtSz-scid mice. Annual Meeting of the American Society of Reproductive Medicine, Toronto, Canada. *Fertil Steril* 1999; (Suppl.):abstract 0-003.

102. Hawkins MM, Draper GJ, Smith RA. Cancer among 1348 survivors of childhood cancer. *Int J Cancer* 1989; **43**:975–978.

103. Li FP, Fine W, Jaffe N, *et al.* Offspring of patients treated for cancer in childhood. *J Natl Cancer Inst* 1979; **62**:1193–1197.

104. Hawkins MM. Pregnancy outcome and offspring after childhood cancer. *Br Med J* 1994; **309**:1034–1040.

105. Grundy R, Gosden RG, Hewitt M, *et al.* Fertility preservation for children treated for cancer (1): scientific advances and research dilemmas. *Arch Dis Child* 2001; **84**:355–359.

106. Grundy R, Larcher V, Gosden RG, *et al.* Personal practice: fertility preservation for children treated for cancer (2): ethics of consent for gamete storage and experimentation. *Arch Dis Child* 2001; **84**:360–362.

107. HFEA Act 1990, Ch. 37. London: The Stationery Office, London.

108. Deech R. Human Fertilisation and Embryology Authority. *Br Med J* 1998; **316**:1095.

109. Anonymous. Gillick v W. Norfolk and Wisbech ANA. *All Engl Law Rep* 1985; 402.

8d

Testicular function

ANGELA B THOMSON, W HAMISH B WALLACE AND CHARLES SKLAR

INTRODUCTION

Tremendous advances in the management of childhood malignancies over the last 30 years mean that the majority of children can realistically hope for long-term survival.[1] With survival rates in excess of 70 per cent, it is estimated that, by the year 2010, one in 250 of the young adult population will be a long-term survivor of childhood cancer.[2] However, the successful treatment of childhood cancer with multiagent chemotherapy, in combination with surgery and or radiotherapy, is associated with significant morbidity in later life.[3] The major challenge faced by pediatric oncologists today is to sustain the excellent survival rates, while striving to improve the quality of life of the survivors.

Testicular dysfunction is well recognized after chemotherapy and radiotherapy treatment for childhood cancer. Cytotoxic agents may cause irreparable damage to the testes with both infertility and hypogonadism reported.[4–15] In contrast to the testicular germinal epithelium, Leydig cells are more resistant to the deleterious effects of chemotherapy and radiotherapy. However, direct irradiation of the testes may cause hypogonadism and testosterone replacement may be required to initiate and sustain pubertal development and normal potency in adulthood.[8–18] After chemotherapy, while overt testosterone deficiency is uncommon, mild Leydig cell dysfunction is increasingly recognized and it is not yet clear whether these patients may benefit from testosterone replacement therapy.[16–18]

While Leydig cell dysfunction is amenable to treatment, damage to the germinal epithelium is usually irreversible and associated with long-lasting or permanent azoospermia.[9,10,14,15] Infertility is a recognized consequence of treatment for childhood cancer. Advances in assisted reproduction techniques have focused attention on preserving gonadal tissue for future use.[19–22] For prepubertal boys, for whom fertility preservation through cryopreservation of semen is not possible, testicular germ cell harvesting and cryopreservation may in the future preserve fertile potential.[23–26] Harvesting, and the potential future use of gonadal tissue, is an exciting area of gamete biology that opens up new and uncharted territory for pediatric oncologists. Many scientific, ethical and legal issues remain to be addressed before techniques to preserve fertility are available.[27] In this subchapter, we review the impact of chemotherapy and radiotherapy treatment of childhood cancer on testicular function, and discuss the merits of androgen replacement therapy and possible options for preservation of fertile potential.

TESTICULAR FUNCTION

The major functions of the male reproductive tract are twofold: (1) to manufacture spermatozoa and deliver these to the female reproductive tract; and (2) to produce male sex steroid hormones, necessary for normal male sexual differentiation during fetal life, puberty, adult male phenotype and behavior, and reproduction.[28,29] The organs

responsible for these functions are: (1) the testes – site of sperm and androgen production; (2) the duct system or transport system; and (3) the accessory glands; for secretion of seminal fluid necessary to support transport and facilitate fertilization. Testicular function is regulated by the anterior pituitary hormones, follicle-stimulating hormone (FSH) and luteinizing hormone (LH), under the controlling influence of hypothalamic gonadotrophin-releasing hormone (GnRH). In turn, the hypothalamic–pituitary–testicular axis is influenced by testicular hormones, completing the negative feedback loop.

Anatomy of the testis

The testes are composed of two structurally distinct but functionally related compartments, the seminiferous tubules and intertubular space, site of spermatogenesis and steroidogenesis, respectively (Figure 8d.1). The intertubular compartment is subdivided into two compartments: the interstitium and intravascular space. The seminiferous tubule, of which there are about 500 in each testis, is a convoluted loop that converges and drains spermatozoa into the rete testis. The tubules are lined by seminiferous epithelium consisting of various types of male germ cells (spermatogenic cells) and a single type of supporting cell, the Sertoli cell. The seminiferous tubules are further subdivided into two compartments, the basal and adluminal compartments, by formation of inter-Sertoli cell tight junctions, which form the blood–testis barrier, and segregate the epithelium into anatomic and physiologic compartments (Figure 8d.1, insert). The two compartments support different stages of spermatogenesis.[28,29]

Spermatogenesis

Spermatogenesis is a complex process by which diploid germ cell spermatogonia undergo proliferation and differentiation into mature haploid spermatozoa.[28] The general organization of spermatogenesis is essentially the same in all mammals and can be divided into phases of development through which all spermatogenic germ cells pass sequentially over time. This highly coordinated process can be divided into three phases: mitotic proliferation of spermatogonial stem cells to yield primary spermatocytes; meiotic maturation of spermatocytes to yield round spermatids; and differentiation of spermatids into mature spermatozoa, known as spermiogenesis. The time taken from division of one stem cell spermatogonia to production of mature spermatozoa varies between species and in humans is determined to be approximately 74 days.

Clearly, male reproduction does not hinge upon an episodic pattern of fertility every 6 weeks or so, but rather, is dependent upon continuous production of mature spermatozoa. Consequently, sperm production is organized spatially and temporally such that rounds of spermatogenesis are initiated at time intervals that are constant and characteristic for each species. There are six stages in humans. To ensure a continuous supply of spermatozoa, each successive segment of the tubule will show a sequential stage of development. It is as if adjacent tubule segments, each containing synchronized populations of spermatogenic stem cells, have entered the cycle slightly out of phase with each other, giving the tubule a helical appearance longitudinally (Figure 8d.2). The resulting appearance is known as the spermatogenic wave.[28,29]

Organization of this highly complex process, both spatially and temporally, is incompletely understood, but there is compelling evidence to suggest that it is attributable to the Sertoli cell, which provides a continuous cytoplasmic network around the tubule that may enable communication and synchronization to occur. The Sertoli cell also spans across the tubule from membrane to lumen, facilitating communication between intratubular space, basal and adluminal compartments. The functions of the Sertoli cell are numerous and include fluid production, phagocytosis of degenerating germ cells, synthesis and secretion of numerous proteins and enzymes, metabolic conversions, and production of known and putative growth factors. The principal role of the Sertoli cell is to support spermatogenesis in response to hormone regulation by FSH and testosterone.[28,29]

Hormone regulation

Testicular function, and ultimately spermatogenesis, is regulated by the anterior pituitary hormones LH and FSH, which are released from the anterior pituitary gland in response to hypothalamic GnRH and modified by various regulatory factors from the testes, namely, testosterone and inhibin. FSH binds exclusively to receptors on the Sertoli cell and stimulates synthesis of androgen receptors, inhibin and activin, which play a mediatory role in spermatogenesis. Testosterone, essential for spermatogenesis, is synthesized and secreted by the Leydig cells in response to stimulation by LH, and passes through the cellular barriers to the Sertoli cell, with a substantial proportion entering the blood and lymphatic system. Testosterone functions primarily as a prohormone, converted to the potent androgen dihydrotestosterone (DHT) via the enzyme 5-α-reductase and to the estrogen, 17-β-estradiol, through the aromatase enzyme. FSH and testosterone act synergistically on Sertoli cells to promote Sertoli cell function and support spermatogenesis because germ cells *per se* do not possess receptors for either hormone.

The mechanism by which spermatogenesis is initiated and sustained is poorly understood, and is likely to involve a number of stimulatory and inhibitory mechanisms. Testosterone exerts a negative feedback regulation

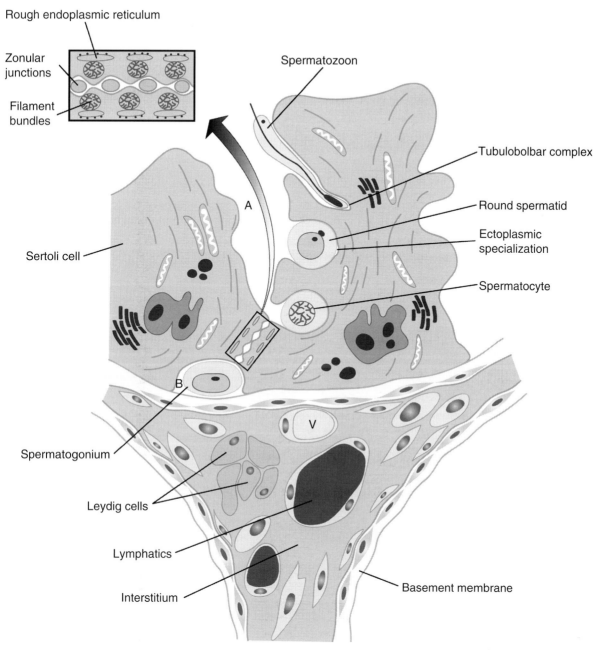

Figure 8d.1 *Cross-section through part of a seminiferous tubule in an adult testis. The testis is divided into two major compartments; the seminiferous tubule and intertubular space. The intertubular space is subdivided into the inerstitum, which includes the lymphatic vessels and Leydig cells, and the vascular compartment (V). The seminiferous tubule is further divided into basal (B) and adluminal (A) compartments. The blood vessels, lymphatics and nerves are contained entirely within the intertubular space, separated from the seminiferous tubules by the basement membrane. Within the tubule, the basal and adluminal compartments are separated by rows of zonular tight and gap junction complexes (see insert), which link adjacent Sertoli cells round the entire circumference of the tubule. The spermatogonia are confined to the basal compartment, while spermatocytes, round and elongating spermatids and spermatozoa are in the adluminal compartment, in intimate contact with the Sertoli cells.*

on the hypothalamic and pituitary hormones. Another such inhibitory mechanism is the regulatory role of the inhibin B. Inhibins are glycoprotein heterodimers composed of an α-subunit and one of two types of β-subunits, either βA (inhibin A) or βB (inhibin B). In males, inhibin B is the major component and the Sertoli cell is the predominant site of its production, although there is some speculation regarding subunit production

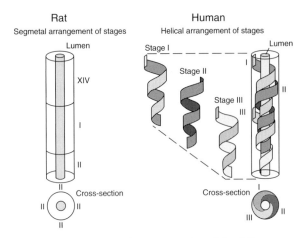

Figure 8d.2 *Diagrammatic representation of the different spatial arrangement of the stages of spermatogenic cycle along a short length of seminiferous tubule in the rat and human. (Modified from Sharpe[28])*

by Leydig and germ cells. Inhibin B, the secretion of which requires the presence of germ cells, mediates non-steroidal negative feedback from the testes, reflecting the number of spermatozoa produced and regulating FSH secretion.[30,31] Inhibin B secretion in the adult requires the presence of intact germ cells[30] and, increasingly, inhibin B is being used as a predictor of germinal epithelial function.

In addition to its mandatory role in spermatogenesis, testosterone has a peripheral role. Testosterone circulates in the plasma, bound largely to plasma proteins (98 per cent), and is converted to the metabolically active hormones, DHT and estradiol. DHT is thought to mediate male sexual differentiation and virilization. Estradiol appears to mediate bone maturation and mineralization, epiphyseal fusion, and negative feedback inhibition of LH and FSH.[28,29]

Puberty

The prepubertal testis has classically been defined as a quiescent organ; however, evidence is emerging to the contrary.[32–34] The development of the testis from the time of fetal differentiation to adulthood is characterized by dramatic morphological and functional changes that lay the groundwork for the onset of spermatogenesis. From birth to puberty the testis has been shown to triple its volume, largely attributable to an increase in seminiferous tubule length.[34] Sertoli cells proliferate intensely and are functionally active during childhood, producing large amounts of anti-Mullerian hormone, throughout the prepubertal period, and inhibin B until the age of 2–4 years.[35] These hormones are believed to modulate the proliferation and differentiation of Leydig cell precursors. Multiplication of early germ cells does occur but

progression beyond the mitotic stage is not supported by the immature Sertoli cells.

At puberty, there is a sleep-entrained increase in the pulsatile secretion of LH and, to a lesser extent, FSH, associated with increased nocturnal plasma testosterone concentrations. With pubertal progression, the increased pulsatile release of gonadotrophins is maintained throughout the day and night, and high concentrations of testosterone are sustained throughout the 24-hour cycle. Spermatogenesis is initiated at puberty as a consequence of increased secretion of FSH. Integral to this is the changing role, and responsiveness of the Sertoli cell. FSH-stimulated maturation of the Sertoli cells to form two compartments and create the blood–testis barrier is essential for the progression of germ cells through meiosis and spermatogenesis. As puberty progresses the responsiveness of the Sertoli cell, and ultimately control of spermatogenesis, shifts from FSH to testosterone.[33,34,36]

INVESTIGATION OF TESTICULAR FUNCTION

Assessment of testicular maturation and function involves pubertal staging, measurement of plasma hormones and semen analysis. Pubertal staging provides important clinical information about both Leydig cell function and spermatogenesis.[37] The development of normal secondary sexual characteristics would imply intact Leydig cell function with normal steroidogenesis. Reduced testicular volume (<12 ml), determined using the Prader orchidometer, is strongly suggestive of impaired spermatogenesis and azoospermia. Hormone analysis requires measurement of basal plasma FSH, LH, testosterone and inhibin B, if available.[38] In prepubertal children, hormone analysis is an unreliable predictor of gonadal damage because the hypothalamic–pituitary–testicular axis is quiescent. In postpubertal boys, elevated LH and diminished testosterone levels would indicate Leydig cell dysfunction. Subtle Leydig cell damage may be manifest by elevated LH with normal serum testosterone levels. Elevated FSH and diminished inhibin B would support impaired spermatogenesis, but semen analysis remains the definitive measure of spermatogenesis (Table 8d.1).

Table 8d.1 *Indicators of testicular function*

Leydig cell dysfunction	Reduced testosterone
	Elevated luteinizing hormone
Germinal epithelial dysfunction	Reduced testicular volume
	Elevated follicle-stimulating hormone
	Low inhibin B
	Impaired spermatogenesis

TESTICULAR DAMAGE

Cytotoxic chemotherapy and radiotherapy may damage the testes at all ages, and result in hormone insufficiency and sterility. However, the full impact of gonadotoxic treatment in prepubertal children is difficult to detect during childhood and may be manifest during puberty as hypogonadism or in adulthood as infertility.[4–15]

There is convincing evidence that the prepubertal testis is susceptible to the toxic effects of radiation and chemotherapy.[7–10,15] In the prepubertal testis, there is a steady turnover of early germ cells, which before the haploid stage is reached, undergo spontaneous degeneration. It is likely that it is this activity that renders the prepubertal testis vulnerable to the deleterious impact of cytotoxic therapy.[7,9,10,28,33,34] Although the exact mechanism is uncertain, it appears to involve a combination of destruction of the proliferating germ cell pool and, where germ cells survive, inhibition of further differentiation.[39]

The mechanism of Leydig cell damage is equally uncertain. Chemotherapy may have a direct cytotoxic effect upon the Leydig cells, or an indirect impact by damaging other cell populations and disrupting paracrine regulation. Radiotherapy may directly destroy the slowly turning over Leydig cells at high doses or, more likely, have an indirect effect due to damage to the vasculature. Radiotherapy damage to the testes is associated with decreased testicular blood flow.[40] Where this is marked, compensatory mechanisms may be insufficient to increase intratesticular testosterone concentrations, resulting in reduced testosterone output. Furthermore, reduction in arterial blood flow into the testes may be associated with a diminished stimulatory effect of LH.[41]

Chemotherapy

GERMINAL EPITHELIAL DAMAGE

Chemotherapy-induced damage to the testicular germinal epithelial has been recognized for many years and was first described in humans by Spitz in 1948.[42] Postmortem examination of testicular tissue from 30 men treated with nitrogen mustard demonstrated complete absence of spermatogenesis and seminiferous tubules lined with Sertoli cells only, in 90 per cent of cases. Since then, a number of agents have been identified as causing testicular damage, including cis-platinum, procarbazine and the alkylating agents, such as chlorambucil and cyclophosphamide (Table 8d.2).[9,10,43–47] Cytotoxic chemotherapy agents may produce longlasting or permanent damage to the germinal epithelium, resulting in oligozoospermia or azoospermia.[9,10,48–52]

The extent of the damage to the testis is dependent upon the agent administered and dose received.[9,10,43,46–52]

Table 8d.2 *Gonadotoxic chemotherapy agents*

Alkylating agents
Cyclophosphamide
Ifosfamide
Nitrosoureas, e.g. BCNU, CCNU
Chlorambucil
Melphalan
Busulphan
Antimetabolites
Cytarabine
Platinum agents
Cis-platinum
Others
Procarbazine

However, as most treatments are delivered as multiagent regimens, often with synergistic toxicity, it can be difficult to determine the specific contribution of each individual agent. The impact of chemotherapy on testicular function has been widely investigated and most clinical studies have focused on combination chemotherapy regimens used in the treatment of hematological malignancies, particularly Hodgkin's disease.[9,10,47–51] Occasionally, chemotherapeutic agents are administered as monotherapy, enabling the direct gonadotoxic effects of the agent to be studied, such as cyclophosphamide treatment of immunologically mediated disease.[46,53]

Combination chemotherapy treatment of Hodgkin's disease with established regimens [mechlorethamine, vinblastine, procarbazine and prednisolone (MVPP), or mechlorethamine, vincristine, procarbazine and prednisolone (MOPP), or chlorambucil, vinblastine, procarbazine and prednisolone (ChlVPP), or cyclophosphamide, vincristine, procarbazine and prednisolone (COPP)] have been reported in a number of studies to result in permanent azoospermia in more than 85 per cent of adult males. The gonadotoxic agents in these regimens are mechlorethamine and procarbazine in MVPP and MOPP, chlorambucil and procarbazine in ChlVPP, and procarbazine and cyclophosphamide in COPP.[9,10,47–50,54] The ABVD combination (Adriamycin, bleomycin, vinblastine and dacarbazine), which contains neither an alkylating agent nor procarbazine, has been shown to be significantly less gonadotoxic, resulting in temporary azoospermia in 33 per cent of patients and oligozoospermia in 21 per cent, with 'full' recovery after 18 months reported in all patients retested.[49] However, the advantage of reduced incidence of azoospermia is offset by the increased potential of cardiac disease owing to anthracycline exposure.

In view of the high chance of azoospermia associated with treatment for Hodgkin's disease, alternating combination chemotherapy regimens, 'hybrid' regimens, have been developed in an attempt to reduce the overall dosage of any one particular agent and potentially reduce

all drug-related side effects. 'Hybrid' regimens, such as alternate cycles of ABVD with cycles of ChlVPP or MOPP, appear to be as effective as single-regimen therapies with respect to cure rates, and will hopefully be less gonadotoxic and cardiotoxic. Fertility is preserved in approximately 50 per cent of men following three cycles of MOPP, in contrast to almost universal azoospermia following six cycles of MOPP.[50] In direct comparison of MOPP treatment with MOPP/ABVD, azoospermia was reported in 100 per cent and 76 per cent of patients, respectively.[55]

A number of other combination chemotherapy regimens have also been studied that do not include procarbazine or chlorambucil, and have generally been shown to be less gonadotoxic. Treatment of 51 men with non-Hogkin's lymphoma (NHL) with CHOP (cyclophosphamide, doxorubicin, vincristine and prednisolone)-based chemotherapy rendered all men azoospermic during treatment, but recovery to normospermia occurred in 67 per cent of patients and oligozoospermia in 5 per cent by 5 years.[56] A number of other regimens have been used successfully to treat NHL and are also associated with a more favorable outcome in terms of testicular function, including MACOP-B or VACOP-B (mechlorethamine, doxorubicin, prednisolone, vincristine, cyclophosphamide and bleomycin, or vinblastine replacing mechlorethamine in the latter),[57] VAPEC-B (vincristine, doxorubicin, prednisolone, etoposide, cyclophosphamide and bleomycin)[58] and VEEP (vincristine, etoposide, epirubicin and prednisolone).[51] The vast majority of men have normal fertility following treatment with the above regimens, which, although containing cyclophosphamide, emphasizes the role of procarbazine in causing irreversible damage to the testicular germinal epithelium.

Bone marrow transplantation (BMT) or peripheral blood stem cell (PBSC) rescue following marrow ablation is increasingly being used to treat a number of hematological and solid malignancies successfully. Testicular dysfunction may follow marrow ablation therapy with total body irradiation (TBI) or high-dose chemotherapy, including cyclophosphamide and busulphan. In a study of 155 patients, aged 13–56 years, undergoing BMT for hematological malignancies or aplastic leukemia, preparative chemotherapy regimens included cyclophosphamide (200 mg/kg) in 109 patients, or busulphan (16 mg/kg) and cyclophosphamide (200 mg/kg) in the remaining 46 patients. Recovery of testicular function, defined by normal FSH and/or sperm production, was assessed at 3 (1–19) years post-treatment. In the group treated with cyclophosphamide only, 67 of the 109 (39 per cent) patients had evidence of recovery, while amongst those who received both agents testicular dysfunction was evident in 38 of 46 (83 per cent).[15] Busulphan was clearly associated with greater gonadotoxicity at those doses. In another study semen analysis in long-term survivors of BMT receiving preconditioning with busulphan

(16 mg/kg) and cyclophosphamide (120 mg/kg) demonstrated sperm production in 21 out of 26 (81 per cent) of patients, 10 of whom were oligozoospermic.[59]

Follow-up of 30 men for a mean of 12.8 years following treatment with cyclophosphamide (total dose 560–840 mg/kg) for childhood nephrotic syndrome, reported azoospermia in 13 per cent, oligozoospermia in 30 per cent and normal semen analysis in the remaining 57 per cent of the men.[46] The threshold for impaired spermatogenesis was a total dose of 10 g. However, when used for the treatment of solid tumors in combination with doxorubicin and dacarbazine, or vincristine, which have not been shown to be gonadotoxic, azoospermia was permanent in 90 per cent of men treated with cyclophosphamide doses >7.5 g/m.[2,60] Management of childhood leukemia, which is the commonest childhood malignancy, is continually evolving and often includes cyclophosphamide or cytarabine. A study of testicular histology in 44 boys treated for ALL demonstrated a 50 per cent reduction in tubular fertility index (TFI) (per centage of tubules containing identifiable spermatozoa), with severe impairment (TFI < 40 per cent) in 18 patients. The severity of the damage was influenced by previous chemotherapy treatment with cyclophosphamide and cytarabine ($>1 \text{ g/m}^2$), whereas the tubular fertility index improved with increasing time from treatment.[61] 'Full' recovery of spermatogenesis was observed in three of seven of the patients with severe depression of TFI followed up for median (range), 10.8 (5.5–15.9) years off treatment.[44] Germinal epithelial damage has also been described following successful treatment for childhood ALL with a modified LSA_2L_2 protocol, which includes treatment with cyclophosphamide and cytarabine.[62] In contrast, normal testicular function was reported in 14 boys successfully treated for ALL with treatment, which did not include either cyclophosphamide or cytarabine.[63] Current treatment of ALL in the UK includes cytarabine (total dose 2 g/m^2 or 4 g/m^2) and cyclophosphamide (total dose 1.2 g/m^2 or 2.4 g/m^2). Although this is unlikely to be sterilizing, long-term follow-up is necessary.

Ifosfamide, an analogue of cyclophosphamide, is another potentially gonadotoxic agent, although limited data describing its effect on testicular function are available. In one study that included six patients treated with ifosfamide-based regimens (total dose/m²: $84–126 \text{ g/m}^2$) for Ewing's sarcoma or rhabdomyosarcoma during childhood and adolescence, only two men had a normal semen analysis, two were oligozoospermic and the remaining two patients were azoospermic.[52]

The value of serum inhibin B in detecting male gonadal dysfunction was studied in 27 postpubertal and 12 pubertal survivors of childhood cancer. Serum inhibin B levels were found to correlate with testicular volume and gonadotrophin concentrations. In the postpubertal group, small testicular volume was strongly correlated with low

inhibin B levels (<42 pg/ml) and inversely related to FSH levels. In all prepubertal survivors, inhibin B levels were greater than 90 pg/ml, except in one patient with testicular cancer, whose inhibin B was barely detectable and FSH was elevated, indicative of testicular damage. Inhibin B appears to be a sensitive marker of germinal epithelial function and may be a tool for evaluation of testicular function in cancer survivors unable to produce semen for analysis.[64]

Where spermatogenesis is preserved, there are very limited data available on the quantity and quality of the sperm produced. Evaluation of testicular function in 33 men who had undergone treatment with multiagent chemotherapy regimens, plus or minus radiotherapy, for a variety of hematological and solid malignancies during childhood, identified two populations of patients, those who were azoospermic and those with preservation of sperm production.[52] Of the 33 men, 30 per cent were azoospermic with raised FSH and undetectable inhibin B concentrations. Azoospermia was present after chemotherapy treatment with ChlVPP for Hodgkin's disease, ifosfamide based therapy for Ewing's sarcoma and radiotherapy treatment with TBI or testicular irradiation for ALL or lymphoma. For the group of patients with preservation of spermatogenesis, sperm concentration was significantly lower compared with a cohort of healthy men, median (interquartile range) 37.1 (19.7–89.9) and 90.7 (50.5–121.5) $\times 10^6$/ml, respectively ($p = 0.002$), with 26 per cent of the men having oligozoospermia. Only 33 per cent of the group had a normal semen analysis as defined by the World Health Organisation criteria.[52]

LEYDIG CELL DAMAGE

The Leydig cells are less vulnerable to the cytotoxic effects of chemotherapy than the sensitive germinal epithelium.[10,43,46–48,53,54] Gonadotoxic chemotherapy agents responsible for germinal epithelial damage may, however, also cause Leydig cell dysfunction. In a study of 30 men treated with cyclophosphamide (2–3 mg/kg body weight/day for a mean of 280, range 42–556, days) for childhood nephrotic syndrome, all men had normal development of secondary sexual characteristics, normal libido and sexual function. All patients demonstrated a significantly raised LH response on stimulation with LH- releasing hormone, in the presence of normal testosterone concentrations, suggesting compensated Leydig cell failure.[46]

Following treatment for Hodgkin's disease with the gonadotoxic regimens, MVPP, MOPP, ChlVPP and COPP, elevated LH (basal and stimulated) are reported in 24–88 per cent of patients.[9,10,45,47,48,54] In the majority (>85 per cent of patients) testosterone levels are within the normal range, indicating compensated Leydig cell dysfunction.

Young boys and adolescent males who receive standard dose cyclophosphamide (200 mg/kg) as conditioning therapy for BMT appear to retain normal Leydig cell function, as evidenced by normal hormone profile and pubertal development in the majority of males.[65] Although the data are limited, Leydig cell function appears to be preserved in most males treated with the combination of busulphan and cyclophosphamide, despite damage to the germinal epithelium.[66]

Assessment of Leydig cell function in long-term survivors of childhood cancer, with and without preservation of sperm production, has shown that serum LH was significantly greater in both the non-azoospermic and azoospermic groups compared with healthy controls (Figure 8d.3). Testosterone concentrations were within normal limits in all three groups with no significant differences between the groups. These findings provide further evidence of the vulnerability of Leydig cells to cytotoxic insult. With increasing time after treatment and increasing age, Leydig cell damage may require consideration of testosterone replacement. Continued long-term, endocrine surveillance of survivors who are infertile after cytotoxic insult would appear to be justified. Furthermore, these studies demonstrate that, even where sperm production is present, subtle Leydig cell damage is likely. This may reflect greater susceptibility of the Leydig cells to cytotoxic insult than was previously appreciated.[52]

Radiotherapy–induced damage

GERMINAL EPITHELIAL DAMAGE

The germinal epithelium is very sensitive to damage from both radiotherapy and chemotherapy. The degree and permanency of radiotherapy-induced testicular damage depends on the treatment field, total dose and fractionation schedule (Table 8d.3).[12–15,67] Doses as low as 0.1–1.2 Gy damage dividing spermatogonia and disrupt cell morphology, resulting in oligozoospermia.[67,68] Following low-dose single-fraction irradiation, complete recovery of spermatogenesis was observed 9–18 months following irradiation with 1 Gy, by 30 months following doses of 2–3 Gy and at 5 years or more in those treated with 4 Gy.[67,68] The germinal epithelium appears to be more susceptible to fractionation of radiotherapy, with doses greater than 1.2 Gy fractionated, resulting in permanent azoospermia.[14]

In a large study, 463 males, mean age 26 (range 11–62) years, received TBI, 10–15.75 Gy, as preparative treatment before BMT for hematological malignancies or aplastic anemia.[15] Assessment of testicular function at mean age 3 (range 1–19) years post-transplant demonstrated impaired testicular function, with normal defined as normal FSH, LH and testosterone concentrations with

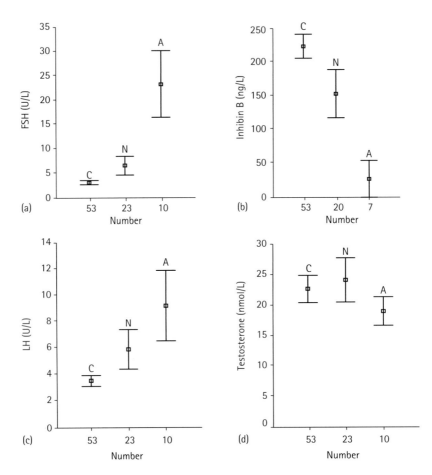

Figure 8d.3 *Comparison of endocrine parameters in azoosphermic and non-azoospermic cancer survivors and control subjects. (a, b) There is an inverse relationship between follicle-stimulating hormone (FSH) and inhibin B levels. Damage to the germinal epithelium, with complete azoospermia, is associated with high FSH levels and almost undetectable inhibin B levels. Even where there is preservation of sperm production, there is endocrine evidence of mild impairment, with significantly elevated FSH and low inhibin B levels compared with the control group. This is in keeping with reduced sperm concentration in the cancer survivors. (c, d) Although all cancer survivors have normal levels of testosterone, luteinizing hormone (LH) levels are significantly greater in both the non-azoospermic and azoospermic patents than in the control population, suggesting mild Leydig cell dysfunction. C, controls; N, non-azoospermia; A, azoospermia.*

evidence of sperm production, in 83 per cent (382 of 463) of subjects.

The effects of irradiation on testicular function were evaluated in 60 long-term survivors of childhood ALL. All patients received 18 or 24 Gy cranial or craniospinal irradiation; groups one and two, and the third group received 12 Gy abdominal irradiation in addition to craniospinal irradiation. Primary germ-cell dysfunction, defined as elevated FSH and/or reduced testicular volume, was significantly associated with the field of radiotherapy. Of the patients who received additional abdominal irradiation, 55 per cent demonstrated evidence of germinal epithelial dysfunction, in contrast to none of the patients treated with cranial irradiation alone. Interestingly, 17 per cent of the group receiving craniospinal irradiation demonstrated evidence of primary germ cell damage,

Table 8d.3 *Radiotherapy-induced damage to the reproductive tract*

Site	Effect
Cranial/total body irradiation	Hypogonadotrophic hypogonadism
Total body irradiation/ pelvic/testes	Germinal epithelium
	>1.2 Gy – azoospermia
	0.1–1.1 Gy – oligoozospermia
	Leydig cells
	>20 Gy – prepubertal
	>30 Gy – postpubertal

indicating that scatter irradiation exposure may also impair testicular function.[69]

Gonadal function was assessed in 15 boys following testicular irradiation for childhood ALL. The dose to the

testes was 12 Gy in 12 boys, 15 Gy in one boy and 24 Gy in the remaining two boys. Azoospermia was observed in all boys.[70]

In a further study, testicular function was investigated in 21 boys, mean age 19.0 years, following TBI and BMT for hematological malignancies at a mean age of 11.3 years, 15 of whom were prepubertal at time of treatment. All boys had reduced testicular volumes (mean 10.5 ml) with elevated basal FSH concentrations, with normalization in only one patient, indicating severe impairment of reproductive function following TBI.[71]

LEYDIG CELL DAMAGE

Leydig cells are more resistant to damage from radiotherapy than the germinal epithelium and progression through puberty with normal potency is common, despite severe impairment of spermatogenesis. Susceptibility to radiation-induced Leydig cell damage appears to be inversely related to age, or sexual maturation, with greater damage following smaller doses in prepubertal boys.[12,13,71–75]

The impact of radiotherapy on testicular function has been studied in children undergoing BMT for leukemia. Seventeen prepubertal boys, aged less than 12 years, received hyperfractionated TBI (total dose 13.75–15 Gy) with a testicular boost of 4 Gy in 16 patients and 12 Gy in the remaining patient. Before undergoing transplantation, all of the boys had received multiagent chemotherapy and, for nine of them, this had included cyclophosphamide. Of the 17 boys, mean age 14 (range 10.4–17.1) years, 14 (82 per cent) entered puberty spontaneously, two were less than 12 years old and prepubertal, and the remaining subject, who had received a 12 Gy testicular boost, required androgen replacement therapy to induce puberty. Although overt Leydig cell failure was rare, 36 per cent of the subjects demonstrated compensated Leydig cell dysfunction. Furthermore, pubertal boys with raised plasma LH concentrations were younger at the time of BMT than pubertal boys with normal levels of LH.[73] Similar reports of increased vulnerability of the young Leydig cell to radiation-induced damage are reported in a number of studies.[65,73–76] Leydig cell function was evaluated in 41 men treated with TBI (12 Gy fractionated or 10 Gy single dose), 6 Gy single dose total lymphoid irradiation or chemotherapy alone at age 7.7 (0.6–13.6) years. Leydig cell dysfunction was reported in ten (24 per cent) of the men, of whom three had complete Leydig cell failure.[76] Testicular irradiation with doses of greater than 20 Gy is associated with Leydig cell dysfunction in prepubertal boys, while Leydig cell function is usually preserved up to 30 Gy in sexually mature males (Table 8d.3).[73–76]

Pubertal development after TBI was investigated in 21 boys treated with allogeneic BMT for hematological malignancies at a mean age 11.3 years. Fifteen of the boys were prepubertal at BMT. Normal development of secondary sexual characteristics was observed in 19 men. The remaining two men with hypogonadism had received an additional boost of testicular irradiation and required androgen supplementation. However, despite clinical evidence of intact Leydig cell function, and normal testosterone levels in all 19 men, LH levels were elevated in the majority of subjects indicating mild Leydig cell dysfunction.[72]

CLINICAL IMPACT OF IMPAIRED TESTICULAR FUNCTION

The clinical implications of frank Leydig cell failure and azoospermia are very clear. The implications of mild/subclinical Leydig cell insufficiency are, however, unclear. The clinical manifestations of Leydig cell dysfunction will inevitably depend upon the age of the child at the time of treatment. Loss of Leydig cell function before the onset of, or during, puberty will be associated with failure to enter puberty spontaneously or arrest of pubertal development. Cytotoxic insult following the development of normal secondary sexual characteristics will manifest clinically as erectile dysfunction, reduced libido, fatigue and mood changes, and biochemically will be associated with decreased bone mineral density, loss of muscle mass and other metabolic disturbances.[16–18]

Leydig cell failure in the prepubertal child will require androgen supplementation for induction and progression of puberty and, in the adult, testosterone replacement. Increasing evidence is emerging that compensated Leydig cell impairment may play an important role in bone mineral density (BMD) and general well-being.[16–18] In the adult male, overt testosterone deficiency is associated with decreased energy level, poor libido, increased incidence of anxiety and depression, altered body composition and reduced BMD. These symptoms, if found in males following chemotherapy, imply mild testosterone deficiency.[16–18] Limited data are available exploring the role of testosterone supplementation in men with compensated Leydig cell dysfunction. In a single-blind randomized study, 35 men (mean age 40.9 years) with mild Leydig cell dysfunction, as defined by raised LH, and low or low normal testosterone level, were identified following treatment with cytotoxic chemotherapy for malignancy. Patients were randomized to receive 12 months treatment with transdermal testosterone or placebo patches. Testosterone levels increased significantly in the testosterone-treated group compared with the placebo group and LH levels returned to normal values in 94 per cent of subjects. However, there were no significant changes in BMD, body composition or lipid profile, apart from a small reduction in low-density lipoprotein (LDL) cholesterol. In terms of quality of life, the only perceived benefit was a marginal

reduction in physical fatigue with no effects on mood or sexual function.[77] Testosterone supplementation for mild hypogonadism appears to be of limited clinical benefit, but further studies are required to further our understanding and define the role of testosterone replacement therapy.

FERTILITY PRESERVATION

Advances in assisted reproduction, and increasing interest in gamete extraction and maturation have focused attention on preserving gonadal tissue from children before sterilizing chemotherapy or radiotherapy, with the realistic expectation that future technologies will be able to utilize their immature gametes. The impetus for preserving gonadal tissue follows on the heels of pioneering experiments in ewes,[78] together with media interest in the report of a successful autologous ovarian graft in a previously oophorectomized female.[79] In addition, live human births have been reported resulting from the transfer of embryos fertilized with immature spermatogenic cells.[80–85] Such issues have inevitably raised questions from parents and oncologists about their possible application in children undergoing cancer therapies.[27,86]

Established practice

CRYOPRESERVATION OF GAMETES

Potential strategies for preservation of male fertility are dependent upon the sexual maturity of the patient. The only established current clinical option for preservation of male fertility is cryopreservation of spermatozoa (Table 8d.4). Spermatozoa are usually obtained from the ejaculate by masturbation but may be obtained using rectal electrostimulation techniques under anesthetic. When it is not possible to obtain an ejaculate, sperm can be retrieved by epididymal aspiration or testicular biopsy in sexually mature men. The onset of spermatogenesis, or spermarche, is difficult to determine. Spermarche is a midpubertal event, preceding the ability to produce an ejaculate, which occurs at a median age of 13.4 years (range 11.7–15.2 years) when median testicular volume is 11.5 (4.7–19.6) ml.[87] Once spermarche is established, studies of serial urine specimens have shown that spermaturia is a variable intermittent process throughout puberty. The detection of sperm in the urine, spermaturia, may provide a valuable clinical tool. Peripubertal males with spermaturia may identify a population of males who are able to produce sperm but not yet mature enough to produce a sample by masturbation. Surgical retrieval of spermatozoa may be considered for this group.

Not infrequently, sperm produced by cancer patients at the time of diagnosis is of poor quality. With advances in assisted reproduction techniques, in particular

Table 8d.4 *Clinical and experimental strategies for preservation of male reproductive function in children undergoing treatment for cancer*

Clinical practice	Experimental strategies
Sperm banking	Cryopreservation of
Ejaculation	testicular tissue
Rectal electrostimulation	Gonadotrophin
Testicular/epididymal aspiration	suppression

intracytoplasmic sperm injection (ICSI), which involves the injection of a single spermatozoan directly into an ooctye, the problems of low numbers and poor motility may be cirvcumvented.[20–22] More recently, a small number of pregnancies have been achieved with ICSI, using immature spermatids and secondary spermatocytes extracted from testicular tissue in men with spermatogenic arrest.[80–85]

Experimental strategies (Table 8d.4)

GONADOTROPHIN SUPPRESSION

One approach to preserving fertile potential was based on the original idea that the prepubertal testis was quiescent and therefore protected from the cytotoxic effects of chemotherapy and radiotherapy. It was hypothesized that suppression of spermatogenesis to render the testes 'prepubertal' might protect the normally rapidly dividing germ cell population from damage. In rats, suppression of hypothalamic–pituitary–gonadal axis by administration of the GnRH analogue, goserelin, before and during chemotherapy with procarbazine, enhanced recovery of spermatogenesis.[88] Similarly, protection of spermatogenesis in rats subjected to treatment with procarbazine, cyclophosphamide and radiotherapy has been demonstrated using a number of hormones, including testosterone alone or in combination with estrogen,[89] GnRH analogues in combination with testosterone[90] or the anti-androgen flutamide.[91,92] Furthermore, recovery from spermatogenic damage in rats induced by radiotherapy or procarbazine treatment has been shown to be enhanced by treatment with GnRH analogues or testosterone, even when administered after the gonadotoxic agent.[88,89] While it has since become clear that the prepubertal testis is susceptible to the deleterious effects of cytotoxic therapy, the mechanisms by which such hormonal manipulation offers protection or enhancement of recovery of spermatogenesis are unclear. If azoospermia following cytotoxic treatment is a consequence of destruction of the rapidly proliferating spermatogonial stem cells, this would result in azoospermia within 12 weeks, the time taken from differentiation of stem cell to mature spermatozoa. Yet, spontaneous recovery of spermatogenesis is reported

after many years of azoospermia. In rats, it has been shown that some stem cells survive cytotoxic therapy and that the resulting azoospermia is a consequence of the inability of those spermatogonia that are present to proliferate and differentiate.[39] Hormonal analysis following irradiation in rats has shown a dramatic increase in intratesticular testosterone levels, and it has been postulated that suppression of the hypothalamic–pituitary–gonadal axis promotes multiplication and differentiation of spermatogonia by lowering intratesticular testosterone.[93,94]

While there is significant evidence for the success of protection/recovery strategies in rats, clinical studies in man have to date been inconclusive.[95–98] In one study where cyclophosphamide was administered as immunosuppressive therapy for nephrotic syndrome in adult men, preservation of fertility was achieved.[95] Of the men who received cyclophosphamide alone, 90 per cent remained azoospermic at 6 months post-treatment, whereas sperm concentrations returned to normal in all five of the men who received testosterone therapy during the immunosuppressive treatment. Other studies have failed to show similar benefits in humans. Suppression of testicular function with a GnRH agonist, alone or in combination with testosterone during gonadotoxic chemotherapy treatment for lymphoma, did not confer any protective benefit or enhance recovery of spermatogenesis.[96,97] In men treated with sterilizing radiotherapy and chemotherapy for childhood cancer, effective gonadotrophin suppression with medroxyprogesterone acetate for at least 3 months did not result in restoration of spermatogenesis.[98] The absence of histological evidence of spermatogonial stem cells in testicular biopsies from these men before and after suppression suggests complete ablation of the germinal epithelium and irreversible infertility. Endocrine manipulation to enhance recovery of spermatogenesis may be successful in patients in whom the testicular insult is less severe and there is preservation of spermatogonial stem cells.

HARVESTING TESTICULAR TISSUE

For prepubertal boys, lacking in haploid gametes, there are no options currently available to preserve fertility and any potential strategies must be considered entirely experimental. In theory, testicular tissue could be removed before the start of treatment and cryopreserved either as a segment of tissue or as isolated germ cells. Following cure from his malignancy, the patient could have the frozen–thawed testicular tissue autografted to the testes. Alternatively, isolated germ cells could be reimplanted into the patient's own testes or these cells could be matured in vitro until they reached a stage sufficiently mature to achieve fertilization with ICSI.

The concept of testicular germ cell transplantation was pioneered by Brinster and colleagues in 1994.[24] Testicular germ cells isolated from mouse testis, and transplanted into the testis of genetically or experimentally sterile mice initiated and sustained normal donor spermatogenesis, restoring fertility and producing healthy offspring.[99] Successful transplantation has also been shown in mouse recipients rendered sterile with the chemotherapeutic agent, busulphan. Interestingly, these experiments also demonstrated both endogenous and donor spermatogenesis simultaneously, indicating that busulphan did not kill all the endogenous stem cells.[24] Subsequent studies have shown that testicular germ cell transplantation can occur through autologous, heterologous (mouse to mouse, rat to rat) or xenologous (hamster, dog, rabbit or rat to mouse) transfer of cells. The site can be heterotopic, as a graft to a non-gonadal site in the recipient, or homotopic when the cells are reintroduced into the testis.[24–26,99–101] In order to develop autologous germ cell transplantation in humans, techniques have to be developed by which human testicular germ cells can be isolated, stored and reintroduced into the testis.

Testicular tissue obtained by testicular biopsy has been successfully cryopreserved with subsequent isolation of spermatozoa from the thawed tissue and successfully used in ICSI.[102,103] These studies have only utilized spermatozoa or immature spermatogenic cells retrieved from tissue post-thaw and it may be that survival of spermatogonial germ cells post-thaw is poor. Furthermore, as there is a more than a theoretical risk of transplanting tumor cells, it is likely that clinical practice will involve enzymatic digestion and isolation of germ cells before cryopreservation rather than autografting testicular tissue.

Transplantation in rodent models has involved only semipurified cell populations of germ cells and somatic cells. For human application, purified stem cell populations would be necessary to ensure that no malignant cells were transferred. The term 'stem cell' is a functional description, given that there are no morphological, antigenic or biochemical criteria by which to identify these cells in vivo or in vitro. Spermatogonial transplantation is the only method at present by which stem-cell presence can be authenticated. In mice, LacZ encodes for the enzyme β-galactosidase, which can be demonstrated histochemically as an intracellular blue reaction product. Effective purification will demand the development of specific antibody probes to differentiate stem cells from other cells. Studies have shown that a number of cell surface antigens are expressed on stem cells, including α-6, β-1 integrin and c-kit, which may enable enrichment using magnetic cell sorting.[104] The major limitation for human application is that these antigens are shared with other progenitor cells, including hematopoietic cells, creating inherent problems in cancer patients.

The highly efficient process of spermatogenesis begins in puberty, although a number of immature spermatogenic cells are described in the prepubertal testis.

It is believed that 10^4 germ cells contain as few as two stem cell spermatogonia capable of self-renewal. With the average number of germ cells in the testis estimated to range between $13-83 \times 10^6$ during childhood, the relatively small numbers of stem cell spermatogonia available poses a challenge for the process of stem-cell isolation.[34] Consequently, there is a need to develop an *in vitro* culture system to augment stem cell numbers following harvesting and isolation. The feasibility of enrichment has been shown by Nagano *et al.* who have maintained mouse stem cells in culture for up to 4 months and the cultured cells initiated successful spermatogenesis following transplantation.[105]

Cryopreservation of spermatozoa and fertilization following thawing are well established. Application of this approach to stem-cell spermatogonia will require modification and optimization of freezing procedures, taking into consideration the inherent biological differences between the immature diploid stem cells and mature gametes.[106] There is thus a need for studies to devise cryopreservation regimens that are applicable to stem cells from the pre-pubertal testis.

FUTURE USE OF CRYOPRESERVED TESTICULAR TISSUE

The future use of testicular germ cells is likely to involve either maturation of the germ cells *in vitro* for use with ICSI or transplantation. Ideally, transplantation would involve injecting preparations of purified germ cells into the testis with restoration of natural fertility. *In vitro* maturation techniques, although still very much in their infancy, would have the advantage of eliminating any risk of transplanting harvested malignant cells back into the patient. Creating an environment *in vitro* to stimulate germ-cell maturation and differentiation into spermatozoa may be the only option for a number of patients where cancer therapy damage has been so extensive that the supporting Sertoli cells would be unable to support spermatogenesis. Attempts to cultivate male germ cells *in vitro* have shown that germ cells can survive several months in culture and are likely to be undergoing cell division.[107] Tesarik reported *in vitro* spermatogenesis and healthy offspring using ICSI. However, the maturation process involved *in vitro* maturation of late stages of spermatogenesis rather than development from germ cells.[107,108]

A number of studies have concentrated on developing the most efficient technique for infusing the stem cells into the testis. The simplest and most effective method of filling the seminiferous tubules *in vitro* proved to be by injection into the rete testis of bull, monkey and man, under ultrasound guidance.[109] These experiments involved injection into partially involuted or prepubertal testes. This eliminates the problems associated with backpressure of fluid in fully active testes, which would otherwise

block the infusion of the cell suspension into the tubules. The development of an animal primate model of autologous germ-cell transplantation has been explored by Schlatt and colleagues.[109,110] Successful *in vivo* rete injections have been performed on cynomolgus monkeys under the guidance of ultrasonography. Injecting the cells into the rete allows a much larger volume to be infused in contrast to the microinjections involved in reinfusing directly into the seminiferous tubules.[109] Using the primate animal model, follow-up studies have explored the feasibility of these techniques for application in oncology patients.[110] Germ cells were retrieved and cryopreserved from the monkeys followed by testicular irradiation (total dose 2 Gy) rendering them azoospermic and mimicking the impact of gonadotoxicity in oncology patients. Subsequent transfer of the germ cells into one of the testis was associated with earlier and better regrowth of the testis and reinduction of spermatogenesis in comparison to the untreated testis with the latter also serving as a measure of the degree of spontaneous recovery of spermatogenesis. However, at the end of the study there was no difference in absolute sperm counts between the testes, highlighting the complex nature of germ cell transplantation and the necessity for further work to perfect this technique for human application.

Immature testicular tissue has been shown to grow and differentiate when grafted into another species.[25] This provides an additional strategy for conserving the male germline and circumvents the risk of reintroducing malignant cells. Clearly, this technique is unlikely to be ethically acceptable and is compromised by the risk of interspecies transfer of potentially pathogenic microorganisms.

Clinical practice for harvesting gonadal tissue

Harvesting and storage of ovarian cortical tissue from girls and young women before gonadotoxic chemotherapy has been available in a number of centers since the mid-1990s and, more recently, a few centers report the storage of testicular tissue.[111] The Royal College of Obstetricians and Gynaecologists has provided a report from a working party on the storage of ovarian and prepubertal testicular tissue. This provides standards for best practice in the cryopreservation of gonadal tissue, including the criteria for providing a service, patient identification and selection, standard operating procedures and requirements for safe storage.[112]

PROGENY

Overall, there are reassuring reports that there is no increased incidence of either congenital abnormalities or

childhood malignancy in children born to long-term survivors of childhood cancer.[113,114] However, these successful pregnancies mostly result from normally achieved conception. We do not know the consequences of circumventing the natural selection processes of normal sexual reproduction using assisted reproduction techniques (ART), nor the effects of ART on the complex cascade of precisely timed molecular interactions of early embryonic development. Continued surveillance of the progeny of survivors of childhood cancer remains essential.[115]

Paternal risk to the offspring

The mutagenic potential of cancer therapy may confer a risk to the fetus conceived using gametes produced after cancer therapy, although current epidemiological data suggest that offspring of cancer survivors do not have an increased incidence of congenital abnormalities or cancer relative to the general population.[113,114] There is at least the hypothetical possibility of injection of abnormal spermatozoa or immature spermatogenic cells carrying abnormal genomic DNA with the potential to increase congenital and other abnormalities amongst offspring.[115,116] Studies in animals have shown that exposure of the male germline to chemotherapy agents may disrupt spermatozoal DNA and result in deleterious effects on embryo development.[117–119] Awareness of the importance of sperm DNA integrity for accurate transmission of genetic material to the offspring has necessitated the development of new techniques to assess sperm characteristics in more detail.[116]

It has become clear that men from subfertility clinic populations, with abnormalities of the conventional criteria of semen quality, also demonstrate elevated levels of damage to the genomic DNA in their gametes. Even amongst normal populations, sperm chromatin damage has been linked with impaired fecundity.[120] It has been shown that sperm DNA damage does not preclude pronucleus formation at ICSI and that abnormal DNA within the male gamete is detectable in the early embryo.[121] Thus far, evidence on the safety of ICSI has been largely based upon its use in populations of men with deficits in spermatogenesis unrelated to potentially mutagenic cancer treatment. This evidence has been broadly reassuring concerning health risks to the offspring, although it is limited by the restricted length of follow-up currently available.[122,123] Studies have shown that, although, by conventional criteria, semen quality is frequently abnormal in long-term survivors of childhood cancer, the sperm produced do not appear to carry a greater burden of damaged DNA (Figure 8d.4).[52] This observation goes some way to providing reassurance about the use of ICSI, which will circumvent the problems associated with severe oligozoospermia and asthenozoospermia, and offer cancer survivors the possibility of paternity in adulthood.

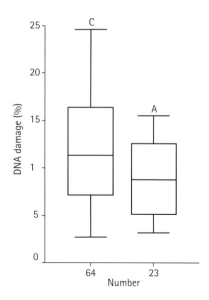

Figure 8d.4 *Sperm DNA integrity in long-term survivors of childhood cancer compared with healthy controls (p = 0.06). The median, interquartile range and maximum and minimum values are shown. C, controls; A, azoospermia.*

Successful pregnancies have been achieved using immature spermatogenic cells, which may add an additional risk to the fetus. Fertilization of oocytes with immature spermatogenic cells, such as round cells and elongated spermatids, which have not yet completed spermatogenesis, must be pursued with caution. The mechanism by which sperm precursor cells activate the oocyte at fertilization is uncertain, but it is speculated that suboptimal oocyte activation may confer poor fertilization, implantation and high early abortion rates.[124] Spermatid transition into spermatozoa is characterized by salient changes in nuclear protein composition.[125] The significance of circumventing these changes is uncertain. Genetic imprinting plays an important role in embryogenesis and in processes leading to the development of pediatric cancers, including Wilms' tumor and embryonal rhabdomyosarcoma, and other human diseases.[126] Although the mechanism involved in genetic imprinting is uncertain, it is likely to involve differences in DNA methylation and requires careful consideration when embarking on germ-cell maturation. Children born following assisted conception using spermatozoa and immature spermatogenic cells require long-term careful monitoring.

ETHICAL ISSUES

Harvesting gonadal tissue and its future use is an exciting new area of gamete biology, which raises a wide range of unresolved ethical and legal dilemmas that must be addressed before embarking on any clinical

program.[27,86,111,114,127] These include issues relating to the safety of the tissue harvesting, subsequent use and possible implications for the progeny, together with the legal constraints enforced by the Human Fertilisation and Embryology Authority (HFEA) relating to gamete storage and manipulation, and the common laws defining validity of consent in the event of any such procedures becoming available. Valid consent is necessary for clinical research, rendering potentially harmful interventions both ethical and legal. To be valid, consent must be informed, voluntarily obtained and given by a competent person. Legal competence for a person to give consent requires that the individual is able to understand the information given to them, believes that this information applies to them, retains it and uses it to make an informed choice. The complex issues of fertility preservation and limited time for discussion imposed by therapeutic imperatives, further fuelled by parental and patient anxieties, will inevitably diminish the validity of such consent. Some of these practical difficulties may be alleviated if obtaining consent is considered as a continuum, which can be divided into two stages, with part one involving harvesting and cryopreservation of the tissue and part two involving subsequent use of the tissue. Issues relating to the use of the tissue in the event of the death of the patient must also be discussed.[27,86]

To further complicate these issues, the legal framework defines who is eligible to give the consent. In the UK, adolescents over the age of 16 years in Scotland, and 18 years in England, may give consent to treatment in accordance with the Family Law Reform Act 1969 s8, while for younger children ('minors') consent is generally obtained by proxy. In exception to this, legally valid consent from 'minors' can be obtained if their doctor considers that they are competent to make an informed and wise decision (Gillick competence).[128] However, the field of assisted reproduction is governed by the statute in the UK and is under the jurisdiction of the HFEA (HFEA Act, 1990), which dictates strict guidelines on the requirements for informed consent with respect to the storage of gametes and embryos, and their subsequent use.[129] The HFEA grants licenses to individuals for certain procedures involving gametes. Proxy consent is specifically excluded and there is a requirement to provide written and verbal information, and an offer of independent counseling. A gamete is defined by the HFEA to be 'a reproductive cell, such as an ovum or spermatozoa, which has a haploid set of chromosomes and which is capable of taking part in fertilization with another of the opposite sex to form a zygote'.[130] In practice, this would mean that non-gametes, or immature germ cells, could be harvested from children, with parental consent, and stored in unlicensed premises. Of course, should this immature material ever be matured to form gametes, the requirements for storage of such material would then fall under the jurisdiction

of the HFEA. In sexually mature boys, sperm may be produced or retrieved surgically, and written consent obtained in accordance with the Gillick principle and cryopreserved in a licensed center.

In December 1999 an international conference was held in Cambridge, the specific aim of which was to develop an ethically acceptable strategy for the practice and research related to preserving fertility in children and adolescents being treated for cancer. From this meeting a consensus statement was drawn up, which made a number of recommendations.[27] Integral to these recommendations were the design and implementation of well-constructed research strategies, confined to a finite number of specialist centers, with centralization of data and rapid dissemination of the results. In turn, these protocols and results should be subject to rigorous review to ensure high standards for collection procedures and storage of material. At both a research and clinical level, this would involve multidisciplinary teamwork with multicenter collaboration, dictating optimum communication to ensure the best interests of the child are met. It was also recommended that prospective studies be set up to gather data on the impact of current treatment strategies on fertility outcomes in prepubertal children treated for cancer to facilitate further our understanding of the gonadotoxic impact of chemotherapy and radiotherapy, in the hope that future treatment regimens may be modified accordingly. The experimental nature of this work makes it essential to ensure that clinical and research practice develops in a phased and coordinated manner.

CONCLUSIONS

As treatment for childhood cancer has become increasingly successful, adverse effects on reproductive function are assuming greater importance. Preservation of fertility before treatment must be considered in all young patients at high risk of subfertility. Limitation of radiation exposure by shielding of the testes should be practiced where possible and sperm banking should be offered to all sexually mature boys at risk of infertility. The rapidly advancing experimental techniques for harvesting of gonadal tissue must be considered and embarked upon without unrealistic expectations, although future utilization of the tissue is unlikely to be realized until the next decade.

Semen can be stored before sterilizing chemotherapy and radiotherapy for use at a later date, thus preserving fertility. Attempts to restore spermatogenesis in azoospermic men, using hormone manipulation have so far been unsuccessful. However, capitalizing on the unique properties of the spermatogonial stem cell, testicular tissue could be harvested before treatment and cryopreserved for use at a later date. The functional capacity of the testes appears to be preserved and autotransplantation of the

stem cells in rats has been shown to reinitiate spermatogenesis and permanently restore fertility. Where fears of reintroducing tumor cells may limit applicability of this approach in humans, *in vitro* maturation and use with assisted reproduction techniques is a realistic alternative.

It is incumbent upon oncologists to facilitate appropriate counselling of patients at risk of subfertility as part of their routine care. The importance of the late effects of treatment are receiving increasing recognition and in the UK strategies for long-term follow-up are currently being explored.[3] Addressing fertility issues at the time of diagnosis of cancer will help young cancer patients and their families to endure their disease and its treatment in a more optimistic light.

KEY POINTS

- Successful treatment of childhood cancer may be associated with impaired testicular function in adulthood.
- The testis is highly susceptible to the toxic effects of radiation and chemotherapy at all ages of life.
- Assessment of testicular maturation and function involves pubertal staging, plasma hormone analysis and semen analysis.
- Total body, pelvic or testicular irradiation may cause testicular damage, and the degree of impairment is related to the radiation dose, fractionation schedule and age at time of treatment.
- Apart from cryopreservation of spermatozoa in the sexually mature male, all alternative strategies remain experimental.
- Best practice in the cryopreservation of gonadal tissue, including the criteria for providing a service, patient identification and selection, standard operating procedures and requirements for safe storage need to be established.
- Concerns that the offspring of patients successfully treated for cancer might have an increased risk of congenital abnormalities and childhood cancer have not been substantiated.

REFERENCES

1. Wallace WHB. Growth and endocrine function following the treatment of childhood malignant disease. In: Pinkerton CR, Plowman PN (eds) *Paediatric oncology: clinical practice and controversies*, 2nd edn. London: Chapman and Hall Medical, 1997:706–731.
2. Bleyer WA. The impact of childhood cancer on the United States and the world. *Cancer* 1990; **40**:355–367.
3. Wallace WHB, Blacklay A, Eiser C, *et al*. Developing strategies for long-term follow up of survivors of childhood cancer. *Br Med J* 2001; **323**:271–274.
4. Waring AB, Wallace WHB. Subfertility following treatment for childhood cancer. *Hosp Med* 2000; **61**:550–557.
•5. Howell SJ, Shalet SM. Testicular function following chemotherapy. *Hum Reprod Update* 2001;**7**:363–369.
6. Howell S, Shalet S. Gonadal damage from chemotherapy and radiotherapy. *Endocrinol Metab Clin North Am* 1998; **27**:927–943.
7. Papadakis V, Vlachopapadopoulou E, van Syckle K, *et al*. Gonadal function in young patients successfully treated for Hodgkin's disease. *Med Pediatr Oncol* 1999; **32**:366–372.
◆8. Chatterjee R, Mills W, Katz M, *et al*. Germ cell failure and Leydig insufficiency in post-pubertal males after autologous bone marrow transplantation with BEAM for lymphoma. *Bone Marrow Transplant* 1994; **13**:519–522.
◆9. Whitehead E, Shalet, SM, Jones PH, *et al*. Gonadal function after combination chemotherapy for Hodgkin's disease in childhood. *Arch Dis Child* 1982; **57**:287–291.
◆10. Mackie EJ, Radford M, Shalet SM. Gonadal function following chemotherapy for childhood Hodgkin's disease. *Med Pediatr Oncol* 1996; **27**:74–78.
◆11. Howell SJ, Radford JA, Ryder WDJ, Shalet SM. Testicular function after cytotoxic chemotherapy: evidence of Leydig cell insufficiency. *J Clin Oncol* 1999; **17**:1493–1498.
12. Sklar CA, Robison LL, Nesbit ME, *et al*. Effects of radiation on testicular function in long-term survivors of childhood acute lymphoblastic leukaemia: a report from the Children Cancer Study Group. *J Clin Oncol* 1990; **8**:1981–1987.
◆13. Leiper AD, Grant DB, Chessells JM. Gonadal function after testicular radiation for acute lymphoblastic leukaemia. *Arch Dis Child* 1986; **61**:53–56.
◆14. Speiser B, Rubin P, Casarett G. Azoospermia following lower truncal irradiation in Hodgkin's disease. *Cancer* 1973; **32**:692–696.
15. Sanders JE, Hawley J, Levy W, *et al*. Pregnancies following high-dose cyclophosphamide with or without high-dose busulfan or total-body irradiation and bone marrow transplantation. *Blood* 1996; **87**:3045–3052.
16. Howell SJ, Radford JA, Adams JE, Shalet SM. The impact of mild Leydig cell dysfunction following cytotoxic chemotherapy on bone mineral density (BMD) and body composition. *Clin Endocrinol* 2000; **52**:609–616.
17. Howell SJ, Radford JA, Smets EMA, Shalet SM. Fatigue, sexual function and mood following treatment of haematological malignancy: the impact of mild Leydig cell dysfunction. *Br J Cancer* 2000; **82**:789–793.
18. Holmes SJ, Whitehouse RW, Clark ST, *et al*. Reduced bone mineral density in men following chemotherapy for Hodgkin's disease. *Br J Cancer* 1994; **70**:371–375.
19. Sanger WG, Olson JH, Sherman JK. Semen cryobanking for men with cancer – criteria change. *Fertil Steril* 1992; **58**:1024–1027.
20. Rosenlund B, Sjoblom P, Tornblom M, *et al*. In vitro fertilization and intracytoplasmic sperm injection in the treatment of infertility after testicular cancer. *Hum Reprod* 1998; **13**:414–418.
21. Aboulghar MA, Mansour RT, Serour GI, *et al*. Fertilization and pregnancy rates after intracytoplasmic sperm injection using ejaculate semen and surgically retrieved sperm. *Fertil Steril* 1997; **68**:108–111.
22. Chen SU, Ho H, Chen HF, *et al*. Pregnancy achieved by intracytoplasmic sperm injection using cryopreserved semen from a man with testicular cancer. *Hum Reprod* 1996; **11**:2645–2647.
•23. Schlatt S, von Schonfeldt V, Schepers AG. Male germ cell transplantation: an experimental approach with a clinical perspective. *Br Med Bull* 2000; **56**:824–836.

◆24. Brinster RL, Zimmermann JW. Spermatogenesis following male germ-cell transplantation. *Proc Natl Acad Sci USA* 1994; **91**:11289–11302.

25. Clouthier DE, Avarbock MR, Maika SD, *et al.* Rat spermatogenesis in mouse testis. *Nature* 1999; **381**:418–421.

◆26. Avarbock MR, Brinster CJ, Brinster RL. Reconstitution of spermatogenesis from frozen spermatogonial stem cells. *Nat Med* 1996; **2**:693–696.

27. Wallace WHB, Walker DA. Conference consensus statement: ethical and research dilemmas for fertility preservation in children treated for cancer. *Hum Fertil* 2001; **4**:69–76.

28. Sharpe, RM. Regulation of spermatogenesis. In: Knobil E, and JD Neill JD (eds) *The physiology of reproduction*, 2nd edn. New York: Raven Press 1994:1363–1419.

29. Johnson MH, Everitt BJ. Testicular function in the adult. *Essential reproduction*, 5th edn. Oxford: Blackwell Sciences 1999: 53–68.

30. Andersson AM, Muller J, Skakkebaek NE. Different roles of prepubertal and postpubertal germ cells and Sertoli cells in the regulation of serum inhibin B levels. *J Clin Endocrinol Metab* 1999; **83**:4451–4458.

31. Anderson RA, Sharpe R. Regulation of inhibin production in the human male and its clinical applications. *Int J Androl* 2000; **23**:136–144.

32. Kelnar CJH, McKinnell C, Walker M, *et al.* Testicular changes during infantile 'quiescence' in the marmoset and their gonadotrophin dependence: a model for investigating susceptibility of the prepubertal human testis to cancer therapy? *Hum Reprod* 2002; **17**:1367–1378.

33. Rey R. The prepubertal testis: a quiescent or a silently active organ? *Histol Histopathol* 1999; **14**:991–1000.

34. Muller J, Skakkebaeck NE. Quantification of germ cells and seminiferous tubules by stereological examination of testicles from 50 boys who suffered from sudden death. *Int J Androl* 1983; **6**:143–156.

35. Andersson AM, Toppari J, Haavisto AM, *et al.* Longitudinal reproductive hormone profile in infants: peak of inhibin B levels in infant boys exceeds levels in adult men. *J Clin Endocrinol Metab* 1998; **83**:675–681.

36. Sklar C. Reproductive physiology and treatment-related loss of sex hormone production. *Med Pediatr Oncol* 1999; **33**:2–8.

37. Tanner JM, Whitehouse RH. Clinical longitudinal standards for height, weight, height, height velocity and stages of puberty. *Arch Dis Child* 1976; **51**:1709.

38. Crofton PM, Evans AEM, Groome NP, *et al.* Inhibin B in boys from birth to adulthood: relationship with age, pubertal stage, follicle-stimulating-hormone and testosterone. *Clin Endocrinol* 2002; **56**:215–221.

39. Kangasniemi M, Huhtanini I, Meistrich ML. Failure of spermatogenesis to recover despite the presence of A spermatogonia in the irradiated LBNF1 rat. *Biol Reprod* 1996; **54**:1200–1208.

40. Wang J, Galil KA, Setchell BP. Changes in testicular blood flow and testosterone production during aspermoatogenesis after irradiation. *J Endocrinol* 1983; **98**:35–46.

41. Setchell BP, Galil KA. Limitations imposed by testicular blood flow on the function of Leydig cells in rats *in vivo*. *Aust J Biol Sci* 1983; **36**:285–293.

42. Spitz S. The histological effects of nitrogen mustards on human tumors and tissues. *Cancer* 1948; **i**:383–398.

43. Wallace WHB, Shalet SM, Crowne EC, *et al.* Gonadal dysfunction due to cis-platinum. *Med Pediatr Oncol* 1989; **17**:409–413.

44. Wallace WHB, Shalet SM, Lendon M, Morris Jones PH. Male fertility in long-term survivors of acute lymphoblastic leukaemia in childhood. *Int J Androl* 1991; **14**:312–319.

45. Chapman RM, Sutcliffe SB, Rees LH, *et al.* Cyclical combination chemotherapy and gonadal function. *Lancet* 1979; **1**:285–289.

46. Watson AR, Rance CP, Bain J. Long-term effects of cyclophosphamide on testicular function. *Br Med J* 1985; **291**:1457–1460.

47. Shafford EA, Kingston JE, Malpas JS, *et al.* Testicular function following the treatment of Hodgkin's disease in childhood. *Br J Cancer* 1993; **68**:1199–1204.

48. Heikens J, Behrendt H, Adriaanse R, Berghout A. Irreversible gonadal damage in male survivors of pediatric Hodgkin's disease. *Cancer* 1996, **78**:2020–2024.

49. Viviani S, Santoro A, Ragni G, *et al.* Gonadal toxicity after combination chemotherapy for Hodgkin's disease: comparative results of MOPP vs ABVD. *Eur J Cancer Clin Oncol* 1985; **21**:601–605.

50. da Cunha MF, Meistrich ML, Fuller LM, *et al.* Recovery of spermatogenesis after treatment for Hodgkin's disease: limiting dose of MOPP chemotherapy. *J Clin Oncol* 1984; **2**:571–575.

51. Hill M, Milan S, Cunningham D, *et al.* Evaluation of the VEEP regimen in adult Hodgkin's disease with assessment of gonadal and cardiac toxicity. *J Clin Oncol* 1995; **13**:387–395.

◆52. Thomson AB, Campbell AJ, Irvine DS, *et al.* Semen quality and spermatozoal DNA integrity in survivors of childhood cancer. *Lancet* 2002; **360**:361–367.

53. Rivkees SA, Crawford JD. The relationship of gonadal activity and chemotherapy-induced gonadal damage. *JAMA* 1988; **259**:2123–2125.

54. Bramswig JH, Heimes U, Heiernann E, *et al.* The effects of different cumulative doses of chemotherapy on testicular function. *Cancer* 1990; **65**:1298–1302.

55. Anselmo AP, Cartoni C, Bellantuono T, *et al.* Risk of infertility in Hodgkin's disease treated with ABVD vs MOPP vs ABVD/MOPP. *Haematologica* 1990; **75**:155–158.

56. Pryzant RM, Meistrich ML, Wilson G, *et al.* Long-term reduction in sperm count after chemotherapy with and without radiation therapy for non-Hodgkin's lymphomas. *J Clin Oncol* 1993; **11**:239–247.

57. Muller U, Stahel RA. Gonadal function after MACOP-B or VACOP-B with or without dose intensification and ABMT in young patients with aggressive non-Hodgkin's lymphoma. *Ann Oncol* 1993; **4**:399–402.

58. Radford JA, Clark S, Crowther D, Shalet SM. Male fertility after VAPEC-B chemotherapy for Hodgkin's disease and non-Hodgkin's lymphoma. *Br J Cancer* 1994; **69**:379–381.

59. Grigg AP, McLachlan R, Zaja J, Szer J. Reproductive status in long-term bone marrow transplant survivors receiving busulfan-cyclophosphamide (120 mg/kg). *Bone Marrow Transplant* 2000; **26**:1089–1095.

60. Meistrich ML, Wilson G, Brown BW, *et al.* Impact of cyclophosphamide on long-term reduction in sperm count in men treated with combination chemotherapy for Ewing and soft tissue sarcomas. *Cancer* 1992; **70**:2703–2712.

61. Lendon M, Hann IM, Palmer MK, *et al.* Testicular histology after combination chemotherapy for acute lymphoblastic leukaemia. *Lancet* 1978; **ii**:439–441.

62. Quigley C, Cowell C, Jiminez M, *et al.* Normal or early development of puberty despite gonadal damage in children treated for acute lymphoblastic leukaemia. *N Engl J Med* 1989; **321**:143–151.

63. Blatt J, Poplack DG, Sherins RJ. Testicular function in boys after chemotherapy for acute lymphoblastic leukaemia. *N Engl J Med* 1981; **304**:1121–2114.

64. Lahteenmaki PM, Toppari J, Roukonen A, *et al.* Low serum inhibin B concentrations in male survivors of childhood malignancy. *Eur J Cancer* 1999; **35**:612–619.

65. Sklar C, Boulad F, Small T, Kernan N. Endocrine complications of pediatric stem cell transplantation. *Front Biosci* 2001; **6**:17–22.

66. Sanders JE, the Seattle Marrow Transplant Team. The impact of marrow transplant preparative regimens on subsequent growth and development. *Semin Haematol* 1991; **28**:244–249.

◆67. Clifton DK, Bremner WJ. The effect of testicular X-irradiation on spermatogenesis in man. A comparison with the mouse. *J Androl* 1983; **6**:387–392.

◆68. Rowley MJ, Leach DR, Warner GA, Heller CG. Effects of graded ionising radiation on the human testis. *Radiat Res* 1974; **59**:665–678.

69. Castillo LA, Craft AW, Kernahan J, *et al*. Gonadal function after 12-Gy testicular irradiation in childhood acute lymphoblastic leukaemia. *Med Pediatr Oncol* 1990; **18**:185–190.

70. Sklar CA, Robison LL, Nesbit ME, *et al*. Effects of radiation on testicular function in long-term survivors of childhood acute lymphoblastic lymphoma leukaemia: a report from the Children Cancer Study Group. *J Clin Oncol* 1990; **8**:1981–1987.

71. Bakker B, Massa GG, Oostdijk W, *et al*. Pubertal development and growth after total-body irradiation and bone marrow transplantation for haematological malignancies. *Eur J Pediatr* 2000; **159**:31–37.

72. Sarafoglou K, Boulad F, Gillio A, Sklar C. Gonadal function after bone marrow transplantation for acute leukaemia during childhood. *J Pediatr* 1997; **130**:210–216.

73. Relander T, Cavallin-Stahl E, *et al*. Gonadal and sexual function in men treated for childhood cancer. *Med Pediatr Oncol* 2000; **35**:52–63.

74. Shalet SM, Tsatsoulis A, Whitehead E, Read G. Vulnerability of the human Leydig cell to radiation damage is dependent upon age. *J Endocrinol* 1989; **120**:161–165.

75. Chatterjee R, Kottaridis PD, McGarrigle HH, *et al*. Patterns of Leydig cell insufficiency in adult males following bone marrow transplantation for haematological malignancies. *Bone Marrow Transplant* 2001; **28**:497–502.

76. Couto-Silva AC, Trivin C, Thibaud E, *et al*. Factors affecting gonadal function after bone marrow transplantation during childhood. *Bone Marrow Transplant* 2001; **28**:67–75.

77. Howell SJ, Radford JA, Adams JE, *et al*. Randomized placebo-controlled trial of testosterone replacement in men with mild Leydig cell insufficiency following cytotoxic chemotherapy. *Clin Endocrinol* 2001; **55**:315–324.

◆78. Gosden RG, Baird DT, Wade JC, Webb R. Restoration of fertility to oopherectomized sheep by ovarian autografts stored at −196°C. *Hum Reprod* 1994; **9**:597–603.

79. Oktay K, Karlikaya G. Ovarian function after transplantation of frozen, banked, autologous ovarian tissue. *N Engl J Med* 2000; **342**:1919.

80. Tesarik J, Mendoza C, Testart J. Viable embryos from injection of round spermatids into oocytes. *N Engl J Med* 1995; **333**:525.

81. Tesarik J, Mendoza C. Spermatid injection into human oocytes. I. Laboratory techniques and special features of zygote development. *Hum Reprod* 1996; **11**:772–779.

82. Fishel S, Green S, Hunter A, *et al*. Human fertilisation with round and elongated spermatids. *Hum Reprod* 1997; **12**:336–340.

83. Sofikitis N, Mantzavinios T, Loutradis D, *et al*. Cytoplasmic injections of secondary spermatocytes for non-obstructive azoospermia. *Lancet* 1998; **351**:1177–1178.

84. Vanderzwalmen P, Zech H, Birkenfield A, *et al*. Intracytoplasmic injection of spermatids retrieved from testicular tissue, influence of testicular pathology, type of selective spermatids and oocyte activation. *Hum Reprod* 1997; **12**:1203–1213.

85. Bernadeu R, Cremades N, Takahashi K, Sousa M. Successful pregnancy after spermatid injection. *Hum Reprod* 1998; **13**:1898–1900.

86. Grundy R, Larcher V, Gosden RG, *et al*. Personal practice: fertility preservation for children treated for cancer (2): ethics of consent for gamete storage and experimentation. *Arch Dis Child* 2001; **84**:360–362.

87. Neilson CT, Skakkebaek NS, Richardson DW. Onset of the release of spermatozoa (spermarche) in boys in relation to age, testicular growth, pubic hair and height. *J Clin Endocrinol Metab* 1986; **62**:532–535.

88. Ward JA, Robinson J, Barrington JA, *et al*. Protection of spermatogenesis in rats from the cytotoxic procarbazine by the depot formulation of Zoladex, a gonadotrophin-releasing hormone agonist. *Cancer Res* 1990; **50**:569–574.

89. Delic JI, Bush C, Peckham MJ. Protection from procarbazine-induced damage of spermatogenesis in the rat by androgen. *Cancer Res* 1986; **46**:1909–1914.

90. Pogach LM, Lee Y, Gould S, *et al*. Partial prevention of procarbazine induced germinal cell aplasia in rats by sequential GnRH antagonist and testosterone administration. *Cancer Res* 1988; **48**:4354–4360.

91. Kangasniemi M, Wilson G, Huhtaniemi I, Meistrich ML. Protection against procarbazine-induced testicular damage by GnRH-agonist and antiandrogen treatment in the rat. *Endocrinology* 1995; **136**:3677–3680.

92. Meistrich ML, Parchuri N, Wilson G, *et al*. Hormonal protection from cyclophosphamide-induced inactivation of rat stem spermatogonia. *J Clin Androl* 1995; **16**:334–341.

◆93. Meistrich ML, Kangasniemi M. Hormone treatment after irradiation stimulates recovery of rat spermatogenesis from surviving spermatogonia. *J Androl* 1997; **18**:80–87.

◆94. Meistrich ML, Wilson G, Huhtaniemi I. Hormonal treatment after cytotoxic therapy stimulates recovery of spermatogenesis. *Cancer Res* 1999; **59**:3557–3560.

◆95. Masala A, Faedda R, Alagna S, *et al*. Use of testosterone to prevent cyclophosphamide-induced azoospermia. *Ann Intern Med* 1997; **126**:292–295.

96. Johnson DH, Linde R, Hainsworth JD, *et al*. Effect of luteinizing hormone releasing hormone agonist given during combination chemotherapy on post-therapy fertility in male patients with lymphoma: preliminary observations. *Blood* 1985; **65**:832–836.

97. Waxman JH, Ahmed R, Smith D, *et al*. Failure to preserve fertility in patients with Hodgkin's disease. *Cancer Chemother Pharmacol* 1987; **19**:159–162.

◆98. Thomson AB, Anderson RA, Irvine DS, *et al*. Investigation of suppression of the hypothalamic–pituitary–gonadal axis to restore spermatogenesis in azoospermic men treated for childhood cancer. *Hum Reprod* 2002; **17**:1715–1723.

99. Brinster RL, Avarbock MR. Germline transmission of donor haplotype following spermatogonial transplantation. *Proc Natl Acad Sci USA* 1994; **91**:11303–11307.

100. Russell LD, Brinster RL. Ultrastructural observations of spermatogenesis following transplantation of rat testis cells into mouse seminiferous tubules. *J Androl* 1996; **17**:615–627.

101. Ogawa T, Dobrinski I, Avarbock MR, Brinster RL. Xenogeneic spermatogenesis following transplantation of hamster germ cells to mouse testes. *Biol Reprod* 1999; **60**:515–521.

102. Hovatta O, Foudila T, Siegberg R, *et al*. Pregnancy resulting from intracytoplasmic injection of spermatozoa from a frozen–thawed testicular biopsy specimen. *Hum Reprod* 1996; **11**:2472–2473.

103. Oates RD, Mulhall J, Burgess C, *et al*. Fertilization and pregnancy using intentionally cryopreserved testicular tissue as the sperm source for intracytoplasmic injection in 10 men with non-obstructive azoospermia. *Hum Reprod* 1997; **12**:734–739.

104. Shinohar T, Avabrock MA, Brinster RL. β_1- and α_6-integrins are surface markers on mouse spermatogonial stem cells. *Proc Natl Acad Sci USA* 1999; **96**:5504–5509.

105. Nagano M, Avarbock MR, Leonida EB, *et al.* Culture of mouse spermatogonial stem cells. *Tissue Cell* 1998; **30**:389–397.

•106. Aslam I, Fishel S, Moore H, *et al.* Fertility preservation of boys undergoing anti-cancer therapy: a review of the existing situation and prospects for the future. *Hum Reprod* 2000; **15**:2154–2159.

107. Tesarik J, Bacheci M, Ozcan C, *et al.* Restoration of fertility by in-vitro spermatogenesis. *Lancet* 1999; **353**:555–556.

108. Tesarik J, Mendoza C, Greco E. In vitro culture facilitates the selection of healthy spermatids for assisted reproduction. *Fertil Steril* 1999; **72**:809–813.

109. Schlatt S, Rosiepen G, Weinbauer GF, *et al.* Germ cell transfer into rat, bovine, monkey and human testes. *Hum Reprod* 1999; **14**:1440–1450.

110. Schlatt S, Foppiani L, Rolf C, *et al.* Germ cell transplantation into X-irradiated monkey testes. *Hum Reprod* 2002; **17**:55–62.

111. Brook PF, Radford JA, Shalet SM, *et al.* Isolation of germ cells from human testicular tissue for low temperature storage and autotransplantation. *Fertil Steril* 2001; **75**:269–274.

112. Royal College of Obstetricians and Gynaecologists. Storage of ovarian and prepubertal testicular tissue: report of a working party. London: Royal College of Obstetricians and Gynaecologists, 2000.

113. Hawkins MM, Draper GJ, Smith RA. Cancer among 1348 survivors of childhood cancer. *Int J Cancer* 1989; **43**:975–978.

•114. Li FP, Fine W, Jaffe N, *et al.* Offspring of patients treated for cancer in childhood. *J Natl Cancer Inst* 1979; **62**:1193–1197.

115. Grundy R, Gosden RG, Hewitt M, *et al.* Fertility preservation for children treated for cancer (1): scientific advances and research dilemmas. *Arch Dis Child* 2001; **84**:355–359.

116. Sun J-G, Jurisicova A, Casper RF. Detection of deoxyribonucleic acid fragmentation in human sperm: correlation with fertilization in vitro. *Biol Reprod* 1997; **66**:602–607.

117. Trasler JM, Hales BF, Robaire B. Paternal cyclophosphamide treatment of rats causes fetal loss and malformations without affecting male fertility. *Nature* 1985; **316**:144–146.

118. Trasler JM, Hales BF, Robaire B. Chronic low dose cyclophosphamide treatment of adult male rats: effects on fertility, progeny outcome and the male reproductive and hematologic systems. *Biol Reprod* 1987; **37**:317–326.

119. Kelly SM, Robaire B, Hales BF. Paternal cyclophosphamide exposure causes decreased cell proliferation in cleavage-stage embryos. *Biol Reprod* 1994; **50**:55–64.

120. Spano M, Bonde JP, Hjollund HI, *et al.* Sperm chromatin damage impairs human fertility. *Fertil Steril* 2000; **73**:43–50.

121. Twigg J, Irvine DS, Aitken R. Oxidative damage to DNA in human spermatozoa does not preclude pronucleus formation at ICSI. *Hum Reprod* 1998; **13**:1864–1881.

122. Bonduelle M, Camus M, De Vos A, *et al.* Seven years of intracytoplasmic sperm injection and follow-up of 1987 subsequent children. *Hum Reprod* 1999; **14**:243–264.

123. Sutcliffe AG, Taylor B, Saunders K, *et al.* Outcome in the second year of life after *in vitro* fertilisation by intracytoplasmic sperm injection: a UK case-control study. *Lancet* 2001; **357**:2080–2084.

124. Sousa M, Mendoza C, Barros A, Tesarik J. Calcium response of human oocytes after intracytoplasmic injection of leukocytes, spermatocytes and round spermatids. *Mol Hum Reprod* 1996; **2**:853–857.

125. Tesarik J, Kopeony V. Nucleic acid synthesis and development of human male pronucleus. *J Reprod Fertil* 1989; **86**:549–558.

126. Hall JG. Genomic imprinting: review and relevance to human diseases. *Am J Hum Genet* 1990; **46**:857–873.

127. Nugent D, Hamilton M, Murdoch A and the BFS Committee. BFS Recommendations for good practice on the storage of ovarian and prepubertal testicular tissue. *Hum Reprod* 2000; **3**:5–8.

128. Anonymous. Gillick v W. Norfolk and Wisbech ANA. *All Engl Law Rep* 1985; 402.

129. HFEA Act 1990, Ch. 37. London: The Stationery Office, 1990.

130. Deech R. Human Fertilisation and Embryology Authority. *Br Med J* 1998; **316**:1095.

8e

Pregnancy outcome

DANIEL M GREEN

INTRODUCTION

The potential of cancer chemotherapeutic agents[1] and high-energy radiation to cause mutations has caused concern among patients and physicians about the possible adverse effects of treatment on pregnancies that occur either during or following treatment for childhood cancer. These effects have been studied in experimental animals. Evidence of an increased risk for adverse pregnancy outcome, as manifested by an increased rate of spontaneous abortion, stillbirth, premature birth, birth defects or cancer in the offspring has been sought in survivor populations.

MUTAGENESIS

Experimental data – radiation

The effect of preconception exposure to irradiation on fertility and progeny of experimental animals was studied in mice. The immature arrested murine oocyte, although highly sensitive to killing by radiation is quite resistant to mutation induction following irradiation.[2] Similarly, the murine spermatogonial stem cell is resistant to mutation induction following single-dose radiation exposures of 108–504 cGy, as measured by preimplantation or postimplantation loss, or the induction of malformations. However, the frequency of induction of malformations is increased in animals exposed to fractionated irradiation.[3]

Experimental data – chemotherapy

Chemotherapeutic agents can be classified as mutagenic or non-mutagenic based upon the results of testing using the Ames Salmonella/microsome assay system. Those agents that are mutagenic in the Ames Salmonella/microsome assay system include doxorubicin (Adriamycin), daunorubicin, cyclophosphamide, ifosfamide, 1-(2-chloroethyl)-3-cyclohexyl-1-nitrosourea (CCNU), 1,3-bis (2-chloroethyl)-1-nitrosourea (BCNU), 5-(3,3-dimethyl-1-triazeno)imidazole-4-carboxamide (DTIC), cis-diamminedichloroplatinum (II) (DDP), chlorambucil, nitrogen mustard, etoposide, and 6-mercaptopurine.[4–11] Procarbazine was classified as a mutagen based upon the results of a modified Salmonella/microsome assay system.[12] Vincristine, vinblastine, methotrexate, 6-thioguanine, l-asparaginase, actinomycin D and cytosine arabinoside are not mutagenic in the Ames Salmonella/microsome assay system.[4,5,6,13] Cyclophosphamide was shown to increase the frequencies of fetal loss and congenital malformations in experimental animals without causing a decrease in fertility.[14]

Human data – radiation exposure

The effects of gamma and neutron radiation on mutation frequency in the offspring of Japanese exposed to the atomic bombs in Hiroshima and Nagasaki have been evaluated in detail using protein electrophoretic mobility and protein activity as measures of mutational effects.[15] No evidence of an effect of radiation on the frequency of mutation in the offspring of proximally exposed subjects

was identified.[16,17] However, using assays of the frequency of mutation of the glycophorin A locus[18,19] or the hypoxanthine-guanine phosphoribosyl transferase (HGPRT) locus,[20] several investigators confirmed that evidence of mutation could be identified many years after exposure to gamma or neutron irradiation. Mutations have been identified in adult cancer patients following treatment with radiation therapy and/or chemotherapy using the HGPRT assay.[21]

The effect of preconception diagnostic gonadal irradiation on the frequency of childhood cancer in the offspring was evaluated in two studies. One study demonstrated a statistically significant increase in the frequency of childhood cancer among the offspring of women who received diagnostic preconception gonadal irradiation,[22] whereas another study found no increase in the risk of childhood cancer among the offspring of men or women who had received diagnostic preconception gonadal irradiation.[23]

Human data – chemotherapy exposure

Several authors reviewed the outcome of pregnancies that occurred while one or more chemotherapeutic agents were being given to the mother.[24–26] Fetal malformations occurred in 19.2 per cent (10 out of 52) of pregnancies in which aminopterin was administered during the first trimester as an abortifacient,[24] 50 per cent (3 out of 6) of fetuses following administration of cyclophosphamide during the first trimester, 50 per cent (1 out of 2) of fetuses following administration of chlorambucil during the first trimester and 9.1 per cent (2 out of 22) of fetuses following administration of bulsulfan during the first trimester.[26] Others reported both normal[27,28] and abnormal[29,30] infants born following treatment with combination chemotherapy during pregnancy for Hodgkin's disease. Multiple congenital anomalies were reported in an infant born following an unsuccessful attempted abortion using methotrexate.[31] An infant born of a woman who received maintenance therapy with methotrexate, 6-mercaptopurine, vincristine and prednisone, followed by reinduction with vincristine, prednisone and doxorubicin during the pregnancy was normal.[32]

PREGNANCY OUTCOME

Most early case series were derived from patient cohorts or convenience samples followed at a single institution. Li et al. reported the outcome of 293 pregnancies in patients or their spouses following treatment for cancer in childhood. There were 242 live births, including one set of twins, 25 spontaneous abortions, 19 induced

abortions, one stillbirth and seven pregnancies in gestation. The male to female (M:F) ratio was 1.09:1.00 for the offspring of the partners of the male survivors and 0.89:1.00 for the offspring of the female survivors. Four offspring (2 per cent) had major anomalies. There was no difference in the survival or the incidence of major or minor anomalies of these offspring compared to their first cousins. Karyotypes were normal in 91.6 per cent (22 out of 24) of the offspring examined.[33,34]

Blatt et al. reported the outcome of pregnancies of 23 women and the wives of seven men following intensive chemotherapy for a variety of malignant diseases. The series included 42 pregnancies, ten of which were terminated electively because of fear of a treatment-related fetal anomaly, two aborted spontaneously, two were in gestation and 28 had been completed with the birth of term singleton infants. No major anomalies were identified in these infants.[35]

Green et al. reported the outcome of 280 pregnancies including 1 stillbirth, 8 premature births and 144 full-term live births reported by 100 pediatric cancer survivors. The spouses of 25 male patients reported 39 births (M:F 0.65:1.00), including one stillbirth. Thirty-five women reported 63 births, including one stillbirth and six premature births (M:F 1.04:1.00). The frequency of congenital anomalies was 3.3 per cent among the liveborn offspring of the female patients and 3.3 per cent among the liveborn offspring of the spouses of the male patients.[36,37] The association of specific chemotherapeutic agents with the occurrence of a congenital anomaly was examined using stepwise logistic regression analysis. The cumulative dosages of doxorubicin, cyclophosphamide, vincristine, procarbazine, chlorambucil, actinomycin D and vinblastine were entered as covariates, with the occurrence of an anomaly as the outcome. There was no relationship between the cumulative dosage of any of these drugs and the occurrence of an anomaly in the offspring. There was no relationship between the number of mutagens (zero, one, two, three, four or more) received by the patient and the occurrence of an anomaly in the offspring.[36]

Studies of pregnancy outcome focused on disease-specific evaluation in those treated for Wilms' tumor, Hodgkin's disease and acute lymphoblastic leukemia. Holmes and Holmes reported that women who received combined modality treatment for Hodgkin's disease were significantly more likely to produce abnormal offspring than female controls.[38] The abnormalities reported included autism and scleroderma, conditions that are not congenital anomalies (Table 8e.1). Simon suggested that studies such as that by Holmes and Holmes should be analyzed in a manner that restricts the comparison of pregnancy outcome to patients with a specific treatment history (such as radiation therapy only) and the patients' siblings, rather than enlarging the

Table 8e.1 *Pregnancy outcome after treatment for Hodgkin's disease: female patients (adult series)*

Study/therapy	Number of pregnancies	Spontaneous abortions	Live births	Congenital abnormalities
Le Floch[68]				
XRT only	6	0	4	0
XRT + Chemo	4	1 (25%)	4	0
Holmes[38,69]				
XRT only	37	3(8%)	34	1 (3%)
XRT + Chemo	14	0	13	2 (15%)
Chemo only	2	0	1	0
McKeen[40]	9	0	8	0
Horning[70]				
XRT only	11	0	9	0
XRT + Chemo	7	0	8[a]	0
Chemo only	10	0	7	0
Andrieu[71]	30	4 (13%)	22[a]	1 (5%)
Whitehead[72]	17	4 (24%)	9	0

Chemo, chemotherapy; XRT, radiation therapy.
[a]One set of twins.

Table 8e.2 *Pregnancy outcome after treatment for Hodgkin's disease: female patients (pediatric series)*

Study/therapy	Number of pregnancies	Spontaneous abortions	Live births	Congenital abnormalities
Donaldson[73]				
XRT only	4	0	2	0
XRT + Chemo	4	0	3	0
Green[74]				
XRT only	22	0	16	1 (5%)
XRT + Chemo	11	2 (18%)	8	1 (9%)

Chemo, chemotherapy; XRT, radiation therapy.

comparison group to include patients with all possible treatment histories.[39]

McKeen *et al.* reported anomalies in 50 per cent (4 out of 8) of live born infants following treatment for Hodgkin's disease at or shortly after conception, compared to 14.7 per cent (5 out of 34) of live born infants conceived following the completion of treatment,[40] suggesting that pregnancies that occur in close temporal relation to treatment are at greater risk of an abnormal outcome. Only two studies reported pregnancy outcome following treatment during childhood or adolescence for Hodgkin's disease (Table 8e.2). The birthweights of infants born to former Hodgkin's disease patients or their spouses were within the normal range. The studies suggest that pregnancies that occur after the completion of therapy of children or adults for Hodgkin's disease do not have an increased risk of an abnormal outcome.

Green *et al.* reported the outcome of 81 pregnancies in 27 women and the spouses of nine men following treatment in childhood for Wilms' tumor. The frequency of spontaneous abortion in this population was not

different from that of the population at large. The birthweights of those infants born of women who had received abdominal irradiation were significantly lower than those of infants born of women treated only with surgery or those of infants born of the spouses of irradiated male patients.[41] The finding of an increased frequency of adverse pregnancy outcomes among irradiated women was confirmed by Li and his colleagues[42] and others.[43,44] Byrne and her colleagues identified bicornuate uterus in two of 26 female Wilms' tumor survivors, and suggested this as a possible cause for reproductive loss in some female Wilms' tumor survivors.[43] Subsequently, Nicholson and his colleagues reported uterine anomalies in 2 of 24 female Wilms' tumor survivors screened with magnetic resonance imaging of the pelvis and pelvic ultrasonography.[45] The frequency of uterine anomalies is significantly higher among female Wilms' tumor survivors than among unselected females.[46,47]

Several normal children have been born of patients successfully treated during childhood for acute lymphoblastic leukemia.[48–50] Ross reported no excess of

spontaneous abortions, stillbirths, or major malformations following the treatment of women with one of several sequential single agent chemotherapy programs for gestational trophoblastic neoplasms.[51]

All prior studies of offspring of survivors of childhood cancer had too few offspring of parents treated with mutagenic chemotherapeutic agents to have sufficient statistical power to exclude an effect of this treatment on pregnancy outcome. The Childhood Cancer Survivor Study (CCSS) is a multi-institutional collaborative study that assembled a cohort of 20 276 five-year survivors of specific childhood cancers treated initially at 25 participating institutions. Pregnancy outcome following the completion of treatment has been evaluated in the members of this cohort.[52]

One thousand nine hundred and fifteen CCSS female participants reported 4029 pregnancies (63 per cent live births, 1 per cent stillbirths, 15 per cent miscarriages, 17 per cent abortions, 3 per cent unknown or in gestation). The gender ratio (M:F) was 1.09:1.0 for the offspring of the female survivors, compared to 1.09:1.0 for the offspring of the female siblings of all the male and female survivors.[53]

Women 15–20, 21–25 and 26–30 years of age were significantly less likely than the female siblings with the same age at pregnancy to have a live birth. Those 21–25 years of age were significantly more likely to have a medical abortion.

There were significantly more miscarriages reported by the survivors of central nervous system tumors, compared to the female siblings [relative risk (RR) 1.65; 95% confidence interval (95% CI) 1.16–2.34; $p = 0.006$). The excess of miscarriages remained significant (RR 1.67; 95% CI 1.17–2.37; $p = 0.004$) when age at start of pregnancy 0–20 years was included in a multivariate model. There were significantly more medical abortions reported by survivors in all diagnostic groups except non-Hodgkin's lymphoma. The excess remained when the variable age at start of pregnancy 0–20 years was included in a multivariate model for patients with leukemia (RR 1.37; 95% CI 1.05–1.78; $p = 0.02$), central nervous system tumors (RR 1.98; 95% CI 1.33–2.95; $p < 0.001$), Hodgkin's disease (RR 1.46; 95% CI 1.12–1.91; $p = 0.005$), Wilms' tumor (RR 1.65; 95% CI 1.04–2.61; $p = 0.03$), soft tissue sarcoma (RR 1.42; 95% CI 1.00–2.01; $p = 0.05$), and bone cancer (RR 1.74; 95% CI 1.28–2.37; $p < 0.001$).

All treatment groups had a lower RR of live birth than did the female siblings. However, there was no significant difference in the RR of a live birth among the various treatment groups.

The RR of miscarriage was 1.33 (95% CI 0.98–1.80; $p = 0.07$) among those treated with cranial irradiation but not spinal irradiation, compared to irradiated survivors who received neither cranial nor spinal irradiation, and

was 1.40 (95% CI 1.02–1.94; $p = 0.04$) among those treated with cranial irradiation but not spinal irradiation compared to those who received no radiation therapy. The RR of miscarriage was 1.60 (95% CI 0.85–3.00; $p = 0.14$) for survivors of acute lymphoblastic leukemia who received cranial irradiation, but not spinal irradiation, compared to those who had received no radiation therapy. The RR of miscarriage was 3.63 (95% CI 1.70–7.78; $p < 0.001$) among those who received cranial and spinal irradiation, compared to those who received no radiation therapy, suggesting that spinal irradiation may adversely impact pregnancy outcome. The RR of miscarriage at less than 12 weeks of gestation was not increased in any of the radiation therapy subgroups evaluated, whereas the RR of miscarriage at 12 or more weeks of gestation was increased in those who had received cranial and spinal radiation therapy (RR 6.10; 95% CI 3.06–12.2; $p < 0.0001$) and those who had received radiation therapy, but neither cranial nor spinal radiation therapy (RR 1.90; 95% CI 1.23–2.95; $p = 0.004$).

Compared to patients who did not receive radiation therapy, the risk of miscarriage was increased among women whose ovaries were included in the radiation therapy field (RR 1.86; 95% CI 0.82–4.18; $p = 0.14$), were near the radiation therapy field (RR 1.64; 95% CI 0.97–2.78; $p = 0.06$), but was not elevated if the ovaries were shielded (RR 0.90; 95% CI 0.23–3.45; $p = 0.86$), compared to patients who did not receive radiation therapy. However, a comparison of the combined group whose ovaries had been in or near the field, or shielded, with those who did not receive radiation therapy showed a significant effect (RR 1.65; 95% CI 1.05–2.59; $p = 0.03$). The relative risk of miscarriage was increased among those whose ovaries were near the radiation therapy field, when compared to the female siblings.

The rate of live birth was not lower and the rate of stillbirth was not higher for the patients treated with any particular chemotherapeutic agent, in comparison to those who had not been treated with the agent. The cumulative doses of several chemotherapeutic agents were divided into tertiles. There was no significant difference in the rate of live birth, miscarriage or medical abortion by tertile.

The offspring of survivors were more likely to weigh less than 2500 g at birth than were the offspring of the female siblings (RR 2.05; 95% CI 1.42–2.95; $p < 0.001$). The effects of offspring gender, maternal smoking or alcohol consumption history were not significant. The offspring of the survivors who received pelvic irradiation were more likely to weigh less than 2500 g at birth than offspring of those who did not receive radiation to the pelvis (RR 1.85; 95% CI 1.07–3.18; $p = 0.03$) (Figure 8e.1). There were no differences in the distributions of birthweights of offspring of survivors who had or had not been treated with an alkylating agent, but the

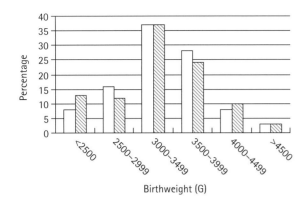

Figure 8e.1 *Offspring of female survivors of childhood cancer: distribution of birthweight by treatment with (hatched columns) or without (open columns) pelvic radiation therapy.*

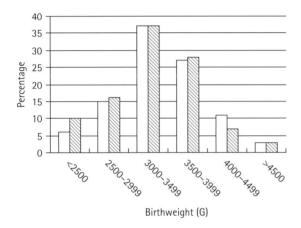

Figure 8e.2 *Offspring of female survivors of childhood cancer: distribution of birthweight by treatment with (hatched columns) or without (open columns) non-alkylating agent chemotherapy.*

offspring of survivors who were treated with a non-alkylating chemotherapeutic agent were more likely to weigh less than 2500 g than were those whose mothers were not so treated (RR 1.80; 95% CI 1.15–2.83; $p = 0.01$) (Figure 8e.2).

When entered into a multivariate model that included live birth number, maternal age category (11–20, 21–20, 31–40), maternal smoking, maternal drinking and maternal education, pelvic radiation therapy increased the RR of birthweight less than 2500 g (RR 2.15; 95% CI 1.24–3.72; $p = 0.007$). Similarly, the RR of birthweight less than 2500 g was increased if the mother received non-alkylating agent chemotherapy (RR 2.31; 95% CI 1.43–3.74; $p = 0.0007$). The relationship of specific non-alkylating agent chemotherapeutic agents was evaluated using this model. The RR was not increased when the agent was actinomycin D (RR 1.19; 95% CI 0.75–1.89; $p = 0.47$), but was increased if the agent was daunorubicin or

doxorubicin (RR 1.92; 95% CI 1.33; 2.78; $p = 0.0005$) or if the agent was any agent other than an alkylating agent, actinomycin D, doxorubicin or daunorubicin (RR 1.73; 95% CI 1.12–2.70; $p = 0.014$). In the model that included pelvic irradiation, alkylating agent, actinomycin D, daunorubicin or doxorubicin, live birth number, maternal age, maternal smoking, maternal drinking and maternal education, the RR of birthweight less than 2500 g was 2.67 (95% CI 1.51–4.75; $p = 0.0008$). Maternal educational level was the only additional significant variable in this model. However, in the model that included daunorubicin or doxorubicin, live birth number, maternal age, maternal smoking, maternal drinking, and maternal educational level, pelvic irradiation (RR 2.55; 95% CI1.45–4.47; $p = 0.001$), daunorubicin or doxorubicin (RR 2.14; 95% CI 1.43–3.21; $p = 0.0002$) and maternal educational level (did not complete high school) (RR 1.97: 95% CI 1.04–3.72; $p = 0.04$) were all significant variables. There was no evidence of a dose–response relationship when doxorubicin or daunorubicin cumulative dose tertile was substituted for the dichotomous drug exposure variable.[53]

A total of 1227 CCSS male participants reported they sired 2323 pregnancies. The sex ratio was 1.0:1.03 for the offspring of the partners of the male patients, compared to 1.24:1.0 among the offspring of the partners of the male siblings ($p = 0.016$). The sex ratio of the offspring, by treatment received was: surgery only, 1.19:1.0 (64:54) (number of male offspring:number of female offspring); radiation therapy only, 1.75:1.0 (7:4); chemotherapy only, 1.0:1.13 (16:18); surgery and radiation therapy, 1.0:1.08 (109:118); surgery and chemotherapy, 1.14:1.0 (124:109); radiation therapy and chemotherapy, 1.07:1.04 (29:27), surgery, radiation therapy and chemotherapy, 1.0:1.22 (199:242); and unknown, 1.05:1.0 (100:95).[54] The RR of a male offspring following treatment with the following chemotherapeutic agents was: BCNU, 0.77 ($p = 0.33$); CCNU, 0.64 ($p = 0.32$); chlorambucil, 2.18 ($p = 0.29$); cyclophosphamide, 1.25; ($p = 0.08$); nitrogen mustard, 0.81 ($p = 0.44$); and procarbazine, 1.02 ($p = 0.93$).

The proportion of pregnancies that resulted in a live birth was significantly lower for the partners of the male survivors than for the partners of the survivors' siblings (RR 0.79; 95% CI 0.65–0.96, $p = 0.016$). There were significantly more medical abortions reported by the partners of the Wilms' tumor patients (RR 2.43; 95% CI 1.35–4.38, $p = 0.003$). Bone cancer patients reported significantly lower rates of live births (RR 0.59; 95% CI 0.44–0.78, $p = 0.0003$), and significantly higher rates of miscarriage (RR 1.58; 95% CI 1.10–2.26; $p = 0.012$) and medical abortion (RR 1.56; 95% CI 1.04–2.33; $p = 0.031$), when compared to the partners of sibling controls. There were no significant differences in the frequency of live birth when the pregnancies of the partners

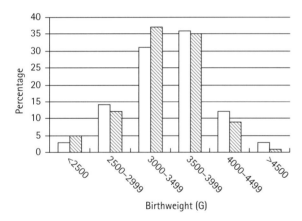

Figure 8e.3 *Offspring of partners of male survivors of childhood cancer: distribution of birthweight by treatment with (hatched columns) or without (open columns) alkylating agent chemotherapy.*

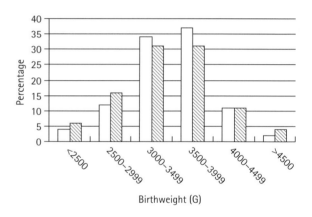

Figure 8e.4 *Offspring of partners of male survivors of childhood cancer: distribution of birthweight by treatment with (hatched columns) or without (open columns) pelvic radiation therapy.*

of the male survivors were compared within the survivor cohort by the survivor's treatment.

The partners of male survivors whose testes were in the radiation therapy field, near the radiation therapy field or were shielded had very few live births. The rate of stillbirth or miscarriage was not increased among the partners of male survivors whose testes were not irradiated or who received no radiation therapy. The frequency of miscarriage among the partners of the male survivors was not increased if the survivor had received cranial irradiation, craniospinal irradiation, spinal irradiation only, no cranial or spinal irradiation or no irradiation.

The rate of live births was significantly lower among the partners of male survivors treated with actinomycin D (RR 0.68; 95% CI 0.49–0.94; $p = 0.02$). The rates of live birth and of stillbirth were not different for offspring of the partners of male survivors treated with any other particular chemotherapeutic agent. The rate of miscarriage was higher for the partners of male survivors treated with >5000 mg/m^2 of procarbazine than for those treated with 0–5000 mg/m^2 of procarbazine (RR 2.44; 95% CI 1.28–4.67; $p = 0.007$). Neither the rate of live birth nor the rate of miscarriage was increased among the offspring of the partners of male survivors treated with cyclophosphamide.

There was no difference in the distribution of birthweights of offspring of the partners of male survivors who had or had not been treated with an alkylating agent (RR 1.62; 95% CI 0.84–3.11; $p = 0.15$) (Figure 8e.3), whose partner smoked during pregnancy (RR 1.64; 95% CI 0.76–3.53; $p = 0.21$), or who had or had not received pelvic irradiation (RR 1.51; 95% CI 0.61–3.74; $p = 0.38$) (Figure 8e.4). The offspring of male survivors who were treated with a non-alkylating agent chemotherapeutic agent (RR 3.03; 95% CI 1.15–7.98;

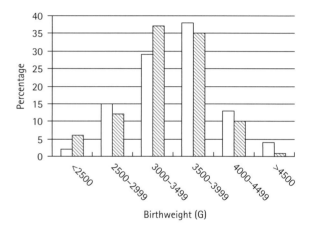

Figure 8e.5 *Offspring of partners of male survivors of childhood cancer: distribution of birthweight by treatment with (hatched columns) or without (open columns) non-alkylating agent chemotherapy.*

$p = 0.025$) (Figure 8e.5) were more likely to weigh less than 2500 g.[54]

Although the CCSS results are the largest series of offspring born to childhood cancer survivors, maternal and offspring medical records were not examined to document maternal pregnancy complications. The National Wilms Tumor Study Group (NWTSG) reported the results of their study of pregnancy outcome after treatment for Wilms' tumor.[55]

The NWTSG patients reported 427 pregnancies of ≥20 weeks gestation. There were one miscarriage, one elective abortion, four stillbirths, 409 liveborn singleton infants and 12 liveborn infants from twin gestation. Medical records of 309 pregnancies of ≥20 weeks duration were reviewed. Complications of pregnancy and labor, including hypertension complicating pregnancy

(ICD 642), early or threatened labor (ICD 644), malposition of fetus (ICD 652), obstructed labor (ICD 660), abnormality of forces of labor (ICD 661) and umbilical cord complications (ICD 663) were examined. None of these was significantly more frequent among the partners of men who were treated with flank radiation, compared to those who were not. However, early or threatened labor ($p = 0.030$) and malposition of the fetus ($p = 0.007$) were more frequent among irradiated women. The trend test result suggested that both complications were more frequent among women treated with higher radiation doses. The odds ratio (OR) of early or threatened labor was 2.36 (95% CI 0.93–6.02) among those who received >2500 cGy, compared to the unirradiated females, and the OR of malposition of the fetus was 6.26 (95% CI 1.50–36.57) among those who received ≥2500 cGy compared to the unirradiated females. The increased risk of malposition of the fetus remained significant in a multivariate model that included gestational age ($p = 0.028$). There was no difference in the frequency of early or threatened labor ($p = 0.676$) or malposition of the fetus ($p = 0.756$) in the group of women treated with actinomycin D only, or vincristine and actinomycin D, compared to the group treated with vincristine, actinomycin D and doxorubicin.

The mean gestational age of the offspring of the irradiated females was 37.23 (±4.00) weeks, compared to 38.47 (±2.95) weeks for those of the unirradiated females ($p = 0.005$). The mean gestational age of the offspring of the irradiated (39.23 ± 2.09 weeks) and that of the offspring of the unirradiated (39.48 ± 1.92 weeks) males did not differ ($p = 0.59$). There was an excess of infants born prior to 36 weeks of gestation to women ($p = 0.0005$), but not to the partners of men, who received flank irradiation. The excess was greatest among those women who had received flank radiation doses exceeding 2500 cGy. The OR of birth prior to 36 weeks of gestation was 4.07 (95% CI 1.74–9.90) among the offspring of the females who received ≥2500 cGy compared to the offspring of the unirradiated females. There was no difference in the percentage of infants born prior to 36 weeks of gestation ($p = 0.322$) in the group of offspring of women treated with actinomycin D only, or vincristine and actinomycin D, compared to the group treated with vincristine, actinomycin D and doxorubicin.

The mean birthweight of the offspring of the irradiated females was 3036 ± 805 g, compared to 3245 ± 620 g for those of the unirradiated females ($p = 0.02$). The mean birthweight of the offspring of the irradiated (3466 ± 451 g) and that of the offspring of the unirradiated (3475 ± 794 g) males did not differ ($p = 0.94$). There was an excess in the percentage of infants with a birthweight less than 2500 g born to women ($p = 0.017$), but not the partners of men, who received flank radiation. The proportion of infants with a birthweight less than 2500 g

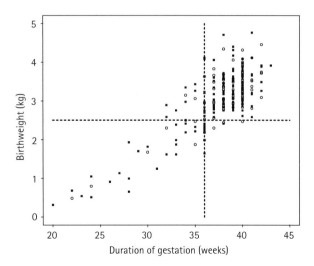

Figure 8e.6 *Graph of birthweight versus gestational age for offspring of unirradiated female (open circle) and irradiated female (solid square) Wilms' tumor patients.*

was greater among the offspring of women who received flank radiation therapy doses greater than 2500 cGy. Most of the low birthweight infants had weights that were appropriate for their gestational age (Figure 8e.6). There was no difference in the percentage of infants with a birthweight less than 2500 g ($p = 0.129$) in the group of offspring of women treated with actinomycin D only or vincristine and actinomycin D, compared to the group treated with vincristine, actinomycin D and doxorubicin.

Effect on birthweight

The offspring of women who received flank irradiation as a component of their protocol therapy for Wilms' tumor were significantly more likely to have a birthweight of less than 2500 g than were those born to women whose protocol treatment for Wilms' tumor did not include flank irradiation. This finding confirms those of several previous studies,[41,42,43,44,56,57] including that of Chiarelli and her colleagues, who reported an increased relative risk of low birthweight offspring among women treated with >2500 cGy of abdominal-pelvic radiation.[57]

The mechanism responsible for low birthweight after pelvic irradiation is unknown. The studies of Critchley and her colleagues suggest that damage to both the uterine vasculature and myometrium contribute. These investigators demonstrated that uterine length was significantly less in ten women with ovarian failure who had been treated with whole-abdomen irradiation. Endometrial thickness did not increase in response to hormone replacement therapy in three women who underwent weekly ultrasound examination. No flow was detectable

with Doppler ultrasound through either uterine artery of five women and through one uterine artery in three additional women.[58,59] Ultrasonographic examination of four women treated with total body irradiation revealed ovarian structures in only two of the four and significantly reduced uterine volume in all four. Three had undetectable uterine blood flow and no significant endometrial tissue. Patients who were treated with total body irradiation prior to puberty had a smaller increase in uterine volume in response to steroid hormone replacement therapy than did those treated after puberty with total body irradiation.[60]

Congenital malformations

The frequency of birth defects has been evaluated in offspring of childhood cancer survivors in several studies. Offspring of survivors of Wilms' tumor [57] and acute lymphoblastic leukemia[61] do not have an increased frequency of major congenital malformations. Dodds and her colleagues, utilizing a case-control study design, did not identify an excess of exposures to radiation therapy, chemotherapy, pelvic radiation therapy or chemotherapy with an alkylating agent among the parents of Ontario children with a reported birth defect compared to control parents whose child did not have a birth defect.[62] Hawkins et al. reported congenital malformations in 3.1 per cent of offspring ($n = 161$) of survivors or their partners exposed to mutagenic therapy (radiation therapy involving direct exposure of the abdomen or gonads or treatment with an alkylating agent) compared to 2.3 per cent of the offspring ($n = 835$) of those not exposed to mutagenic therapy.[63] Byrne et al. reported a cytogenetic syndrome in 0.2 per cent, a single gene disorder in 0.6 per cent and a simple malformation in 2.7 per cent of 2198 offspring of childhood cancer survivors or their partners, compared to a cytogenetic syndrome in 0.1 per cent, a single gene disorder in 0.2 per cent and a simple malformation in 2.8 per cent of 4544 offspring of the survivors' siblings or their partners ($p = 0.3$).[64]

Twenty of 309 singleton infants for whom medical records were reviewed had a total of 32 congenital malformations. Twelve had a single congenital malformation, five had two, two had three and one had four congenital malformations. Congenital malformations were more frequent among the offspring of women who received flank radiation therapy ($p = 0.054$). No such increase was observed for irradiated males ($p = 1.0$). There was no difference in the percentage of infants with no versus one or more congenital anomalies ($p = 0.757$) in the group of offspring of women treated with actinomycin D, only or vincristine and actinomycin D,

compared to the group treated with vincristine, actinomycin D and doxorubicin.[55]

Cancer in offspring

The offspring of former pediatric cancer patients may be at increased risk of developing cancer during childhood or adolescence due either to genetic factors and/or germline mutations produced by the treatment of the parent. An evaluation of the incidence of childhood cancer in 2308 offspring of survivors of childhood and adolescent cancer, and 4719 offspring of the former patients' sibling controls revealed no difference in the frequency of childhood cancer between the two groups. The reported frequencies were 0.30 per cent among the offspring of the former patients and 0.23 per cent among the offspring of the sibling controls.[65] Hawkins and his colleagues reported that the frequency of childhood cancer among the 1199 offspring of survivors with a primary diagnosis other than retinoblastoma was 0.17 per cent[66] and was 0.50 per cent among 5629 offspring of survivors with a primary diagnosis other than retinoblastoma identified by the Nordic countries cancer registries.[67]

Former pediatric cancer patients who have familial cancer phenotypes, such as bilateral retinoblastoma, neurofibromatosis, nevoid basal cell carcinoma syndrome or familial polyposis coli, are at increased risk of having affected offspring and should be counseled regarding this risk.

RECOMMENDATIONS

Many former patients are concerned that their offspring may be either at increased risk of having a congenital anomaly or developing childhood cancer. The available data suggest that offspring born following treatment for childhood cancer are not at increased risk for either of these outcomes. However, large numbers of offspring of former pediatric cancer patients have only recently become available for study. Former patients should be encouraged to participate in studies designed to evaluate pregnancy outcome and the health of their progeny. Such studies are necessary to provide the data necessary for these former patients to make informed decisions regarding childbearing. Women whose treatment for Wilms' tumor included abdominal irradiation do have an increased risk of giving birth to a premature or small for gestational age infant, and should have close obstetrical observation. Former patients who have a familial predisposition to childhood cancer, such as neurofibromatosis, bilateral retinoblastoma or nevoid basal cell carcinoma syndrome, should be counseled appropriately regarding the risk of cancer in their offspring.

KEY POINTS

- The proportion with a birthweight less than 2500 g is greater for offspring of female survivors who received radiation therapy that included the pelvis than among the survivors' female siblings.
- The male : female ratio is reversed among the offspring of male survivors of childhood cancer compared to the ratio of the offspring of their male siblings.
- The frequency of childhood cancer is not increased among the offspring of survivors of childhood cancer who do not have a recognized genetic condition, such as familial retinoblastoma, neurofibromatosis or Li–Fraumeni syndrome.
- The frequency of chromosomal abnormalities, single gene defects and congenital malformations is not increased among the offspring of survivors of childhood cancer.

REFERENCES

1. Sieber SM, Adamson RH. Toxicity of antineoplastic agents in man: Chromosomal aberrations, antifertility effects, congenital malformations and carcinogenic potential. *Adv Cancer Res* 1975; **22**:57–155.
2. Russell WL. Mutation frequencies in female mice and the estimation of genetic hazards of radiation in women. *Proc Natl Acad Sci USA* 1977; **74**:3523–3527.
3. Kirk KM, Lyon MF. Induction of congenital malformations in the offspring of male mice treated with x-rays at pre-meiotic and post-meiotic stages. *Mutation Res* 1984; **125**:75–85.
4. Matheson D, Brusick D, Carrano R. Comparison of the relative mutagenic activity for eight antineoplastic drugs in the Ames Salmonella/microsome and TK ± mouse lymphoma assays. *Drug Chem Toxicol* 1978; **1**:277–304.
5. Benedict WF, Baker MS, Haroun L, *et al.* Mutagenicity of cancer chemotherapeutic agents in the Salmonella/microsome test. *Cancer Res* 1977; **37**:2209–2213.
6. Seino Y, Nagao M, Yahagi T, *et al.* Mutagenicity of several classes of antitumor agents to Salmonella typhimurium TA98, TA100, and TA92. *Cancer Res* 1978; **38**:2148–2156.
7. Auletta AE, Martz AG, Parmar AS. Mutagenicity of nitrosourea compounds for Salmonella typhimurium: Brief communication. *J Natl Cancer Inst* 1978; **60**:1495–1497.
8. Franza BR Jr, Oeschger NS, Oeschger MP, Schein PS. Mutagenic activity of nitrosourea antitumor agents. *J Natl Cancer Inst* 1980; **65**:149–154.
9. Anderson D, Styles JA. The bacterial mutation test. *Br J Cancer* 1978; **37**:924–930.
10. Matney TS, Nguyen TV, Connor TH, *et al.* Genotoxic classification of anticancer drugs. *Terato Carcino Mutagen* 1985; **5**:319–328.
11. Nguyen TV, Theiss JC, Matney TS. Exposure of pharmacy personnel to mutagenic antineoplastic drugs. *Cancer Res* 1982; **42**:4792–4796.
12. Puyeo C. Natulan induces forward mutations to L-arabinose resistance in Salmonella typhimurium. *Mutation Res* 1979; **67**:189–192.
13. Yajima N, Knodo, K, Morita K. Reverse mutation tests in Salmonella typhimurium and chromosomal aberration tests in mammalian cells in culture on fluorinated pyrimidine derivatives. *Mutation Res* 1981; **88**:241–254.
14. Trasler JM, Hales BF, Robaire B. Paternal cyclophosphamide treatment of rats causes fetal loss and malformations without affecting male fertility. *Nature* 1985; **316**:144–146.
- 15. Schull WJ. *Effects of atomic radiation. A half-century of studies from Hiroshima and Nagasaki*. New York: Wiley-Liss, Inc, 1995:243–271.
16. Neel JV, Satoh C, Goriki K, *et al.* Search for mutations altering protein charge and/or function in children of atomic bomb survivors: Final report. *Am J Hum Genet* 1988; **42**:663–676.
17. Neel JV, Satoh C, Hamilton HB, *et al.* Search for mutations affecting protein structure in children of atomic bomb survivors: preliminary report. *Proc Natl Acad Sci USA* 1980; **77**:4221–4225.
18. Langlois RG, Bigbee WL, Kyoizumi S, *et al.* Evidence for increased somatic cell mutations at the glycophorin A locus in atomic bomb survivors. *Science* 1987; **236**:445–448.
19. Kyoizumi S, Nakamura N, Hakoda M, *et al.* Detection of somatic mutations at the glycophorin A locus in erythrocytes of atomic bomb survivors using a single beam flow cytometer. *Cancer Res* 1989; **49**:581–588.
20. Hakoda M, Akiyama M, Kyoizumi S, *et al.* Increased somatic cell mutant frequency in atomic bomb survivors. *Mutation Res* 1988; **201**:39–49.
21. Albertini RJ. Somatic gene mutations in vivo as indicated by the 6-thioguanine-resistant T-lymphocytes in human blood. *Mutation Res* 1985; **150**:411–422.
22. Shlono PH, Chung CS, Myrianthopoulos NC. Preconception radiation, intrauterine diagnostic radiation and childhood neoplasia. *J Natl Cancer Inst* 1980; **65**:681–686.
23. Kneale GW, Stewart AM. Pre-conception x-rays and childhood cancers. *Br J Cancer* 1980; **41**:222–226.
24. Nicholson HO. Cytotoxic drugs in pregnancy. *J Obstet Gynaecol Brief Comm* 1968; **75**:307–312.
25. Sokal JE, Lessmann EM. Effects of cancer chemotherapeutic agents on the human fetus. *JAMA* 1960; **172**:1765–1771.
26. Sweet DL, Kinzie J. Consequences of radiotherapy and antineoplastic therapy for the fetus. *J Reprod Med* 1976; **17**:241–246.
27. Daly H, McCann SR, Hanratty TD, Temperley IJ. Successful pregnancy during combination chemotherapy for Hodgkin's disease. *Acta Haematol* 1980; **64**:154–156.
28. Nisce LZ, Tome MA, He S, *et al.* Management of coexisting Hodgkin's disease and pregnancy. *Am J Clin Oncol* 1986; **9**:146–151.
29. Garrett MJ. Teratogenic effect of combination chemotherapy. *Ann Intern Med* 1974; **80**:667(Letter).
30. Thomas PRM, Peckham MJ. The investigation and management of Hodgkin's disease in the pregnant patient. *Cancer* 1976; **38**:1443–1451.
31. Milunsky A, Graef JW, Gaynor MF. Methotrexate-induced congenital malformations. *J Pediatr* 1968; **72**:790–795.
32. Dara P, Slater LM, Armentrout SA. Successful pregnancy during chemotherapy for acute leukemia. *Cancer* 1981; **47**:845–846.
33. Li FP, Jaffe N. Progeny of childhood cancer survivors. *Lancet* 1974; **2**:707–709.
34. Li FP, Fine W, Jaffe N, *et al.* Offspring of patients treated for cancer in childhood. *J Natl Cancer Inst* 1979; **62**:1193–1197.

35. Blatt J, Mulvihill JJ, Ziegler JL, *et al*. Pregnancy outcome following cancer chemotherapy. *Am J Med* 1980; **69**:828–832.

36. Green DM, Zevon MA, Lowrie G, *et al*. Congenital anomalies in children of patients who received chemotherapy for cancer in childhood and adolescence. *N Engl J Med* 1991; **325**:141–146.

◆37. Green DM, Fiorello A, Zevon MA, *et al*. Birth defects and childhood cancer in offspring of survivors of childhood cancer. *Arch Pediatr Adolesc Med* 1997; **151**:379–383.

38. Holmes GE, Holmes FF. Pregnancy outcome of patients treated for Hodgkin's disease. *Cancer* 1978; **41**:1317–1322.

39. Simon R. Statistical methods for evaluating pregnancy outcomes in patients with Hodgkin's disease. *Cancer* 1980; **45**:2890–2892.

40. McKeen EA, Mulvihill JJ, Rosner F, Zarrabi MH. Pregnancy outcome in Hodgkin's disease. *Lancet* 1979; **2**:590(Letter).

41. Green DM, Fine WE, Li FP. Offspring of patients treated for unilateral Wilms' tumor in childhood. *Cancer* 1982; **49**:2285–2288.

42. Li FP, Gimbrere K, Gelber RD, *et al*. Outcome of pregnancy in survivors of Wilms' tumor. *JAMA* 1987; **257**:216–219.

43. Byrne J, Mulvihill JJ, Connelly RR, *et al*. Reproductive problems and birth defects in survivors of Wilms' tumor and their relatives. *Med Pediatr Oncol* 1988; **16**:233–240.

44. Hawkins MM, Smith RA. Pregnancy outcomes in childhood cancer survivors: probable effects of abdominal irradiation. *Int J Cancer* 1989; **43**:399–402.

45. Nicholson HS, Blask AN, Markle BM, *et al*. Uterine anomalies in Wilms' tumor survivors. *Cancer* 1996; **78**:887–891.

46. Byrne J, Nussbaum-Blask A, Taylor WS, *et al*. Prevalence of Mullerian duct anomalies detected at ultrasound. *Am J Med Genet* 2000; **94**:9–12.

47. Byrne J, Nicholson HS. Excess risk for Mullerian duct anomalies in girls with Wilms tumor. *Med Pediatr Oncol* 2002; **38**:258–259.

48. Lilleyman JS. Male fertility after successful chemotherapy for lymphoblastic leukaemia. *Lancet* 1979; **2**:1125 (Letter).

49. Moe PJ, Lethinen M, Wegelius R, *et al*. Progeny of survivors of acute lymphocytic leukemia. *Acta Paediatr Scand* 1979; **68**:301–303.

50. Nesbit ME, Krivit W, Robison L, Hammond D. A follow-up report of long-term survivors of childhood acute lymphoblastic or undifferentiated leukemia. *J Pediatr* 1979; **95**:727–730.

51. Ross GT. Congenital anomalies among children born of mothers receiving chemotherapy for gestational trophoblastic neoplasms. *Cancer* 1976; **37**:1043–1047.

52. Robison LL, Mertens AC, Boice JD, *et al*. Study design and cohort characteristics of the childhood cancer survivor study: a multi-institutional collaborative project. *Med Pediatr Oncol* 2002; **38**:229–239.

◆53. Green DM, Whitton JA, Stovall M, *et al*. Pregnancy outcome of female survivors of childhood cancer. A report from the Childhood Cancer Survivor Study. *Am J Obstet Gynecol* 2002; **187**:1070–1080.

◆54. Green DM, Whitton JA, Stovall M, *et al*. Pregnancy outcome of partners of male survivors of childhood cancer. A report from the Childhood Cancer Survivor Study. *J Clin Oncol* 2003; **21**:716–721.

◆55. Green DM, Peabody EM, Nan B, *et al*. Pregnancy outcome after treatment for Wilms tumor. A report from the National Wilms Tumor Study Group. *J Clin Oncol* 2002; **20**:2506–2513.

56. Garber JE, Lynch EA, Meadows AT, *et al*. Pregnancy outcome after therapy of childhood cancer. *Proc Am Soc Clin Oncol* 1990; **9**:290 (abstract).

57. Chiarelli AM, Marrett LD, Darlington GA. Pregnancy outcomes in females after treatment for childhood cancer. *Epidemiology* 2000; **11**:161–166.

◆58. Critchley HOD, Wallace WHB, Shalet SM, *et al*. Abdominal irradiation in childhood: the potential for pregnancy. *Br J Obstet Gynecol* 1992; **99**:392–394

59. Critchley HOD. Factors of importance for implantation and problems after treatment for childhood cancer. *Med Pediatr Oncol* 1999; **33**:9–14.

60. Bath LE, Critchley HOD, Chambers SE, *et al*. Ovarian and uterine characteristics after total body irradiation in childhood and adolescence: response to sex steroid replacement. *Br J Obstet Gynaecol* 1999; **106**:1265–1272.

61. Kenney LB, Nicholson HS, Brasseux C, *et al*. Birth defects in offspring of adult survivors of childhood acute lymphoblastic leukemia. A Children's Cancer Group/National Institutes of health report. *Cancer* 1996; **78**:169–176.

62. Dodds L, Marrett LD, Tomkins DJ, *et al*. Case-control study of congenital anomalies in children of cancer patients. *Br Med J* 1993; **307**:164–168.

63. Hawkins MM. Is there evidence of a therapy-related increase in germ cell mutation among childhood cancer survivors? *J Natl Cancer Inst* 1991; **83**:1643–1650.

◆64. Byrne J, Rasmussen SA, Steinhorn SC, *et al*. Genetic disease in offspring of long-term survivors of childhood and adolescent cancer. *Am J Hum Genet* 1998; **62**:45–52.

◆65. Mulvihill JJ, Connelly RR, Austin DF, *et al*. Cancer in offspring of long-term survivors of childhood and adolescent cancer. *Lancet* 1987; **2**:813–817.

◆66. Hawkins MM, Draper GJ, Smith RA. Cancer among 1,348 offspring of childhood cancer. *Int J Cancer* 1989; **43**:975–978.

◆67. Sankila R, Olsen JH, Anderson H, *et al*. Risk of cancer among offspring of childhood cancer survivors. *N Engl J Med* 1998; **338**:1339–1344.

68. LeFloch O, Donaldson SS, Kaplan HS. Pregnancy following oophoropexy and total nodal irradiation in women with Hodgkin's disease. *Cancer* 1976; **38**:2263–2268.

69. Holmes GE. Personal communication, 1987.

70. Horning SJ, Hoppe RT, Kaplan HS, Rosenberg SA. Female reproductive potential after treatment for Hodgkin's disease. *N Engl J Med* 1981; **304**:1377–1382.

71. Andrieu JM, Ochoa-Molina ME. Menstrual cycle, pregnancies and offspring before and after MOPP therapy for Hodgkin's disease. *Cancer* 1983; **52**:435–438.

72. Whitehead E, Shalet SM, Blackledge G, *et al*. The effect of combination chemotherapy on ovarian function in women treated for Hodgkin's disease. *Cancer* 1983; **52**:988–993.

73. Donaldson SS, Kaplan, HS. A survey of pediatric Hodgkin's disease at Stanford University: Results of therapy and quality of survival. In: Rosenberg SA, Kaplan HS (eds) *Malignant lymphomas. etiology, immunology, pathology, treatment*. New York: Academic Press, 1982:571–590.

74. Green DM, Hall B. Pregnancy outcome following treatment during childhood or adolescence for Hodgkin's disease. *Pediatr Hematol Oncol* 1988; **5**:269–277.

Musculoskeletal complications

Osteoporosis

BERNADETTE MD BRENNAN

INTRODUCTION

As a result of modern treatment protocols, the majority of children with cancer will now survive to adulthood and, in particular, patients with acute lymphoblastic leukemia (ALL), who form a significant proportion of this cohort of survivors. Therefore, the long-term complications of their treatment have become increasingly important. Furthermore, because of the ability to treat children with ALL successfully from the 1970s onwards, a significant proportion of this cohort are now reaching their 30th and 40th decade, so the specific issue of bone health needs to be addressed.

Bone mineral measurement, or bone densitometry, has gained importance in the diagnosis and management of patients with metabolic bone disease, such as osteoporosis. Osteoporosis is a systemic skeletal disease characterized by low bone mass and microarchitectural deterioration of bone tissue, with a consequent increase in bone fragility and susceptibility to fracture. For a 50-year-old Caucasian woman, the risk of hip fracture in her remaining lifetime is approximately 16 per cent; therefore, any underlying condition or treatment that increases this risk will have a significant impact on the bone morbidity of that individual, increasing the risk of fracture and the consequent demands on the health service. For each standard deviation (SD) decrease in femoral bone density in women, there is a 2.6-fold increase in the risk of fracture. In other words, a woman whose hip bone density is 1 SD below the mean for her age is about seven times more likely to have a hip fracture than a woman whose bone density is 1 SD above the mean, mean being zero SD.[1]

NORMAL ACCRETION OF BONE MASS

Normal bone has two main components, trabecular (cancellous) and cortical (compact) bone. Where these two types of bone are combined, at various sites, it is known as integral bone. In the skeleton, bone remodeling is a tightly controlled process that occurs at the bone surface and results in bone turnover. Bone formation occurs only in areas of previously resorbed bone. The remodeling cycle consists of an activated phase, followed by bone resorption, a reversal phase, followed by bone formation, and a resting phase.[2] Normally bone formation and resorption are coordinated and in balance, but in conditions of persistently increased bone resorption or decreased bone formation, reduced bone mineral density (BMD) and hence osteoporosis occurs. During childhood, volumetric BMD is in the main unchanged, but bone height increases and hence growth occurs.[3] At puberty, marked changes in the skeleton occur, which include ossification and growth. If the rate of bone mineralization and bone mass accretion is reduced during puberty, peak bone mass, which is attained postpuberty, is reduced, which predicts for osteoporosis and fractures later in life .[4] In young women, bone mineral accretion begins at the onset of puberty and continues until the age of 16 years, or 2 years postmenses and in men until the age of 20 years.[5,6]

Approximately 80 per cent of the total skeleton is composed of cortical bone, the rest is trabecular bone. Bone turnover is much slower in cortical bone. Trabecular bone has a large surface composed of connecting plates of bone containing multiple holes, giving it a porous appearance. It is within trabecular bone that many of the active metabolic processes concerning bone formation occur, with bone turnover about eight times greater than that of cortical bone. Certain regions of the skeleton are rich in trabecular bone; including vertebrae, femoral necks and distal radii and, as a result of its metabolic activity, trabecular bone is more readily effected by pathological conditions. Therefore, it is not surprising that pathological conditions often manifest as fractures of vertebrae, hip and wrist.

There are four types of cells present in bone: osteoblasts, osteoclasts, resting surface cells and osteocytes. Osteoblasts cover the surface of trabecular bone and are mainly responsible for new bone formation and its active mineralization. They become incorporated into the mineralized bone matrix and lose many of their organelles to become osteocytes, or lose their polyhedral shape to become resting surface cells. Osteocytes are small cells that lie in lacunae filled by interstitial fluid surrounded by mineralized bone matrix. The function of the fluid is to allow transfer of metabolites to and from the mineralized matrix. It is believed that, through this route, osteocytes may play a role in matrix metabolism. The cells responsible for bone resorption are osteoclasts, which are thought to originate from the hemopoietic stem cells. Resorption of bone is necessary for bone remodeling (replacement of old matrix by new) and the maintenance of serum calcium levels. The development and modeling of bone is a process that is controlled by hormones and growth factors, including growth hormone (GH), sex steroids, insulin growth factor 1 and 2 (IGF-1 and 2), transforming growth factor β (TGF-β), and certain bone morphogenic proteins (BMPs). The increase in GH, IGF-1 and sex steroids during puberty are important for skeletal development, and hence bone growth and increased bone mineral deposition. The latter is due to the increase in osteoblastic numbers and activity. The accumulation in bone mass increases by approximately 4–6-fold over a 3-year period in girls and a 4-year period in boys during puberty.[7] This increase is measurable in bone in the lumbar spine and femoral neck, areas that are richer in the more metabolically active trabecular bone. Once peak bone mass is obtained, an equilibrium of activity is reached by the osteoblasts and osteoclasts, and is responsible for the maintenance of skeletal structure.

From an inorganic perspective, bone is composed of osteoid and minerals (mainly phosphate and calcium). Collagen, along with several other matrix materials, forms the base upon which calcium and phosphate are deposited. The primary collagen in bone is type 1, although there are 15 other different types of collagen also present.

FACTORS AFFECTING BONE MINERALIZATION AND THE ATTAINMENT OF PEAK BONE MASS

Apart from hormonal influences, other factors are important for the attainment of peak bone mass.

Genetic

Genetic factors have a very large influence on the attainment of peak bone mass. Women whose mothers develop postmenopausal osteoporosis are more likely to develop clinically significant bone disease in adulthood. The BMD of children closely resembles that of their parents and that of identical twins correlates more closely than that of non-identical twins.

Body mass

Increased mechanical loading on the skeleton as a result of increased body mass is associated with increased bone mass. Young and colleagues, however, using the twin model, showed that lean body mass rather than fat mass was the more important determinant of bone mass in girls and young women.[8]

Calcium intake

During childhood and adolescence supplements of dietary calcium increase areal BMD. Elegant experiments using twin pairs to exclude genetic influence have shown that, at least in prepubertal children, the administration of calcium supplements was beneficial to the skeleton.[9] Calcium supplementation also benefits adolescent girls regardless of their pubertal status.[10] In a more recent study mean bone mineralization and bone area continued to increase significantly in cohorts who had previously received calcium supplementation, even though it had been stopped for at least 3.5 years at the time of assessment.[11]

ASSESSMENT OF BONE MINERALIZATION

Bone mineral measurement, or bone densitometry, is used to give information on the fracture risk for a specific skeletal site and can be used to estimate the rate of bone loss. Assessment of BMD can be evaluated by different methods including single-photon absorptiometry (SPA), dual-photon absorptiometry (DPA), single X-ray absorptiometry (SXA), dual X-ray absorptiometry (DXA), and quantitative computed tomography (QCT).

Bone mineral status can be expressed as crude bone mineral mass in grams, mineral mass adjusted for projected bone area – areal BMD ($g/cm^{2)}$, or mineral mass, adjusted for the bone volume – volumetric BMD (g/cm^3). Volumetric BMD is measured by QCT and is not subject to the confounding effect of bone size. Using QCT, it has been shown that there is no difference in vertebral bone densitometry between boys and girls once pubertal status has been taken into account,[3] and is stable throughout childhood until it increases at puberty. Furthermore, because it images in a cross-sectional plane, QCT is unique among methods of measurement in providing separate estimates of trabecular and cortical bone BMD. Until recently, the method has been used with commercial computed tomography (CT) scans to assess BMD of the vertebrae with an effective radiation dose equivalent of 60 μSv. This radiation dose is much higher than other methods for measuring BMD and hence has precluded its use in children. Recently, however, peripheral QCT (pQCT) has become available with commercial CT scanners to assess total and trabecular BMD at the distal forearm. Radiation exposure is 3 μSv and hence this low dose makes it suitable for use in growing children.

The most widely used method for BMD assessment is DXA with an effective radiation dose of 1–3 μSv, which measures integral bone. This gives areal BMD (BMD_A) obtained by dividing bone mineral contents (BMC) by bone area. In growing subjects, BMC and BMD_A both increase with increasing height, even when the bone mineral volumetric density remains unaltered.[12] Therefore, any condition or treatment that leads to 'small bones' can give a falsely low BMD_A.

FACTORS IN CHILDHOOD CANCER AND ITS TREATMENT THAT MAY AFFECT BONE MINERALIZATION

The disease itself

Skeletal abnormalities have been described in association with ALL, including osteoporosis,[13,14] vertebral compression factors[13–19] and juxtametaphyseal lucent bands or 'leukemic lines' in long bones.[13,15] Halton and colleagues examined BMD using DXA in children with ALL at diagnosis and found it to be reduced with an altered mineral hemostasis.[20] This study implicated the leukemic process as a causative factor in the altered vitamin D metabolism and skeletal abnormalities that are present in some children with ALL at diagnosis.[20] A further study assessing BMD at diagnosis in children with ALL and other cancers demonstrated no decrease in volumetric BMD at the time of diagnosis compared to controls.[21] This differs from Halton and colleagues, possibly due to the use of

apparent volumetric BMD by Arikoski and colleagues adjusting for any effect of small bone size, which would give a false impression of a reduced BMD at diagnosis.[21] In Halton's study, this adjustment was not made.[20]

Chemotherapy and steroids

Glucocorticoids are integral in the treatment of childhood ALL and lymphoma, either as prednisolone or, more recently, dexamethasone. The later drug is also used throughout childhood cancer treatment either as an antiemetic or for tumor-associated edema. Glucocorticoids enhance bone resorption and decrease bone formation. Consequently, they decrease bone mass and increase the risk of fractures.[22] The increased bone resorption is in part the result of a decrease in intestinal calcium resorption and an increase in the urinary excretion of calcium. *In vivo*, glucocorticoids inhibit intestinal calcium transport, opposing the effects of vitamin D, but the mechanism has yet to be established. Serum levels of vitamin D metabolites in patients receiving glucocorticoids are virtually normal and glucocorticoids induce the expression of calbindin-D28K, a protein involved in intestinal calcium transport.[23–25] Glucocorticoids have an acute stimulatory effect on bone resorption *in vitro* but, in long-term cultures, they are an inhibitory.[26] The stimulation may be due to an increase in osteoclast activity and is in accordance with the effects observed *in vivo*. The mechanism of this increased activity is not known, although it could involve the induction of interleukin 6 (IL-6) receptors in skeletal cells.[27] IL-6 is a cytokine known to induce osteoclast recruitment and to play a central role in bone resorption.[28]

The predominant result of glucocorticoid excess is impairment of bone formation and is associated with a decrease in serum levels of osteocalcin, a marker of osteoblastic function.[29] In the main, this is due to the direct effect of glucocorticoids on cells of osteoblastic lineage but an additional component could be due to indirect mechanisms, such as inhibition of gonadotrophin and sex steroid production.[22] Glucocorticoids have a paradoxical effect on bone cell function, inducing the differentiation of pre-osteoblastic cells, the formation of multilayered bone nodules that eventually mineralize and inhibit specific aspects of the differentiated function of osteoblasts.[30] Glucocorticoids decrease cell replication, depleting a cell population capable of synthesizing bone collagen, and repress type 1 collagen gene expression by the osteoblast by decreasing the rate of transcription and destabilizing α_1 I collagen mRNA.[31] As type 1 collagen is the major structural protein of the bone matrix, a decrease in its expression and an increase in its degradation are critical to the inhibitory actions of glucocorticoids on bone matrix and bone mass.

In patients chronically exposed to excessive amounts of glucocorticoids, osteoporosis is observed. Analysis of biopsies from patients on glucocorticoids reveals decreased bone matrix apposition rate, decreased trabecular volume and increased bone resorption.[23,32,33] Aaron and colleagues also showed, using histomorphometric analysis, a decline in all aspects of bone formation, except for the calcification front.[34] Osteoblastic function and number are altered, and the cells becoming spindle shaped and attenuated. This results in a decrease in trabecular bone volume but not in trabecular number.[34–36] Excess glucocorticoids result in decreased BMD, 30–50 per cent of patients developing vertebral fractures.[22,32] This loss in BMD is greater in trabecular than cortical bone; consequently, they have greater bone mineral loss in the vertebral spine. Partial or total restoration of bone mass can result from discontinuation of glucocorticoids.[37,38]

Studies in patients with Cushing's syndrome show marked osteopenia prior to therapy for the glucocorticoid excess equally severe in the lumbar spine and in the femoral neck.[39] In a preliminary report, Mercado-Asis and colleagues showed that the decrease in BMD was more severe in pediatric than in adult patients with Cushing's syndrome.[40] This is in agreement with the observations that very young patients receiving glucocorticoid therapy lose bone mass more rapidly than older patients.[41]

Clinical studies in children with ALL on long-term methotrexate demonstrated evidence of osteoporosis and osteoporotic fractures.[42–45] Furthermore, Nesbit and colleagues demonstrated abnormalities in calcium metabolism with increased excretion of urinary calcium in a similar cohort of children with bone abnormalities.[46] Methotrexate is known to affect calcium excretion in the urine and stool[47] and, although all patients would have also received prednisolone, their osteopathy was attributed to the methotrexate. Further evidence for methotrexate-induced osteopathy comes from studies where methotrexate has been used without steroids.[48] In this study, a high incidence of osteopathy was reported in infants with brain tumors who received high cumulative methotrexate doses of between 20–135 g/m^2 without steroids.

In animal models (Wistar Lewis rats), Friedlaender and colleagues evaluated the effects of antineoplastic drugs (doxorubicin and methotrexate) on intact bone in order to elucidate their effects on bone remodeling.[49] Short-term administration of methotrexate caused a 26.9 per cent reduction in net trabecular bone volume and doxorubicin an 11.5 per cent decrease. Both drugs significantly and profoundly diminished bone formation rates by nearly 60 per cent.

Finally, a study assessing BMC of two groups of patients with osteosarcoma treated with high and low doses of methotrexate demonstrated only in the group receiving high-dose methotrexate a significant loss in BMC compared to controls.[50]

Growth hormone deficiency

The endocrine system is particularly sensitive to cancer therapies. Long-term survivors of childhood cancer who receive cranial irradiation have lower than predicted height, with growth hormone deficiency (GHD) as the most frequent endocrine deficiency observed.[51] Until recently, the majority of children with ALL have received low-dose cranial irradiation (18–24 Gy) and a significant proportion of brain tumors also receive radiotherapy, the resultant GHD in a proportion of these children must be considered as a factor for any potential alteration in bone mineral status. Many studies have looked at children with GHD and the effect on bone mass,[52–54] showing it to be significantly reduced compared with normal control subjects. However, the techniques used for these observations (SPA, DPA) in growing children are complicated by the influence of size of the subject on these methods. As these measurements provide an index of the amount of bone mineral per unit length, it is dependent on both the width and the depth of the bone, and increases with an increase in the size of the bone. Thus, measurements may be reduced in children with untreated GHD as a consequence of the small stature of these patients.

Degerblad and colleagues reported that adults with childhood-onset GHD have reduced forearm cortical and integral bone mass, as measured by SPA, compared with men and women of approximately the same age.[55] However, this group did not comment on the statistical significance of the findings, and the number of subjects in this study was small. Subsequent studies of adults with childhood onset of GHD have also reported a significant reduction in bone mass.[56–60] Kaufman and colleagues reported a 20–30 per cent reduction in BMD in the forearm and between 9 and 19 per cent reduction in the lumbar spine.[57] Hyer et al. studied five adults with childhood-onset GHD who had not previously received treatment with GH, and demonstrated a significant reduction in DXA measurement of the lumbar spine, femoral neck and Ward's triangle BMD compared with a small number of healthy controls.[56] The study, however, had small numbers of subjects. De Boer's study[60] is significant in that it reported on 70 men with childhood-onset GHD showing a significant decrease in BMD (corrected for estimated bone volume) in lumbar spine and femoral neck.

Sex steroid deficiency

Ovarian failure can be expected following childhood cancer treatment, if the ovary is irradiated either directly, as in pelvic or total body irradiation, or as a result of scatter following spinal radiotherapy. Adult women with ovarian failure develop osteopenia. Bone mass is reduced after the menopause,[61] following bilateral oophorectomy,[62]

and in women with premature ovarian failure following chemotherapy for treatment of Hodgkin's disease.[63,64] However, in women with premature ovarian failure following cytotoxic chemotherapy alone for hematological malignancies, BMD may be affected less. Howell and colleagues describe such a scenario, where BMD was not significantly reduced in the lumbar spine, hip or forearm despite a mean duration of amenorrhea of 49 months.[65] Therefore, the cause of the ovarian dysfunction is important in determining the impact on the skeleton. Following treatment for childhood cancer that results in ovarian failure, estrogen replacement for normal pubertal development and subsequent complete hormone replacement postpuberty will usually occur. Therefore, we cannot assume that this cohort will have reduced BMD, assuming they have no other confounding factor to reduce it. The effect of ovarian failure secondary to childhood cancer treatment on bone mineralization, however, has not as yet been addressed.

Hypogonadism in males following childhood cancer is only likely to occur following irradiation (XRT) to the testes and in doses such as those used to treat leukemic relapse (24 Gy). So far, following chemotherapy alone or with total body irradiation (TBI) as part of pretransplant conditioning, significant hypogonadism has not been reported. Again it is likely that testosterone deficiency in this scenario is corrected to allow for pubertal development and with full replacement therapy thereafter. In young men with idiopathic hypogonadotrophic hypogonadism, bone mass is reduced;[66] this also occurs in men who have been castrated.[67] Hypogonadism in males and its effect on bone mineral density following childhood cancer treatment, however, has not been addressed and, almost certainly, this would be a difficult study to perform, as the hypogonadism is unlikely to occur in isolation without other factors that may affect bone mineralization.

BONE MINERAL DENSITY AFTER ALL

Several factors must be considered. First, up to 1990 the majority of children with ALL in the UK, and prior to this throughout Europe and the USA, would have received cranial XRT as central nervous system (CNS) prophylaxis. Hence a significant proportion will have reduced GH secretion either throughout childhood[68,69] or, indeed, when they reached adulthood.[70] Furthermore, as previously discussed, GH status affects bone mineralization with GHD leading to reduced BMD.[59] In modern treatment for ALL, the majority of children will not receive cranial XRT but glucocorticoids continue to be used, especially dexamethasone, which may have more glucocorticoid potency, and overall chemotherapy, including methotrexate, is more intensified. Second, not all studies

assessing BMD in either children or adults following childhood ALL treatment have taken into account bone size, or height and its effect on BMD. Hence the method of assessment of BMD or the adjustment of the BMD for the height of the individual is important in considering the significance of any results obtained.

In the early literature of bone mineral status following childhood ALL, several studies have looked at bone mass in childhood.[71–75] Gilsanz and colleagues assessed 42 children treated for childhood ALL 3–4 years after completion of chemotherapy (mean age 11.77 ± 0.53 years).[72] The major advantage of this study was the use of QCT, which avoids the effect of bone size on the BMD results. Bone mineral volumetric density of the lumbar spine measured with QCT was significantly reduced but was heavily influenced by a large proportion of the cohort who had received cranial XRT. The bone mass was less in those treated with cranial XRT (mean z score -0.93; $n = 29$) than in the non-irradiated group (mean z score 0.21; $n = 13$). The bone mass, however, was not related to the dose of cranial XRT (18 Gy vs. 23 Gy vs. 25 Gy), sex or pubertal status at follow-up. In a second study, Nussey and colleagues assessed BMD in a cohort of 64 survivors of childhood malignancy.[73] In a subgroup of 43 survivors of ALL, all had received cranial XRT and only a smaller subgroup ($n = 14$) had not received GH therapy. They were thought to be GHD and were found to have a significant reduction in BMD, implying GHD is a major contributor to their reduced BMD. A further subgroup of ALL survivors who had received GH therapy had a BMD no different from the control group. The definition of GHD in this cohort, however, was clinically determined in the majority. Furthermore, their analysis was complicated by including spinal BMD data from patients who had received spinal irradiation, which is a known independent cause of osteopenia. An earlier study by Leeuw and colleagues assessed bone mineral content in 19 children with ALL during their therapy using SPA.[74] The sparcity of details in this study make it difficult to assess the results, but they again concluded that the distribution of the results of the BMC assessments was not as expected in healthy children and was decreased compared to the normal controls. They did not find, however, an association between the decreased BMC, and duration or intensity of treatment received by the children.

Henderson and colleagues measured BMD of the lumbar spine in 60 patients age 5.5–20.1 years (mean 12.4 years), who had no known disease 1.0–14.5 years (mean, 4.3 years) after completing treatment for a malignancy.[75] The cohort included 30 children treated for ALL, of whom 14 received cranial XRT. The age-normalized BMD findings (z scores) were correlated with multiple variables, including measures of growth and nutrition, type of malignancy and various treatments, including use of steroids, methotrexate or cranial XRT. BMD was

normal in most patients with a mean z score of -0.28 ± 0.14 ($\pm$SE). Only 8 per cent of the patients were more than 2 SDs below the age-matched normal BMD. Weight z score was the major determinant of BMD z score. Calcium intake and height z score were also important variables. Bone density z scores tended to be lower in those who received cranial XRT, but the difference did not reach statistical significance. They concluded that most survivors of childhood malignancies would not be left with a clinically significant deficit in BMD. It is significant that the study by Henderson demonstrates the influence of height z scores as a determinant of BMD.[75] This again emphasized that the techniques used for the assessment of BMD (SPA, DXA) in most of the studies so far are influenced by the size of the bone, as these measurements provide an index of the amount of bone mineral per unit length, which is obviously dependent on both the width and the depth of the bone.

These early studies suggest BMD is reduced in children following childhood ALL but, apart from Gilsanz's study, reduced bone size may have led to falsely low BMD, as BMD was not expressed as crude bone mineral mass, or adjusted for height or bone area. Three further studies by Nysom et al.,[76] Warner et al.[77] and Brennan et al.[78] either include volumetric BMD methods, such as QCT,[78] or adjust BMD for bone size.[76,77] Furthermore, they include large numbers of participants and, in some studies, assess BMD after final height has been achieved.

Nysom and colleagues studied 95 survivors of childhood ALL who were in first remission and at a median age 16.2 years at the time of the study (range 6.1–34.2 years).[76] None had been irradiated outside the cranial field. Adjusted for sex and age, the mean whole body bone mineral content (BMC) and BMD_A were both significantly reduced (0.4 SDs less than the predicted mean value). This was mainly caused by reduced bone mass in the 33 participants who were aged 19 years or older at follow-up. In these young adults, the mean height for age, bone area for height and BMC for bone area were all significantly reduced. This indicated that the reduced whole body bone mass was caused by both reduced bone size and reduced size adjusted bone mass. Reduced bone size was related to previous cranial XRT. Reduced size-adjusted bone mass was not significantly related to age at diagnosis or follow-up, length of follow-up, cranial XRT, cumulative dose of methotrexate or corticosteroids, or endocrine status at follow-up. In participants less than 19 years at assessment (62 patients), the average whole body bone mass did not differ significantly from that of controls but patients had significantly less lumbar spine mass than controls. Cranial XRT did have an effect in this group, as whole body bone mass was significantly less in the irradiated group. Impaired attainment of peak bone mass is likely after cranial XRT for childhood ALL, because GHD of childhood onset impairs accretion of bone mass.[57,60]

The role of GH status and its possible causative role in reduced BMD following childhood ALL was addressed in our study.[78] BMD was assessed in a cohort of 31 (16 males) adults who had received cranial XRT in childhood as part of their treatment for ALL. Their GH status had been previously determined using an insulin stress test and arginine stimulation test. Furthermore, BMD assessment included QCT. There was a significant reduction in vertebral trabecular BMD (median z score -1.25, $p < 0.001$), in lumbar spine integral BMD (median z score -0.74, $p = 0.001$), in forearm cortical BMC (median z score -1.35, $p < 0.001$), and less so in femoral neck integral BMD (median z score -0.43, $p = 0.03$). There was no significant difference among the GH status groups for the following BMD measurements: vertebral trabecular BMD, lumbar spine integral BMD or femoral neck integral BMD ($p = 0.8$, $p = 0.96$ and $p = 0.4$, respectively). There was only a marginal significant difference for BMD at the wrist between GH status groups ($p = 0.04$). There was no correlation between the BMD measurements with time since or age at diagnosis. Possible explanations included a direct effect of chemotherapy, steroids, or both, on bone during childhood and hence an effect of the accretion of bone mass. The numbers of patients with severe GHD, however, was small (eight) and hence this may explain why we were not able to show an effect of reduced GH secretion on BMD.

A further causative factor in reduced BMD following childhood ALL may be reduced physical activity. The development of skeletal mass in healthy children has been associated with activity pattern.[79] Warner and colleagues explored the role of physical activity on bone mass in survivors of childhood ALL and the effect of various chemotherapeutic agents.[77] This group also appreciated the effect of body size on the interpretation of bone mineral data. By multiple regression analysis, they derived predictive equations for BMC using measurements made in healthy sibling controls with BMC as the dependent variable and bone area (BA), age, height, weight, pubertal stage and sex as the independent variables. The measurement BMC was expressed as a percentage of the predictive value (per cent BMC), hence the measurement per cent BMC at each site for the normal controls was 100 per cent. Despite no significant reduction in per cent BMC for the whole body in children treated for ALL, per cent BMC was reduced at the spine compared with controls [92.4 (8.0) per cent vs. 100.4 (9.7) per cent, respectively; $p < 0.005$] and at the hip compared with both other malignancies and controls [89.0 (11.5) per cent vs. 96.1 (11.7) per cent and 100.4 (9.2) per cent, respectively; $p < 0.0005$]. Increasing length of time of therapy was associated with a significant increase in per cent BMC at both the spine and the hip. Both exercise capacity and level of physical activity were correlated with per cent BMC at the hip ($r = 0.44$, $p < 0.001$; and $r = 0.29$, $p < 0.01$,

respectively). Interestingly, there was no correlation between per cent BMC and cumulative corticosteroid dosage at any site but there was correlation with the number of weeks of oral methotrexate.

Similar studies of BMD assessment in ALL survivors either in childhood[21,79,80] or in adults[81,82] in whom all had received cranial XRT as part of their childhood ALL treatment have demonstrated reduced BMD, but most studies can only hypothesize about the underlying cause. The most recent study by Kaste and colleagues examined BMD in a large cohort (141) and used QCT, a volumetric assessment of BMD. BMD was significantly reduced (mean z score −0.78 SD) and again cranial XRT is implicated.[80]

Other groups have performed prospective studies in order to tease out causative factors in treatment.[83,84] In both studies, BMD decreased significantly during treatment, which did not include cranial XRT. However, methotrexate, corticosteroids and decreased physical activity were all implicated. These later studies still suggest that, although cranial XRT has been omitted for the majority in modern ALL treatment protocols, reduced BMD will still occur in the majority of survivors.[83,84] Larger cohort cross-sectional studies refute this.[85,86] Kadan-Lottick and colleagues examined whole-body areal BMD using DXA in 75 subjects, currently (31 per cent) or previously treated for childhood ALL. Sixty-six (88 per cent) individuals had received dexamethasone as part of their treatment regimen. Overall, the mean whole body BMD z score was normal (+0.22 ± 0.96). Furthermore, patients further out from the end of treatment had a significantly higher BMD z score.

Whole-body BMD may be normal despite significantly abnormal regional BMD in ALL survivors[76,77] and does not give information on the metabolically active bone (trabecular bone) in areas such as wrist and spine. This has been specifically addressed in our recent study (unpublished). We assessed volumetric BMD using peripheral QCT in 58 children who had been treated for ALL without cranial XRT with a mean time of 4.5 years since completion of treatment. All patients were at least 1 year since the completion of treatment. Total (integral bone) distal radial BMD was normal [mean z score 0.32 (±0.95) SD] but mean distal radial trabecular z score was reduced [mean z score −0.66 (±0.86) SD]. Analysis as yet does not support Kadan-Lottick and colleagues finding that the greater time out from treatment the better the BMD.[85] The acute and long-term consequences of these findings and risk of fractures are yet to be determined.

BMD following other childhood cancers

Much of the work has focused on survivors of ALL as the clinical impression of increased fractures appeared to be greater in this group. However, other studies have addressed BMD in non-ALL patients, including brain tumors[73, 87,88] and various other solid tumors.[75,77,84] Not all studies demonstrate a reduction in BMD[77] and, in some studies, reduced bone mass was confined to subgroups of patients, such as those with growth hormone insufficiency who had not received adequate substitution therapy.[73] In most studies, however, the numbers of specific tumor types or similar treatments are too small to explore any meaningful causative factors or, indeed, assess whether BMD is truly reduced or not.

One study explores the role of ifosfamide as a potential causative factor for decreased BMD.[89] Ifosfamide is increasingly being used to treat solid tumors in childhood, and is standard therapy in soft tissue and in some bone sarcomas. The effect of ifosfamide on renal phosphate loss and hypercalciuria is well reported.[90] Therefore, de Schepper and colleagues[89] assessed BMD and bone mineral metabolism in 13 children 3 months or more after completion of cytotoxic chemotherapy that included ifosfamide. Mean (SD) BMD of the children was −0.88 (1.44) and three children had osteopenia, i.e. BMD z score < −2SD. They concluded that BMD was normal in most patients. Although the numbers are small, the results, I believe, are not normal and further studies with larger numbers could explore this.

FUTURE CONSIDERATIONS

The literature so far from cross-sectional studies following childhood ALL treatment, including cranial XRT, demonstrates significant reduction in regional BMD but, as this cohort gets older, we need to assess its significance and their risk of fractures, in particular at the hip. There is now an emerging body of evidence that BMD may not be reduced following childhood ALL; if cranial XRT is omitted or if BMD is reduced, it improves with time since completion of treatment. This needs to be confirmed by serial assessment of BMD with time in this cohort after the completion of treatment.

It is not clear that reduced BMD is an important late effect in other cancers with the exception of those patients whose GH secretion is reduced by cranial XRT. However, the long-term effects of ifosfamide on bone needs further research. Hypogonadism following childhood cancer and its effect on BMD has not been explored and, in particular, the effectiveness of sex steroid replacement in this cohort and the suitability of preparations used, such as hormone replacement therapy in young women that is designed for postmenopausal women.

As yet, no interventional studies with such treatment for osteoporosis as biphosphates have been performed either in children or adults following childhood cancer treatment. This next step should only be considered if we

truly have evidence emerging of increased fractures rather than cross-sectional data as BMD z scores. Intervention, however, with weight-bearing exercise could be considered and may benefit other late effects, such as obesity.

KEY POINTS

- Many factors may affect bone mineralization in the growing child, including the disease itself or the treatment received.
- Bone size must be taken into account when assessing bone mineral density (BMD), in particular when using non-volumetric methods.
- Chemotherapy implicated in poor bone mineralization includes steroids, methotrexate and possibly anthracyclines, such as doxorubicin.
- Irradiation indirectly causing growth hormone deficiency or sex steroid deficiency will also contribute to reduced BMD.
- The main disease groups who may have reduced BMD includes those treated for ALL with cranial XRT and brain tumors with growth hormone secretion abnormalities, usually as a result of cranial irradiation.
- Modern ALL treatment, which does not include cranial irradiation, may not lead to a reduced BMD.

REFERENCES

1. Cummings SR, Black DM, Nevitt MC, et al. Bone density at various sites for prediction of hip fractures. Lancet 1993; 341:72–75.
2. Baron R. Anatomy and ultrastructure of bone In: Farus MJ (ed.) Primer on metabolic diseases and disorders of mineral metabolism, 2nd edn. New York: Raven Press, 1993;3–9.
◆3. Gilsanz V, Gibbens DT, Roe TF, et al. Vertebral bone density in children: effect of puberty. Radiology 1988; 166:847–850.
4. WHO Technical Report Series. Assessment of fracture risk and its application to screening for postmenopausal osteoporosis: report of a World Health Organization Study Group. Geneva: World Health Organisation, 1994.
5. Bonjour JP, Thientz G, Buchs B, et al. Critical years and stages of puberty for spinal and femoral bone mass accumulation during adolescence. J Clin Endocrinol Metab 1991; 73:555–563.
6. Glastre C, Braillon P, David L, et al. Measurement of bone mineral content of the lumbar spine by dual energy x-ray absorptiometry in normal children: correlations with growth parameters. J Clin Endocrinol Metab 1990; 70:1330–1333.
7. Bonjour JP, Theintz G, Law F, et al. Peak bone mass. Osteoporosis Int 1994; 1:S7–13.
8. Young D, Hopper JL, Nowson CA, et al. Determinants of bone mass in 10 years old to 26 year old females–a twin study. J Bone Mineral Res 1995; 10:558–567.
9. Johnston CC Jr, Miller JZ, Slemenda CW, et al. Calcium supplementation and increases in bone mineral density in children. N Engl J Med 1992; 327:82–87.
10. Lloyd T, Andon MB, Rollings N, et al. Calcium supplementation and bone mineral density in adolescent girls. JAMA 1993; 270:841–844.
11. Bonjour JP, Chevalley T, Ammann P, et al. Gain in bone mineral mass in prepubertal girls 3.5 years after discontinuation of calcium supplementation: a follow-up study. Lancet 2001; 358:1208–1212.
12. Prentice A, Parsons TJ, Cole TJ. Uncritical use of bone mineral density in absorptiometry may lead to size-related artefacts in the identification of bone mineral determinants. Am J Clin Nutr 1994; 60:837–842.
13. Silverman FN. The skeletal lesions in leukemia: clinical and roentgenographic observations in 103 infants and children, with a review of the literature. Am J Radiol 1948; 59:819–844.
14. Samuda GM, Cheng MY, Yeung CY. Back pain and vertebral compression: an uncommon presentation of childhood acute lymphoblastic leukemia. J Pediatr Orthoped 1987; 7:175–178.
15. Baty JM, Vogt EC. Bone changes of leukemia in children. Am J Rhematol 1935; 34:310–314.
16. Epstein BS. Vertebral changes in childhood leukemia. Radiology 1957; 68:65–69.
17. Cohn SL, Morgan R, Mallette LE. The spectrum of metabolic bone disease in lymphoblastic leukemia. Cancer 1987; 59:346–350.
18. Newman AS, Melhorn DK. Vertebral compression in childhood leukemia. Am J Dis Child 1987; 125:863–865.
19. Masera G, Carnelli V, Ferrari M, et al. Prognostic significance of radiological bone involvement in childhood acute lymphoblastic leukemia. Arch Dis Child 1977; 52:530–533.
20. Halton JM, Atkinson SA, Traher L, et al. Mineral homeostasis and bone mass at diagnosis in children with acute lymphoblastic leukemia. J Pediatr 1995; 126:557–564.
21. Arikoski P, Komulainen J, Riikonen P, et al. Alterations in bone turnover and impaired development of bone mineral density in newly diagnosed children with cancer: a 1-year prospective study. J Clin Endocrinol Metab 1999; 84:3174–3181.
22. Lukert BP, Raisz LG. Glucocorticoid-induced osteoporosis: pathogenesis and management. Ann Intern Med 1990; 112:352–364.
23. Hahn TJ, Halstead LR, Teitelbaum SL, Hahn BH. Altered mineral metabolism in glucocorticoid-induced osteopenia: effect of 25-hydroxyvitamin D administration. J Clin Invest 1979; 64:655–665.
24. Morris HA, Need AG, O'Loughlin PD, et al. Malabsorption of calcium in corticosteroid-induced osteoporosis. Calcified Tiss Int 1990; 46:305–308.
25. Corradino R, Fullmer CS. Positive cotranscriptional regulation of intestinal calbindin-D_{28K} gene expression by 1,25-dihydroxyvitamin D_3 and glucocorticoids. Endocrinology 1991; 128:944–950.
26. Gronowicz G, McCarthy MB, Raisz LG. Glucocorticoids stimulate resorption in fetal rat parietal bones in vitro. J Bone Mineral Res 1990; 5:1223–1230.
27. Geisterfer M, Richards CD, Gauldie J. Cytokines oncostatin M and interleukin 1 regulate the expression of the IL-6 receptor (gp80, gp130). Cytokine 1995; 7:503–509.
28. Jilka RL, Hangoc G, Girasole G, et al. Increased osteoclast development after Estrogen loss: Mediation by interluekin-6. Science 1992; 257:88–91.
29. Peretz A, Praet JP, Bosson D, et al. Serum osteocalcin in the assessment of corticosteroid induced osteoporosis. Effect of long and short term corticosteroid treatment. J Rhematol 1989; 16:363–367.
30. Bellows CG, Aubin JE, Heersche JNM. Physiological concentrations of glucocorticoids stimulate formation of bone

nodules from isolated rat calvaria cells *in vitro*. *Endocrinology* 1987; **121**:1985–1992.

31. Delany A, Gabbitas B, Canalis E. Cortisol down-regulates osteoblast α1 (1) procollagen mRNA by transcriptional and post-transcriptional mechanisms. *J Cell Biochem* 1995; **57**:488–494.

• 32 Reid IR, Grey AB. Corticosteroid osteoporosis. *Bailliere Clin Rheumatol* 1993; **7**:573–587.

33. Jowsey J, Riggs BL. Bone formation in hypercortisonism. *Acta Endocrinol* 1970; **68**:21–28.

34. Aaron JE, Francis RM, Peacock M, Makins BM. Contrasting microanatomy of idiopathic and corticosteroid-induced osteoporosis. *Clin Orthoped* 1989; **243**:294–305.

35. Dempster D, Arlot M, Meunier P. Mean wall thickness and formation periods of trabecular bone packets in corticosteroid-induced osteoporosis. *Calcified Tiss Int* 1983; **35**:410–417.

36. Chappard D, Legrand E, Basle MF, *et al*. Altered trabecular architecture induced by corticosteroids: a bone histomorphometric study. *J Bone Mineral Res* 1996; **11**: 676–681.

37. Polock NA, Eisman JA, Dunstan CR, *et al*. Recovery from steroid-induced osteoporosis. *Ann Int Med* 1987; **107**:319–323.

38. Lufkin EG, Watner HW, Beigs Trath E. Reversibility of steroid-induced osteoporosis. *Am J Med* 1988; **85**:887–888.

39. Hermus A-DR, Smals AG, Swinkels LM, *et al*. Bone mineral density and bone turnover before and after surgical cure of Cushing's syndrome. *J Clin Endocrinol Metab* 1995; **80**:2859–2865.

40. Mercado-Asis L, Leong G, Reynolds J, *et al*. Bone mineral density in adult and pediatric patients with endogenous Cushing syndrome. *Programme 76th Meeting of the Endocrine Society* 1994:1569.

41. Rüegsegger P, Medici T, Anliker M. Corticosteroid-induced bone loss: a longitudinal study of alternate day therapy in patients with bronchial asthma using quantitative computed tomography. *Eur J Clin Pharmacol* 1983; **25**:615–620.

42. Ragab AH, Frech RS, Vietti TJ. Osteoporotic fractures secondary to methotrexate therapy of acute leukemia in remission. *Cancer* 1970; **25**:580–585.

43. O'Regan S, Melhorn DK, Newman AJ. Methotrexate-induced bone pain in childhood leukemia. *Am J Dis Child* 1973; **125**:489–490.

44. Stanisavljevic S, Babcock AL. Fractures in children treated with methotrexate for leukemia. *Clin Orthopaed Related Res* 1997; **125**:139–144.

45. Schwartz A, Leonidas JC. Methotrexate osteopathy. *Int Skeletal Soc* 1984; **11**:13–16.

46. Nesbit M, Krivit W, Heyn R, Sharp H. Acute and chronic effects of methotrexate on hepatic, pulmonary, and skeletal systems. *Cancer* 1976; **37**:1048–1054.

47. Nevinny MB, Krent MS, Moore EW. Metabolic studies on the effect of methotrexate. *Metabolism* 1965; **14**:135–139.

48. Meister B, Gassner I, Streif W, *et al*. Methotrexate osteopathy in infants with tumors of the central nervous system. *Med Pediatr Oncol* 1994; **23**:493–496.

49. Friedlaender GE, Tross RB, Doganis AC, *et al*. Effects of chemotherapeutic agents on bone. *J Bone Joint Surg* 1984; **66A**:602–607.

50. Grundi S, Butturini L, Ripamonti C, *et al*. The effects of methotrexate (MTX) on bone: a densitometric study conducted on 59 patients with MTX administered at different doses. *Ital J Orthopaed Traumatol* 1988; **14**:227–231.

• 51. Murray RD, Brennan BMD, Rahim A, Shalet SM. Survivors of childhood cancer: long-term endocrine and metabolic problems dwarf the growth disturbance. *Acta Paediatr Suppl* 1999; **433**:5–12.

52. Shore RM, Chesney RW, Mazess RB, *et al*. Bone mineral status in growth hormone deficiency. *J Pediatr* 1980; **96**:393–396.

53. Zamboni G, Antoniazzi F, Radetti G, *et al*. Clinical and laboratory observations: effects of two different regimens of recombinant human growth hormone therapy on the bone mineral density of patients with growth hormone deficiency. *J Pediatr* 1991; **119**:483–485.

54. Saggese G, Baroncelli GI, Bertelloni S, *et al*. Effects of long term treatment with growth hormone on bone and mineral metabolism in children with growth hormone deficiency. *J Pediatr* 1993; **122**:37–45.

55. Degerblad M, Almkvist O, Grunditz R, *et al*. Physical and psychological capabilities during substitution therapy with recombinant growth hormone in adults in the growth hormone deficiency. *Acta Endocrinol* 1990; **123**:185–193.

56. Hyer SL, Rodin DA, Tobias JH, *et al*. Growth hormone deficiency during puberty reduces adult bone mineral density. *Arch Dis Child* 1992; **67**:1472–1474.

57. Kaufman JM, Taelman P, Vermeulen A, Vandeweghe M. Bone mineral status in growth hormone-deficient males with isolated and multiple pituitary deficiencies of childhood onset. *J Clin Endocrinol Metab* 1992; **74**:118–123.

58. Amato G, Carella C, Fazio S, *et al*. Body composition, bone metabolism, and heart structure and function in growth hormone (GH)-deficient adults before and after GH replacement therapy at low doses. *J Clin Endocrinol Metab* 1993; **77**:1671–1676.

59. O'Halloran DJ, Tsatsoulis A, Whitehouse RW, *et al*. Increased bone mineral density after recombinant human growth hormone (GH) therapy in adults with isolated GH deficiency. *J Clin Endocrinol Metab* 1993; **76**:1344–1348.

◆60. De Boer H, Blok GJ, Van Lingen A, *et al*. Consequences of childhood-onset growth hormone deficiency for adult bone mass. *J Bone Mineral Res* 1994; **9**:1319–1326.

61. Rigg BL, Melton LJ. Evidence of two distinct syndromes of involutional osteoporosis. *Am J Med* 1983; **75**:899–901.

62. Richelson LS, Wahner HW, Melton LJ, Riggs BL. Relative contributions of aging and estrogen deficiency to postmenopausal bone loss. *N Engl J Med* 1984; **311**:1273–1275.

63. Redman JR, Bajorunas DR, Wong G, *et al*. Bone mineralization in women following successful treatment of Hodgkin's disease. *Am J Med* 1988; **85**:65–72.

64. Kreuser ED, Felsenberg D, Behles C, *et al*. Long-term gonadal dysfunction and its impact on bone mineralization in patients following COPP/ABVD chemotherapy for Hodgkin's disease. *Ann Oncol* 1992; **3**(Suppl.4):105–110.

65. Howell SJ, Berger G, Adams JE, Shalet SM. Bone mineral density in women with cytotoxic-induced ovarian failure. *Clin Endocrinol* 1998; **49**:397–402.

66. Finkelstein JS, Klibanski A, Neer RM, *et al*. Increases in bone density during treatment of men with idiopathic hypogonadotropic hypogonadism. *J Clin Endocrinol Metab* 1989; **69**:776–783.

67. Stepan JJ, Lachman M, Zverina J, *et al*. Castrated men exhibit bone loss: effect of calcitonin treatment on biochemical indices of bone remodeling. *J Clin Endocrinol Metab* 1989; **69**: 523–527.

68. Kirk JA, Stevens MM, Menser MA, *et al*. Growth failure and growth-hormone deficiency after treatment for acute lymphoblastic leukemia. *Lancet* 1987; **i**:190–193.

69. Crowne EC, Moore C, Wallace WHB, *et al*. A novel variant of growth hormone (GH) insufficiency following low dose cranial irradiation. *Clin Endocrinol* 1992; **36**:59–68.

70. Brennan BMD, Rahim A, Mackie EM, *et al*. Growth hormone status in adults treated for acute lymphoblastic leukemia in childhood. *Clin Endocrinol* 1998; **48**:777–783.

71. Atkinson SA, Fraher L, Gundberg CM, *et al*. Mineral homeostasis and bone mass in children treated for acute lymphoblastic leukemia. *J Pediatr* 1989; **114**:793–800.

◆72. Gilsanz V, Carlson ME, Roe TF, Ortega JA. Osteoporosis after cranial irradiation for acute lymphoblastic leukemia. *J Pediatr* 1990; **117**:238–244.

73. Nussey SS, Hyer SL, Brada M, Leiper AD. Bone mineralization after treatment of growth hormone deficiency in survivors of childhood malignancy. *Acta Paediatr Suppl* 1994; **399**:9–14.

74. Leeuw JA, Piers DA, Kamps WA. Osteoporosis in children with leukemia: a potentially debilitating anomaly. *Haematol Blood Transfusion* 1990; **33**:580–582.

75. Henderson RC, Madsen CD, Davis C, Gold SH. Bone density in survivors of childhood malignancies. *J Pediatr Hematol Oncol* 1996; **18**:367–371.

◆76. Nysom K, Holm K, Michaelsen KF, *et al.* Bone mass after treatment for acute lymphoblastic leukemia in childhood. *J Clin Oncol* 1998; **16**:3752–3760.

◆77. Warner JT, Evans WD, Webb DKH, *et al.* Relative osteopenia after treatment for acute lymphoblastic leukemia. *Pediatr Res* 1999; **45**:544–551.

◆78. Brennan BMD, Rahim A, Adams JA, *et al.* Reduced bone mineral density in young adults following cure of acute lymphoblastic leukemia in childhood. *Br J Cancer* 1999; **79**:1859–1863.

79. Slemenda CW, Miller JZ, Hui SL, *et al.* Role of physical activity in the development of skeletal mass in children. *J Bone Mineral Res* 1991; **6**:1227–1233.

◆80. Kaste SC, Jones-Wallace D, Rose SR, *et al.* Bone mineral decrements in survivors of childhood acute lymphoblastic leukemia: frequency of occurrence and risk factors for their development. *Leukemia* 2001; **15**:728–734.

81. Aisenberg J, Hsieh K, Kalaitzoglou G, *et al.* Bone mineral density in young adult survivors of childhood cancer. *J Pediatr Hematol Oncol* 1998; **20**:241–245.

82. Hoorweg-Nijman JJG, Kardos G, Roos JC, *et al.* Bone mineral density and markers of bone turnover in young adult survivors of childhood lymphoblastic leukemia. *Clin Endocrinol* 1999; **50**:237–244.

83. Arikoski P, Komulainen J, Riikonen P, *et al.* Impaired development of bone mineral density during chemotherapy: a prospective analysis of 46 children newly diagnosed with cancer. *J Bone Mineral Res* 1999; **14**:2002–2009.

84. Boot AM, van den Heuvel-Eibrink MM, Hahlen K, *et al.* Bone mineral density in children with acute lymphoblastic leukemia. *Eur J Cancer* 1999; **35**:1693–1697.

85. van der Sluis IM, van den Heuvel-Eibrink MM, Hahlen K, *et al.* Bone mineral density, body composition, height in long-term survivors of acute lymphoblastic leukemia in childhood. *Med Pediatr Oncol* 1999; **35**:415–420.

◆86. Kadan-Lottick N, Marshall JA, Baron AE, *et al.* Normal bone mineral density after treatment for childhood acute lymphoblastic leukemia diagnosed between 1991 and 1998. *J Pediatr* 2001; **138**:89–904.

87. Mithal NP, Almond MK, Evans K, Hoskin PJ. Reduced bone-mineral density in long-term survivors of medulloblastoma. *Br J Radiol* 1993; **66**:814–816.

88. Barr RD, Simpson T, Webber CE, *et al.* Osteopenia in children surviving brain tumors. *Eur J Cancer* 1998; **34**:873–877.

89. de Schepper J, Hachimi-Idrissi S, Louis O, *et al.* Bone metabolism and mineralisation after cytotoxic chemotherapy including ifosfamide. *Arch Dis Child* 1994; **71**:346–348.

90. Skinner R, Pearson ADJ, Price L, *et al.* Nephrotoxicity associated with ifosfamide. *Arch Dis Child* **71**:346–348.

9b

Bone and collagen turnover

PATRICIA M CROFTON

INTRODUCTION

Children with cancer are exposed to multiple risk factors for the development of osteoporosis. These include the disease process itself, radiotherapy, chemotherapy, poor nutrition and lack of physical activity. Any combination of these factors may result in osteopenia, failure to attain optimal peak bone mass and predisposition to later osteoporosis. Retrospective studies have confirmed that many adult survivors of childhood cancer have low bone mass (see Chapter 9a). However, these outcome studies, valuable in themselves, cannot dissect out the causes of the osteopenia. Furthermore, treatment protocols are constantly being refined and improved; retrospective outcome studies can only address the effects of earlier, often heterogeneous protocols, many of which have since become obsolete. For example, current protocols for acute lymphoblastic leukemia (ALL) now employ less cranial irradiation but more intensive chemotherapy than previously.

To gain insight into the causes and mechanisms of osteopenia in children treated for cancer, several complementary approaches are required. Each of these has advantages and potential pitfalls. In clinical studies on children with cancer, bone mineral density (BMD) is clearly the most relevant outcome measure, but there may be methodological difficulties in interpreting areal BMD measurements in children (or adults) whose treatment has resulted in impaired growth, delayed puberty and reduced final height, owing to the confounding effects of bone size. Mathematical adjustment for bone size may undercompensate or overcompensate for these effects. Changes in BMD can only be assessed at 6-monthly or yearly intervals, which may be too infrequent to determine which phases of treatment have the most deleterious effect. There is little information on bone turnover from histomorphometry in children because of the obvious ethical difficulties in carrying out repeated invasive bone biopsies and uncertainties regarding the optimal site. Clinical studies employing serial measurements of biochemical markers of bone metabolism and selected hormones may dissect out the dynamic effects of each phase of treatment on whole body bone turnover and give insight into mechanisms but cannot give information on particular bone sites, nor can they definitively separate out individual versus synergistic effects of each component of a multidrug regimen. Serial histomorphometry in animal models is useful in studying the effects of individual drugs on bone in the intact organism but requires caution in extrapolating to human children, particularly with regard to dosage. Recently, studies on cultured human bone cells have enabled researchers to tease out the effects of individual drugs and hormones at cellular level, alone or in combination. However, the behavior of cultured bone cell lines may sometimes diverge from that of true osteoblasts, and may not fully reflect the mineral milieu and complex hormonal and paracrine interactions of the intact organism. All these approaches are therefore complementary and together have helped to increase our understanding of the causes of osteopenia in survivors of childhood cancer.

Table 9b.1 *Some biochemical markers of bone and collagen turnover[a]*

Marker name	Sample type	Marker of
Bone formation		
Procollagen type I C-terminal (PICP) and N-terminal (PINP) propeptides	Plasma	Type I collagen synthesis (bone and soft tissue) and Osteoblast, early proliferative phase
Bone-specific alkaline phosphatase (ALP)	Plasma	Osteoblast, maturation phase
		Hypertrophic chondrocytes of epiphyseal growth plate
Osteocalcin (bone gla protein)	Plasma	Osteoblast, mineralization phase
Bone resorption		
Cross-linked telopeptide of type I collagen (ICTP)	Plasma	Breakdown of type I collagen
Acid phosphatase	Plasma	Osteoclast (non-specific)
Pyridinoline	Urine	Breakdown of mature, cross-linked collagen
Deoxypyridinoline	Urine	Breakdown of mature bone collagen
N-telopeptide of type I collagen (NTX)	Urine	Breakdown of type I collagen
Hydroxyproline	Urine	Collagen turnover (insensitive, non-specific for bone)

[a]Only those markers that have been included in this chapter are listed.

BIOCHEMICAL MARKERS OF BONE AND COLLAGEN TURNOVER

The main markers of bone and collagen turnover that have been used in studies of children with cancer are listed in Table 9b.1. The C-terminal and N-terminal propeptides of type I procollagen (PICP and PINP) are released into the circulation during synthesis of type I collagen, and are principally markers of proliferative osteoblasts and of bone collagen matrix formation, although lesser amounts may emanate from soft tissue (Table 9b.1).[1] Bone-specific alkaline phosphatase (ALP) and osteocalcin are markers of the mature osteoblast in its successive differentiating and mineralising phases.[2] All three markers, therefore, reflect different aspects of bone formation. Bone ALP is also found in the hypertrophic chondrocytes of the epiphyseal growth plate but contribution to circulating levels from this source is currently unknown. Bone ALP and osteocalcin change more slowly than PICP in response to disease and therapeutic interventions, but are more bone-specific.

Of the plethora of markers of bone resorption (Table 9b.1), urinary deoxypyridinoline is the most bone-specific but, because of its wide intraindividual biological variation in children,[3] it has proved a less useful marker of bone resorption in many clinical situations than a plasma-based marker, the cross-linked telopeptide of type I collagen (ICTP).

Many of these markers have been validated in adults by bone histomorphometry and calcium kinetics.[4–9] Cross-sectional studies in normal children have demonstrated wide interindividual variation in all markers of bone and collagen turnover, with a pattern during infancy, childhood and adolescence that mirrors the childhood growth curve and reflects the active processes of bone formation and resorption during growth.[1] Good age- and sex-specific reference data that are appropriate to the laboratory method used and the population studied are essential when judgements are made about whether or not a bone marker level is 'normal'. Because of the wide reference ranges, these markers are most useful when measured serially with each child acting as his/her own control.

EFFECT OF DISEASE PROCESS ON MINERAL, BONE AND COLLAGEN TURNOVER

Acute lymphoblastic leukemia

At diagnosis, plasma calcium, magnesium and phosphate are normal in children with ALL, although there may be increased urinary excretion of calcium.[10,11] Parathyroid hormone (PTH) and 25-hydroxyvitamin D (25OHD) levels are relatively normal.[10–12] 1,25-dihydroxyvitamin D ($1,25(OH)_2D$) has been variously reported to be either undetectable[10,11] or normal[12] in most children presenting with ALL. The discrepancies may have partly or wholly arisen from differences in the analytical methods used and the populations studied, and from the appropriateness of literature-based reference ranges to these particular populations and methods.

PICP, PINP, osteocalcin, and total or bone ALP are all low at diagnosis compared with age- and sex-matched healthy children, indicating decreased bone formation (Table 9b.2).[10–15] These children also have low levels of the resorption markers, ICTP and urinary pyridinoline and deoxypyridinoline,[10,12–15] confirming a low bone turnover state caused by the disease itself. Insulin-like growth factor 1 (IGF-1), IGF binding protein 3 (IGFBP-3)

Table 9b.2 *Markers of bone formation, bone resorption and the growth hormone axis at diagnosis, and before treatment in children with acute lymphoblastic leukemia*

Bone formation	Bone resorption	GH axis	Reference
Osteocalcin ↓↓ Total ALP ↓	Ur Dpd ↓	–	10, 15
–	–	IGF-1 ↓↓ IGFBP-3 ↓↓ IGFBP-2 ↑↑	16
PICP ↓↓ PINP ↓↓	ICTP ↓↓	–	13
PICP ↓↓ Bone ALP ↓↓	ICTP ↓ Ur Pyd ↓↓ Ur Dpd ↓↓	IGF-1 ↓↓ IGFBP-3 ↓ IGFBP-2 ↑↑ Ur GH ↑↑	14
PICP ↓ Osteocalcin ↓↓ Total ALP ↓	ICTP ↓	IGF-1 ↓↓ IGFBP-3 ↔	12

ALP, alkaline phosphatase; Dpd, deoxypyridinoline; GH, growth hormone; ICTP, cross-linked telopeptide of type I collagen; IGF, insulin-like growth factor; IGFBP, insulin-like growth factor binding protein; PICP, procollagen type I C-terminal propeptide; PINP, procollagen type I N-terminal propeptide; Pyd, pyridinoline; Ur, urine; ↔ normal compared with reference group; ↓ significantly low compared with healthy controls; ↓↓ markedly low (below the reference range or more than 1.5 SDs below the mean for age- and sex-matched healthy children); ↑↑ markedly high (more than 2SDs above the mean for age- and sex-matched healthy children).

and growth hormone binding protein (a measure of growth hormone receptor status) are also low at diagnosis, whereas urinary growth hormone and IGFBP-2 are increased, suggesting a growth hormone-resistant state.[12,14,16] Strong positive correlations between IGFBP-3 and IGF-1, PICP and bone ALP are consistent with a pivotal role for IGFBP-3 in controlling IGF-1 bioavailability, and hence bone formation.[14]

Solid tumors

In children with solid tumors (including lymphomas but excluding ALL), bone formation markers (PICP and bone ALP) were low at diagnosis relative to age- and sex-matched healthy children, while the bone resorption marker, ICTP, was relatively normal,[17] suggesting an imbalance between bone formation and breakdown. IGF-1 was low while IGFBP-2 was high. In general, the abnormalities were qualitatively similar to those observed in children with ALL[14] but less marked.

Mixed cancers

In a mixed group of children with leukaemias (15), lymphomas (12) and solid tumors (19), plasma calcium,

phosphate, magnesium and, to a lesser extent, PTH were significantly low at diagnosis compared with normal values.[18] Osteocalcin was also relatively low and PICP very low, while the bone resorption marker, ICTP, was slightly high, suggesting an imbalance between bone collagen synthesis and degradation. Separate data for the different diagnostic groups were not reported.

EFFECT OF TREATMENT ON BONE, MINERAL AND COLLAGEN TURNOVER

Radiotherapy

It is well-recognized that spinal irradiation causes direct, dose-dependent damage to vertebrae but it may take months or years for this to become evident.[19] Probably because of this long time lag, there have been few studies of the direct effects of irradiation on bone and collagen turnover. One study in young rats in which doses of 0.5–8 Gy were applied to the left hind leg, using the contralateral leg as a control, showed only a very transient, dose-dependent lowering effect on metaphyseal bone ALP.[20] Irradiation (0–6 Gy) of cultured mouse osteoblasts demonstrated decreased cell proliferation and dose-dependent, sustained reduction in collagen synthesis,[21] but the relevance to intact humans is uncertain. In humans, trabecular bone turnover in the vertebrae is probably the largest contributor to circulating markers of bone turnover. However, the gap in our knowledge concerning the effects of spinal irradiation on overall bone turnover in growing children is unlikely to be remedied because spinal irradiation is now largely avoided in modern treatment protocols.

Cranial irradiation appears to have little immediate effect on markers of bone formation and resorption (unpublished observations). Indirect adverse effects of cranial irradiation on BMD have been demonstrated, mediated through adverse effects on growth hormone and sex hormone secretion, and manifested mainly during puberty.[22–31] These studies have generally been retrospective outcome studies because of delayed effects, long time scales, wide normal ranges for BMD in puberty and difficulty in pinpointing when these sometimes subtle processes begin. Although growth hormone deficiency in children is associated with low levels of markers of bone and collagen turnover,[32–39] there is overlap with the normal range. There is, therefore, unlikely to be a role for these markers either in diagnosing GH deficiency or, because of the confounding effects of altered growth, in delineating its effects on bone.

Chemotherapy: specific agents

In recent years, there has been a shift away from cranial irradiation, with its long-term effects on growth and

Table 9b.3 *Effects of glucocorticoids on bone*

Bone formation	Bone resorption	Effect on bone markers
Osteoblast proliferation ↓	Osteoclast production ↓	PICP ↓
Type I collagen synthesis ↓	Osteoclast apoptosis ↔	Bone ALP ↓ or ↔ or ↑
Osteoblast differentiation ↑	Bone resorption ↓	Osteocalcin ↓↓
Osteoblast apoptosis ↑	Renal reabsorption of calcium ↓	ICTP ↓
Histomorphometric variables ↓	Intestinal absorption of calcium ↓	Ur Pyd ↓
	PTH ↑ (secondary to calcium effects)	Ur Dpd ↓

ALP, alkaline phosphatase; Dpd, deoxypyridinoline; ICTP, cross-linked telopeptide of type I collagen; PICP, procollagen type I C-terminal propeptide; PTH, parathyroid hormone; Pyd, pyridinoline; Ur, urine; ↓, decreased; ↑, increased; ↔, no change; ↓↓, markedly decreased.

BMD, and towards more intensive chemotherapy protocols, especially in the treatment of ALL. This has resulted in renewed attention being paid to possible adverse effects of chemotherapy on bone and bone metabolism. Most information is available for glucocorticoids and methotrexate, but other agents may also be implicated in adverse effects on bone and certain drug combinations may have synergistic or protective effects.

GLUCOCORTICOIDS

The adverse effects of glucocorticoids on bone and growth are well known. They have been shown to have a wide range of complex and diverse effects on bone (Table 9b.3). *In vitro*, they have a dose-dependent inhibitory effect on osteoblast proliferation and type I collagen synthesis, and promote osteoblast differentiation.[40–46] Enhanced osteoblast differentiation may lead to increased expression of ALP, as collagen synthesis is down-regulated.[47] By contract, osteocalcin synthesis is strongly inhibited by glucocorticoids, although the consequences *in vivo* are uncertain.[48]

In animal models, high-dose glucocorticoid treatment results in a decrease in bone density, trabecular narrowing, decreased serum osteocalcin, a decrease in histomorphometric variables of bone formation and an increase in osteoblast apoptosis, with reversal of these effects after weaning off steroids.[49,50] Decreased trabecular width is consistent with incomplete cavity repair. Bone biopsies taken from patients on long-term glucocorticoid treatment reveal decreased bone matrix apposition rates, decreased trabecular volume and increased osteoblast apoptosis.[45,49]

Some glucocorticoid effects may be mediated through decreased IGF-1 synthesis in osteoblasts, where IGF-1 has an autocrine role in increasing type I collagen synthesis,

matrix apposition rates and bone formation.[45] Coculture of osteoblasts with IGF-1 can partially reverse the inhibitory effects of glucocorticoids on osteoblast proliferation.[46]

It has recently been demonstrated that 11β-hydroxysteroid dehydrogenase is present in human osteoblasts, where it is regulated by a number of factors likely to be present in the bone microenvironment.[48] This enzyme alters the balance between active cortisol and inactive cortisone and may modulate some or all of the actions of glucorticoids *in vivo*.

Glucorticoid effects on osteoclasts and collagen degradation are more controversial. It has been widely assumed that these agents promote bone degradation because of the increased urinary calcium excretion observed in patients on long-term treatment. However, this may be largely due to a direct inhibitory effect on the renal tubular reabsorption of calcium.[51] A similar inhibitory effect on intestinal calcium absorption may result in a negative calcium balance. It has been demonstrated that parathyroidectomy prevents excessive bone resorption in patients treated with glucocorticoids,[45] suggesting that secondary hyperparathyroidism may be the main mechanism whereby excessive bone loss may occur in some patients on long-term glucocorticoid therapy. In animal models, glucocorticoid treatment results in decreased osteoclast production and impaired bone resorption, but no effect on osteoclast apoptosis.[49,50,52]

A number of clinical studies have demonstrated that infants and children treated with glucorticoids show dose-related suppression of all circulating markers of collagen formation and resorption, with rapid recovery – sometimes to supraphysiological levels – after stopping treatment.[53–56] This confirms that, in children, glucorticoids suppress both collagen synthesis and its degradation.

METHOTREXATE

There have been several reports of bone pain, osteoporosis, fractures and impaired bone healing in children with ALL treated under earlier protocols that employed methotrexate as the sole chemotherapeutic agent.[57–60] These children had normal growth.[60] Histomorphometric studies in rats have demonstrated that methotrexate treatment results in osteopenia, markedly reduced trabecular bone volume, low rates of bone formation and mineral apposition, but marked increases in osteoclast surface and osteoclast number.[61–63] Markers of bone formation (total ALP and osteocalcin) and the calcium content of their ashed femurs were lower in methotrexate-treated compared with control rats, although hydroxyproline excretion (an insensitive, non-specific marker of bone resorption) was similar in the two groups.[62] The adverse histomorphometric effects persisted long after cessation of treatment, with no signs of recovery.[63]

A series of *in vitro* studies have shed further light on the processes involved, although some of the evidence is conflicting. Methotrexate treatment of cultured human osteoblasts derived from trabecular bone resulted in a strong, dose-dependent inhibition of cell proliferation, but did not affect ALP or osteocalcin expression.[64] The authors concluded that methotrexate is a potent inhibitor of osteoblast proliferation but does not affect basal osteoblast phenotypic expression. Another study, employing cultured osteoblasts and osteoclast-like cells derived from neonatal mouse calvariae, found that, although osteoblast cell number was unaffected by methotrexate, osteocalcin production and matrix calcification were reduced in a dose-dependent fashion.[65] Osteoclast-like cell numbers and expression of acid phosphatase (an osteoclast marker) were not significantly affected by methotrexate. These authors concluded that methotrexate might interfere with the ability of the osteoblast to calcify matrix, possibly through defective osteocalcin production. A recent study, employing several bone cell lines that express different stages of the osteoblast phenotype, has established that the precise effect of methotrexate depends on maturation stage of the osteoblast.[66] In immature osteoblasts, methotrexate suppressed ALP activity in a dose-dependent manner and impaired calcified nodule formation, whereas in mature osteoblasts ALP was only suppressed at high doses of methotrexate.

IFOSFAMIDE

Following the first description of hypophosphatemic rickets in children treated with ifosfamide,[67] the phosphaturic effect of this drug has become well recognized. Ifosfamide affects bone indirectly through altered renal handling of phosphate rather than through a direct toxic effect on bone and, in severe cases, may result in a full-blown Fanconi syndrome with the development of rickets.[68–71] Risk factors include younger age and higher cumulative doses of ifosfamide.[72] Kother and coworkers have studied 11 children with cancer treated with chemotherapy that included ifosfamide.[73] Although they found a decrease in serum phosphate and osteocalcin during chemotherapy, associated with low fractional reabsorption of phosphate and aminoaciduria, all of these normalized after cessation of treatment. The low osteocalcin was felt to be a secondary consequence of phosphate loss. Other studies on larger groups of patients have indicated that impaired phosphate reabsorption and Fanconi syndrome may persist in a substantial proportion of patients followed up for 5 years after completion of chemotherapy[72] or even develop progressively after completion of treatment.[74] It is now common practice to monitor plasma phosphate and the renal threshold for phosphate reabsorption as part of the long-term follow-up of survivors of childhood cancer treated with high-dose ifosfamide.

CISPLATIN

Children treated with cisplatin all show significant and progressive decreases in plasma magnesium, with around half of all cisplatin-treated children developing overt hypomagnesemia.[75,76] This is due to nephrotoxicity, resulting in urinary magnesium wasting. Persistent hypomagnesemia after stopping chemotherapy has been reported in about a third of treated children, unrelated to the total dose of cisplatin received.[75,77] However, a more recent, larger study of 46 survivors of childhood cancer, investigated more than 3 years after stopping treatment, found plasma magnesium levels similar to controls.[78] Severe magnesium depletion has been shown to have adverse effects on osteoblastic activity and bone formation in some animal models.[79] In humans, severe hypomagnesemia may impair both PTH secretion and skeletal responsiveness to PTH, resulting in secondary hypocalcemia. However, the clinical significance of milder degrees of hypomagnesemia is questionable. There have been no published reports of bone turnover in children treated with cisplatin.

OTHER CHEMOTHERAPY AGENTS, ALONE OR IN COMBINATION

Doxorubicin treatment for 5 days profoundly decreases bone formation in rats, resulting in moderately decreased trabecular bone volume even over this short period.[61] Similar studies in animal models have not been performed for most other chemotherapeutic agents.

A series of elegant experiments has recently been carried out to investigate the effects of a wide range of chemotherapy agents on cultured human osteoblast-like cells.[80] The choice of drugs tested was determined by current UK treatment protocols for ALL. Cell numbers were reduced in a dose-dependent fashion by all chemotherapeutic agents tested (Table 9b.4) and a variety of dose–response curves were observed. Chemotherapy may reduce cell numbers by various mechanisms, including loss of proliferative ability and increased apoptosis. Reductions in osteoblast-like cell numbers were comparable to those observed in leukemic cells when the same agents were used in similar concentrations. Immature osteoblast-like cells (osteosarcoma and osteoprogenitor cell lines) were more chemosensitive than more highly differentiated osteoblast-like cells derived from bone explants from children. Interestingly, although treatment with dexamethasone alone had a mildly suppressive effect on cell numbers (Table 9b.4), preincubation with dexamethasone had a partially protective effect when these cells were subsequently treated with other chemotherapeutic agents. This partially protective effect was presumably mediated by the known effects of glucocorticoids in down regulating osteoblast proliferation and up regulating differentiation to a more mature chemotherapy-resistant phenotype. A further report has suggested that certain drug

combinations (vincristine/asparaginase, etoposide/ daunorubicin, cytarabine/etoposide) may inhibit bone cell proliferation to a greater extent than the individual drugs alone.[81] Similar studies of other chemotherapeutic agents

Table 9b.4 *Effect of chemotherapeutic agents used in treatment of childhood cancer on human osteoblast-like cell (MG63) numbers. Data taken from Davies et al.[80]*

Chemotherapy agent	Concentration[a] (mol/L)	Reduction in cell number[b] (%)
Vincristine	10^{-9}	50
Daunorubicin	10^{-8}	90
Methotrexate	10^{-7}	70
Cytarabine	10^{-7}	50
Etoposide	10^{-6}	40
Thioguanine	10^{-5}	30
Mercaptopurine	10^{-5}	20
Asparaginase	0.5^c	–
Dexamethasone	10^{-8}	10
Prednisolone	10^{-6}	10

[a]Minimum concentration of chemotherapy agents at which a significant decrease of osteoblast-like cell numbers occurs.
[b]Approximate degree of suppression of osteoblast-like cell numbers at a standardized drug dosage of 10^{-5} mol/l, expressed as a percentage compared with control values.
[c]Expressed as units/ml.

used in the treatment of solid tumors have not yet been performed.

These experiments demonstrate that bone cell culture studies are a powerful tool for investigating the effects of individual chemotherapeutic agents, alone or in combination. However, caution must be exercised in uncritically extrapolating these results to clinical practice. Cultured bone cells may differ from normal osteoblasts in several important respects. For example, in osteosarcoma cell lines, there is deregulation of the normal sequential pattern of gene expression, often resulting in simultaneous expression of ALP and osteocalcin, while cells are actively proliferating.[2] Furthermore, in the intact organism, there may be many other mineral, endocrine, paracrine and autocrine factors, such as growth factors and cytokines, that may modulate the effects of cytotoxic drugs on bone.

Clinical studies in children with ALL

Changes in markers of bone turnover and hormones affecting bone and mineral metabolism before, during and after chemotherapy are summarized in Table 9b.5.

INDUCTION AND/OR FIRST INTENSIFICATION

In a longitudinal study of Finnish children with ALL, employing a 6-week induction regimen comprising

Table 9b.5 *Summary of changes in bone markers before, during and after completion of chemotherapy in children with acute lymphoblastic leukemia*

Markers	Diagnosis	Induction/first intensification	Maintenance/ continuing phase	After completion
Bone formation				
PICP	Low	Further decrease	Normal	Normal
PINP	Low	Further decrease	Normal	–
Osteocalcin	Low	Further decrease	Low or normal[a]	Normal
Bone ALP	Low	Transient increase → decrease	Low	Increase to normal
Bone resorption				
ICTP	Low	Slight increase[b] or further decrease[c]	Normal	Normal
Ur Pyd	Low	Remained low or decreased further	–	–
Ur Dpd	Low	Remained low	–	–
Ur NTX	–	–	High	–
Hormones				
IGF-1	Low	Increase → normal	Normal	Normal
PTH	Normal	Slight increase	Normal	Normal
25OHD	Normal	–	Normal	Normal
1,25(OH)$_2$D	Normal or ?very low[d]	?very low[d]	?very low[d]	Normal or ?very low[d]

ALP, alkaline phosphatase; Dpd, deoxypyridinoline; ICTP, cross-linked telopeptide of type I collagen; IGF-1, insulin-like growth factor 1; NTX, N-telopeptide of type I collagen; 1,25(OH)$_2$D, 1,25-dihydroxyvitamin D; 25OHD, 25-hydroxyvitamin D; PICP, procollagen type I C-terminal propeptide; PINP, procollagen type I N-terminal propeptide; PTH, parathyroid hormone; Pyd, pyridinoline; Ur, urine.
[a]Discrepant results in successive Canadian studies.[11,84]
[b]Finnish protocol (including prednisone and methotrexate).
[c]UK protocol (including prednisolone but no systemic methotrexate).
[d]Canadian studies only.[10,11,15,84]

prednisone, methotrexate, vincristine, asparaginase and doxorubicin, PICP and PINP declined further from levels that were already low before treatment began, indicating further suppression of type I collagen synthesis and bone matrix formation.[13] ICTP, a marker of bone resorption that was low before treatment began, increased slightly during this period, although it remained low compared with published age-related reference data.

A similar longitudinal study was conducted in the UK on children following UKALL XI protocols.[14] The induction regimen (weeks 1–5) comprised prednisolone, asparaginase and vincristine, and was followed by a first intensification (week 6) that included prednisolone, vincristine, daunorubicin, etoposide, cytarabine and thioguanine. As in the Finnish study, PICP levels decreased further compared with already low levels before treatment began (Figure 9b.1). Bone ALP increased transiently, then decreased. This is consistent with the known effects of glucocorticoids in down regulating osteoblast proliferation (PICP) and enhancing osteoblast differentiation (bone ALP). The subsequent decrease in bone ALP was presumably caused by an overall reduction in the population of osteoblasts and their precursors. In contrast to the Finnish study, ICTP declined further during induction and first intensification, and urinary deoxypyridinoline, another specific marker of bone resorption, remained low. This difference may be tentatively ascribed to the use of prednisolone (suppressing bone resorption) without methotrexate in the UK protocol in contrast to the opposing effects of oral methotrexate (enhancing bone resorption) and prednisone (suppressing bone resorption) in the Finnish protocol. Urinary growth hormone decreased, whereas IGF-1 and IGFBP-3 increased during this period, implying restoration of growth hormone sensitivity. The effect of chemotherapy on markers of bone turnover was independent of its effects on IGF-1 and IGFBP-3, which normalized over this period (Figure 9b.1), suggesting a direct effect at target tissue level rather than mediated through the growth hormone-IGF-1 axis. During this period, the children demonstrated decreased height and negative lower leg growth.

A Canadian report on children treated according to Dana Farber Cancer Institute protocols 87 001 or 91 001 demonstrated that the induction phase of chemotherapy (which, like the Finnish and UK protocols, included high-dose steroids) was also associated with further suppression of osteocalcin and pyridinoline excretion.[15]

In both Finnish and UK studies, there was a rapid increase in markers of bone collagen formation (PICP, P1NP) in the 2 weeks after stopping glucocorticoid treatment, indicating a resumption of osteoblast proliferation (Figure 9b.1).[13,14] ICTP and urinary deoxypyridinoline also increased dramatically, consistent with enhanced bone turnover. These changes preceded resumption of lower leg growth.[14]

HIGH–DOSE METHOTREXATE

In the UK study, children with ALL who had been randomized to receive systemic high-dose methotrexate as central nervous system (CNS) prophylaxis in weeks 9, 11 and 13 were compared with a matching group who did not.[14] PICP and bone ALP were significantly lower and

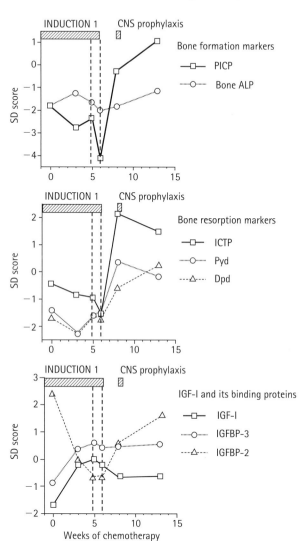

Figure 9b.1 *Changes in markers of bone formation, bone resorption and the growth hormone–IGF-1 axis in 22 newly-diagnosed children with acute lymphoblastic leukemia. First 5 weeks: induction of remission. The dashed lines indicate first intensification (1), completed in week 6. Weeks 7 and 8 were free of chemotherapy. CNS-directed treatment commenced in week 9. Markers are expressed as mean SD scores in relation to age- and sex-matched reference groups. The hatched bar indicates prednisolone treatment. ALP, alkaline phosphatase; CNS, central nervous system; Dpd, deoxypyridinoline; ICTP, cross-linked telopeptide of type I collagen; IGF-1, insulin-like growth factor 1; IGFBP-2/-3, insulin-like growth factor binding protein 2/3; PICP, procollagen type I C-terminal propeptide; Pyd, pyridinoline; Ur, urine. Data redrawn from Crofton et al.[14]*

ICTP was significantly higher in the children who received high-dose methotrexate. This is consistent with the reduced osteoblast proliferation and expression of PICP and ALP observed in earlier cell culture and animal model studies. Although evidence from these earlier studies for an effect of methotrexate on osteoclast function was conflicting, this clinical study confirms that high-dose methotrexate not only impairs bone formation but also enhances bone degradation in children.

THIRD INTENSIFICATION

In the UKALL-XI protocols, some patients were randomized to receive a third intensification block of chemotherapy, starting in week 35 and lasting 8 weeks. Third intensification comprised dexamethasone, asparaginase and vincristine followed by cytarabine, thioguanine and cyclophosphamide, a different combination of drugs from those used in the first two intensifications. A small study of nine children treated with third intensification compared with nine children treated with maintenance chemotherapy over the same period demonstrated marked reductions in PICP, bone ALP and ICTP in response to dexamethasone, indicating an overall suppression of bone turnover, but a return to baseline after dexamethasone was stopped and other drugs started.[82] The lack of catch-up in the collagen markers after stopping dexamethasone contrasts with their previous dramatic catch-up during the two chemotherapy-free weeks that followed first intensification (see above, Figure 9b.1). This discrepancy may be attributable to treatment with cytarabine and thioguanine during the latter part of third intensification: both of these drugs have been demonstrated to have toxic effects on the osteoblast *in vitro* (see above).[80]

MAINTENANCE/CONTINUING CHEMOTHERAPY

In the Finnish study, maintenance chemotherapy was instituted from week 7 of treatment and markers of collagen turnover continued to be measured up to week 12.[13] Maintenance chemotherapy comprised methotrexate alone (low-risk patients), or methotrexate, cytarabine, purinethol and cyclophosphamide (intermediate risk), or methotrexate, cytarabine, 6-mercaptopurine and cyclophosphamide (high risk). During this early period on maintenance chemotherapy, PICP, PINP and ICTP increased to normal or near-normal levels. Whether collagen turnover markers differed among treatment groups was not reported.

Children treated according to UK protocols were studied throughout their second year of chemotherapy while they were receiving a continuing chemotherapy regimen of monthly vincristine and prednisolone, weekly methotrexate and daily mercaptopurine.[83] Growth was normal. PICP, ICTP and IGF-1 did not change over this period and did not differ significantly from age- and sex-matched

controls. However, bone ALP (a more specific marker of bone formation than PICP) remained significantly low compared with age-matched controls. The low bone ALP observed at diagnosis and throughout chemotherapy is evidence that children with ALL experience a prolonged period (at least 2 years) of suboptimal bone formation. The main culprit is likely to be methotrexate. Prednisolone/vincristine are administered less frequently than methotrexate during continuing maintenance chemotherapy and, in cell-culture experiments, concomitant prednisolone administration may protect osteoblasts from the cytotoxic effects of vincristine (see above).[80]

Canadian studies have focused largely on various aspects of mineral balance. An early cross-sectional study was carried out on children following Boston protocols 81-001 and 85-001 during maintenance chemotherapy comprising, over 3-weekly cycles: prednisone (5 days), 6-mercaptopurine (14 days), vincristine (once) and methotrexate (weekly).[84] Around half the children were reported to have mild hypomagnesemia, hypomagnesiuria, ionic hypocalcemia and hypercalciuria. Total ALP was low-normal. Osteocalcin (the only bone-specific marker measured) was low and correlated with plasma magnesium. Administration of oral magnesium to a subgroup of hypomagnesemic children resulted in an increase in plasma magnesium, ionized calcium and osteocalcin into the normal range. PTH was normal but $1,25(OH)_2D$ was undetectable in almost all patients.

This preliminary Canadian study was followed by a prospective longitudinal cohort study (measurements at 6-monthly intervals) on children following the Dana Farber Cancer Institute protocol 87-001, employing a similar regimen during the maintenance phase.[11,15] Fractures occurred in around 20 per cent of children over this period, associated with progressive decreases in lumbar spine BMD in postpubertal (but not prepubertal) children. This study confirmed mild hypomagnesemia compared with a small group of age-matched controls. Dietary intake and absorption of magnesium were adequate but there may have been a mild excessive renal loss, exacerbated by aminoglycoside antibiotics during episodes of febrile neutropenia. The clinical significance of the mild hypomagnesaemia is unclear. In contrast to the earlier study, ionized calcium, osteocalcin and PTH were normal and were apparently unaffected by magnesium supplementation. $1,25(OH)_2D$ was again reported as subnormal in more than 70 per cent children, although 25OHD levels were normal. This is a puzzling finding as $1,25(OH)_2D$ is required for full osteocalcin expression by the osteoblast.[2] Deficiency usually results in high ALP and low osteocalcin,[1] together with secondary hyperparathyroidism. Instead, osteocalcin was high-normal, total ALP low-normal and PTH normal. Since the remarkably low levels of $1,25(OH)_2D$ had been present at diagnosis, had continued unchanged throughout treatment and persisted after

completion of treatment,[84] their relevance to calcium balance and bone turnover at diagnosis and during treatment must be questioned. Urinary excretion of N-telopeptide of collagen (a marker of bone resorption) was apparently increased in nearly 60 per cent children by the end of treatment but this may have been an artefact of its expression in relation to urinary creatinine, which may be lower in children with ALL than in normal healthy children.

A mixed cross-sectional and semi-longitudinal study from the Netherlands reported the effects of chemotherapy protocol ALL-8 (Dutch Childhood Leukaemia Study Group) on bone turnover in 32 children.[12] Protocol ALL-8 resembles the Berlin–Frankfurt–Münster (BFM)–ALL 90 protocol and encompasses a wide range of chemotherapy agents (including glucocorticoids and methotrexate) in the induction phase and low-dose methotrexate and mercaptopurine during maintenance therapy. Detailed changes through chemotherapy cannot be ascertained because of limitations in study design and relatively infrequent sampling intervals. However, patients treated for 6 months or longer had levels of PICP, osteocalcin, ICTP, IGF-1 and IGFBP-3 that were higher than patients studied at diagnosis and not significantly different from controls.

POSTCHEMOTHERAPY

A small cohort of seven children was studied at completion of chemotherapy according to UK protocols and followed up for 1–3 months after stopping treatment.[83] PICP and ICTP were normal compared with age- and sex-matched controls while on treatment and did not change after treatment was completed. There was evidence of a contribution to circulating PICP arising from soft tissue collagen synthesis in addition to the contribution from bone. By contrast, bone ALP was low on treatment and increased in all patients after stopping treatment. There was, therefore, evidence of short-term recovery of osteoblast function after stopping chemotherapy.

Atkinson and coworkers studied a cohort of 16 children with ALL treated according to Boston protocols 81-001 and 85-001 during maintenance chemotherapy and again more than 6 months after completion of chemotherapy.[84] In terms of mineral balance, plasma and urinary magnesium increased to normal values, while urinary calcium excretion decreased to normal values after cessation of treatment. Osteocalcin increased from low to normal values, while total ALP (a crude, non-specific marker of bone formation) increased from low-normal to high-normal values. Overall, the study confirmed osteoblast recovery in the medium term.

In a cross-sectional study of 21 survivors of ALL, who had been treated with a variety of chemotherapy regimens (all including methotrexate) according to Italian Association of Pediatric Hematology and Oncology protocols between 6 months and 2 years previously, PICP,

osteocalcin, bone ALP, calcium, phosphate, magnesium, 25OHD and 1,25(OH)$_2$D were all normal.[85] PTH and calcitonin were slightly lower than in controls. The explanation for this is uncertain and the clinical significance, if any, unclear. This study confirmed normal bone formation and normal mineral metabolism after completion of maintenance chemotherapy.

Similarly, in a small group of survivors of ALL treated by chemotherapy alone according to the Dutch ALL-8 protocol (comprising a wide range of chemotherapy agents, including glucocorticoids and methotrexate) and studied 1 year after completion of treatment, calcium, phosphate, PICP, osteocalcin, total ALP, ICTP, PTH and 1,25(OH)$_2$D were all normal.[12]

Other retrospective studies have been conducted on adult survivors of childhood ALL treated with a mixture of protocols that included glucocorticoids, vincristine, methotrexate and cranial irradiation. In a UK study, osteocalcin and ICTP were similar to age- and BMI-matched young adult controls,[86] implying normal bone turnover despite inclusion in the study of some GH-deficient and GH-insufficient patients. Similarly, in a Netherlands study, PICP, bone ALP, ICTP and urinary calcium excretion were all similar to age- and sex-matched controls.[87] This was despite evidence of impaired GH secretion and low IGF-1 in several of the patients, presumably attributable to the cranial irradiation most of them had received.

Clinical studies in children with solid tumors

A study on 25 children with solid tumors (five with lymphomas) demonstrated that bone ALP increased gradually through the first few cycles of intensive blocks of chemotherapy, but remained low relative to age- and sex-matched healthy children.[17] Samples collected immediately prior to each block of chemotherapy showed a gradual increase in PICP from low levels at diagnosis to normal levels within the first few cycles. Preblock ICTP also rose to high-normal over the same period. IGF-1 increased gradually to normal, while IGFBP-2 decreased to high-normal levels. PICP and ICTP showed a cyclical pattern, decreasing markedly immediately after each block of intensive chemotherapy but recovering between blocks. This pattern was attributed to the high-dose dexamethasone administered as an antiemetic in conjunction with each chemotherapy block, causing marked suppression of collagen turnover. Some children with lymphoma did not receive high-dose dexamethasone as an antiemetic but did receive prednisolone as part of their chemotherapy: these children had an identical cyclical pattern in their collagen markers. The marked cyclical changes in collagen turnover associated with the widespread use of high-dose steroids as antiemetic therapy

tend to obscure any separate underlying effect of the chemotherapy blocks themselves. However, there was some evidence that the intermittent blocks of intensive chemotherapy used to treat solid tumors may have resulted in a moderate excess of bone collagen degradation over synthesis throughout treatment. The relatively low levels of bone ALP also suggests an adverse effect on osteoblast maturation that, in some children, persisted throughout treatment.

Clinical studies in children with mixed cancers

Arikoski and coworkers studied a group of 46 children, comprising 15 with leukemias (11 with ALL), 12 with lymphomas and 19 with solid tumors, who were followed up for 6 months from diagnosis.[18] Children with leukemias were treated with chemotherapy alone according to the protocols of the Nordic Society of Pediatric Hematology and Oncology. Patients with solid tumors were treated according to various international protocols. Most of the children with leukemias or lymphomas, but only around one-third of the patients with solid tumors received glucocorticoids or methotrexate. An overlapping cohort of 28 children (10 ALL, 18 solid tumors) was followed up for 1 year.[88] Some of these children also received radiotherapy to various sites. In a further cross-sectional study, this Finnish group measured bone turnover markers after completion of chemotherapy in 22 children with ALL and 26 children with other malignancies.[89]

The low levels of PICP and osteocalcin observed at diagnosis did not change during the first month of treatment but increased thereafter to reach normal levels after 6 months.[18] The slightly high ICTP at diagnosis increased further during this period. This apparent continued excess of bone resorption over bone formation coincided with a decrease in apparent volumetric BMD in the femoral neck and, to a lesser degree, the lumbar spine. There was no correlation between individual biochemical markers and percentage change in BMD at the two sites. However, there was a correlation between the cumulative dose of methotrexate and ICTP at 6 months, suggesting that this agent may be causally implicated in the apparent excess of bone resorption.

In the overlapping cohort of patients with ALL and solid tumors studied over 1 year of chemotherapy, similar changes in bone markers were reported over the first 6 months of treatment, with little further change in the markers between 6 months and 1 year.[88] The slightly low 25OHD reported at diagnosis (taking into account seasonal variation) did not change during the 1 year follow-up and was probably a result of nutritional deficits and reduced sunlight exposure. 1,25(OH)$_2$D (relatively normal at diagnosis) also changed little after 1 year. PTH

(low-normal at diagnosis) increased significantly during treatment but whether it exceeded normal values in any patient was not reported. At diagnosis, BMD values in the femoral neck and lumbar spine were similar to controls. After 1 year of treatment BMD had decreased in the femoral neck and was correlated with osteocalcin at diagnosis, suggesting that, over this longer time scale, the early deficit in bone mineralization reflected by osteocalcin may have been linked to the later outcome of reduced bone mass acquisition at this site. In this report, BMD in the lumbar spine did not change significantly over 1 year of chemotherapy in the group as a whole but was nevertheless correlated with PICP measured at 1 year, suggesting a relationship between rates of bone collagen synthesis, reflected by PICP, and BMD outcome at the lumbar spine.

In the separate group of children with cancer studied cross-sectionally around 1 month after completion of chemotherapy, PICP, osteocalcin and total ALP were similar to published reference data but ICTP was slightly increased, possibly indicating a slight excess of bone resorption.[89] The authors speculated that a possible explanation may have been decreased physical activity associated with disease and hospitalization. Plasma calcium, 25OHD and 1,25(OH)$_2$D were modestly low compared with literature-based reference values. PTH was generally normal.

In these heterogenous groups of children with cancer, there was, therefore, evidence that low bone formation at diagnosis was corrected within 6 months of starting treatment, whereas the apparent slight excess of bone resorption persisted throughout treatment. A mild deficit in vitamin D may have contributed to hypocalcemia in some patients but, in the absence of apparent secondary hyperparathyroidism, it is unlikely that this had a major impact on bone resorption. It was not possible to tease out the relative contributions of chemotherapy and radiotherapy to the observed effects of treatment on bone turnover and BMD.

Bone marrow transplants

There are no published data on the effects of bone marrow transplants on bone turnover in children. A prospective longitudinal study on adults undergoing bone marrow transplant for hematological malignancies found that osteocalcin and bone ALP decreased progressively, with a nadir 2–3 weeks after marrow infusion, while ICTP increased over the same period.[90] None of the markers regained baseline levels over the 12 weeks of the study. Various myeloablative regimens were employed, all involving high-dose chemotherapy and around half involving total body irradiation. Regimens that included glucocorticoids resulted in a lower level of osteocalcin (the synthesis of which is specifically inhibited by glucocorticoids), but

no difference in bone ALP or ICTP compared with non-glucocorticoid regimens. The authors speculated that myeloablative therapy may damage osteoprogenitor cells and that some of the inhibition of osteoblast function and stimulation of bone resorption may be mediated by cytokine release. A more recent prospective longitudinal study of adults undergoing bone marrow transplants for hematological diseases confirmed that osteocalcin decreased to a nadir 3 weeks after marrow transplant but recovered to basal levels by 3 months.[91] ICTP increased to a maximum at 4 weeks, decreasing more gradually to reach basal levels after 1 year post-transplant. There was no difference in marker response between patients who had total body irradiation as part of the myeloablative regimen and those who did not. This evidence of a relatively prolonged excess of bone resorption over formation, apparently largely attributable to high-dose chemotherapy, was associated with a decline in BMD of the lumbar spine and proximal femoral head over the 1 year of follow-up. Such studies have not been replicated in children, but it seems likely that bone marrow transplant would also result in adverse effects on bone formation and resorption in children.

NUTRITION

Children with malnutrition have decreased rates of bone formation and increased rates of bone resorption.[92] Adolescent patients with anorexia nervosa have relatively normal levels of bone formation markers (PICP and osteocalcin) but high levels of bone resorption markers (ICTP and deoxypyridinoline).[93] In severely malnourished young children, PICP, bone ALP, IGF-1 and IGFBP-3 are low, but increase during nutritional rehabilitation, while ICTP and IGFBP-2 are high and decrease during refeeding.[94] Many of these responses are apparently mediated through IGF-1 and its binding proteins. There is, therefore, mounting evidence that malnutrition in children may result in impaired bone and collagen formation, and increased bone collagen degradation. In children with malignancies, poor nutrition at diagnosis, during intensive chemotherapy and during episodes of febrile neutropenia may contribute to some of the observed abnormalities of bone and collagen turnover, but it may well be impossible to design studies that can tease out these effects.

PHYSICAL ACTIVITY

Although the beneficial effects of physical activity on bone mass are well recognized, few studies have examined its effects on markers of bone turnover in children. In healthy peripubertal girls, bone markers (PINP, bone ALP, osteocalcin and ICTP) were not apparently directly related to physical activity but did account for a small, but significant proportion of the variation in bone mass acquisition at the femoral neck and lumbar spine over 1 year of follow-up.[95] Although it is well known that immobilization may result in marked bone loss, there is little or no published evidence for its effects on markers of bone turnover in children. The existing evidence of a direct effect of physical activity on markers of bone turnover is, therefore, weak. Children with cancer may have low levels of physical activity and periods of immobilization in hospital. No studies have specifically addressed the question of whether this reduced physical activity in children with cancer may contribute to the low bone turnover observed in most patients at diagnosis, to the marked changes in bone markers observed during intensive chemotherapy or to the slight chronic excess of bone resorption compared with formation observed during the less intensive phases of chemotherapy in some studies.

CONCLUSIONS

Most clinical studies have concentrated on children with ALL, since these form a homogeneous group treated according to standardized intensive chemotherapy protocols. There are fewer reports for children with solid tumors or mixed cancers, and these are more difficult to interpret because of the variety of different primary cancers and of treatment regimens.

At diagnosis, children with ALL have growth hormone resistance and low rates of bone turnover likely to be caused by the disease itself. Chemotherapy affects bone directly at target tissue level rather than through the growth hormone–IGF-1 axis. During induction of remission, markers of bone formation are further suppressed, while markers of bone resorption either remain suppressed or increase slightly, depending on the exact chemotherapy protocol used. This further suppression of bone turnover is likely to be due to glucocorticoids: when these are stopped, bone turnover increases dramatically. High-dose methotrexate, used during CNS prophylaxis, impairs bone formation and enhances bone resorption. During less intensive maintenance/continuing phases of chemotherapy, both growth and collagen turnover are relatively normal but low bone ALP levels indicate a chronic deficit in osteoblastic function, which subsequently returns to normal after completion of chemotherapy. Although there is no evidence of any long-term persistence of abnormalities in bone turnover, the early marked suppression of bone turnover coupled with evidence of abnormal osteoblast function throughout the 2 years of chemotherapy may contribute to the increased fracture rate and decline in BMD SD scores reported in some studies. Evidence for possible influences of vitamin D and its

metabolites on bone mineralization in children with ALL is conflicting, while the clinical significance of mild hypomagnesemia is doubtful. The contribution of nutritional deficits, periods of hospitalization and low physical activity to the changes in bone turnover observed have not been ascertained, but are likely to have only a modest modulating influence.

Children with solid tumors and lymphomas have low rates of bone formation but relatively normal rates of bone resorption at diagnosis. Although bone formation increases during the first few months of chemotherapy, so does bone resorption and an apparent imbalance between formation and resorption persists throughout treatment. The clinical significance of this imbalance and how it may contribute to bone acquisition and peak bone mass over the longer term are at present unclear.

Studies in animal models that are designed to assess the effects of individual chemotherapy agents on bone have largely been restricted to glucocorticoids and methotrexate. Recent *in vitro* bone cell culture studies have demonstrated that a wide range of other chemotherapy agents may also have adverse effects on osteoblasts and that some drug combinations may have synergistic effects, whereas glucorticoids may partially protect osteoblasts by down regulating proliferation and accelerating differentiation. Further studies into detailed mechanisms and reversibility are awaited.

KEY POINTS

- Children with acute lymphoblastic leukemia (ALL) have very low rates of bone formation and variably low rates of bone resorption at diagnosis.
- Periods of intensive chemotherapy in children treated for ALL are associated with further suppression of bone formation and continued low bone resorption, probably largely due to their glucocorticoid component.
- High-dose methotrexate impairs bone formation and enhances bone resorption.
- Children with ALL have evidence of impaired osteoblast function throughout treatment.
- In children with ALL, osteoblast function returns to normal after completion of chemotherapy.
- Children with solid tumors have low rates of bone formation but normal rates of bone resorption at diagnosis.
- In children with solid tumors, both bone formation and bone resorption increase during treatment, but the slight imbalance between the two persists.
- Both the underlying disease process and chemotherapy affect bone turnover in children with cancer, and both are likely to contribute to reduced net bone mass acquisition during treatment.

REFERENCES

● 1. Crofton PM, Kelnar CJH. Bone and collagen markers in paediatric practice. *Int J Clin Pract* 1998; **52**:557–565.
● 2. Stein GS, Lian JB, Owen TA. Relationship of cell growth to the regulation of tissue-specific gene expression during osteoblast differentiation. *FASEB J* 1990; **4**:111–123.
3. Shaw NJ, Dutton J, Fraser WD, Smith CS. Urinary pyridinoline and deoxypyridinoline excretion in children. *Clin Endocrinol* 1995; **42**:607–612.
4. Delmas PD, Malaval L, Arlot ME, Meunier PJ. Serum bone gla-protein compared to bone histomorphometry in endocrine diseases. *Bone* 1985; **6**:339–341.
5. Eastell R, Delmas PD, Hodgson SF, *et al*. Bone formation rate in older normal women: concurrent assessment with bone histomorphometry, calcium kinetics, and biochemical markers. *J Clin Endocrinol Metab* 1988; **67**:741–748.
6. Eastell R, Hampton L, Colwell A, *et al*. Urinary collagen crosslinks are highly correlated with radioisotopic measurements of bone resorption. In: Christiansen C, Overgaard K (eds) *Osteoporosis.* Copenhagen: Osteopress ApS, 1990:469–470.
7. Delmas PD, Schlemmer A, Gineyts E, *et al*. Urinary excretion of pyridinoline crosslinks correlates with bone turnover measured on ileac crest biopsy in patients with vertebral osteoporosis. *J Bone Miner Res* 1991; **6**:639–644.
8. Eriksen EF, Charles P, Melsen F, *et al*. Serum markers of type I collagen formation and degradation in metabolic bone disease: correlation with bone histomorphometry. *J Bone Miner Res* 1993; **8**:127–132.
9. Charles P, Mosekilde L, Risteli L, *et al*. Assessment of bone remodeling using biochemical indicators of type I collagen synthesis and degradation: relation to calcium kinetics. *Bone Miner* 1994; **24**:81–94.
10. Halton JM, Atkinson SA, Fraher L, *et al*. Mineral homeostasis and bone mass at diagnosis in children with acute lymphoblastic leukemia. *J Pediatr* 1995; **126**:557–564.
11. Halton JM, Atkinson SA, Fraher L, *et al*. Altered mineral metabolism and bone mass in children during treatment for acute lymphoblastic leukemia. *J Bone Miner Res* 1996; **11**:1774–1783.
12. Boot AM, van den Heuvel-Eibrink MM, Hählen K, *et al*. Bone mineral density in children with acute lymphoblastic leukaemia. *Eur J Cancer* 1999; **35**:1693–1697.
13. Sorva R, Kivivuori S-M, Turpeinen M, *et al*. Very low rate of type I collagen synthesis and degradation in newly diagnosed children with acute lymphoblastic leukemia. *Bone* 1997; **20**:139–143.
◆ 14. Crofton PM, Ahmed SF, Wade JC, *et al*. Effects of intensive chemotherapy on bone and collagen turnover and the growth hormone axis in children with acute lymphoblastic leukemia. *J Clin Endocrinol Metab* 1998; **83**:3121–3129.
15. Atkinson SA, Halton JM, Bradley C, *et al*. Bone and mineral abnormalities in childhood acute lymphoblastic leukemia: influence of disease, drugs and nutrition. *In J Cancer* 1998; (Suppl. 11):35–39.
16. Mohnike KL, Kluba U, Mittler U, *et al*. Serum levels of insulin-like growth factor-I, -II and insulin-like growth factor binding proteins -2 and -3 in children with acute lymphoblastic leukaemia. *Eur J Pediatr* 1996; **155**:81–86.
17. Bath LE, Crofton PM, Evans AEM, *et al*. Bone turnover and growth during and after chemotherapy in children with solid tumours. *Pediatr Res* (in press).
18. Arikoski P, Komulainen J, Riikonen P, *et al*. Impaired development of bone mineral density during chemotherapy: a prospective analysis of 46 children newly diagnosed with cancer. *J Bone Miner Res* 1999; **14**:2002–2009.

19. Neuhauser EB, Wittenborg MH, Berman CZ, Cohen J. Irradiation effects of roentgen therapy on the growing spine. *Radiology* 1952; **59**:637–650.
20. Engström H, Turesson I, Waldenström J. The effect of 50 kV X-ray irradiation on the alkaline phosphatase activity of growing rat bone. *Int J Radiat Biol* 1981; **40**:659–663.
21. Gal TJ, Munoz-Antonia T, Muro-Cacho CA, Klotch DW. Radiation effects on osteoblasts *in vitro*: a potential role in osteoradionecrosis. *Arch Otolaryngol Head Neck Surg* 2000; **126**:1124–1128.
22. Shalet SM, Beardwell CG, Pearson D, Morris Jones PH. The effect of varying doses of cerebral irradiation on growth hormone production in childhood. *Clin Endocrinol* 1976; **5**:287–290.
23. Ahmed SR, Shalet SM, Beardwell CG. The effects of cranial irradiation on growth hormone secretion. *Acta Paediatr Scand* 1986; **75**:255–260.
24. Kirk JA, Raghupathy P, Stevens MM, *et al.* Growth failure and growth-hormone deficiency after treatment for acute lymphoblastic leukaemia. *Lancet* 1987; **i**:190–193.
25. Cicognani A, Cacciari E, Vecchi V, *et al.* Differential effects of 18- and 24-Gy cranial irradiation on growth rate and growth hormone release in children with prolonged survival after acute lymphocytic leukemia. *Am J Dis Child* 1988; **142**:1199–1202.
26. Lannering B, Rosberg S, Marky I, Moëll C. *et al.* Reduced growth hormone secretion with maintained periodicity following cranial irradiation in children with acute lymphoblastic leukaemia. *Clin Endocrinol* 1995; **42**:153–159.
27. Gilsanz V, Carlson ME, Roe TF, Ortega JA. Osteoporosis after cranial irradiation for acute lymphoblastic leukemia. *J Pediatr* 1990; **117**:238–244.
28. Nussey SS, Hyer SL, Brada M, Leiper AD. Bone mineralization after treatment of growth hormone deficiency in survivors of childhood malignancy. *Acta Paediatr* 1994; (Suppl. 399): 9–14.
29. Arikoski P, Komulainen J, Voutilainen R, *et al.* Reduced bone mineral density in long-term survivors of childhood acute lymphoblastic leukemia. *J Pediatr Hematol Oncol* 1998; **20**:234–240.
30. Arikoski P, Komulainen J, Riikonen P, *et al.* Reduced bone density at completion of chemotherapy for a malignancy. *Arch Dis Child* 1999; **80**:143–148.
31. Warner JT, Evans WD, Webb DK, *et al.* Relative osteopenia after treatment for acute lymphoblastic leukemia. *Pediatr Res* 1999; **45**:544–551.
32. Johansen JS, Jensen SB, Riis BJ, *et al.* Serum bone gla protein: a potential marker of growth hormone (GH) deficiency and the response to GH therapy. *J Clin Endocrinol Metab* 1990; **71**:122–126.
33. Trivedi P, Risteli J, Risteli L, *et al.* Serum concentrations of the type I and III procollagen propeptides as biochemical markers of growth velocity in healthy infants and children with growth disorders. *Pediatr Res* 1991; **30**:276–280.
34. Kanzaki S, Hosoda K, Moriwake T, *et al.* Serum propeptide and intact molecular osteocalcin in normal children and children with growth hormone (GH) deficiency: a potential marker of bone growth and response to GH therapy. *J Clin Endocrinol Metab* 1992; **75**:1104–1109.
35. Sartorio A, Conti A, Monzani M. New markers of bone and collagen turnover in children and adults with growth hormone deficiency. *Postgrad Med J* 1993; **69**:846–850.
36. Kubo T, Tanaka H, Inoue M, *et al.* Serum levels of carboxyterminal propeptide of type I procollagen and pyridinoline crosslinked telopeptide of type I collagen in normal children and children with growth hormone (GH) deficiency during GH therapy. *Bone* 1995; **17**:397–401.
37. Fujimoto S, Kubo T, Tanaka H, *et al.* Urinary pyridinoline and deoxypyridinoline in healthy children and in children with growth hormone deficiency. *J Clin Endocrinol Metab* 1995; **80**:1922–1928.

38. Marowska J, Kobylinska M, Lukaszkiwicz J, *et al.* Pyridinium crosslinks of collagen as a marker of bone resorption rates in children and adolescents: normal values and clinical application. *Bone* 1996; **19**:669–677.
39. Tobiume H, Kanzaki S, Hida S, *et al.* Serum bone alkaline phosphatase isoenzyme levels in normal children and children with growth hormone (GH) deficiency: a potential marker for bone formation and response to GH therapy. *J Clin Endocrinol Metab* 1997; **82**:2056–2061.
●40. Cutroneo KR, Rokowski R, Counts DF. Glucocorticoids and collagen synthesis: comparison of *in vivo* and cell culture studies. *Collagen Rel Res* 1981; **1**:557–568.
41. Canalis E. Effect of glucocorticoids on type I collagen synthesis, alkaline phosphatase activity, and deoxyribonucleic acid content in cultured rat calvariae. *Endocrinology* 1983; **112**:931–939.
●42. Oikarinen AI, Uitto J, Oikarinen J. Glucocorticoid action on connective tissue: from molecular mechanisms to clinical practice. *Med Biol* 1986; **64**:221–230.
●43. Delaney AM, Dong Y, Canalis E. Mechanisms of glucocorticoid action in bone cells. *J Cell Biochem* 1994; **56**:295–302.
44. Delaney AM, Gabbitas BY, Canalis E. Cortisol down regulates osteoblast alpha 1 (I) procollagen mRNA by transcriptional and posttranscriptional mechanisms. *J Cell Biochem* 1995; **57**:488–494.
●45. Canalis E. Mechanisms of glucocorticoid action in bone: implications to glucocorticoid-induced osteoporosis. *J Clin Endocrinol Metab* 1996; **81**:3441–3447.
46. Jonsson KB, Frost A, Larsson R, *et al.* A new fluorometric assay for determination of osteoblastic proliferation: effects of glucocorticoids and insulin-like growth factor-I. *Calcif Tissue Int* 1997; **60**:30–36.
47. Kasperk C, Schneider U, Sommer U, *et al.* Differential effects of glucocorticoids on human osteoblastic cell metabolism *in vitro*. *Calcif Tissue Int* 1995; **57**:120–126.
●48. Cooper MS, Hewison M, Stewart PM. Glucocorticoid activity, inactivity and the osteoblast. *J Endocrinol* 1999; **163**:159–164.
49. Weinstein RS, Jilka RL, Parfitt AM, Manolagas SC. Inhibition of osteoblastogenesis and promotion of apoptosis of osteoblasts and osteocytes by glucocorticoids. *J Clin Invest* 1998; **102**:274–282.
50. Silvestrini SG, Ballanti P, Patacchioli FR, *et al.* Evaluation of apoptosis and the glucocorticoid receptor in the cartilage growth plate and metaphyseal bone cells of rats after high-dose treatment with corticosterone. *Bone* 2000; **26**:33–42.
51. Gennari C. Glucocorticoid induced osteoporosis. *Clin Endocrinol* 1994; **41**:273–274.
52. Defranco DJ, Lian JB, Glowacki J. Differential effects of glucocorticoid on recruitment and activity of osteoclasts induced by normal and osteocalcin-deficient bone implanted in rats. *Endocrinology* 1992; **131**:114–121.
53. Hyams JS, Moore RE, Leichtner AM, *et al.* Relationship of type I procollagen to corticosteroid therapy in children with inflammatory bowel disease. *J Pediatr* 1988; **112**:893–898.
54. Wolthers OD, Juul A, Hansen M, *et al.* The insulin-like growth factor axis and collagen turnover during prednisolone treatment. *Arch Dis Child* 1994; **71**:409–413.
55. Birkebæk NH, Esberg G, Andersen K, *et al.* Bone and collagen turnover during treatment with inhaled dry powder budesonide and beclomethasone dipropionate. *Arch Dis Child* 1995; **73**:524–527.
56. Crofton PM, Shrivastava A, Wade JC, *et al.* Effects of dexamethasone treatment on bone and collagen turnover in preterm infants with chronic lung disease. *Pediatr Res* 2000; **48**:155–162.
57. Ragab AH, Frech RS, Vietti TJ. Osteoporotic fractures secondary to methotrexate therapy of acute leukemia in remission. *Cancer* 1970; **25**:580–585.

58. Nesbit M, Krivit W, Heyn R, Sharp H. Acute and chronic effects of methotrexate on hepatic, pulmonary, and skeletal systems. *Cancer* 1976; **37**:1048–1054.

59. Stanisavljevic S, Babcock AL. Fractures in children treated with methotrexate for leukemia. *Clin Orthop* 1977; **125**:139–142.

60. Schwartz AM, Leonidas JC. Methotrexate osteopathy. *Skel Radiol* 1984; **11**:13–16.

♦ 61. Friedlaender GE, Tross RB, Doganis AC, *et al*. Effects of chemotherapeutic agents on bone. I. Short-term methotrexate and doxorubicin (adriamycin) treatment in a rat model. *J Bone Joint Surg* 1984; **66**:602–607.

♦ 62. May KP, West SG, McDermott MT, Huffer WE. The effect of low-dose methotrexate on bone metabolism and histomorphometry in rats. *Arthritis Rheum* 1994; **37**:201–206.

♦ 63. Wheeler DL, Vander Griend RA, Wronski TJ, *et al*. The short- and long-term effects of methotrexate on the rat skeleton. *Bone* 1995; **16**:215–221.

64. Scheven BAA, van der Veen MJ, Damen CA, *et al*. Effects of methotrexate on human osteoblasts *in vitro*: modulation by 1,25-dihydroxyvitamin D_3. *J Bone Miner Res* 1995; **10**:874–880.

65. May KP, Mercill D, McDermott MT, West SG. The effect of methotrexate on mouse bone cells in culture. *Arthritis Rheum* 1996; **39**:489–494.

66. Uehara R, Suzuki Y, Ichikawa Y. Methotrexate (MTX) inhibits osteoblastic differentiation *in vitro*: possible mechanism of MTX osteopathy. *J Rheumatol* 2001; **28**:251–256.

67. Skinner R, Pearson ADJ, Price L, *et al*. Hypophosphataemic rickets after ifosfamide treatment in children. *Br Med J* 1989; **298**:1560–1561.

68. Burk CD, Restaino I, Kaplan BS, Meadows AT. Ifosfamide-induced renal tubular dysfunction and rickets in children with Wilms tumor. *J Pediatr* 1990; **117**:331–335.

69. Pratt CB, Meyer WH, Jenkins JJ, *et al*. Ifosfamide, Fanconi's syndrome, and rickets. *J Clin Oncol* 1991; **9**:1495–1499.

♦ 70. Skinner R, Sharkey IM, Pearson AD, Craft AW. Ifosfamide, mesna, and nephrotoxicity in children. *J Clin Oncol* 1993; **11**:173–190.

71. Segal LS, Palumbo RC, Robertson WW. The development of rickets as a complication of chemotherapy for the treatment of Wilms' tumor. *Orthopedics* 1995; **18**:261–264.

♦ 72. Loebstein R, Atanackovic G, Bishai R, *et al*. Risk factors for long-term outcome of ifosfamide-induced nephrotoxicity in children. *J Clin Pharmacol* 1999; **39**:454–461.

73. Kother M, Schindler J, Oette K, Berthold F. Abnormalities in serum osteocalcin values in children receiving chemotherapy including ifosfamide. *In Vivo* 1992; **6**:219–221.

74. Rossi R, Pleyer J, Schafers P, *et al*. Development of ifosfamide-induced nephrotoxicity: prospective follow-up in 75 patients. *Med Pediatr Oncol* 1999; **32**:177–182.

75. Ariceta G, Rodriguez-Soriano J, Vallo A, Navajas A. Acute and chronic effects of cisplatin therapy on renal magnesium homeostasis. *Med Pediatr Oncol* 1997; **28**:35–40.

♦ 76. Lajer H, Daugaard G. Cisplatin and hypomagnesemia. *Cancer Treat Rev* 1999; **25**:47–58.

77. Brock PR, Koliouskas DE, Barratt TM, *et al*. Partial reversibility of cisplatin nephrotoxicity in children. *J Pediatr* 1991; **118**:531–534.

♦ 78. von der Weid NX, Erni BM, Mamie C, *et al*. Cisplatin therapy in childhood: renal follow up 3 years or more after treatment. Swiss

Pediatric Oncology Group. *Nephrol Dial Transplant* 1999; **14**:1441–1444.

● 79. Wallach S. Effects of magnesium on skeletal metabolism. *Magnes Trace Elem* 1990; **9**:1–14.

♦ 80. Davies JH, Evans BAJ, Jenney MEM, Gregory JW. In vitro effects of chemotherapeutic agents on human osteoblast-like cells. *Calcif Tissue Int* 2002; **70**:408–415.

♦ 81. Davies JH, Evans BAJ, Jenney MEM, Gregory JW. In vitro effects of combination chemotherapy on osteoblasts: implications for osteopenia in childhood malignancy. *Bone* 2002; **31**:319–326.

82. Crofton PM, Ahmed SF, Wade JC, *et al*. Effects of a third intensification block of chemotherapy on bone and collagen turnover, insulin-like growth factor I, its binding proteins and short-term growth in children with acute lymphoblastic leukaemia. *Eur J Cancer* 1999; **35**:960–967.

83. Crofton PM, Ahmed SF, Wade JC, *et al*. Bone turnover and growth during and after continuing chemotherapy in children with acute lymphoblastic leukemia. *Pediatr Res* 2000; **48**:490–496.

84. Atkinson SA, Fraher L, Gundberg CM, *et al*. Mineral homeostasis and bone mass in children treated for acute lymphoblastic leukemia. *J Pediatr* 1989; **114**:793–800.

85. Praticò G, Caltabiano L, Ragusa R, *et al*. Bone metabolism in childhood acute lymphoblastic leukemia off-therapy. *Int J Pediatr Hematol Oncol* 1998; **5**:437–442.

86. Brennan BM, Rahim A, Adams JA, *et al*. Reduced bone mineral density in young adults following cure of acute lymphoblastic leukaemia in childhood. *Br J Cancer* 1999; **79**:1859–1863.

87. Hoorweg-Nijman JJG, Kardos G, Roos JC, *et al*. Bone mineral density and markers of bone turnover in young adult survivors of childhood lymphoblastic leukaemia. *Clin Endocrinol* 1999; **50**:237–244.

♦ 88. Arikoski P, Komulainen J, Riikonen P, *et al*. Alterations in bone turnover and impaired development of bone mineral density in newly diagnosed children with cancer: a 1-year prospective study. *J Clin Endocrinol Metab* 1999; **84**:3174–3181.

89. Arikoski P, Kröger H, Riikonen P, *et al*. Disturbance in bone tunover in children with a malignancy at completion of chemotherapy. *Med Pediatr Oncol* 1999; **33**:455–461.

● 90. Carlson K, Simonsson B, Ljunghall S. Acute effects of high-dose chemotherapy followed by bone marrow transplantation on serum markers of bone metabolism. *Calcif Tissue Int* 1994; **55**:408–411.

91. Kang MI, Lee WY, Oh KW, *et al*. The short-term changes of bone mineral metabolism following bone marrow transplantation. *Bone* 2000; **26**:275–279.

92. Abrams SA, Silber TJ, Esteban NV, *et al*. Mineral balance and bone turnover in adolescents with anorexia nervosa. *J Pediatr* 1993; **123**:326–331.

93. Stefanis N, Mackintosh C, Abraha HD, *et al*. Dissociation of bone turnover in anorexia nervosa. *Ann Clin Biochem* 1998; **35**:709–716.

94. Doherty CP, Crofton PM, Sarkar MAK, *et al*. Malnutrition, zinc supplementation and catch-up growth: changes in insulin-like growth factor I, its binding proteins, bone formation and collagen turnover. *Clin Endocrinol* 2002; **57**:391–399.

95. Lehtonen-Veromaa M, Mottonen T, Irjala K, *et al*. A 1-year prospective study on the relationship between physical activity, markers of bone metabolism, and bone acquisition in peripubertal girls. *J Clin Endocrinol Metab* 2000; **85**:3726–3732.

Limb salvage and spinal surgery

HANNAH MORGAN AND ERNEST U CONRAD III

HISTORICAL PERSPECTIVES: DIAGNOSTIC DECADES VS. CHEMOTHERAPY AND IMAGING

The first reports of limb-sparing surgical procedures for malignant bone tumors occurred in Europe and North America in the 1930s with studies conducted by and reported on by Drs Lexer, Albee, and Phemister.[1] While interest in more aggressive surgical techniques slowly developed, the next several decades saw an emphasis on the need for better diagnostic imaging and pathology evaluations for various musculoskeletal tumors. Assessing malignant from 'benign aggressive' bone tumors remained a challenge. Radiographic and pathologic techniques improved dramatically over the next 3–4 decades, allowing surgeons to become more selective about using procedures that would preserve greater postoperative function for patients.

Major surgical events in the 1970s and 1980s revolved around the institution of chemotherapy before and after surgery. Neoadjuvant preoperative chemotherapy, as it is known today, was first instituted at Memorial-Sloan Kettering in 1971 with the introduction of methotrexate chemotherapy for osteosarcoma[2,3,5] At that time, the institution of chemotherapy for osteosarcoma was much debated for several decades until it became a widely supported technique for the treatment of osteosarcoma.[4,5] Subsequently, effective chemotherapy for Ewing's sarcoma and soft-tissue sarcomas in children became popular, and allowed more conservative surgical procedures. Several decades of surgical experience were required before surgeons recognized the beneficial effects of preoperative chemotherapy on the primary tumor, the most significant of which was the ability to resect tumors with closer surgical margins. The issue of adequate or acceptable surgical margins for malignant tumors became possible because of improvements in imaging (magnetic resonance imaging; MRI) and pathology, and because of the efficacy of neoadjuvant chemotherapy. The correlation of surgical specimens and histologic response to preoperative imaging remains a challenging task for surgeons and oncologists, and the precise nature and extent of surgical margins remains a significant challenge for even the most disciplined surgeons.

SURGICAL INDICATIONS FOR AMPUTATION VS. LIMB SALVAGE

A multi-institutional study published in 1979 demonstrated the lack of significant risk of tumor recurrence for limb salvage surgery over amputation for the treatment of osteosarcoma.[6,7] The study showed that a limb-sparing surgery did not result in a higher tumor recurrence versus amputations. Many variables influence the decision for limb-salvage surgery.[8] Indications for limb-salvage surgery include the following.

Adequate skin and soft-tissue for wound coverage after resection

Adequate skin or soft-tissue coverage arises as a surgical issue most commonly as a result of a poorly placed surgical biopsy incision. Rarely does a pediatric sarcoma present with extensive dermal involvement, although extensive, deep, intramuscular tumor involvement also affects skin viability. Problems arise most commonly for the surgeon at time of resection, when an inexperienced surgeon has executed the initial sarcoma biopsy. Documented biopsy complications have actually increased over the last 20 years, despite published series that recognize problems with biopsies performed by inexperienced surgeons.[9] In addition to biopsy complications, patients suffering a local recurrence of their tumors typically have soft-tissue or skin-coverage problems contributing to their likelihood for subsequent amputation.

Lack of involvement of the major neurovascular structures

As a general rule, a patient is a candidate for limb-salvage surgery when there is no tumor involvement of the major neurovascular bundle at the time of initial presentation. Exceptions to that rule are patients who have isolated tumor involvement of a major artery or nerve, who might be managed with an arterial or nerve resection and reconstruction. It is unusual for a tumor to invade a major artery without also involving the vein because those two structures are typically adjacent. Major vein resections with reconstructions, as a general rule, are not effective in the vast majority of patients because of the high likelihood of thromboses and failures. Any major nerve involvement by tumor, such as of the sciatic nerve, has traditionally been considered to be a contraindication to limb salvage owing to the difficulty in re-enervation of those defects with nerve grafts. Patients presenting with definite nerve deficits secondary to tumor involvement will usually require resections of those nerves. Primary involvement of a major neurovascular bundle at presentation is, in general, an unusual finding.

Reconstructable and stable osseous construct

As a general rule, the reconstruction of bony resections for osseous sarcomas may be accomplished with either cadaveric allografts or metallic implants. Indications for allograft reconstructions typically involve 'intercalary' or diaphyseal segments that do not involve a joint surface. In the past, 'osteochondral allografts' used in reconstructing joint or osteochondral segments have not shown adequate success for lower-extremity reconstructions because of the poor viability of the transplanted cartilaginous joint surfaces. Ligamentous instability in allograft transplants also creates problems. Osteochondral reconstructions of the upper extremity still remain a reasonable alternative for upper extremity tumors. Postoperatively, metallic-joint reconstructions may bear weight sooner than osseous constructs because they do not require the bony healing required by their allograft counterpart. The vast majority of sarcoma surgeons now find the best alternative for reconstruction after osteochondral resection to be a metallic total joint implant because of its superior function, faster rehabilitation and fewer complications. Exceptions to this rule include younger patients and upper extremity resections.

Compliant reasonable patient

Limb-salvage patients need to understand the functional limitations after limb-salvage surgery. They must also understand the need for prolonged orthopedic follow-up. In order to achieve a successful limb-salvage procedure, patients need to be able to work with physical therapy postoperatively to achieve an acceptable range of motion and strength. Postoperative rehabilitation for limb-salvage patients involves partial weight-bearing and extensive work on range of motion for at least 3–6 months, depending on the type of reconstruction. Patients also need to restrict recreational activities and understand the reason for such restrictions, depending on the type of reconstruction. Long-term, yearly orthopedic follow-up is also an important patient obligation.

INITIAL BIOPSY

Biopsy techniques

Biopsy for sarcomas remains a challenging but important procedure. Both soft-tissue and osseous sarcomas are best managed with an open incisional biopsy. Primary tumor excision prior to chemotherapy is not the technique preferred by most sarcoma surgeons for pediatric sarcomas. In children, the biopsy is almost always carried out in the operating room or under sedation/anesthesia within the radiology department. The vast majority of tumors are managed with an open incisional biopsy under a general anesthetic to determine the pathological diagnosis, but also to provide tumor specimens for biologic studies. The need for tissue for biologic studies has stimulated most surgeons to prefer an open incisional biopsy over tru-cut needle techniques. Occasionally, a computed tomography (CT)-guided needle biopsy under sedation will be preformed for the diagnosis of a pelvic or spinal tumor.

LIMB-SALVAGE TECHNIQUES

Limb-salvage surgery may be carried out for tumors of soft tissue, bone or lesions that may involve both soft tissue and bone.

Soft-tissue resections

Soft-tissue sarcomas represent the majority of all pediatric sarcoma resections. They typically do not involve an osseous resection. The tumor status (i.e. 'contaminated' vs. 'uncontaminated') surgical margins of soft-tissue resections remain a significant surgical/pathological documentation challenge. That challenge can only be met by a coordinated effort between surgeon and pathologist. The challenge is significant because it requires both the assessment of a margin and the anatomic location of that margin. It is mandatory for surgeons to anatomically label a specimen at the time of resection to aid in specimen orientation with the pathologist. Routine, coordinated, joint review of those specimens by all team members is advisable.

Surgical margins have traditionally been described by the Enneking system[10] as 'wide' (>1.0 cm) through normal tissue, 'marginal' (1–3 mm) through inflammatory tissue or 'contaminated' through tumor tissue. Whether resections are microscopically or grossly contaminated is a description of arguable significance.[11,12] Contaminated margins should be considered for re-excision if the surgeon can locate them and if major anatomic structures are

not involved. Radiation therapy is considered an important preoperative, postoperative or intraoperative adjuvant for local control. Pathologic evaluation of surgical margins via intraoperative frozen section is of limited value in assessing margins. The best information on surgical margins is provided by well-documented, final, surgical margins.

Osseous extremity resections and reconstructions

Osseous reconstructions of the extremities are common surgical procedures for osseous sarcomas. Approximately 90–95 per cent of the pediatric patients in our clinic with high-grade sarcomas are managed with a limb-salvage procedure.[6,14] They may be appropriately and simply categorized as those that involve a joint surface, 'osteochondral' resections (Figure 9c.1), and those that involve the diaphysis, or 'intercalary' resections (Figure 9c.2). Intercalary resections that are distal in the femur and close to the femoral condyles are sometimes referred to as 'condyle-sparing' resections.

Intercalary and condyle-sparing resections (Figure 9c.1a, b) are best reconstructed with cadaveric allografts because they spare the adjacent joint. These grafts work well in this situation because they have the ability to heal at the osseous interface. On the other hand, cadaveric allografts have problems because they are not viable and are at risk of fracture, or may be associated with delayed bony union (12–24 months).[15] Metallic intercalary reconstructions also exist but are less popular.

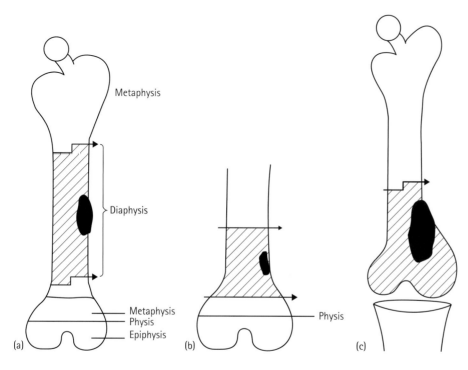

Figure 9c.1 *(a) Intercalary resection; (b) condyle-sparing resection; and (c) osteoarticular resection.*

'Osteoarticular' or joint resections (Figure 9c.1c) are usually reconstructed with cemented or uncemented metallic implants. These implants typically resemble a modular total knee or total hip with a metallic segment that replaces the resected shaft (Figure 9c.2). These implants function relatively well. The need to revise this type of reconstruction occurs in approximately 30–40 per cent of patients at 10 years.[16,17] Stem loosening is the main reason for revision of such a reconstruction. The need for amputation due to failure should be low (5 per cent or less) and occurs primarily because of local tumor recurrence.

Arthrodesis almost always represents an alternative to osteoarticular joint reconstructions. This is true for the shoulder, hip and knee. Arthrodesis may represent the preferred reconstructive alternative for the ankle, wrist and lesser joints. While an awkward alternative to arthroplasty, arthrodesis can represent a lasting durable construct.

Limb salvage at different anatomic sites

DISTAL FEMUR

This is the most common location with the most active growth plate in the leg (i.e. 1 cm/year until age 14 years in females or 16 years in males). The greatest mechanical stress in the leg occurs at this site. Compensating for leg-length discrepancies is an important issue in children under the age of 12 years.

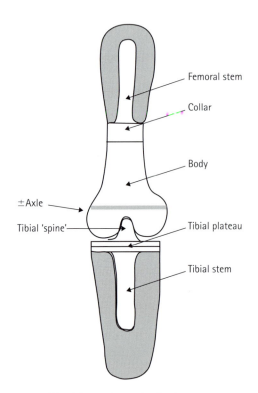

Figure 9c.2 *Distal femoral resection implant components.*

PROXIMAL TIBIA

This is the second most common location for an onco-logic 'total knee' and usually involves reconstruction of the distal femur with a total-knee arthroplasty. Attachment of the patellar (quadriceps) tendon occurs at the proximal tibia (i.e. tibial tubercle) and represents a challenge at that attachment.

PROXIMAL HUMERUS

Three-fourths of the growth of the arm occurs at the proximal humeral growth plate. Achieving good function of the rotator cuff (abductors of the arm) is also a major challenge. Osteochondral allografts are a good reconstructive technique in this location because of the rotator cuff tendinous attachments on the allograft.[18] Large tumors of the proximal humerus can be resected with only a minimal humeral reconstruction and preservation of the neurovascular bundle. This procedure is called a scapulohumeral resection or Tikhoff–Linberg resection.[19] It is an excellent compromise to shoulder amputation for large shoulder tumors that have extensive soft-tissue involvement and difficulties with shoulder reconstruction. A typical Tikhoff–Linberg resection results in a flail shoulder with a functional elbow and ipsilateral hand.

DISTAL TIBIA

Osteoarticular resections here have not traditionally been reconstructed with metallic joints in the distal tibia because of the lack of a reliable total-ankle replacement.[20] These patients are best reconstructed with a distal tibial allograft and an ankle fusion, as arthroplasty at this site has been fraught with complications. Many distal tibial tumors are managed with below-knee amputation.

PROXIMAL FEMUR

There is little growth potential at the proximal femoral epiphysis but reattaching the gluteal muscles at the greater trochanter is important, and acetabular procedures in young patients may result in hip dysplasias in patients under the age of 12 years.

DISTAL HUMERUS

This is an unusual site and probably best reconstructed with an osteochondral allograft, although total-elbow metallic implants are also an option, as is amputation. Very little longitudinal growth occurs at this site, but total-elbow arthroplasties are relatively risky.

PELVIS

Pelvic resections can be categorized into three types: posterior iliac or Type I; acetabular or Type II; and anterior obturator resections or Type III. These resection types are illustrated in Figure 9c.3.[21–23] Pelvic resections for pediatric

sarcomas are more complicated because of more complex bony anatomy, adjacent major nerves (sciatic and femoral) and vessels (common and internal/external iliac), and pelvic contents (i.e. bowel and bladder).

Soft-tissue resections do not require the extensive reconstruction of osseous pelvic tumors but are still a surgical challenge, especially when located inside the pelvis. Reconstruction choices following osseous pelvic resections include: no reconstruction (i.e. a 'flail' pelvis), iliofemoral or ischiofemoral arthrodesis, or arthroplasty with or without pelvic allograft. Pelvic allograft reconstruction can give excellent function, but must be considered carefully regarding adequate tumor margins and the risk of orthopaedic problems following reconstruction (Figure 9c.3).

The complication rate for pelvic procedures is high (30–60 per cent), but tumor control is reasonable, and function is vastly superior to pelvic amputations. Pelvic procedures involve the risk of a large blood loss and perioperative mortality not associated with extremity procedures.

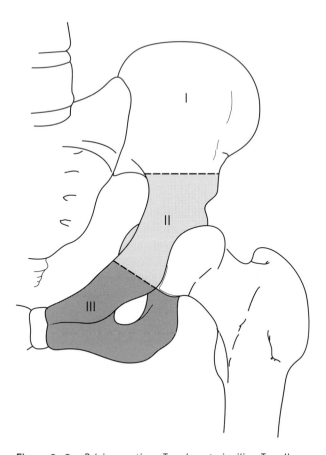

Figure 9c.3 *Pelvic resections: Type I, posterior iliac; Type II, acetabular; Type III, anterior obturator. (Reproduced from Conrad EU III, Springfield D, Peabody TD. Pelvis. In: Simon MA, Springfield D (eds) Surgery for bone and soft-tissue tumors. Philadelphia: Lippincott-Raven, 1998:323–341.)*

Leg-lengthening techniques

Pediatric osseous resections are reconstructed with relative ease compared to the challenge of achieving lengthening of those constructs in the growing child. Those challenges can be categorized into three groups of variable difficulty based on their respective ages (Table 9c.1).

Children can be categorized according to their growth potential as those under 6 years of age, those between 6 and 12 years of age, and those over the age of 12 years. Those over 12 years are a relatively minor problem with 2 cm of growth in girls and 4 cm in boys. Those between 6 and 12 years of age will have anywhere from 2 to 10 cm of growth remaining, and those patients under the age of 6 years will have at least 8–10 cm of growth remaining.[24] Patients under the age of 6 years are a major challenge for leg lengthening because of the need to lengthen the leg by 8–10 cm. In some cases, this represents approximately 50 per cent of the leg length at presentation. Achieving that goal has a high complication rate (100 per cent) and is an unattractive prospect for most families after chemotherapy and limb salvage.

Respective growth of the different anatomic sites is summarized in Table 9c.2. General rules for growth in children are fairly reliable. The proximal humerus and the distal femur both grow at a rate of approximately 1 cm per year, while the other ends of the femur and humerus have less than half that amount of growth. Another good general rule is that girls experience most of their growth by the age of 14 years, boys by the age of 16 years.

There are three basic methods for solving growth discrepancies with limb-sparing surgery: Amputation or rotationplasty,[25] expandable prosthesis (i.e. total-knee arthroplasty that allows lengthening),[26] and Ilizarov techniques and premature growth arrest. Solving extremity length discrepancies by amputation is a realistic approach

Table 9c.1 *Distal femoral growth potential[a]*

Age (years)	Girls	Boys
Under 6	8 cm	10 cm
6–12	2–8 cm	4–10 cm
12–16	2 cm	4 cm

[a] Based on the premise that distal femoral growth equals 1 cm per year until age 14 years in females and age 16 years in males.

Table 9c.2 *Percentage relation growth/bony site*

Bone	Proximal	Distal
Humerus	50%	20%
Femur	30%	70%
Tibia	55%	45%

for children under the age of 10 years with greater growth potential. Expandable implants can be lengthened mechanically with a turnbuckle-type device, by modular segment exchange or by electromagnetic field. All of these techniques are very experimental with high risks for failure and multiple revisions.[27] Osseous lengthenings are similarly complicated and difficult to utilize in tumor patients.

AMPUTATION TECHNIQUES

Amputation surgery for sarcomas remains the traditional gold standard.[7] It is a technique that is especially effective for young children under the age of 10 years because of the challenge of leg growth. It is also the most reliable way to achieve local tumor control after an initial attempt at limb salvage has failed with a local recurrence. Patients who do not have the more delicate limb-sparing procedures do not have to be as cautious with their recreational activities.

Patients treated with amputations do, however, struggle with rehabilitation issues of their own. The patients usually require 6 weeks postoperatively before their first prosthetic fitting. Walking begins 6–8 weeks postoperatively, and walking without crutches on the new leg is not achieved for another 2–3 months. Proficiency in walking requires a total of 3–6 months after surgery. Amputation patients also struggle with various issues, such as stump pain and mechanical-alignment issues. A 'new leg' or prosthesis is required approximately every 2 years for active adolescents. Excellent Internet sites designed for patients by patients for various types of amputations now exist.

Lower-extremity amputations vs. rotationplasty

The following amputation sites and associated issues are listed by their prevalence.

DISTAL FEMUR OR AKA (ABOVE-KNEE AMPUTATION)

This is the most common amputation in the sarcoma setting and it requires a residual femoral length of 12–14 cm for good function. The longer the osseous stump, the stronger the patient's function.

THROUGH-KNEE AMPUTATION VS. VAN NES ROTATIONPLASTY

This is a very suitable amputation for younger children because it avoids bony overgrowth after amputation, and the patient tolerates putting weight on the ends of the femoral condyles. This ability to bear weight easily and directly on the femoral condyles is a great advantage.

The Van Nes rotationplasty involves a resection of a distal femoral segment with reattachment of the remaining tibia in a rotated position. Rotating the tibia 180° places the foot backwards and converts the ankle to the level of the knee, thus forming a functional knee joint.[25,28]

PROXIMAL TIBIAL, OR BKA (BELOW-KNEE AMPUTATION)

This requires a minimum of 12–14 cm for good fit and function. Patients with adequate tibial growth for strength will have excellent function. Patients with at least a midtibial length will be able to participate in sports as teenagers. Function is excellent, and losing your foot and ankle is only a relatively minor functional hardship. The emotional issues still abound, however. It is helpful to show these patients and their families other patients who have previously been treated with a BKA; they will be surprised at the 'normal' appearance of BKA patients and their high level of function.

FOOT OR SYME'S AMPUTATION

Amputations and disarticulations of the ankle or foot are also extremely functional for patients. They require specially fitted shoe prostheses to ambulate well. Their level of function is very high and they are frequently able to ambulate at home without their prostheses or shoes.

PROXIMAL FEMUR AND PELVIC AMPUTATION

Proximal thigh amputations involve amputations proximal to the medial thigh level. Adequate femoral length is required in order to have enough strength to make use of a proximal-thigh prosthesis. This usually requires 12–14 cm of the proximal femur. The shorter the remaining femoral segment, the more difficult prosthetic fitting, and the more difficult the prosthetic usage will be.

An amputation through the hip joint is referred to as a hip disarticulation. An amputation through the pelvis is referred to as a hemipelvectomy. A patient treated with either of these procedures may still use a prosthesis, but it is not efficient mechanically. Young patients will use hemipelvectomy prostheses on a daily basis until they reach an older age (30–40 years), when it may be used only occasionally.

Upper-extremity amputations

FOREQUARTER OR SHOULDER AMPUTATIONS

In general, losing your upper extremity is a greater emotional loss than losing your lower extremity, and it can be a significant challenge for even the most well-adjusted patient. Large proximal humeral tumors that involve the scapula will require an amputation proximal to the shoulder

joint, or a forequarter amputation. Smaller humeral tumors requiring amputation may be managed with a shoulder disarticulation. The scapular muscle powers prosthetic fittings after a shoulder disarticulation, and patients can benefit from those prostheses. Forequarter amputations do not have functional prostheses because of the loss of scapular muscles, but they do routinely use a shoulder 'bump' for clothing.

ABOVE-ELBOW, BELOW-ELBOW AND HAND AMPUTATIONS

Above-elbow, below-elbow and hand amputations are unusual. Prosthetic fittings are mechanical (hook), or myo-electric, which is very expensive and requires extensive training. Most patients recover very quickly from these procedures, and there are now excellent Internet sites for these patients.

SURGICAL COMPLICATIONS

Surgical complications that interfere with the resumption of chemotherapy should be a relatively rare event with the vast majority of sarcoma patients. Chemotherapy delays greater than 6 weeks may have a deleterious effect on patient outcome. Surgical complications that delay chemotherapy more than 4–6 weeks should be rarely encountered. More difficult surgical procedures, such as those involving the pelvis, sacrum or spine, will be more likely to involve such delays.

Acute postoperative complications

Acute surgical complications occur in the first 6 weeks and can have serious effect in delaying postoperative chemotherapy. For that reason, these problems should be dealt with quickly. Complications resulting in a delay of chemotherapy longer than 4–6 weeks are serious potential problems and should be rare occurrences ($>$10 per cent).

DRAINING WOUND OR WOUND NECROSIS

If serous wound drainage lasts longer than 5–7 days or there is wound necrosis, patients should be taken back to the operating room for a wash out and/or wound revision. Marginal flap necrosis can usually be revised easily with a surgical debridement, closure and a rapid recovery.

WOUND INFECTION

As a general rule, positive wound cultures require a wash out plus 6 weeks of intravenous antibiotics, depending on the extent or depth of the infection. Treating early wound infection with a surgical wash out and intravenous antibiotics may prevent an infected implant or graft that would necessitate removal.

PERIOPERATIVE WOUND BLEEDING

This is a very unusual event. Patients should be embolized acutely within 3–4 hours, or returned to the operating room within 4–6 hours!

ARTERIAL INJURY

This injury should be recognized acutely in the operating room at the time of the procedure. Recognize, evaluate and treat acutely within 1–2 hours, or subsequent amputation is very likely.

VENOUS OBSTRUCTION

Do not treat surgically. This requires anticoagulation.

MAJOR NERVE PROBLEMS

Nerve injuries usually represent a stretch injury or neuropraxia. Management usually involves observation, then a nerve study, if no improvement is shown at 6 weeks postoperatively. If the surgeon is worried about a possible nerve laceration, then the surgical site should be explored acutely.

LOSS OF FIXATION OR BONY PROBLEMS

Surgeon should revise or observe depending on the details and the postoperative chemotherapy schedule.

Chronic/late postoperative complications

Surgical complications that occur late (i.e., after the six-week postoperative interval), can have their own effect on postoperative functional outcomes, and may necessitate subsequent surgical procedures. Some of these chronic or late effects are given below.

LATE INFECTION

Take the patient to the operating room for cultures and wash out. Start intravenous antibiotics and decide on options in a delayed fashion, depending on the chemotherapy schedule and extent of the infection.

DELAYED UNION OF ALLOGRAFT

If the patient shows no radiographic evidence of bony union at 6–8 months postoperatively, he or she will require autogenous bone grafting, or revision of fixation. Allografts typically take a long time to heal (6–12 months). Autogenous bone grafting, or revision of fixation, should be considered at 8–12 months, if bony union has not occurred.

KNEE STIFFNESS AFTER ARTHROPLASTY

The best recommendation in this situation is to avoid joint stiffness in the early postoperative period with closed

operative manipulation at 6 weeks postoperatively and continued physical therapy. CPM (continuous passive motion) machines can be effective for knee patients, especially during postoperative chemotherapy. Late stiffness that is unresponsive to physical therapy may be an indication for a surgical release.

POSTOPERATIVE PAIN

Consider the cause of the patient's postoperative pain. Is it mechanical, muscular, neurogenic or vascular? Usually, postoperative pain in this setting is muscular in etiology. Manage the pain with anti-inflammatories, if the patient is off chemotherapy, in addition to pain medication or narcotics. Continue physical therapy if at all possible.

PERIPROSTHETIC OR ALLOGRAFT FRACTURE

Prosthetic, periprosthetic or graft fractures should be revised surgically within 1–2 weeks unless the patient is on chemotherapy – an unusual scenario – when fixation will have to wait an appropriate surgical interval. Rather than discontinuing chemotherapy, brace the site and select an appropriate later time to revise between chemotherapy cycles.

LEG-LENGTH DISCREPANCY

Leg-length discrepancies in children following limb-sparing surgery that involves sacrifice of a growth plate should involve arrest of the contralateral growth plate in an actively growing child. That procedure should occur within 1 year of the initial procedure in order to minimize any leg-length discrepancy. Lengthening of the involved extremity is typically carried out at the surgical resection in order to provide a 1–2-year period of time before leg-length discrepancies occur.

Leg-length discrepancies are most significant in children under the age of 10, of intermediate significance in children between the age of 10 and 12 years, and minimally significant in teenagers over the age of 12 years. Females, as a general rule, do not have significant growth after the age of 14 and males after the age of 16.[24]

The most active growth plates (distal femur and proximal humerus) grow at rates of approximately 1 cm per year.

SPINAL DEFORMITIES FOLLOWING TREATMENT OF CHILDHOOD TUMORS

Primary spinal neoplasms arising from the mesenchymal elements of the spinal column are relatively rare in children and account for only a small proportion (1–5 per cent) of pediatric tumors. Other malignancies, such as abdominal or retroperitoneal neoplasms, like Wilms'

Table 9c.3 *Spinal tumors: age distribution*

Diagnosis	Age (years)	Spinal location
Neuroblastoma	0–6	Thoracic
Astrocytoma	6–12	Thoracolumbar
Sarcoma	12–20	Thoracolumbar

tumor, may affect the spine secondarily. The effects of these tumors on spinal growth and the consequences of their treatment may be severe. The character and degree of deformity are determined by the age of the child, type of tumor and the treatment employed.[29]

Intramedullary spinal cord tumors in children tend to have characteristic age distributions. Neuroblastomas, malignant neoplasms derived from primitive neural crest cells, predominate in younger children, typically those under 6 years of age (Table 9c.3). The peak age at presentation is approximately 18 months. Spinal neuroblastomas typically are found in the distribution of the sympathetic ganglia in a paramidline position. Presenting signs and symptoms may include weakness, neurological deficit, pain, palpable mass, spinal deformity and, in some cases, system effects, such as fever or weight loss. Therapy is usually based on the age of the patient and the stage of disease and typically involves surgery with or without radiation therapy. In disseminated cases, chemotherapy and more aggressive radiotherapy may be considered.[30,32]

Astrocytomas found in the pediatric population tend to occur in a slightly older population, with a mean age of 7 years and an age range of 6–12 years. These are also malignant tumors, but 80–85 per cent have low-grade histology and behavior. Motor weakness, gait deterioration and spinal deformity may be seen at initial presentation. The treatment of low-grade astrocytomas is usually surgical and an intramedullary spinal resection is often possible. Radiation therapy has some benefit in the treatment of astrocytoma, but is frequently used in the adjuvant setting following surgery or local recurrence. For malignant astrocytomas, surgical debulking followed by total neuraxis radiation and possible chemotherapy has been recommended. The survival rate of low-grade lesions is approximately 60 per cent, but is much worse in patients with malignant, high-grade lesions.[33]

Sarcomas may develop in the mesenchymal tissues of the spine but are less frequently seen than in the extremities. Spinal sarcoma patients are typically adolescents, and are less common than those with neuroblastoma and astrocytoma tumors. Primary lymphoma of the spine is also seen in adolescents. Pain is a more frequent initial symptom in this group. The typical location of sarcomas is in the lumbosacral spine, which contrasts with neuroblastoma and astrocytoma, more frequently found in the

thoracic or cervical regions. Therapy consists of neoadjuvant and adjuvant chemotherapy, and surgical resection. Patients rarely present with acute spinal compromise and are best managed initially with biopsy and chemotherapy, followed by resection. Overall 5-year survival is 50 per cent.[29]

In addition to early neurologic injury that may develop from the effects of the tumor itself or from surgical treatment, late spinal deformity not infrequently affects patients with spinal cord neoplasms. The risk of deformity is indirectly related to patient age. The type and severity of deformity depend on the age of the child, the size and anatomical location of the lesion, and the treatment regimen. Surgical resection of tumors can lead to spinal deformity, if stabilizing structures are disrupted. In 1983, Denis [31]developed a three-column model of the spine to aid in predicting instability after spinal injury: the anterior column includes the anterior half of the vertebral body, the middle column includes the posterior vertebral body and post, longitudinal ligament, and the posterior column is made of all the bony and soft tissues of the posterior arch, including the facet joints and laminae.

This anatomical model of Denis can also be used to predict deformity patterns that occur after surgical treatment of spinal tumors. For instance, neuroblastomas and astrocytomas tend to occur in young children in the thoracic and cervical spinal regions. Removal of posterior spinal elements is often necessary to gain adequate exposure of the lesion; the loss of these structures allows increased spinal flexion (kyphosis), which in turn transmits the spinal load more anteriorly. When the axis of flexion is anterior, more tensile stress is placed on the remaining posterior stabilizing structures, as well as compression stress on the anterior vertebral bodies and, over time, a permanent kyphotic deformity may develop. Scoliosis may also develop in addition to kyphosis, especially if a unilateral facet joint is destabilized or radiation therapy fields are asymmetric. Spinal nerve root injury owing to tumor involvement or to treatment may also result in muscle imbalance, which may aggravate any scoliosis. Spondylolisthesis, a condition in which one vertebra slips forward on another, can also occur after facet injury or after excessive release of posterior stabilizing structures. With multilevel or thoracolumbar laminectomy, spinal column deformity develops in over 30 per cent of patients. Typically, more severe deformities develop in younger children who are skeletally immature.[32–35]

Radiation therapy may lead to the late development of spinal deformity. If the radiation field is symmetric, then the main effect will be an overall decrease in spinal height. If the physeal plates are damaged asymmetrically, then scoliosis, kyphosis or kyphoscoliosis may develop. Spinal osteonecrosis secondary to vascular injury and contracture of paraspinal muscles from radiation effects also contribute to abnormal spinal growth and development.[35]

Treatment of spinal deformities that develop after treatment for pediatric spine tumors again depends on the severity of the disease as well as the age of the child. Mild deformities in older children may be observed with serial examinations and radiographs. In patients who are very young or in whom a progressive or significant deformity develops, surgical stabilization may be undertaken. Bracing is rarely effective except perhaps in the immediate postoperative period after spinal tumor resection.

The most successful management of spinal deformities is prevention. Newer surgical techniques limit the osseous extent of laminectomy exposure, which results in much greater spinal stability and less subsequent deformity. Preservation of the facets joints posteriorly is a critical and relatively new concept. If an extensive exposure does need to be performed, immediate spinal stabilization should be considered. Radiation should be avoided when possible, especially in younger children. If used, the treatment field should be symmetrical and physes should be shielded when allowed. Fractionation and decreased total doses may also minimize the injury from radiation treatment. Patients and their families should be educated about the risk of developing spinal deformities and follow-up should be prolonged, as deformities can develop as late as 7 years post-treatment.

LATE EFFECTS AND LONG-TERM FOLLOW-UP

Both amputation and limb-salvage patients have significant problems long after successful surgical procedures.[36,37] Amputees never escape the need for new prostheses. Limb-spared patients are reconstructed with implants that have a 10-year failure rate of 30–40 per cent requiring future orthopaedic revisions, or allograft constructs that have a 25–30 per cent rate of delayed union. All of these patients require regular orthopaedic follow-up throughout adulthood.[8] The medical and oncologic complications of chemotherapy and radiation therapy are obviously additional long-term significant issues for these patients.

After the completion of chemotherapy, adolescent limb-salvage patients still require careful orthopedic follow-up. Girls under the age of 14 years and boys under the age of 16 years require yearly radiographic leg-length studies to follow potential leg-length discrepancies in addition to X-rays of their grafts or implants to detect the possibility of delayed union or fracture (grafts) or stem loosening (implants). While late infections are not common, they do occur in 5–10 per cent of different sites depending on the procedure and the implant. After 10 years of follow-up, patients may be followed at 2–3-year intervals. Orthopedic complications after 3–5 years occur in 30–50 per cent of patients.

Following these patients is extremely important, both emotionally and physically.[37] While limb-sparing procedures are successful most of the time, they do demand follow-up for the rest of the patients' lives.

Long-term outcome assessment is an important tool for both patients and their treatments. Many patients will require medical treatment for associated problems or chronic pain. The orthopedic surgeon performing limb salvage should play an active role with these follow-up issues.[8]

KEY POINTS

- Surgical indications for limb salvage involve tumor response to chemotherapy.
- Sarcoma biopsies require experience and expertise.
- Patient rehabilitation and expectations are a key to success.
- Long-term (ten-year) orthopedic follow-up is important for limb-salvage patients.
- Pediatric patients under age 12 have significant extremity growth issues.
- Amputation or rotationplasty is optimal under age ten.
- Limb-salvage complications must not delay chemotherapy.
- Spinal tumors are high risk for tumor recurrence and spinal deformity.

REFERENCES

1. Phemister DB. Conservative bone surgery in the treatment of bone tumors [as reprinted from *SGO* 1940; 70:355]. *CORR* 1986; **204**:4–8.
2. Meyers PA, Heller G, Healey J, *et al*. Chemotherapy for non-metastatic osteogenic sarcoma: the Memorial-Sloan Kettering experience. *J Clin Oncol* 1992; **10(1)**:5–15.
◆3. Rosen G, Marcove RC, Caparros B, *et al*. Primary osteogenic sarcoma: the rationale for preoperative chemotherapy and delayed surgery. *Cancer* 1979; **43(6)**:2163–2177.
◆4. Link MP, Goorin AM, Horowitz M, *et al*. Adjuvant chemotherapy for high-grade osteosarcoma of the extremity: updated results of the Multi-Institutional Osteosarcoma Study. *Clin Orthop* 1991; **270**:8–14.
5. Goorin AM, Abelson HT, Frei E. Osteosarcoma: fifteen years later. *N Engl J Med* 1985; **313(26)**:1637–1643.
6. Rougraff BT, Simon MA, Kneisl JS, *et al*. Limb salvage compared with amputation for osteosarcoma of the distal end of the femur: a long-term oncological, functional, and quality of life study. *J Bone Joint Surg [Am]* 1994; **76(5)**:649–656.
◆7. Simon MA, Aschliman M, Thomas N, *et al*. Limb salvage versus amputation for osteosarcoma of the distal end of the femur. *J Bone Joint Surg [Am]* 1986; **68(9)**:1331–1337.

●8. Simon MA. Current concepts review: limb salvage for osteosarcoma. *J Bone Joint Surg [Am]* 1988; **70(2)**:307–310.
◆9. Mankin HJ, Mankin CJ, Simon MA. The hazards of the biopsy, revisited: members of the Musculoskeletal Tumor Society. *J Bone Joint Surg [Am]* 1996; **78(5)**:656–663.
10. Enneking WF, Spannier SS, Goodman MA. A system for the surgical staging of musculoskeletal sarcomas. *Clin Orthop* 1980; **153**:106–120.
11. Simon MA, Enneking WF. The management of soft-tissue sarcomas of the extremities. *J Bone Joint Surg [Am]* 1976; **58(3)**:317–327.
◆12. Rydholm A, Rooser B. The surgical margin in soft-tissue sarcoma. *J Bone Joint Surg [Am]* 1989; **71(9)**:1429–1430.
13. Enneking WF, Dunham W, Gebhardt MD, *et al*. A system for the functional evaluation of reconstructive procedures after surgical treatment of tumors of the musculoskeletal system. *Clin Orthop* 1993; **286**:241–246.
◆14. Schuetze SM, Rubin BP, Vernon C, *et al*. Positron emission tomography response predicts survival in soft tissue sarcoma. Currently submitted to *Clinical Orthopaedics and Related Research*, 2003.
15. Dubousset J, Missenard G, Kalifa CH. Management of osteogenic sarcoma in children and adolescents. *Clin Orthop* 1991; **270**:52–59.
◆16. Malawer MM, Chou LB. Prosthetic survival and clinical results with use of large-segment replacements in the treatment of high-grade bone sarcomas. *J Bone Joint Surg [Am]* 1995; **77(8)**:1154–1165.
◆17. Eckardt JJ, Eilber FR, Rosen G, *et al*. Endoprosthetic replacement for stage IIB osteosarcoma. *Clin Orthop* 1991; **270**:202–213.
18. Malawer MM. Tumors of the shoulder girdle: technique of resection and description of a surgical classification. *Orthop Clin North Am* 1991; **22(1)**:7–35.
19. Linberg BE. Interscapulo-thoracic resection for malignant tumors of the shoulder joint region. *J Bone Joint Surg* 1928; **10**:344–349, or *Clin Orthop* 1999; **358**:3–7.
20. Zwart HJ, Taminiau AH, Schimmel JW, *et al*. Kotz modular femur and tibial replacement: 28 cases followed for 3 (1–8) years. *Acta Orthop Scand* 1994; **65(3)**:315–318.
21. Aho AJ, Ekfors T, Dean PB, *et al*. Incorporation and clinical results of large allografts of the extremities and pelvis. *Clin Orthop* 1994; **307**:200–213.
22. Campanacci M, Capanna R. Pelvis resection: the Rizzoli experience. *Orthop Clin North Am* 1991; **22(1)**:65–86.
23. Conrad EU III, Springfield D, Peabody TD. Pelvis. In: Simon MA, Springfield D (eds.) *Surgery for bone and soft-tissue tumors*. Philadelphia: Lippincott-Raven Publishers, 1998:323–341.
24. Moseley CF. Growth. In: Lovell WW, Winters RB (eds) *Pediatric orthopaedics*, 2nd edn. Philadelphia: JB Lippincott, 1986:27–39.
25. Kotz R, Salzer M. Rotation-plasty for childhood osteosarcoma of the distal part of the femur. *J Bone Joint Surg [Am]* 1982; **64(7)**:959–969.
26. Kenan S, Bloom N, Lewis MM. Limb sparing surgery in skeletally immature patients with osteosarcoma: The use of the expandable prosthesis. *Clin Orthop* 1991; **270**:223–230.
27. Gonzalez-Herrant P, Burgos-Flores J, Ocete-Guzman JG, *et al*. The management of limb-length discrepancies in children after treatment of osteosarcoma and Ewing's sarcoma. *J Pediatr Orthop* 1995; **15(5)**:561–565.
28. Jacobs PA. Limb salvage and rotationplasty for osteosarcoma in children. *Clin Orthop* 1984; **188**:217–222.
29. Conrad EU, Olszewski AD, Berger M, *et al*. Pediatric spine tumors with spinal cord compromise. *J Pediatr Orthop* 1992; **12(4)**:454–460.
◆30. Katzenstein HM, Kent P, London WB, *et al*. Treatment and outcome of 83 children with intraspinal neuroblastoma: the

Pediatric Oncology Group experience. *J Clin Oncol* 2001; **19(4)**:1047–1055.

31. Denis F. The three-column spine and its significance in the classification of acute thoracolumbar spinal injuries. *Spine* 1983; **8(8)**:817–831.

◆32. Mayfield JK, Riseborough EJ, Jaffee N, *et al*. Spinal deformity in children treated for neuroblastoma: the effect of radiation and other forms of treatment. *J Bone Joint Surg [Am]* 1981; **63A(2)**:183–193.

33. Houten JK, Weiner HL. Pediatric intramedullary spinal cord tumors: special considerations. *J Neuro Oncol* 2000; **47(3)**:225–230.

34. Papagelopoulos PJ, Peterson HA, Ebersold MJ, *et al*. Spinal column deformity and instability after lumbar or thoracolumbar laminectomy for intraspinal tumors in children and young adults. *Spine* 1997; **22(4)**:442–451.

35. Makipernaa A, Heikkila JT, Merikanto J, *et al*. Spinal deformity induced by radiotherapy for solid tumors in childhood: a long-term follow up study. *Eur J Pediatr* 1993; **152(3)**:197–200.

36. Sugarbaker PH, Barafsky I, Rosenberg SA, *et al*. Quality of life assessment of patients in extremity sarcoma clinical trials. *Surgery* 1982; **91(1)**:17–23.

37. Weddington WW Jr, Seagraves KB, Simon MA. Psychological outcome of extremity sarcoma survivors undergoing amputation or limb salvage. *J Clin Oncol* 1985; **3(10)**:1393–1399.

10

Bone marrow transplantation

RODERICK SKINNER AND ALISON D. LEIPER

INTRODUCTION

The number of hemopoietic stem cell transplants (HSCTs) performed in children has increased greatly over the last two decades. Since 1993, over 3000 pediatric autologous and allogeneic HSCTs have been reported to the United Kingdom Children's Cancer Study Group (UKCCSG) Bone Marrow Transplant (BMT) Registry, with approximately 300–350 performed annually since 1995 (personal communication, Dr J Cornish on behalf of UKCCSG BMT Registry). Data from the International Bone Marrow Transplant Registry (IBMTR) shows that the number of allogeneic HSCTs in children and adolescents (below 21 years of age) has increased since the early 1990s, with an average of about 2000 transplants per year since 1995 (2002 IBMTR/ABMTR Summary Slides, State-of-the-Art in Blood and Marrow Transplantation). It is estimated that registrations to the IBMTR account for about 40 per cent of HSCTs performed worldwide, thereby implying that approximately 5000 allogeneic HSCTs are performed annually in this age group.

The increase in HSCT activity in children has been particularly evident in allogeneic transplantation for serious hematological disease (both malignant and non-malignant), facilitated by rapid developments in the use of alternative donors [e.g. unrelated donors (URDs) and mismatched related donors (RDs), including haploidentical RDs] and stem cell sources [e.g. umbilical cord blood (UCB) and peripheral blood stem cells (PBSCs)].

Autologous transplantation has also evolved rapidly, with considerably increased use of PBSC transplants in several high-risk solid malignancies. At the same time, many new prophylactic and therapeutic strategies in supportive care have been introduced and refined, contributing to improved transplant-related mortality (TRM) in both allogeneic and autologous HSCTs. It is hoped that lower TRM ultimately will result in higher long-term survival. Data from the UKCCSG BMT Registry shows that the 6-month survival after allogeneic HSCT for acute lymphoblastic leukemia (ALL) was 73 per cent between 1993 and 1995 and 85 per cent between 1997 and 1999 for HLA-identical RD transplants, and 70 per cent and 80 per cent, respectively, for URD transplants during the same time periods, suggesting reduced TRM. The 5-year event-free survival (EFS) after allogeneic HSCT for ALL in second remission (the commonest single indication for pediatric HSCT during the 1990s) is currently 54 per cent for RDs and 45 per cent for URDs. Children undergoing allogeneic HSCT for the other main hematological indications, principally ALL in first remission, acute or chronic myeloid leukemia, and aplastic anemia, have a 5-year EFS of between 40 and >80 per cent, depending on the disease and the donor type. Those receiving autologous BMTs or PBSC transplants for solid tumors have a 5-year EFS of up to 50 per cent, depending on the disease (personal communication, Dr J Cornish on behalf of UKCCSG BMT Registry). Similarly, a large prospective study by a multicenter group, representing over 90 per cent of pediatric

transplants performed for malignant disease in Italy, reported a 3-year EFS of 45 per cent in 636 consecutive children transplanted for acute leukemia between 1990 and 1997.[1] Most leukemic relapses after HSCT occur within 2 years of transplant, so patients remaining disease-free at this time have a high expectation of cure.

Therefore, the number of HSCTs performed in children has increased over the last decade and a substantial proportion of these patients will become long-term survivors. Unfortunately, survivors of HSCT have a high risk of late toxicity, which may be considerable for some children.

WHY ARE THE LATE ADVERSE EFFECTS OF HSCT IN CHILDREN IMPORTANT?

Although some children treated by HSCT display few or even no discernable chronic adverse consequences of treatment, the majority suffer from some late side effects. However, this frequency of late toxicity is not surprising when viewed in the context of the indications for which HSCT is often performed. The majority of these children have poor risk (e.g. metastatic solid tumors) or advanced disease (e.g. relapsed leukemia), and many have been extensively pretreated with chemotherapy and sometimes radiotherapy. For such children, while HSCT is usually considered to offer the best and sometimes the only realistic hope of cure, the intensity of 'conditioning' chemoradiotherapy treatment, given immediately prior to HSCT, inevitably leads to a considerable risk of late toxicity. Autologous HSCT involves the delivery of high-dose chemotherapy, sometimes with additional radiotherapy, prior to infusion of autologous stem cells. Allogeneic HSCT also employs high-dose chemoradiotherapy, but its potential late morbidity is increased greatly by additional specific complications, especially those related to total body irradiation (TBI) or to chronic graft-versus-host disease (cGvHD). The large majority of publications of late adverse effects after HSCT, as reported in this chapter, have studied BMT recipients rather than patients who have received transplants from other stem cell sources (e.g. UCB, PBSC). Although it is likely that late adverse effects will be broadly comparable between these different patients groups, further research is necessary in survivors of UCB and PBSC transplants.

In general, most of the late adverse effects of chemotherapy and radiotherapy in pediatric BMT patients are the same as those seen in children receiving similar treatments in the conventional (i.e. non-BMT) setting. However, such side effects may be additive. For example, the clinical features observed in many children with late renal toxicity after BMT suggest radiation nephritis, but the doses delivered with TBI (up to 12–14 Gy) are well below the radiation tolerance of the kidney (20–25 Gy).

It appears that additional chemotherapy administered with TBI lowers the renal radiation tolerance.[2,3] Furthermore, renal tubular toxicity may be exacerbated when the chemotherapy in question is nephrotoxic in its own right (e.g. cisplatin).[4] Furthermore, the frequency and severity of toxicity after BMT may be much greater than that seen following conventional treatment strategies. The very high risk of primary gonadal failure, leading to infertility, after TBI given as part of conditioning treatment for allogeneic BMT for relapsed leukemia contrasts sharply with the potential but relatively low risk of subfertility seen after contemporary treatment protocols for newly diagnosed standard risk ALL or acute myeloid leukemia (AML).

In addition, many other factors may contribute to the late morbidity seen in survivors of BMT. Particularly in the case of certain inherited disorders (e.g. thalassemia, Hurler's disease), the underlying disease may itself leave a long-term legacy in the form of considerable organ damage, which may cause significant disability. Treatment received prior to BMT may result in substantial chronic adverse effects (e.g. nephrotoxicity due to ifosfamide and/or cisplatin in certain solid tumors) before transplant, and may prime patients for even more severe toxicity after BMT. Numerous other treatments used frequently in BMT patients, including several drugs important in many aspects of supportive care, and surgical procedures, may lead to important late adverse consequences in their own right, which again may be additive in effect. Examples include drugs used for GvHD treatment or prophylaxis (corticosteroids, other immunosuppressive agents), anti-infective drugs (especially aminoglycoside antibiotics, amphotericin), and resection of lung tissue in invasive pulmonary aspergillosis.

Therefore, long-term survivors of pediatric BMT are vulnerable to a different range of late adverse effects, which overlaps with but also extends considerably beyond those chronic toxicities seen in children with malignant disease treated without BMT. Both the nature and the severity of late toxicity in BMT patients may lead to substantial chronic morbidity, with considerable implications for their quality of life. Moreover, with ever greater awareness of the potential late adverse consequences of BMT in children, there is an increasing need for the development of strategies to offer optimum care and long-term follow-up of this very high-risk patient group.

A number of comprehensive and up to date reviews of the late adverse effects of BMT in children have been published recently.[5–10] The intention of this chapter is to summarize the various types of late adverse effects that survivors of BMT may experience, and to provide pertinent examples of their wide ranging nature and severity. Particular emphasis is given to those complications that are much more common or severe in, or indeed unique to, allogeneic BMT recipients. Several of the procedural

complications of BMT are effectively confined to allogeneic BMT recipients (e.g. the many consequences of cGvHD), or much commoner in this group than in autologous BMT recipients (e.g. delayed immune reconstitution and its complications). There are often important differences between autologous and allogeneic recipients in the type of adverse effects experienced. For example, when considering second malignancies after BMT, AML and myelodysplasia are predominantly seen in autologous recipients whose transplanted marrow stem cells have often been exposed to extensive prior chemotherapy, while lymphoproliferative disease is essentially only seen in the setting of the intense immunosuppression caused by allogeneic transplantation.[11]

The importance of the numerous other factors influencing the nature and severity of late adverse effects post-BMT will be mentioned where appropriate, especially the impact of the original diagnosis, other medical problems (e.g. infections), treatment received prior to BMT, and other concurrent treatments used during BMT.

LATE ADVERSE EFFECTS OF BMT IN CHILDREN DUE TO CONDITIONING TREATMENT

The late adverse effects of autologous and many of those of allogeneic BMT in children are primarily due to conditioning chemotherapy and radiotherapy. Many of these complications are qualitatively similar to those observed in non-BMT patients. To avoid repetition, they are not discussed in detail in this chapter. Instead, they are listed in Table 10.1, which details the nature and clinical consequences of these events, and provides cross-references to the organ/system-based chapters in this book where greater detail is available. This table highlights the breadth of these toxicities and provides representative estimates of their frequency in selected patient groups, thereby illustrating the scale of the concerns facing long-term survivors of BMT performed in childhood.

The majority of contemporary pediatric autologous BMT procedures are performed in children with high-risk or relapsed solid tumors. However, autologous BMT was performed relatively frequently for children with poor-risk hematological malignancies until the early 1990s, and is still performed in such patients in some centers, particularly in certain countries. The nature and frequency of late adverse effects after autologous BMT inevitably differs to some extent between these two patient groups owing to the different primary treatments given before BMT.

Most children receiving conventional treatment for cancer and leukemia do not receive multiple modalities of treatment that are likely to cause additive toxicity, since care is usually taken in protocol design to avoid concurrent or sequential use of agents with similar late toxicities. Unfortunately, owing to the intensive treatment required, this is not necessarily feasible in patients undergoing BMT, particularly autologous transplants. For example, some patients with solid malignancies may receive anthracyclines during primary treatment, and radiotherapy to a field involving the thorax during primary or relapse therapy, or, in some instances, TBI as part of conditioning therapy prior to BMT. Children with leukemia undergoing BMT may receive anthracyclines during initial and secondary treatment, and then TBI and high-dose cyclophosphamide during conditioning treatment. The cardiotoxicity of anthracyclines is well known,[12] as is the potentially harmful effect of radiation to the left hemithorax.[13] Additionally, although not as well recognized, the high-dose cyclophosphamide used during conditioning treatment prior to BMT appears to be acutely cardiotoxic in its own right, although it is less clear whether it contributes to chronic cardiac impairment in BMT recipients.[14,15]

SELECTED LATE ADVERSE EFFECTS OF BMT IN CHILDREN – COMPLEX PRESENTATIONS AND MULTIFACTORIAL ETIOLOGY

Pulmonary

Pulmonary toxicity is a common cause of morbidity post-BMT and, unfortunately, is still a leading cause of death, especially after allogeneic BMT. It provides an excellent example of the variety of complex presentations of late toxicity that may be observed and of the multiple factors that may contribute to such toxicity.

Chronic pulmonary toxicity may be classified broadly as either *obstructive* or *restrictive* in nature. Restrictive disease may include isolated abnormalities in gas transfer [manifest by reduced diffusion capacity (transfer factor)] or a classical restrictive defect with reduced lung volumes.[16] Up to 20 per cent of BMT recipients develop *symptomatic* chronic pulmonary toxicity[17] but relatively little information is available concerning the frequency of pulmonary symptoms in those patients transplanted in childhood. Nevertheless, fewer children than adults appear to develop clinically overt, especially obstructive, disease. Pleural effusions have been described as a very rare manifestation of serositis in cGvHD, usually presenting within a year of BMT, although later onset has been described.[18,19]

However, pulmonary function testing has revealed a high incidence of asymptomatic abnormalities. In a cross-sectional study of 52 children 3–11 years after autologous (19 patients) or allogeneic (33 patients) BMT for leukemia, 38 per cent showed varying degrees of

Table 10.1 Selected late adverse effects of bone marrow transplantation in children due primarily to previous and/or conditioning chemotherapy and radiotherapy

Organ/system/Toxicity Primary causative treatment(s)[a]	Other potential risk factors	Clinical features and consequences	Frequency[b]	Impact of allogeneic BMT[c]	Comments	Cross-references
Neurological toxicity Before or during BMT: • Chemotherapy (CT) – methotrexate (systemic or intrathecal) • Cranial radiotherapy (RT)[d]	• Prolonged immunosuppression increases risk of CNS infection, especially with opportunistic organisms	• 'Leucoencephalopathy' – variable symptoms/signs • Vascular episodes – cerebrovascular accidents, vasculitis, 'migraine-like' episodes • Infections – meningitis or focal disease; wide variety of causative organisms • CNS tumors – gliomas, lymphomas, meningiomas (attributed to RT); see 'Secondary malignancy'	• 'Leucoencephalopathy' – 7% in patients receiving both CNS-directed treatment pre-BMT (RT and/or intrathecal CT) and intrathecal methotrexate post-BMT[71] • CNS infections – 7% (adults)[72] • CNS tumors – risk increases with time post-BMT, overall incidence 46 times expected[73]	Link suggested[74,75] between cGvHD and: • Vasculitic syndromes • Polymyositis • Myasthenia gravis • Peripheral neuropathy	Note probable additive effect of multiple episodes of CNS-directed treatment, including CT plus RT, or two episodes of RT	2a
Neuropsychological toxicity Before or during BMT: • Chemotherapy – methotrexate (systemic or intrathecal), busulphan • Cranial radiotherapy[d]	• Higher cumulative RT doses, especially prior cranial RT followed by TBI • Young age at treatment (especially less than 3 years) • Female gender • Longer duration of follow-up	• Wide range and severity of neuropsychological functional impairment – memory, attention, intelligence, visual-spatial, verbal skills, fine motor skills, educational achievement • Cognitive function may deteriorate gradually over 10 years or more • Impaired psychosocial function	Patients receiving 2 RT treatments (i.e. cranial RT + TBI, or 2 episodes of cranial RT): • Impaired memory – 46%[76] • Impaired verbal comprehension – 50%[76] • Need for formalized extra educational support – 36%[76] Patients receiving ≤ 1 RT treatment: • No measurable cognitive deficit in CT alone or CT + TBI groups, but sporadic cases of substantial toxicity[69] • Variable IQ changes from pre- to 1 year post-BMT – no change[69], 20% fell ≥ 10 points[77], 44% fell ≥ 2 SEs[78] • Fall ≥ 2 SEs in adaptive behavior scale – 39%[7]	cGvHD may have further profound effects on psychosocial adaptation post-allogeneic BMT	Note additive effects of multiple treatment episodes(as for neurological toxicity), aggravated by shorter intervals between episodes	2b

(continued)

Table 10.1 (continued)

Organ/system/Toxicity Primary causative Treatment(s)	Other potential risk factors	Clinical features and consequences	Frequency[b]	Impact of allogeneic BMT[c]	Comments	Cross-references
Dental/oral toxicity Before or during BMT: • Chemotherapy • Radiotherapy to field including jaws[d]	• Young age at treatment • Prior RT	Dental: • Root – hypoplasia • Teeth – microdontia, enamel hypoplasia, dental aplasia • Impaired craniofacial skeletal growth (primarily due to RT) Oral: • Xerostomia due to reduced saliva formation • Oral/salivary gland tumors – see 'Secondary malignancy'	• Root hypoplasia – 94%[79] • Microdontia – 75%[79] • Enamel hypoplasia – 44%[79] • Dental aplasia – 56%[79] • Impaired craniofacial skeletal growth – 100%[80] • Xerostomia, reduced salivary flow rate – 43%[81] NB All above figures relate to TBI, and are higher than after chemotherapy only[79–81] • Oral/salivary gland tumor – overall incidence 500– >2500 times expected[73]	1. Xerostomia linked with radiotherapy to field including salivary glands (usually TBI) and/or cGvHD[81, 82] 2. Secondary malignancy related to radiotherapy (usually TBI) and/or cGvHD[38]	Unclear (due to conflicting evidence) whether risk of caries is increased	7d
Visual/ocular toxicity Before BMT: • Previous radiotherapy to field including eyes[d] During BMT: • Radiotherapy to field including eyes[d] • ?Chemotherapy • Corticosteroids	• High dose/dose rate and/or unfractionated TBI (cataracts) • Prolonged use of steroids (cataracts)	Anterior segment: • Posterior subcapsular cataract • Keratoconjunctivitis sicca, with reduced tear secretion, leading to corneal/conjunctival ulceration/ scarring Posterior segment: • Chorioretinitis (viral e.g. CMV, VZV; toxoplasmosis)	• Cataract – 5.5% (no RT),[83] up to 34% (fractionated TBI),[84] up to 100% (unfractionated TBI)[83] • Keratoconjunctivitis sicca – 6%[84] • Chorioretinitis – rare (<1%) after 1 year post-BMT[85]	1. Keratoconjunctivitis sicca associated with cGvHD, but can occur in unaffected patients[84] 2. Uncertain if cGvHD, or its treatment with corticosteroids, is an independent risk factor for cataract development	Latent period before cataract formation (classically 3–4 years) may be longer after fractionated TBI, not yet clear whether this will increase ultimate incidence	2c
Auditory toxicity Before or during BMT: • Platinum agents • Aminoglycosides • Radiotherapy to field including ears[d]	• Younger age at treatment increases risk of impaired speech development	• Sensorineural hearing impairment • Impaired speech development	• Variable, but high in vulnerable patient groups, e.g. hearing loss at speech frequencies in young children treated with platinum agents or aminoglycosides before and during BMT – 22–82%[86,87]			2d

Organ toxicity	Risk factors	Clinical manifestations	Incidence	Comments	Caveats	
Cardiotoxicity	Before or during BMT: • Chemotherapy – principally anthracyclines, but also high-dose cyclophosphamide and other alkylating agents • Radiotherapy to a field including heart[d] • Pre-EMT iron overload in thalassaemia • Sepsis	• ECG abnormalities including arrythmias • Myocardial toxicity ranging from subclinical damage (e.g. echocardiographic) to clinical cardiac failure • Pericardial disease, including effusions • Valvular disease	• ECG abnormalities – 16%[88] • Subclinical left ventricular impairment – 25%[89] • Abnormal exercise testing – 74%[88] • Cardiomyopathy – 7%[90] • Cardiac failure – 3%[7] • Incidence of very late toxicity not yet known	Pericardial effusions related to cGvHD in some patients[20]	Not yet proven that BMT causes additional cardiac impairment in children who have already received cardiotoxic treatment	4a 4b
Nephrotoxicity	Before or during BMT: • Chemotherapy – especially platinum agents, ifosfamide • Radiotherapy to fields including kidneys[d] Before, during or after BMT: • Nephrotoxic anti-infective agents • Sequelae of acute renal failure during BMT • Hepatic veno-occlusive disease • ?Young age	• ?Glomerular hyperfiltration • Radiation nephritis – chronic renal (glomerular) impairment, hypertension, anemia, hematuria + hemolysis (in acute form) • Proximal tubular impairment • Isolated hypertension	• Subclinical glomerular impairment – 28%[91,92] • Subclinical tubular impairment – 45%[4] • Subacute radiation nephritis – 46%[3] • Hypertension – 16%[92] • Chronic renal failure – up to 28%[92,93] depending on criteria • End-stage renal failure – rare	1. cGvHD may present rarely with proteinuria, or even nephrotic syndrome[94,95] 2. Additive effect of nephrotoxic immunosuppressive agents, especially cyclosporin A and tacrolimus[92]	Acute presentation of renal toxicity (up to 1 year post-BMT), presumably due to radiation nephritis, may resemble hemolytic uremic syndrome (HUS)	6a, 6b
Endocrine toxicity	Before and during BMT: • Radiotherapy to field including affected gland[d] • Chemotherapy (including busulphan and cyclophosphamide, BuCy) • Unfractionated TBI	Pituitary: • Growth hormone – see 'Growth impairment' • No conclusive evidence of TSH, ACTH, LH/FSH, prolactin deficiency post-BMT Thyroid: • Hypothyroidism (often compensated), may be transient • Hyperthyroidism reported after neck RT, not yet described after TBI • Thyroid tumors – see 'Secondary malignancy' Adrenal: • No conclusive evidence of cortisol deficiency post-BMT	• Hypothyroidism – compensated more common than overt; fractionated TBI – 25%, mostly compensated, may be transient; unfractionated TBI – 58%, overt in 15%[96]; clinical symptoms – 1.1% (adults)[97] • Thyroid tumors (adenomas, carcinomas) – overall incidence 125 times expected[73] • Metabolic syndrome – 39%; type 2 diabetes – 17% (single report)[98] • Type 1 and 2 diabetes mellitus – 8% (single report)[99]	Autoimmune disturbances, including thyroid disease but also diabetes, described particularly in patients with cGvHD[50]	1. Longer term studies required, especially after fractionated TBI 2. Uncertain whether occurrence of metabolic syndrome post-BMT is related to GH deficiency	8a, 8b

(continued)

Table 10.1 (continued)

Organ/system/Toxicity Primary causative treatment(s)[a]	Other potential risk factors	Clinical features and consequences	Frequency[b]	Impact of allogeneic BMT[c]	Comments	Cross-references
		Pancreas: • Metabolic syndrome – hyperinsulinemia, impaired glucose tolerance, hypertriglyceridemia, ± hypertension, ± obesity • Type 1 diabetes mellitus • Type 2 diabetes mellitus				
Growth impairment Before and during BMT: • Radiotherapy – TBI, total lymphoid irradiation (TLI), cranial, craniospinal • Chemotherapy Before, during and after BMT: • Corticosteroids	• Younger age (<6 years) at BMT • Underlying diagnosis, e.g. thalassemia (iron overload) • Chronic illness • High total RT dose (especially >1 RT episode); unfractionated TBI • Growth hormone deficiency • ?Poor nutrition • Constitutional bone marrow failure syndromes (e.g. Fanconi anemia)	• Short stature due to growth impairment • Skeletal disproportion • Reduced bone mineral density in adulthood due to GH deficiency • Adult GH deficiency syndrome	• Short stature (final height below −2 standard deviation scores) – 21% of mixed pediatric population (80% of whom received RT during prior or conditioning treatment)[100] • Mean final height loss (SDS) of −1.17 in males, −0.56 in females; greatest loss (−2.07) after prior cranial RT and unfractionated TBI[100] • Mean final height loss (SDS) greater with younger age at TBI, −3.49 if <6 years at BMT, −1.92 if 6–12 years, −0.37 if 12–15 years[10] • Final height loss after TBI (14 patients) – males 8.6 cm, females 7.9 cm; but not significantly different from target height[101]	1. Association with cGvHD and prolonged use of steroids 2. In general, patients with major postallogeneic BMT complications suffer greater degrees of impaired growth[102]	Not possible to predict precisely the impact of GH treatment on final height in children with TBI-associated GH deficiency; prospective randomized controlled trials, with follow-up to final height, are not yet available	
Reproductive toxicity Before and during BMT: • Radiotherapy to field including gonads (and uterus in females)[d] • Chemotherapy, especially	• Older age at BMT • Gender • High total RT dose; unfractionated TBI • Total dose of	• Delayed/arrested puberty • Impaired fertility • Requirement for hormone replacement treatment in adult life in those patients with Leydig	Males: • Delayed puberty after fractionated TBI, requiring HRT – 7%[103] • Overt Leydig cell failure,		1. Longer follow-up needed to assess full impact of reproductive	8c, 8d, 8e

alkylating agents, e.g. high-dose cyclophosphamide (HD Cy), BuCy, melphalan (males)	alkylating agents (i.e. including prior treatment)	cell or ovarian failure Males: • Leydig cell dysfunction – low testosterone, raised gonadotrophins • Germ cell failure – azoospermia/ oligospermia Females: • Ovarian failure – amenorrhea, low estradiol, raised gonadotrophins • Pregnancy may occur, but uterine damage may lead to miscarriage, or premature delivery and low birthweight, especially if prepubertal at BMT • Even if ovarian recovery occurs, early menopause may follow	requiring HRT – 70%,[103] increasing with age (Dr A. Leiper, unpublished observations) • Germ cell failure – recovery reported, even after TBI, but conception rare, 24% after HD Cy, 7% after BuCy, 1% after TBI[104] Females: • Delayed menarche after fractionated TBI, requiring HRT – 44%[103] • Overt ovarian failure, requiring HRT – recovery may occur after HD Cy (54%), but only rarely after TBI (10%), very rarely after BuCy (1%)[104] • Pregnancy – 24% after HD Cy, 1% after TBI, 0% after BuCy[104]	toxicity 2. Fertility preservation techniques under active investigation	
Musculoskeletal toxicity Before or during BMT: • Chemotherapy, especially methotrexate (reduced bone mineral density, BMD) • Cranial radiotherapy, leading to endocrinopathy (reduced BMD) During BMT: • Radiotherapy to field including affected bone (AVN and OC)[d] Before, during or after BMT: • Corticosteroids (AVN, ?reduced BMD)	• Older age (>16 years), rare <10 years age (AVN) • Male gender (AVN) • GH deficiency, hypogonadism (reduced BMD)	Muscular: See 'Neurological toxicity' Skeletal: • Avascular necrosis (AVN) – hip most commonly affected, often bilaterally • Osteochondroma (OC) – often multiple, malignant change rare • Reduced BMD • Others – including slipped epiphysis, scoliosis	• Avascular necrosis – 0.6% at 5 years in patients <16 years age at BMT[105] • Osteochondroma – 26%[106] • Reduced BMD – varies considerably with methodology, especially choice of controls; whole body bone mass only minimally reduced compared to similar childhood ALL survivors treated without BMT,[107] but BMD reduced more in 10 children (using age but not height-matched controls) than in 13 adults[108]	Association with GvHD and hence steroid usage (AVN, BMD in adult studies) Important need for long-term prospective studies of BMD with appropriate age-/height-matched controls	9a, 9b, 9c
Secondary malignancy Before or during BMT: • Chemotherapy, especially	• Young age • Cranial	• Solid tumors – late onset, median 4–8 years post-BMT; brain	• Solid tumors – risk increases with time, cumulative 4% at	1. Prognosis of secondary 1. Note influence of cGvHD (especially in	3a, 3b

(continued)

Table 10.1 (continued)

Organ/system/Toxicity Primary causative treatment(s)[a]	Other potential risk factors	Clinical features and consequences	Frequency[b]	Impact of allogeneic BMT[c]	Comments	Cross-references
alkylating agents, topoisomerase II inhibitors (especially epipodophyllotoxins) • Radiotherapy	radiotherapy, especially in younger children • High RT dose	and thyroid tumors especially common in young (<5 years age) recipients of cranial RT • Acute myeloid leukemia/myelodysplasia – early onset, median 2½ years post-BMT, often associated with cytogenetic abnormalities, especially deletions or monosomy of chromosomes 5 or 7	10 years, 11% at 15 years post-BMT; greater increased relative risk compared to normal population (60 times expected at >10 years)[73] • AML/MDS – predominantly occur after autologous BMT; very rare in children (age >35 years at BMT is a recognized risk factor)[109]	skin and oral tumors), immunosuppressive treatment and prior diagnosis of Fanconi anemia in allogeneic BMT 2. Post-transplant lymphoproliferative disease, often EBV-related, usually donor-derived, occurs in severely immunosuppressed (often mismatched) allogeneic BMT patients – usually early-onset (<1 year post-BMT)[11]	malignancy post-BMT is variable, but often poor 2. Lympho-proliferative disease may be treated by donor-derived cytotoxic T lymphocytes	

[a]Note that the etiology of late adverse effects is often multifactorial.

[b]The figures given for the frequency of the particular toxicities listed in this table are approximate and representative, and may vary considerably with study methodology (cross-sectional, prospective cohort, etc.) and the patient group (diagnosis, age at and type of BMT, presence of risk factors, etc.). Many studies include both allogeneic and autologous BMT recipients, and some include adult patients.

[c]This column highlights additional toxicity due to specific complications of allogeneic BMT (discussed in more detail in 'Selected late adverse effects of BMT in children – complex presentations and multifactorial etiology' in this chapter).

[d]Including TBI.

ACTH, adrenocorticotrophin; AML, acute myeloid leukemia; AVN, avascular necrosis; BMD, bone mineral density; BMT, bone marrow transplantation; BuCy, busulphan and cyclophosphamide; cGvHD, chronic graft-versus-host disease; CMV, cytomegalovirus; CNS, central nervous system; CT, chemotherapy; EBV, Epstein–Barr virus; ECG, electrocardiogram; GH, growth hormone; HD Cy, high-dose cyclophosphamide; HRT, hormone replacement therapy; LH/FSH, luteinizing hormone/follicle-stimulating hormone; MDS, myelodysplasia; OC, osteochondroma; RT, radiotherapy; SDS, standard deviation scores; TBI, total body irradiation; TSH, thyroid-stimulating hormone; VZV, Varicella zoster virus.

restrictive pulmonary disease, with an isolated diffusion defect in 15 per cent and a restrictive pattern in 23 per cent.[16] A longitudinal study of 25 patients followed up for 4–13 (median 8) years after allogeneic BMT performed in childhood revealed a low transfer factor in 20 per cent, and restrictive lung volume patterns in 40 per cent.[20] Prospective studies of children undergoing autologous BMT show that most long-term survivors have evidence of restrictive deficits (reduced lung volumes and/or diffusion capacity), although the presence of pre-BMT abnormalities in some patients demonstrates the relevance of prior treatment.[21,22] Most children in these studies were asymptomatic, reflecting the considerable pulmonary functional reserve in children, but the high frequency of subclinical abnormalities raises concerns about long-term pulmonary outcome in later life.

The frequency and severity of pulmonary impairment varies with time after BMT. Several longitudinal studies have shown initial reductions in lung volumes and diffusion capacity in the first few months after BMT, followed by partial but often incomplete improvement by 1 year, leaving persisting abnormalities in 40–100 per cent of long-term survivors.[20,21] A few studies have reported further reductions in lung volumes later after BMT.[21]

Many classifications of pulmonary disease early and late post-BMT have been described, including entities defined by clinical and laboratory (e.g. microbiological, histological) findings, such as idiopathic pneumonia syndrome, and others.[23–25] However, the clinical spectrum of chronic obstructive and restrictive non-infective pulmonary disease seen post-BMT is perhaps best encompassed within the late-onset pulmonary syndrome (LOPS). The predominant symptoms are usually breathlessness and cough, but wheezing and occasionally fever may occur.[17,26] Clinical examination, which often reveals crackles and wheezes, and chest radiography, are frequently non-discriminatory, but high-resolution computed tomography scanning may offer a useful indication of the extent and severity of disease.[26]

Classification of the varied histological abnormalities underlying LOPS incorporates bronchiolitis obliterans (BO), bronchiolitis obliterans with organizing pneumonia (BOOP), interstitial pneumonia (lymphocytic or non-classifiable) and diffuse alveolar damage (DAD).[26] Although it is often difficult to relate the clinical features to specific histological diagnoses, it is possible to discern certain associations, particularly the remorseless obstructive disease associated with BO, and the link between cGvHD and both BO and BOOP.[24,25]

Many risk factors have been determined or suggested for late pulmonary complications after BMT. Although there is disagreement between published pediatric studies, restrictive disease has usually been attributed to prior or conditioning chemotherapy (especially bleomycin, busulphan or methotrexate) and radiotherapy (including TBI), and may be exacerbated by cGvHD. Obstructive disease, although rarer in children, appears to be associated with allogeneic, particularly mismatched, BMTs and the development of GvHD.[27] Pulmonary infections before or after BMT may increase the risk of restrictive and perhaps obstructive disease in children, while surgical removal of lung tissue may aggravate the effects of pulmonary toxicity post-BMT.

Late pulmonary infections, especially pneumococcal, but also with other encapsulated bacteria and occasionally opportunistic organisms (e.g. fungi, *Pneumocystis*), occur mainly but not exclusively in the context of cGvHD and immunosuppressive treatment.[28,29]

Management of established chronic pulmonary disease is difficult. Immunosuppressive treatment may be tried, particularly in cases associated with cGvHD, but convincing evidence of efficacy is lacking. Although stabilization may occur, chronic pulmonary disease does not appear to demonstrate any significant reversibility in the absence of treatment. Although the only effective method of prevention is to avoid or reduce known risk factors, it is sensible to minimize exacerbation of existing pulmonary disease by extrinsic factors including smoking.

Gastrointestinal

Chronic gastrointestinal complications post-BMT occur principally in the context of cGvHD. Non-specific features of nausea, vomiting and diarrhea may occur, while more rarely, esophageal stricture may cause dysphagia, and intestinal or pancreatic disease may result in malabsorption.[30–32] Peritoneal effusion has been reported very rarely.[18] A complete symptomatic response to immunosuppressive treatment was seen in 59 per cent of 17 children with chronic intestinal GvHD.[31]

Hepatic

Chronic hepatic disease post-BMT is primarily due to cGvHD or to the sequelae of viral hepatitis (especially hepatitis B and C) in countries where these infections are prevalent. Hepatic cGvHD is rare in most groups of children undergoing BMT, presenting with clinical and biochemical features of cholestasis, which may progress to severe intrahepatic small bile duct damage and loss.[33] Recently, it has been recognized that cGvHD may rarely present with a late onset of acute non-infectious hepatitis.[34] Hepatitis C usually causes chronic hepatitis in long-term survivors of BMT, with a risk of cirrhosis, although severe liver disease is rare.[35] Hepatitis B may cause few problems in those patients no longer on immunosuppressive treatment.[35] Iron overload owing to multiple blood transfusions before and during BMT may contribute to liver dysfunction.[36]

Dermatological

Chronic skin disease post-BMT is predominantly due to cGvHD, manifest by erythema, hypopigmentation and/or hyperpigmentation, poikiloderma and lichenoid lesions, progressing to sclerodermatous skin involvement with joint contractures in severe disease.[37]

Secondary malignancies of the skin may occur and analysis of data from 19 229 BMT recipients (median age 25.5 years at BMT between 1964 and 1992) showed that the relative risk of developing skin melanoma was 5.0, while the development of squamous cell carcinoma of the skin was correlated with cGvHD.[38]

Hematological

Chronic immune-mediated cytopenias may occur late after BMT.[39,40] Although transient in some patients, they may be associated with cGvHD and are sometimes refractory to treatment. Recently, telomere shortening has been described in peripheral blood leukocytes from pediatric BMT recipients, raising the theoretical concern that this may predispose to the development of clonal hematological disorders (e.g. myelodysplasia) later in life.[41] However, the degree of telomere shortening, and hence its clinical significance, remains uncertain.[42]

Immunological

Although adequate phagocyte (including neutrophil) numbers and function are usually restored within the first few months post-BMT, recovery of lymphocyte numbers and function takes much longer.[43,44] Absolute total lymphocyte and B cell numbers reached low normal levels in 68–77 per cent of 22 children by 6 months after BMT (utilizing HLA identical donors in 21 patients) for hematological malignancy, but T-cell recovery was much slower with normal numbers in only 32 per cent.[45] As previously documented in adults, CD4+ helper T cells recovered even more slowly, attaining low normal numbers in only 10 per cent of children by 6 months. There was no evidence of peripheral blood expansion of CD45RO+/CD4+ and CD7−CD4+ 'memory' helper T cells after engraftment had occurred, and thymic-dependent production of CD45RA+/CD4+ 'naive' helper T cells was very slow.[45] These observations do not support previous beliefs that immune recovery post-BMT might be qualitatively and quantitatively superior in children compared to adults. The increasing use of considerably mismatched donors (e.g. haploidentical RDs) in pediatric HSCT, with the consequent increased risks of GvHD and graft rejection, implies that significant immunodeficiency post-HSCT is likely to become more common, owing to both intensive immunosuppressive prophylaxis (including marrow T-cell depletion) and treatment, and the increased delays in immune reconstitution associated with mismatched transplants.

Despite improved strategies to allow earlier diagnosis and treatment of a wide variety of infections post-HSCT, fatal late infections still occur in patients with delayed immune reconstitution, and in some cases may even be increasing owing to rising numbers of extremely immunosuppressed patients. For example, the diagnosis was established more than 6 months after allogeneic BMT in two of six adult patients with adenoviral disease, which is associated with high mortality.[46] Likewise, late invasive pneumococcal infection occurred up to 15 years post-BMT in a large prospective study, with an incidence of 8.6 out of 1000 transplants and a mortality rate of 18 per cent.[47] The incidence was higher (18.9 out of 1000 allogeneic BMTs) in patients with cGvHD. Although antibiotic prophylaxis (commonly with penicillin) is usually recommended post-HSCT, it does not offer complete protection against pneumococcal infection.[47]

It is increasingly recognized that the slow pace of immune reconstitution in HSCT recipients (especially allogeneic) places them at increased risk from vaccine-preventable infections, and the use of a formal reimmunization program, with appropriate precautions, is now recommended post-HSCT.[48, 49]

Disordered immune recovery may occur after autologous and especially allogeneic BMT, leading to autoimmune manifestations, including myasthenia gravis and immune-mediated cytopenias, particularly in the context of cGvHD. Other autoimmune illnesses, especially thyroid disease, but also including diabetes and hepatitis, are reported.[50]

CHRONIC GRAFT–VERSUS–HOST DISEASE

Although cGvHD is fortunately rarer in pediatric BMT recipients than in adults, it may be particularly troublesome in older children and adolescents. Indeed, some pediatric series have reported a significant incidence of cGvHD, and it is likely that its frequency will rise with the increasing use of mismatched or unrelated donors. For example, Matthes-Martin[51] reported that, of 73 children surviving 1 year after allogeneic BMT performed at a median age of 7.9 years at a single center, 27 per cent had cGvHD (extensive in 85 per cent), and a further 4 per cent developed it over the next 2 years. The development of cGvHD may have a considerable adverse impact on the quality of long-term survivorship for several reasons. Its multisystem nature may lead to an extensive variety of persistent and disabling symptoms, which are frequently difficult to control effectively. Intensive immunosuppression, often with multiple agents, is often required, but

Table 9d.2 *Clinical manifestations of chronic graft versus host disease complicating bone marrow transplantation in children[52]*

Peripheral nervous system – myasthenia gravis,[a] peripheral neuropathy

Skin – lichenoid and/or sclerodermatous lesions[b]

Oral – xerostomia (see Table 9d.1), lichenoid and/or atrophic lesions

Ocular – keratoconjunctivitis sicca (see Table 9d.1)

Pulmonary – obstructive airways disease[b]

Renal – proteinuria, nephrotic syndrome[94,95]

Hepatic – cholestatic damage[b]

Gastrointestinal – nausea, vomiting, esophageal strictures, diarrhea, malabsorption (intestinal or pancreatic)[b]

Musculoskeletal – polymyositis, sclerodermatous joint contractures[b]

Serosal – pericardial, pleural and/or peritoneal effusions[18]

Hematological – immune-mediated[a] cytopenias[b]

Immunological – delayed immune reconstitution, increased risk of late infections[b]

Autoimmunity – hypothyroidism and hyperthyroidism, other rare diseases[b]

Secondary malignancies – possible association with squamous carcinoma of buccal cavity and skin[38]

Adverse effects of immunosuppressive treatment, e.g. further increased risk of infections; nephrotoxicity due to cyclosporin A or tacrolimus; contribution of corticosteroids to numerous toxicities, including cataracts, avascular necrosis, growth impairment

[a] May be regarded as further examples of autoimmunity.
[b] See text.

this treatment itself carries considerable risk of morbidity or death due to infection.[52] Ultimately, of the 155 children transplanted in the Matthes-Martin report, 9 per cent died from cGvHD or associated late infections.[51]

Table 10.2 illustrates the complexity and numerous manifestations of this adverse effect of allogeneic BMT in children. Further details are provided elsewhere in this section, and in Table 10.1.

LATE MORBIDITY AND MORTALITY

Unsurprisingly, given the original indication for transplantation, and the frequency and severity of many of the potential late complications, it has been questioned whether BMT confers a normal life span after the initial high-risk period.[53] Socie compared the mortality rates of 6691 allogeneic BMT recipients listed in the IBMTR, who had remained free of their original disease for 2 years post-BMT, with those of an age-, sex- and nationality-matched control population.[54] The median (range) age at BMT was 25 (<1–69) years. All BMTs were performed for leukemia or aplastic anemia between 1980 and 1993. Although the probability of living for a further 5 years (once 'disease-free' at 2 years post-BMT) was 89 per cent, the mortality remained higher than the control population until 6 years post-BMT for aplastic anemia, and until at least 9 years for leukemia.[54] However, the commonest cause of death in those patients transplanted for leukemia was, in fact, recurrent leukemia, despite being disease free at 2 years. Nevertheless, in patients transplanted for aplastic anemia, cGvHD was the commonest cause of death, while in all patients combined, 23 per cent of deaths were due to other causes (most commonly infection not related to GvHD, secondary malignancy or organ failure).

The overall burden of late morbidity in survivors of BMT is likely to impact on the quality of survival. This was investigated in detail by the Great Ormond Street team who examined concurrent combinations of late sequelae.[55,56] A cohort of 83 patients surviving at least 3 years after BMT (autologous in 22, or using allogeneic HLA-identical sibling donors in 61) performed in childhood (mean age 6.8 years) for acute leukemia was evaluated at a median of 7.9 (range 3.5–16.9) years post-BMT. Retrospective case-note review of organ toxicity, growth and endocrine development, neuropsychological function, schooling and employment, second malignant neoplasms and late deaths was performed. However, fertility was not assessed. The median age of evaluation was 14.9 (4.8–30.2) years. BMT was performed in first remission in 52 per cent. Prior cranial, testicular or ocular radiotherapy had been given to 33 per cent, 12 per cent and 2 per cent, respectively. Late sequelae were very common: 93 per cent of survivors had one or more, while 73 per cent had at least three.

The average number of adverse complications per survivor was 3.7, but those receiving TBI (67 patients) had a higher burden of morbidity (5.0 late sequelae per survivor) than those receiving chemotherapy (busulphan and cyclophosphamide) alone (2.3 late sequelae per survivor), although the latter group included fewer children of pubertal age at evaluation. The complications were categorized into mild, moderate and severe, and the frequency of each of these categories in the TBI and chemotherapy alone groups is shown in Table 10.3. Morbidity was higher in the irradiated group, owing to a greater frequency of moderate and severe sequelae (cataracts, growth impairment, thyroid dysfunction, cardiotoxicity and secondary neoplasia). There were nine late deaths (11 per cent of patients surviving at 3 years post-BMT), occurring at a mean of 6.9 years post-BMT, owing to relapsed leukemia in three patients, secondary malignancy in three, cGvHD in two and pneumonitis in one. Overall (including nonfatal cases), secondary neoplasia and chronic GvHD both occurred in 6 per cent of survivors.[55,56]

Clearly, although the long-term results of BMT have improved greatly, and should continue to do so as safer but effective conditioning regimens, and improved infection

Table 9d.3 *Categorization and frequency of late sequelae in 83 patients who underwent bone marrow transplantation (BMT) for acute leukemia in childhood[55,56]*

(a) *Categorization of late sequelae of BMT according to severity*

Mild	Moderate	Severe
Exostoses	Growth and endocrine dysfunction[a]	Life-threatening conditions
Vitiligo	Cognitive deficits	Severe disability
Minor audiological deficits (audiogram)	Cataracts	Secondary malignant neoplasms
Dental	Clinical deafness	
Nasolachrymal duct obstruction	Cardiotoxicity	
	Reduced glomerular filtration rate	
	Osteoporosis	

[a]Infertility is *not* included.

(b) *Frequency of late sequelae of BMT, categorized according to severity and the type of conditioning received*

Severity	Total body irradiation	Busulphan and cyclophosphamide
Mild	49%	47%
Moderate	94%	53%
Severe	31%	23%

and GvHD prophylaxis regimens are developed, late toxicity needs to be reduced further before the procedure can be considered to normalize life expectancy completely.

QUALITY OF LIFE

The quality of life (QoL) following BMT performed during childhood has become a topic of considerable relevance as a natural corollary to considering the life span of long-term survivors. In general terms and using non-specific measures, survivors of BMT function well and show good social reintegration. Out of patients assessed in Socie's IBMTR study,[54] and those in a second large study conducted by the European Group for Blood and Marrow Transplantation (EBMT), consisting of a mixed cohort of 477 adults and 321 children surviving at least 5 years from BMT for malignant or non-malignant disorders,[57] 85–93 per cent of those tested had normal or minimally reduced performance scores (Karnofsky >90 per cent). Other small, exclusively pediatric studies are in agreement.[58–61] The presence of cGVHD has an adverse impact on performance,[57] particularly when still active 1–2 years post-BMT.[54]

As a measure of social reintegration, over 95 per cent of the combined 113 patients of school age (or older) included in Matthes-Martin's[51] and Schmidt's[61] studies resumed school or work. This compares favorably to reports from mixed adult and pediatric studies, with 83–90 per cent returning to school or employment in the EBMT study,[57] and in a study of 212 adults and children transplanted for aplastic anemia in Seattle.[62]

The few formal QoL studies that exist in children are small, including between 28 and 98 patients[50,58,62,63] but several additional adult studies contain childhood populations. Overall, there is general agreement that younger patients have good self-evaluation of their QoL.

The historical method of health-related QoL (HRQL) assessment in children, based on proxy reporting (usually by parents), has major disadvantages in that parental ratings may be significantly lower than the children's self-evaluation.[65] The Spanish collaborative GETMON (Grupo Espanol de Transplante de Medula Osea en el Nino) study is, therefore, useful, in that it investigated survivors of childhood autologous and allogeneic BMT performed for neoplastic disease, who were >17 years of age at assessment and able to answer a QoL telephone questionaire without parental intervention. The 98 disease-free survivors, whose minimum survival was 3 years, valued their QoL more highly than the healthy control group. Although they had more concerns than their peers about physical appearance, education and work opportunities, they identified fewer problems regarding relationships with family and friends, sleep, depression and leisure opportunities.[59]

Not all of the predominantly adult studies share this optimism.[66] However, poorer QoL and performance appear to be correlated with the development of cGvHD in both adults and children.[51,54,57,61,66] Other factors associated with poorer QoL include the presence of late sequelae and older age at BMT performed in adulthood.[61,66] The correlation with older age is unsurprising in view of the increased frequency of cGvHD in adults compared to pediatric BMT recipients.[61] Other factors may exert a negative influence on QoL, such as a short interval from BMT (less than 5 years),[66] although Matthes-Martin observed no difference in QoL between patients more than and those less than 3 years post-BMT performed in childhood.[51] Significant gender differences have been noted in certain aspects of QoL and pyschosocial adjustment in several predominantly adult studies.[57,66,67]

Pre-BMT levels of family cohesion and child adaptive functioning may have considerable influence on QoL and behavioral adjustment after BMT, at least in the short term.[68] Recently, a much larger prospective longitudinal study documented broadly similar findings.[69] This study assessed psychosocial (and cognitive) functioning in 153

children and adolescents both pre-BMT and at 1 year post-BMT, and additionally at 2 years in 74. Psychosocial evaluation concluded that not only was the prevalence of behavioral and social problems low, with stability of function over time, but that pre-BMT functioning was strongly predictive of later functioning. The results of cognitive testing are detailed in Table 10.1 (see 'Neuropsychological toxicity').

As a rule, despite the considerable morbidity suffered, children appear to experience superior QoL when compared to the adult BMT population, at least partly due to the lower frequency of cGvHD. Further large prospective pediatric studies are urgently needed before the true picture can emerge.

CONCLUSIONS

Although the long-term survival of patients undergoing HSCT is improving, the burden of chronic treatment-related morbidity remains considerable. Indeed, as more children undergo HSCT and more survive the potentially lethal early complications, the number of patients at risk of late adverse effects is increasing steadily. Other factors, particularly the rapidly expanding role of highly aggressive HSCT strategies in poor-risk patients, often using very high-dose chemoradiotherapy conditioning or increasingly mismatched donors, have contributed to the emergence of a cohort of survivors with considerable chronic organ damage due to previous treatment, conditioning chemoradiotherapy, cGvHD or all of these. These adverse effects are often particularly prominent and potentially most devastating in those children transplanted in the first few years of life, especially those who have received radiotherapy (e.g. cranial radiotherapy before or TBI during HSCT). There is an urgent need to reduce the frequency and severity of such toxicity so that future patients with these poor-risk diseases may be treated successfully without such a high risk of chronic morbidity.

It is pertinent to remember that relapsed disease remains the commonest cause of failure of BMT in children. Overall, more children succumb to the underlying disease process (both malignant and non-malignant) or its complications (e.g. infection) than die from the transplant process itself.[70] Therefore, the development of chemotherapy and radiotherapy conditioning regimens that maximize efficacy and minimize toxicity carries a very high priority. Likewise, the reduction of the burden of cGvHD by improved prophylaxis and treatment strategies is of paramount importance, as long as it is not at the cost of reducing the potentially curative graft versus leukemia effect.

However, pending these improvements, the need to treat poor-risk patients with BMT highlights the paucity of effective non-BMT treatments. Indeed, in future years, we should hope that the most fundamental means of reducing chronic morbidity from BMT will be to improve the curative potential of conventional primary treatment, thereby reducing the need for high-risk and intensive BMT approaches with their associated toxicity.

ACKNOWLEDGEMENTS

Data from the UKCCSG BMT Registry and the Statistical Center of the IBMTR is quoted with kind permission.

KEY POINTS

- Nearly all children treated by bone marrow transplantation (BMT) will experience at least one late adverse effect of treatment.
- Late adverse effects of BMT are very diverse and may involve any body system or tissue.
- There are many potential causes of late adverse effects after BMT, including high-dose chemotherapy and radiotherapy conditioning treatment, graft-versus-host disease (GvHD), the consequences of the underlying disease, its previous treatment and other supportive therapy, resulting in considerable potential for additive toxicity.
- There are important differences in the range of late adverse effects seen after autologous and allogeneic BMTs.
- Some late adverse effects of BMT (e.g. pulmonary toxicity) are potentially fatal.
- Chronic GvHD is a very important multisystem complication of BMT, which may cause considerable morbidity or even death.
- The increasing incidence of secondary malignant disease with time after BMT, with no plateau yet apparent, is of great concern.
- Despite the frequency and potential severity of late adverse effects, most survivors of BMT performed in childhood report good quality of life.

REFERENCES

1. Balduzzi A, Valsecchi MG, Silvestri D, et al. Transplant-related toxicity and mortality: an AIEOP prospective study in 636 pediatric patients transplanted for acute leukemia. Bone Marrow Transplant 2002; 29:93–100.
2. Cohen EP, Lawton CA, Moulder JE. Bone marrow transplant nephropathy: radiation nephritis revisited. Nephron 1995; 70:217–222.

3. Tarbell NJ, Guinan EC, Niemeyer C, *et al.* Late onset of renal dysfunction in survivors of bone marrow transplantation. *Int J Radiat Oncol Biol Phys* 1988; **15**:99–104.

4. Patzer L, Ringelmann F, Kentouche K, *et al.* Renal function in long-term survivors of stem cell transplantation in childhood. A prospective trial. *Bone Marrow Transplant* 2001; **27**:319–327.

●5. Boulad F, Sands S, Sklar C. Late complications after bone marrow transplantation in children and adolescents. *Curr Probl Pediatr* 1998; **28**:277–297.

●6. Brennan BMD, Shalet SM. Endocrine late effects after bone marrow transplant. *Br J Haematol* 2002; **118**:58–66.

●7. Leiper AD. Non-endocrine late complications of bone marrow transplantation in childhood: Part I. *Br J Haematol* 2002; **118**:3–22.

●8. Leiper AD. Non-endocrine late complications of bone marrow transplantation in childhood: Part II. *Br J Haematol* 2002; **118**:23–43.

●9. Sanders J. Late effects after bone marrow transplant. In: Schwartz CL, Hobbie WL, Constine LS, Ruccione KS (eds) *Survivors of childhood cancer. Assessment and management,* 1st edn. St Louis: Mosby, 1994:293–318.

10. Sanders JE. Growth and development after hematopoietic cell transplantation. In: Thomas ED, Blume KG, Forman SJ (eds) *Hematopoietic cell transplantation,* 2nd edn. Malden: Blackwell Science, 1999:764–775.

●11. Deeg HJ, Socie G. Malignancies after hematopoietic stem cell transplantation: many questions, some answers. *Blood* 1998; **91**:1833–1844.

12. Hale JP, Lewis IJ. Anthracyclines: cardiotoxicity and its prevention. *Arch Dis Child* 1994; **71**:457–462.

13. Billingham ME, Bristow MR, Glatstein E, *et al.* Adriamycin cardiotoxicity: endomyocardial biopsy evidence of enhancement by irradiation. *Am J Surg Path* 1977; **1**:17–23.

14. Goldberg MA, Antin JH, Guinan EC, Rappeport JM. Cyclophosphamide cardiotoxicity: An analysis of dosing as a risk factor. *Blood* 1986; **68**:1114–1118.

15. Kupari M, Volin L, Suokas A, *et al.* Cardiac involvement in bone marrow transplantation: electrocardiographic changes, arrhythmias, heart failure and autopsy findings. *Bone Marrow Transplant* 1990; **5**:91–98.

◆16. Cerveri I, Zoia MC, Fulgoni P, *et al.* Late pulmonary sequelae after childhood bone marow transplantion. *Thorax* 1999; **54**:131–135.

17. Schwarer AP, Hughes JMB, Trotman-Dickenson B, *et al.* A chronic pulmonary syndrome associated with graft-versus-host disease after allogeneic marrow transplantation. *Transplantation* 1992; **54**:1002–1008.

18. Seber A, Khan SP, Kersey JH. Unexplained effusions: association with allogeneic bone marrow transplantation and acute or chronic graft-versus-host disease. *Bone Marrow Transplant* 1996; **17**:207–211.

19. Toren A, Nagler A. Massive pericardial effusion complicating the course of chronic graft-versus-host disease (cGvHD) in a child with acute lymphoblastic leukemia following allogeneic bone marrow transplantation. *Bone Marrow Transplant* 1997; **20**:805–807.

◆20. Nysom K, Holm K, Hesse B, *et al.* Lung function after allogeneic bone marrow transplantation for leukaemia or lymphoma. *Arch Dis Child* 1996; **74**:432–436.

21. Neve V, Foot ABM, Michon J, *et al.* Longitudinal clinical and functional pulmonary follow-up after megatherapy, fractionated total body irradiation, and autologous bone marrow transplantation for metastatic neuroblastoma. *Med Pediatr Oncol* 1999; **32**:170–176.

22. Arvidson J, Bratteby L-E, Carlson K, *et al.* Pulmonary function after autologous bone marrow transplantation in children. *Bone Marrow Transplant* 1994; **14**:117–123.

23. Clark JG, Hansen JA, Hertz MI, *et al.* Idiopathic pneumonia syndrome after bone marrow transplantation. *Am Rev Respir Dis* 1993; **147**:1601–1606.

●24. Afessa B, Litzow MR, Tefferi A. *Bronchiolitis obliterans* and other late onset non-infectious pulmonary complications in hematopoietic stem cell transplantation. *Bone Marrow Transplant* 2001; **28**:425–434.

25. Quabeck K. The lung as a critical organ in marrow transplantation. *Bone Marrow Transplant* 1994; **14**(Suppl, 4):S19–S28.

◆26. Palmas A, Tefferi A, Myers JL, *et al.* Late-onset noninfectious pulmonary complications after allogeneic bone marrow transplantation. *Br J Haematol* 1998; **100**:680–687.

◆27. Schultz KR, Green GJ, Wensley D, *et al.* Obstructive lung disease in children after allogeneic bone marrow transplantation. *Blood* 1994; **84**:3212–3220.

28. Soubani AO, Miller KB, Hassoun PM. Pulmonary complications of bone marrow transplantation. *Chest* 1996; **109**:1066–1077.

29. Engelhard D. Bacterial and fungal infections in children undergoing bone marrow transplantation. *Bone Marrow Transplant* 1998; **21**(Suppl. 2):S78–S80.

30. McDonald GB, Sullivan KM, Schuffler MD, *et al.* Esophageal abnormalities in chronic graft-versus-host disease in humans. *Gastroenterology* 1981; **80**:914–921.

31. Patey-Mariaud de Serre N, Reijasse D, Verkarre V, *et al.* Chronic intestinal graft-versus-host disease: clinical, histological and immunohistochemical analysis of 17 children. *Bone Marrow Transplant* 2002; **29**:223–230.

32. Akpek G, Valladares JL, Lee L, *et al.* Pancreatic insufficiency in patients with chronicgraft-versus-host disease. *Bone Marrow Transplant* 2001; **27**:163–166.

33. McDonald GB, Shulman HM, Sullivan KM, Spencer GD. Intestinal and hepatic complications of human bone marrow transplantation. Part II. *Gastroenterology* 1986; **90**:770–784.

34. Strasser SI, Shulman HM, Flowers ME, *et al.* Chronic graft-versus-host disease of the liver: presentation as an acute hepatitis. *Hepatology* 2000; **32**:1265–1271.

35. Locasciulli A, Nava S, Sparano P, Testa M. Infections with hepatotropic viruses in children treated with allogeneic bone marrow transplantation. *Bone Marrow Transplant* 1998; **21**(Suppl. 2):S75–S77.

36. McKay PJ, Murphy JA, Cameron S, *et al.* Iron overload and liver dysfunction after allogeneic or autologous bone marrow transplantation. *Bone Marrow Transplant* 1996; **17**:63–66.

37. Sullivan KM, Shulman HM, Storb R, *et al.* Chronic graft-versus-host disease in 52 patients: adverse natural course and successful treatment with combination immunosuppresion. *Blood* 1981; **57**:267–276.

38. Curtis RE, Rowlings PA, Deeg HJ, *et al.* Solid cancers after bone marrow transplantation. *N Engl J Med* 1997; **336**:897–904.

39. Barge AJ, Johnson G, Witherspoon R, Torok-Storb B. Antibody-mediated marrow failure after allogeneic bone marrow transplantation. *Blood* 1989; **74**:1477–1480.

40. Klumpp TR, Block CC, Caligiuri MA, *et al.* Immune-mediated cytopenia following bone marrow transplantation. Case reports and review of the literature. *Medicine* 1992; **71**:73–83.

41. Wynn R, Thornley I, Freedman M, Saunders EF. Telomere shortening in leucocyte subsets of long-term survivors of allogeneic bone marrow transplantation. *Br J Haematol* 1999; **105**:997–1001.

42. Rufer N, Brummendorf TH, Chapuis B, *et al.* Accelerated telomere shortening in hematological lineages is limited to the first year following stem cell transplantation. *Blood* 2001; **97**:575–577.

43. Foot ABM, Potter MN, Donaldson C, *et al.* Immune reconstitution after BMT in children. *Bone Marrow Transplant* 1993; **11**:7–13.

44. Lenarsky C. Mechanisms in immune recovery after bone marrow transplantation. Management of posttransplant immune deficiency. *Am J Pediatr Hematol Oncol* 1993; **15**:49–55.

45. de Vries E, van Tol MJD, Langlois van den Bergh R, *et al.* Reconstitution of lymphocyte subpopulations after paediatric bone marrow transplantation. *Bone Marrow Transplant* 2000; 25:267–275.

46. Chakrabarti S, Mautner V, Osman H, *et al.* Adenovirus infections following allogeneic stem cell transplantation: incidence and outcome in relation to graft manipulation, immunosuppression, and immune recovery. *Blood* 2002; 100:1619–1627.

47. Engelhard D, Cordonnier C, Shaw PJ, *et al.* Early and late invasive pneumococcal infection following stem cell transplantation: a European Bone Marrow Transplantation survey. *Br J Haematol* 2002; 117:444–450.

48. Singhal S, Mehta J. Reimmunization after blood or marrow stem cell transplantation. *Bone Marrow Transplant* 1999; 23: 637–646.

49. Skinner R, Cant A, Davies G, *et al.* Immunisation of the immunocompromised child. *Best Practice Statement.* London: Royal College of Paediatrics and Child Health, 2002.

50. Sherer Y, Shoenfeld Y. Autoimmune diseases and autoimmunity post-bone marrow transplantation. *Bone Marrow Transplant* 1998; 22:873–881.

51. Matthes-Martin S, Lamche M, Ladenstein R, *et al.* Organ toxicity and quality of life after allogeneic bone marrow transplantation in pediatric patients: a single centre retrospective analysis. *Bone Marrow Transplant* 1999; 23:1049–1053.

52. Sullivan KM, Agura E, Anasetti C, *et al.* Chronic graft-versus-host disease and other late complications of bone marrow transplantation. *Semin Hematol* 1991; 28:250–259.

53. Thomas ED. Does bone marrow transplantation confer a normal life span? *N Engl J Med* 1999; 341:50–51.

54. Socie G, Stone JV, Wingard JR, *et al.* Long-term survival and late deaths after allogeneic bone marrow transplantation. Late Effects Working Committee of the International Bone Marrow Transplant Registry. *N Engl J Med* 1999; 341:14–21.

55. Pitcher L, Chessels J, Veys P, *et al.* Late effects of bone marrow transplantation for childhood leukaemia – the medical cost of cure (Abstract 3). *Bone Marrow Transplant* 1998; 21(Suppl. 2):S81.

56. Pitcher L, Chessells JM, Hann IM, Leiper AD. Evaluation of late morbidity in patients undergoing bone marrow transplantation for leukaemia in childhood (Abstract P-259). *Med Pediatr Oncol* 1999; 33:251.

57. Duell T, van-Lint MT, Ljungman P, *et al.* Health and functional status of long-term survivors of bone marrow transplantation. *Ann Intern Med* 1997; 126:184–192.

58. Balduzzi A, Gooley T, Anasetti C, *et al.* Unrelated donor marrow transplantation in children. *Blood* 1995; 86:3247–3256.

59. Badell I, Igual L, Gomez P, *et al.* Quality of life in young adults having received a BMT during childhood: a GETMON study. *Bone Marrow Transplant* 1998; 21(Suppl. 2):S68–S71.

60. Gordon BG, Warkentin PI, Strandjord SE, *et al.* Allogeneic bone marrow transplantation for children with acute leukemia: long-term follow up of patients prepared with high dose cytosine arabinoside and fractionated total body irradiation. *Bone Marrow Transplant* 1997; 20:5–10.

61. Schmidt GM, Niland JC, Forman SJ, *et al.* Extended follow-up in 212 long-term allogeneic bone marrow transplant survivors. Issues of quality of life. *Transplantation* 1993; 55:551–557.

62. Deeg HJ, Leisenring W, Storb R, *et al.* Long-term outcome after marrow transplantation for severe aplastic anemia. *Blood* 1998; 91:3637–3645.

63. Kanabar DJ, Attard-Montalto S, Saha V, *et al.* Quality of life in survivors of childhood cancer after megatherapy with autologous bone marrow rescue. *Pediatr Hematol Oncol* 1995; 12:29–36.

64. Nespoli L, Verri AP, Locatelli F, *et al.* The impact of paediatric bone marrow transplantation on quality of life. *Qual Life Res* 1995; 4:233–240.

65. Parsons SK, Barlow SE, Levy SL, *et al.* Health-related quality of life in pediatric bone marrow transplant survivors: according to whom? *Int J Cancer* 1999; (Suppl. 12):46–51.

66. Chiodi S, Spinelli S, Ravera G, *et al.* Quality of life in 244 recipients of allogeneic bone marrow transplantation. *Br J Haematol* 2000; 110:614–619.

67. Heinonen H, Volin L, Uutela A, *et al.* Gender-associated differences in the quality of life after allogeneic BMT. *Bone Marrow Transplant* 2001; 28:503–509.

68. Barrera M, Boyd-Pringle LA, Sumbler K, Saunders F. Quality of life and behavioural adjustment after pediatric bone marrow transplantation. *Bone Marrow Transplant* 2000; 26:427–435.

69. Kupst MJ, Penati B, Debban B, *et al.* Cognitive and psychosocial functioning of pediatric hematopoietic stem cell transplant patients: a prospective longitudinal study. *Bone Marrow Transplant* 2002; 30:609–617.

70. Bosi A, Laszlo D, Labopin M, *et al.* Second allogeneic bone marrow transplantation in acute leukemia: results of a survey by the European Cooperative Group for Blood and Marrow Transplantation. *J Clin Oncol* 2001; 19:3675–3684.

71. Thompson CB, Sanders JE, Flournoy N, *et al.* The risks of central nervous system relapse and leukoencephalopathy in patients receiving marrow transplants for acute leukemia. *Blood* 1986; 67:195–199.

72. Padovan CS, Yousny TA, Schleuning M, *et al.* Neurological and neuroradiological findings in long-term survivors of allogeneic bone marrow transplantation. *Ann Neurol* 1998; 43:627–633.

73. Socie G, Curtis RE, Deeg HJ, *et al.* New malignant diseases after allogeneic marrow transplantation for childhood acute leukemia. *J Clin Oncol* 2000; 18:348–357.

74. Padovan CS, Bise K, Hahn J, *et al.* Angiitis of the central nervous system after allogeneic bone marrow transplantation? *Stroke* 1999; 30:1651–1656.

75. Patchell RA. Neurological complications of organ transplantation. *Ann Neurol* 1994; 36:688–703.

76. Christie D, Battin M, Leiper AD, *et al.* Neuropsychological and neurological outcome after relapse of lymphoblastic leukaemia. *Arch Dis Child* 1994; 70:275–280.

77. Phipps S, Dunavant M, Srivastava DK, *et al.* Cognitive and academic functioning in survivors of pediatric bone marrow transplantation. *J Clin Oncol* 2000; 18:1004–1011.

78. Kramer JH, Crittenden MR, DeSantes K, Cowan MJ. Cognitive nd adaptive behavior 1 and 3 years following bone marrow transplantation. *Bone Marrow Transplant* 1997; 19:607–613.

79. Nasman M, Forsberg CM, Dahllof G. Long-term dental development in children after treatment for malignant disease. *Eur J Orthod* 1997; 19:151–159.

80. Dahllof G, Forsberg CM, Ringden O, *et al.* Facial growth and morphology in long-term survivors after bone marrow transplantation. *Eur J Orthod* 1989; 11:332–340.

81. Dahllof G, Bagesund M, Ringden O. Impact of conditioning regimens on salivary function, caries-associated microorganisms and dental caries in children after bone marrow transplantation. A 4-year longitudinal study. *Bone Marrow Transplant* 1997; 20:479–483.

82. Woo S-B, Lee SJ, Schubert MM. Graft-vs.-host disease. *Crit Rev Oral Biol Med* 1997; 8:201–216.

83. Calissendorff BM, Bolme P. Cataract development and outcome of surgery in bone marrow transplanted children. *Br J Ophthalmol* 1993; 77:36–38.

84. De-Marco R, Dassio DA, Vittone P. A retrospective study of ocular side effects in children undergoing bone marrow transplantation. *Eur J Ophthalmol* 1996; 6:436–439.

85. Coskuncan NM, Jabs DA, Dunn JP, *et al.* The eye in bone marrow transplantation. VI. Retinal complications. *Arch Ophthalmol* 1994; 112:372–379.

86. Parsons SK, Neault MW, Lehmann LE, *et al.* Severe ototoxicity following carboplatin-containing conditioning regimen for autologous marrow transplantation for neuroblastoma. *Bone Marrow Transplant* 1998; 22:669–674.

87. Liesner RJ, Leiper AD, Hann IM, Chessells JM. Late effects of intensive treatment for acute myeloid leukemia and myelodysplasia in childhood. *J Clin Oncol* 1994; 12:916–924.

◆88. Eames GM, Crosson J, Steinberger J, *et al.* Cardiovascular function in children following bone marrow transplant: a cross-sectional study. *Bone Marrow Transplant* 1997; 19:61–66.

◆89. Pihkala J, Saarinen UM, Lundstrom U, *et al.* Effects of bone marrow transplantation on myocardial function in children. *Bone Marrow Transplant* 1994; 13:149–155.

90. Leung W, Hudson MM, Strickland DK, *et al.* Late effects of treatment in survivors of childhood acute myeloid leukemia. *J Clin Oncol* 2000; 18:3273–3279.

91. Kist-van Holthe JE, van Zwet JML, Brand R, *et al.* Bone marrow transplantation in children: Consequences for renal function shortly after and 1 year post-BMT. *Bone Marrow Transplant* 1998; 22:559–564.

◆92. Van Why SK, Friedman AL, Wei LJ, Hang R. Renal insufficiency after bone marrow transplantation in children. *Bone Marrow Transplant* 1991; 7:383–388.

93. Frisk P, Bratteby LE, Carlson K, Lonnerholm G. Renal function after autologous bone marrow transplantation in children: a long-term prospective study. *Bone Marrow Transplant* 2002; 29:129–136.

94. Oliveira JSR, Bahai D, Franco M, *et al.* Nephrotic syndrome as a clinical manifestation of graft-versus-host disease (GVHD) in a marrow transplant recipient after cyclosporine withdrawal. *Bone Marrow Transplant* 1999; 23:99–101.

95. Gomez-Garcia P, Herrera-Arroyo C, Torres-Gomez A, *et al.* Renal involvement in chronic graft-versus-host disease: a report of two cases. *Bone Marrow Transplant* 1988; 3:357–362.

◆96. Thomas BC, Stanhope R, Plowman PN, Leiper AD. Endocrine function following single fraction and fractionated total body irradiation for bone marrow transplantation in childhood. *Acta Endocrinol* 1993; 128:508–512.

97. Al-Fiar FZ, Colwill R, Lipton JH, *et al.* Abnormal thyroid stimulating hormone (TSH) levels in adults following allogeneic bone marrow transplants. *Bone Marrow Transplant* 1997; 19:1019–1022.

98. Taskinen M, Saarinen-Pihkala UM, Hovi L, *et al.* Impaired glucose tolerance and dyslipidaemia as late effects after bone-marrow transplantation in childhood. *Lancet* 2000; 356:993–997.

99. Traggiai C, Stanhope R, Nussey S, Leiper AD. Diabetes mellitus after bone marrow transplantation in chidhood. *Med Pediatr Oncol* 2003; 40:128–129.

◆100. Cohen A, Rovelli A, Bakker B, *et al.* Final height of patients who underwent bone marrow transplantation for hematological disorders during childhood: a study by the Working Party for Late Effects – EBMT. *Blood* 1999; 93:4109–4115.

101. Holm K, Nysom K, Rasmussen MH, *et al.* Growth, growth hormone and final height after BMT. Possible recovery of irradiation-induced growth hormone insufficiency. *Bone Marrow Transplant* 1996; 18:163–170.

102. Adan L, de Lanversin M-L, Thalassinos C, *et al.* Growth after bone marrow transplantation in young children conditioned with chemotherapy alone. *Bone Marrow Transplant* 1997; 19:253–256.

◆103. Sarafoglou K, Boulad F, Gillio A, Sklar C. Gonadal function after bone marrow transplantation for acute leukemia during childhood. *J Pediatr* 1997; 130:210–216.

◆104. Sanders JE, Hawley J, Levy W, *et al.* Pregnancies following high-dose cyclophosphamide with or without high-dose busulfan or total-body irradiation and bone marrow transplantation. *Blood* 1996; 87:3045–3052.

◆105. Socie G, Cahn JY, Carmelo J, *et al.* Avascular necrosis of bone after allogeneic bone marrow transplantation: analysis of risk factors for 4388 patients by the Societe Francaise de Greffe de Moelle (SFGM). *Br J Haematol* 1997; 97:865–870.

106. Harper GD, Dicks-Mireaux C, Leiper AD. Total body irradiation-induced osteochondromata. *J Pediatr Orthop* 1998; 18:356–358.

◆107. Nysom K, Holm K, Michaelsen KF, *et al.* Bone mass after allogeneic BMT for childhood leukaemia or lymphoma. *Bone Marrow Transplant* 2000; 25:191–196.

108. Bhatia S, Ramsay NK, Weisdorf D, *et al.* Bone mineral density in patients undergoing bone marrow transplantation for myeloid malignancies. *Bone Marrow Transplant* 1998; 22:87–90.

109. Bhatia S, Ramsay NKC, Steinbuch M, *et al.* Malignant neoplasms following bone marrow transplantation. *Blood* 1996; 87:3633–3639.

11

Cutaneous complications

E CLAIRE BENTON AND MICHAEL J TIDMAN

INTRODUCTION

Children treated for cancers of all types frequently develop cutaneous complications related either to therapy or to the disease process itself. Radiation therapy and chemotherapy both have a variety of well-recognized short-term side effects, including direct toxicity to the skin and its appendages as well as the cutaneous complications of treatment-related immune suppression. Those patients who develop severe neutropenia or lymphopenia during therapy are particularly at risk of a wide spectrum of opportunistic bacterial, viral and fungal infections.

However, the long-term consequences of childhood cancer and its therapy are less well described. We will consider late complications as those occurring 3 months or more after cessation of active treatment, and will also include signs that could herald relapse or progression of the underlying cancer.

The categories to be described include:

- cutaneous infections related to a relative state of immunosuppression;
- graft-versus-host disease following bone marrow transplantation;
- acquisition of cutaneous disease as a result of allografting;
- adverse effects of irradiation or drugs, including ongoing medication;
- cutaneous or mucosal tumors related to previous chemotherapy or irradiation;
- cutaneous signs of disease recurrence or progression, including malignant infiltrates of the skin and paraneoplastic phenomena.

With survival rates for childhood cancers now being overall in the region of 75 per cent,[1] the long-term consequences of these diseases and their treatments need to be documented so that appropriate strategies for monitoring patients into adult life can be devised, and rapid treatment offered when appropriate. Parallels can be drawn with recipients of organ allografts whose ongoing immunosuppressed state predisposes them both to long-term infective and malignant complications.[2]

INFECTIONS

Human papillomavirus infection

Viral warts caused by the human papillomavirus (HPV) are very common, affecting around 10 per cent of the population at any one time. Their incidence has been reported as up to 25 per cent of children in some epidemiological studies, with hand warts being ten times as common as plantar warts, although any body site may be involved. HPV infections are generally self-limiting, spontaneous resolution occurring in 65 per cent of children in 2 years and up to 95 per cent in 5 years.[3] However, resolution is dependent on an intact immune system, in particular the TH1 response. Patients with persistent immune impairment as a result of disease or its treatment may have extensive warts that are recalcitrant to standard therapies. Their incidence in children after organ transplantation was found to be over 50 per cent.[2] A similar problem is seen especially in children after treatment of hematological malignancies for which high-dose chemotherapy regimes, often including systemic

steroids, are employed. However, no data are available on precise incidence. Although some warts improve spontaneously after cessation of chemotherapy, others may persist for months or years, and can be a cause of discomfort and concern.

Their appearance depends on the infecting HPV type and the anatomical site, but essentially they consist of discrete hyperkeratotic papules or plaques with characteristic thrombosed capillaries visible as black dots after paring the wart with a scalpel blade (Figure 11.1, Plate 4). Viral warts can occur on the oral and occasionally the genital mucosa, a site where there may be possible long-term risks of neoplastic change. Hughes *et al.*[4] demonstrated a significantly increased incidence of cervical intraepithelial neoplasia in women previously treated for Hodgkin's disease. Patients who continue on oral cyclosporin therapy to control graft-versus-host disease are also at risk. Regular cervical cytology and possible colposcopic examination should be considered for such patients in late teenage years and beyond.

Treatment of cutaneous warts should initially comprise standard topical therapies with salicylic acid, glutaraldehyde or formalin creams or gels (although these are not suitable for facial or mucosal warts), with the addition of regular liquid nitrogen cryotherapy for older children who are able to tolerate the discomfort of this procedure.

Therapies for patients with recalcitrant warts, such as intralesional interferon or bleomycin, or immunotherapy by induction of contact allergic hypersensitivity to diphencyprone, are only suitable for adults.[5]

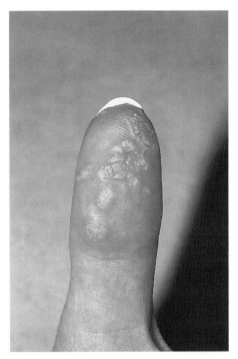

Figure 11.1 *Persistent mosaic viral wart in a young woman after treatment for Hodgkin's disease.*

Molluscum contagiosum

This is a common pox virus infection in children. Individual lesions comprise a pink or flesh-colored papule with an umbilicated center and vary in size from 1 to 5 mm diameter. They will usually resolve spontaneously within months, leaving small, pale, 'pock-like' atrophic scars. Impairment of the TH1 immune response may predispose to the development of extensive lesions that resolve only on restoration of normal immunity.[6] Molluscum contagiosum has been described in patients receiving donor lymphocyte infusions for maintenance of remission in leukemia following bone marrow transplantation.[7] They are often disseminated in the immunosuppressed, probably because there is a reservoir of viral particles in adjacent histologically normal skin.[8] It is important to differentiate molluscum from cryptococcal infection occurring in the presence of persistent severe immunosuppression, as they may have a similar clinical appearance. Treatment comprises traumatizing individual lesions by squeezing with fine forceps or freezing with liquid nitrogen. Application of a topical antibiotic will prevent secondary infection and there is some evidence that topical cidofovir may be of benefit.[9]

Herpes virus infections

Both herpes simplex and herpes zoster infections are more likely to cause problems during active treatment of a cancer but, when immunosuppression is protracted, persistent infection can occur, usually manifesting as indolent ulcers (Figure 11.2, Plate 5). This may be difficult to diagnose and, if suspected, a skin biopsy for histology and viral culture may be necessary to confirm the diagnosis. Response to treatment with acyclovir is usually good but a prolonged course of therapy may be necessary. Acyclovir-resistant herpes infections can occur in the presence of severe immunosuppression.[10]

Yeast infections

Mucocutaneous candidiasis is predominantly a complication observed during active treatment of cancer (Figure 11.3, Plate 6), when it can become systematized. It may also occur with ongoing immunosuppressive therapy or treatment-induced diabetes. Careful attention should be paid to oral hygiene, and nystatin suspension or oral fluconazole used to treat the infection.

Tinea versicolor is caused by the overgrowth of a skin commensal, *Pityrosporum furfur*. It presents as reddish brown, scaly macules on the trunk and proximal parts of the limbs. Characteristically the affected areas become pale after sun exposure. It is uncommon in children but may be seen in young adults with ongoing

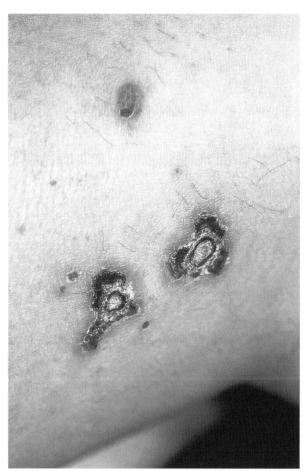

Figure 11.2 *Indolent ulcers caused by persistent* Herpes zoster *infection in an immunosuppressed patient.*

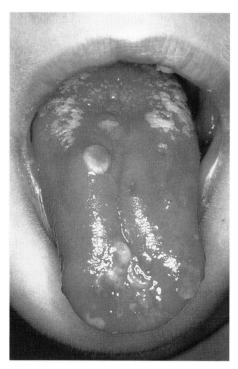

Figure 11.3 *Oral candidiasis in a leukemic child. (Photograph courtesy of Dr H. Wallace.)*

immunosuppression, such as cyclosporin therapy.[11] The diagnosis is confirmed by examining skin scrapings prepared in potassium hydroxide solution for spores and hyphae. It can be treated by application of a solution of selenium sulfide 1 per cent to a wet skin for 15 minutes before rinsing off and subsequent application of clotrimazole cream to any remaining areas. Systemic itraconazole may be helpful for extensive involvement.

Proliferation of other skin commensal mites, such as *Demodex folliculorum* and *Demodex brevis*, will cause an itchy, papular, erythematous dermatitis, which has been described in children treated for acute lymphoblastic leukemia. It responds to the application of 5 per cent permethrin cream.[12]

Dermatophyte infections

These are caused by a group of fungi that invade the hair, skin and nails. Anthropophilic types spread between persons, whereas the zoophilic types are acquired from animals. The commonest clinical presentation is with interdigital maceration ('athlete's foot'), which may then spread to the plantar or dorsal surfaces of the foot, and in some cases the nails. If the infection is present at the time of cancer treatment, the immunosuppression resulting from chemotherapy may result in dissemination of the fungus to other skin sites, where it takes on a characteristic annular configuration (ringworm). Occasionally, deep dermal invasion of the fungus can occur in the severely immunosuppressed.[13] Scalp involvement may result in a large inflammatory mass (kerion) with resultant hair loss and scarring. Zoophilic infections, such as *Microsporum canis* from cats and dogs or *Trichophyton verrucosum* from cattle may vary in appearance from scaly pink macules to inflammatory plaques with peripheral pustulation and scaling. The diagnosis can be confirmed by direct microscopy and culture of skin scrapings, nail clippings or plucked hairs. Examination under ultraviolet (Wood's) light will reveal a green fluorescence with *Microsporum canis* infection. Treatment with systemic antifungal agents, either griseofulvin or terbinafine, is indicated unless the infection is localized to the toe webs, when topical clotrimazole will suffice.

Bacterial infections

Bacterial infections of the skin with *Staphylococcus* or *Streptococcus* may be more common during chemotherapy-induced neutropenia, and children who have spent prolonged periods in hospital during treatment of cancer may acquire nasal or cutaneous staphylococcal carriage.

Impetigo or folliculitis can arise as a result, and antibacterial solutions containing chlorhexidine 1 per cent or benzalkonium chloride 1 per cent can be used for skin cleansing as well as mupirocin cream to eliminate nasal bacterial carriage. Indolent ulcers (ecthyma) secondary to staphylococcal or streptococcal infection may need to be differentiated from ecthyma gangrenosum caused by pseudomonas infection[14] or atypical herpes virus infections. Topical antibacterial agents, such as fusidic acid or mupirocin, can be used for localized involvement, but systemic antibiotics are required for widespread infections.

Cellulitis caused by streptococcal infection requires a portal of entry, such as a breach in the skin, and may be more common during episodes of neutropenia. Spreading areas of tender erythema and edema, sometimes with peripheral blistering and accompanied by pyrexia and malaise, characterize the disease that responds to intravenous phenoxymethylpenicillin and flucloxacillin.

Infestations

Scabies, caused by a skin infestation with the mite *Sarcoptes scabeii*, is common amongst schoolchildren. In the period following cancer chemotherapy when a child's immune response may not have recovered completely, there will be a greater risk of acquiring the infestation. Onset of itching is delayed for several weeks after exposure and is typically nocturnal. It may, however, be less apparent in the immunosuppressed, so the diagnosis can initially be overlooked. The clinical signs include a non-specific excoriated, sometimes pustular, eruption on the trunk and limbs, but the pathognomonic feature is the linear burrow usually detected on the wrists or finger webs (Figure 11.4, Plate 7). In the immunosuppressed, burrows and mites may be numerous and widespread, so-called crusted or Norwegian scabies.[15] Scabies infestation has been mistaken for seborrheic dermatitis of the scalp in children with acute lymphoblastic leukemia.[16]

Treatment involves the application of either permethrin cream for 8 hours or malathion lotion for 24 hours, and should be repeated 1 week later. Both the patient and all close contacts should be treated. Application is to all body sites, including the scalp in the very young and the immunosuppressed. Crotamiton cream can be used to control postscabetic itch, which may persist for several weeks after treatment.

GRAFT-VERSUS-HOST DISEASE

The clinical and histological features produced when immunocompetent cells of donor tissue react with the tissues of an immunosuppressed graft recipient are described as graft-versus-host disease (GvHD). Essential

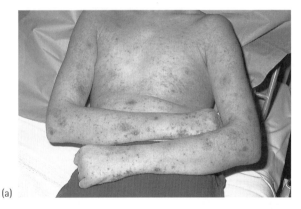

(a)

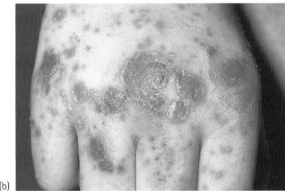

(b)

Figure 11.4   *(a) Impetiginized scabies infestation in an immunosuppressed child. (b) Close up of hands showing multiple burrows. (Photographs courtesy of Dr H. Wallace.)*

conditions permitting the occurrence of the graft-versus-host response are:[17]

1 profound depression of the recipient's cellular immune response;
2 receipt of an allograft of lymphoid immuno-competent cells; and
3 recognition by the allograft of foreign antigens in the host tissue.

The reaction is more likely to occur in the presence of major HLA differences between donor and host, but can occur even when HLA types are identical, for example, in cases of identical twins. The reaction was first described in 1916 and since the 1960s has been reported as an important complication of allogeneic bone marrow transplantation.[18]

Pathogenesis

The donor T lymphocytes interact with recipient histocompatibility antigens to which they become sensitized. These then differentiate and mount an attack on recipient cells producing the clinical signs of graft-versus-host disease. The onset of GvHD is determined by the time between the graft infusion and subsequent lymphocyte

proliferation and differentiation. The target organs are skin, gastrointestinal tract and lung, which all share exposure to endotoxins and bacterial products that can trigger and amplify local inflammation. Those tissues all have a large proportion of antigen-presenting cells that may enhance the graft-versus-host reaction. In addition, other infections, such as cytomegalovirus (CMV), herpes virus or Epstein–Barr virus, may trigger or aggravate GvHD. Chronic disease is thought to result from the generation of autoreactive T-cell clones derived from the engrafted donor lymphoid stem cells, which differentiate within the recipient. The sclerotic changes observed in chronic GvHD result from the effects of cytokines on collagen synthesis.

Pathological features in the skin

These changes are classified into four grades (Table 11.1). The earliest change is perivascular cuffing of lymphocytes around dilated blood vessels with swollen endothelial cells, and this is followed by a mild to moderate lymphocytic infiltrate involving the upper dermis up to the dermoepidermal junction and associated with epidermal basal cell vacuolation. As the disease becomes established, more extensive basal cell vacuolation occurs with disruption of the basement membrane, lymphocyte migration into the epidermis and the development of spongiotic changes (Figure 11.5a, Plate 8a). Single cell necrosis occurs throughout the epidermis. In full thickness GvHD, the epidermis separates at the dermoepidermal junction with widespread desquamation and necrosis of the overlying epidermis (Figure 11.5b, Plate 8b).

Chronic GvHD is characterized by a hyperkeratotic, atrophic epidermis with thickening of the basement membrane and condensed homogeneous connective tissue in the upper dermis, where there are thickened hyalinized collagen bundles and destruction of adnexal structures.

Clinical features of GvHD in the skin

The acute disease is typically seen around the time of hemopocitic recovery 10–14 days after transplantation,

but can vary from 5 to 60 days post-transplant. It starts as a maculopapular eruption, commonly on the palms and soles, and may sometimes mimic eczema.[19] In severe forms, erythroderma with extensive blistering and desquamation as seen in toxic epidermal necrolysis can occur and may be accompanied by fever, and gastrointestinal and liver function abnormalities. The differential diagnosis of acute GvHD includes radiation and drug reactions, palmar and plantar erythrodysesthesia, and exanthematous eruptions associated with hepatitis C or CMV viremia. Not all cases progress to the chronic form but those that do will have first manifested changes of acute GvHD.

Chronic disease is characterized by pigmentation, sclerotic skin and a lichen planus-like rash, including a reticulate white streaking of the buccal mucosa, gingiva, tongue and palate. Polygonal purplish papules with Wickham's striae often occur in a reticulate distribution, suggesting a relationship to the underlying vascular network. Follicular lesions of lichen plano-pilaris may be an early manifestation and the Koebner phenomenon can occur, with localization of lesions to sites of epidermal

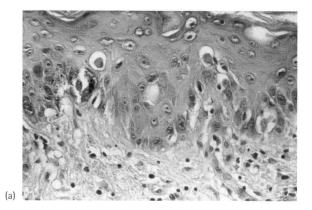
(a)

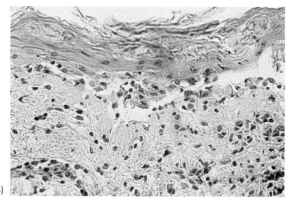
(b)

Figure 11.5 *(a) Grade 2 graft-versus-host disease (GvHD) with basal cell vacuolation and single death together with a lymphocytic infiltrate. (b) Grade 3/4 GvHD showing subepidermal split and necrosis of the overlying epidermis. (Photographs courtesy of Dr K. McLaren.)*

Table 11.1 *Pathological changes in graft-versus-host disease*

Grade	Definition
1	Focal or diffuse vacuolation of the basal epidermal cells
2	Vacuolar alteration of basal epidermal cells: spongiosis and dyskeratosis of epidermal cells
3	Formation of subepidermal cleft in association with spongiosis and dyskeratosis
4	Complete loss of epidermis

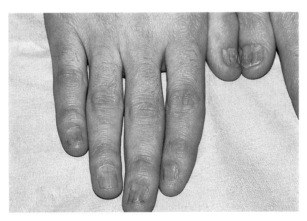

Figure 11.6 *Nail changes in chronic graft-versus-host disease.*

damage. Scarring alopecia and dystrophy of nails characterized by pterygium formation have been reported (Figure 11.6, Plate 9). Hyperpigmentation in a perifollicular or reticulate distribution can predate the appearance of sclerotic change and is thought to represent postinflammatory change. It is usually confined to sites of lichenoid or sclerodermatous change, although diffuse melanoderma as a consequence of graft-versus-host disease has been reported.[20] There are some similarities between the clinical manifestations of chronic graft-versus-host disease and dyskeratosis congenita,[21] and the latter diagnosis should be excluded.[22]

Sclerosis of the skin, which is characterized clinically by a firm indurated texture, is a late manifestation of GvHD, and can be localized or progress to extensive scleroderma resulting in flexion deformities, limitation of movement and ulceration over pressure points. Xerostomia and xerophthalmia have been reported, and there may be features in common with other connective tissue disorders. Patients with chronic GvHD have persistent immune defects and are, therefore, more prone to a variety of bacterial, fungal and viral infections.

Treatment

Since 1980, cyclosporin has replaced methotrexate for the prophylaxis and treatment of GvHD and, although cyclosporin does not reduce its incidence, it does reduce the severity. The cutaneous side effects of cyclosporin include hypertrichosis and gum hypertrophy. Chronic GvHD is treated with cyclosporin and corticosteroids. PUVA photochemotherapy (administration of psoralen followed by UVA exposure)[23] may be helpful for progressive disease but can predispose to skin malignancy in later life.[24] Important aspects of disease management include control of secondary infection and regular physiotherapy.

ADOPTIVE TRANSFER OF SKIN DISORDERS WITH BONE MARROW TRANSPLANTATION

The potential for transfer of a variety of cutaneous disorders by means of bone marrow transplantation should be considered and the recipient counseled about this. Psoriasis, considered to be a condition of abnormal keratinocyte proliferation induced by T lymphocytes, has been reported to develop in bone marrow allograft recipients with no previous history of the condition. It has also occurred within a short time following marrow transplantation from sibling donors who have been psoriasis sufferers.[25,26] Resolution of severe psoriasis in bone marrow allograft recipients has been reported after transplantation from non-psoriatic donors.[27–29] Although those case reports relate to adults, it seems likely that similar potential will apply to children.

The transfer of atopic tendencies with bone marrow has also been reported in two separate cases of young boys with acute leukemia who received transplants from their siblings. In the first case,[30] a 9-year-old recipient, who had acute lymphocytic leukemia, had no history of atopy before transplantation, but within 6 months developed a very similar pattern of food allergy to the donor, his atopic brother.

The second case report was of a 5-year-old boy with acute lymphoblastic leukemia, who after marrow allografting, developed severe atopic dermatitis associated with the same pattern of food allergy as his donor sister. Allergen avoidance enabled control of his eczema.[31] The passive transfer within bone marrow of immunologically primed memory cells is a possible explanation. Transfer of another autoimmune condition, vitiligo, following allogeneic bone marrow transplantation for non-Hodgkin's lymphoma has been recorded in an adult.[32]

The development of Addison's disease 10 years after a successful bone marrow transplant has been reported in a boy with the Wiskott–Aldrich syndrome, which is associated with a predisposition to lymphoreticular malignancies.[33] The patient presented with cutaneous and mucosal hyperpigmentation, fatigue, polyuria and diarrhea. Adrenal antibodies were detected in the patient. However, cotransplantation of an autoimmune adrenal insufficiency appears to have been excluded and, therefore, this may have been a chance association.

ADVERSE EFFECTS OF DRUGS AND RADIATION

Chemotherapeutic drugs used in the short- and long-term may cause a variety of unwanted cutaneous effects, which may be not only uncomfortable and psychologically distressing, but also require to be distinguished from other complications of the treatment of childhood

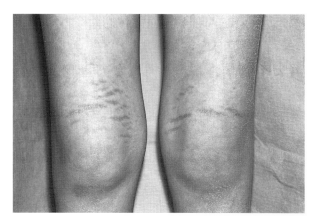

Figure 11.7 *Striae distensae over the knees associated with long-term corticosteroid therapy. (Photograph courtesy of Dr H. Wallace.)*

cancers, such as GvHD and infections. Mucocutaneous reactions to chemotherapy have recently been reviewed.[34]

Systemic corticosteroid therapy is frequently necessary and in the medium to long-term may result in a number of adverse effects on the skin.[35] One of the more distressing for adolescent children is steroid-induced acne, which tends to be more monomorphic than acne vulgaris. The mechanism for this is uncertain but systemic corticosteroids appear to induce cornification in the upper part of the pilosebaceous duct. Another concerning side effect is the development of striae distensae (Figure 11.7, Plate 10) particularly on the trunk. Systemic steroids may also cause cutaneous thinning, resulting in telangiectasia, easy bruising and purpura, hypertrichosis and redistribution of body fat, resulting in truncal adiposity, buffalo hump and moon face.

Alopecia is one of the commonest and most distressing side effects associated with many cytotoxic agents. There are two principal patterns of alopecia: anagen effluvium and telogen effluvium. Hair loss in anagen effluvium is a direct result of depressed mitotic activity in hair matrix cells, resulting in either the production of a defective weakened hair shaft, which breaks easily with normal hair care, or no hair at all. Anagen effluvium normally starts early in chemotherapy and usually resolves once chemotherapy is completed, although this cannot be guaranteed. Occasionally, hair may regrow with a changed texture or color. The hair loss associated with telogen effluvium occurs up to several months after a precipitating event, usually the acute illness associated with the onset of malignancy, or the severe stress surrounding the illness. Spontaneous regrowth with time is the norm.

Numerous cancer chemotherapeutic agents have the potential for inducing hyperpigmentation that may involve the skin, mucous membranes, hair and nails. The mechanism is undetermined but occasionally external factors seem to play a part. The hyperpigmentation may be restricted to areas of skin occluded by tape, electrocardiograph pads or elastic bandages, suggesting that drug excreted in sweat on to an occluded skin surface may result in a direct toxic effect on underlying melanocytes.[36] Gradual resolution usually occurs.

Nail changes including diffuse, transverse or longitudinal bands of pigmentation and leuconychia have been reported with chemotherapeutic agents, sometimes in association with other nail abnormalities, such as Beau's lines, onycholysis and shedding of the nails.[34]

Hyperpigmentation of the buccal mucous membranes, gingiva, tongue, conjunctiva and genital mucous membranes may occasionally occur as a result of cancer chemotherapy.

Ulceration of mucous membranes, particularly those of the mouth, is an important cause of morbidity in cancer chemotherapy. The most common mechanism is a direct toxic effect of the drug on mucous membranes. Bone marrow suppression predisposing to infection and hemorrhage may also be associated with ulceration as a result of infection by normal oral flora or secondary viral infections, particularly with Herpesvirus hominis and Herpesvirus varicellae.

Stomatitis may also be commoner in children than adults because of the higher mitotic index of their oral epithelium.[34] The discomfort of stomatitis may be a limiting factor in administration of chemotherapy. Oral hygiene should be encouraged before and during periods of chemotherapy, and symptomatic measures, such as analgesia and the use of topical mucosal coating agents, may be helpful.

Acral erythema (palmo-plantar syndrome or erythrodysesthesia) is an acute response to chemotherapy. It is primarily a condition of adults, with relatively few cases documented in children.[37,38] It is characterized by an uncomfortable burning sensation that is associated with swelling of the fingers and hands, and may be difficult to distinguish from acute GvHD disease. Activities such as walking or handling objects may be compromised. This condition tends to settle when chemotherapy is stopped but recurrences may occur if chemotherapy is resumed.

Extravasation of certain chemotherapeutic drugs during intravenous administration may result in localized damage, and eventual necrosis and ulceration of the tissues. If left untreated, long-term damage to underlying tendons, nerves and vessels may occur, necessitating surgical intervention.

A number of chemotherapeutic agents, including methotrexate and cyclophosphamide, can have phototoxic effects. Such reactions, resembling sunburn, occur principally on sun-exposed regions and are acute consequences of treatment that will resolve within a few weeks. However, resulting hyperpigmentation may persist for several months. Photo-onycholysis may also occur but will slowly grow out.

Other acute problems associated with chemotherapy include hypersensitivity reactions, flushing, an eruption of lymphocyte recovery, neutrophilic eccrine hidradenitis and eccrine squamous syringometaplasia.

The long-term cutaneous consequences of radiation therapy include atrophy, fibrosis and telangiectasia. Certain chemotherapeutic agents may increase the toxicity of radiotherapy if administered within 1 week of each other. Such radiation enhancement results in an exaggerated early inflammatory reaction, which may cause blistering, necrosis or ulceration, usually settling to leave some postinflammatory hyperpigmentation or, with severe reactions, depigmentation. It is likely that radiation enhancement increases the long-term damage caused by radiotherapy. Radiation recall is the phenomenon of an inflammatory reaction developing in a previously irradiated site as a result of the administration of a chemotherapeutic drug.[34] Radiation damage may be recalled by chemotherapy months to years after the initial radiotherapy and usually occurs very shortly after administration of the incriminated drug. The radiation recall reaction usually settles within a few weeks of stopping chemotherapy.

CUTANEOUS TUMORS

The risk of a second malignancy in those treated for childhood cancer is much greater than in a control population, rising with the passage of time, and, generally, second tumors carry a relatively high mortality. Malignant melanoma and non-melanoma skin cancer together represent a high percentage (10–20 per cent) of second tumors,[39–42] and factors contributing to this probably include reduced immunosurveillance as the result of chemotherapy and the direct toxic effects of radiotherapy plus subsequent exposure to natural ultraviolet radiation. It therefore follows that children who have completed chemotherapy and radiotherapy should be subject to long-term surveillance of their skin, and that they and their parents should be carefully counseled regarding measures to protect against undue sun exposure. Such measures should include advice on the wearing of appropriate outdoor clothing (wide-brimmed hat, long shirt-sleeves, long trousers and tightly woven white material) and the application of suitable sun-screening agents, which confer protection against the ultraviolet A and B ranges of the electromagnetic spectrum when the climatic conditions demand. Modification of outdoor behavior, such as avoiding direct exposure to strong sunlight, should also be encouraged.

Several studies have confirmed that compared with age-matched controls, children undergoing chemotherapy for hematological malignancy are at greater risk of subsequent development of melanocytic nevi,[43–45] which are more likely to occur in less common sites, such as palms and soles.[46]

A large number of melanocytic nevi is a very important risk factor for malignant melanoma;[47] thus, it seems reasonable to advise that individuals who do develop numerous moles should be subject to particular scrutiny, perhaps with a photographic record. However, a large study from Australia did not confirm a significant increase in overall density of melanocytic nevi in pediatric oncology patients, but did show that significantly more had atypical or acral nevi compared to a control population.[48]

One patient in this study developed a malignant melanoma 13 years following chemotherapy and radiotherapy for a rhabdomyosarcoma. Malignant melanoma has also been recorded on the scalp in childhood after cranial irradiation for acute lymphocytic leukemia.[49]

The administration of human growth hormone has been shown to cause melanocytic nevi to grow faster and to result in a reversible stimulation of nevus cells,[50] raising concern about the potential for an increased risk of malignant melanoma in survivors of childhood neoplasia treated with this. In a study of a population of children with secondary growth hormone deficiency, as the result of chemotherapy or radiotherapy for intracranial tumors, human growth hormone therapy was associated with increased numbers of large nevi, although this was not statistically significant.[51]

Non-melanoma skin cancer is very uncommon in childhood. The risk of basal cell carcinoma developing over the succeeding two decades is increased in areas of previous irradiation, especially on the scalp, a site affected by cranial irradiation in the treatment of acute lymphocytic leukemia.[52–54]

These tumors may appear innocuous, are often associated with normal hair growth and, therefore, hidden from view,[55] highlighting the importance of clinical monitoring and the necessity of obtaining histological evaluation of lesions developing within areas of previous irradiation. Radiotherapy during childhood results in atrophic skin in 30 per cent of cases,[56] but the development of basal cell carcinomas may occur in the absence of clinical or histological changes of radiodermatitis. The factors that seem to influence the development of non-melanoma skin cancer include the total accumulated dose of radiation, multiple small-dose treatments, a fair skin coloring, exposure to sunlight and radiation treatment at an early age.[55]

Photochemotherapy (PUVA) is used for the treatment both of GvHD and the rare cases of cutaneous T-cell lymphoma that occur in childhood.[57] This modality of therapy in children may predispose to the development of basal cell carcinomas in later life.[58]

Primary cutaneous lymphoid malignancies are a rare group of disorders comprising approximately 2 per cent of all lymphomas. About 80 per cent of these are of T-cell

origin with the rest being primary cutaneous B-cell lymphomas. Many run an indolent course but it is important to be aware of possible progression of these disorders later in life. Two types in particular have been reported in children: mycosis fungoides and lymphomatoid papulosis. Mycosis fungoides is the more common of these and often commences as atrophic telangiectatic, or occasionally hypopigmented patches, which may progress to infiltrated plaques and, in a few, to the tumor stage.[59] Such patients require monitoring for evidence of later disease progression.[60] Lymphomatoid papulosis is a chronic relapsing and remitting disorder of the skin, which is now considered to be a low-grade CD30-positive cutaneous T-cell lymphoma. It is characterized by crops of pinkish papules and nodules, and occasionally necrotic ulcers, but these are always self-limiting. Progression to systemic lymphoma occurs in less than 10 per cent of adult cases and, although this has not been reported in children, it is nevertheless prudent to keep such patients under supervision into adult life.[61] At this stage there appear to be no reliable predictive factors for disease progression.

CUTANEOUS SIGNS OF DISEASE PROGRESSION OR RELAPSE

Rarely, the skin of children is directly involved in the malignant process, particularly infiltration by leukemic cells or lymphoma occurring either during the initial presentation or later, when it may herald disease relapse.[62,63]

Development of cutaneous nodules, either flesh-colored or duskily erythematous (Figure 11.8, Plate 11), may occur and these may be purpuric if there is a coexisting hemorrhagic diathesis. A skin biopsy for histological evaluation is mandatory if a malignant infiltrate is suspected.

Paraneoplastic phenomena may also present in the skin. Pyoderma gangrenosum and acute febrile neu-

trophilic dermatosis (Sweet's syndrome), although rare in children, have both been reported in association with childhood leukemia. Graham et al.[64] reviewed a series of 46 childhood cases of pyoderma gangrenosum: compared with adults, the distribution of lesions more often involved the head and neck, and the main associated disorders were inflammatory bowel disorders followed by leukemia. The diagnosis is generally a clinical one with pustular lesions progressing to ulcers with a typical cribriform edge. Histological examination of a skin biopsy may exclude alternative diagnoses but is not always diagnostic of pyoderma gangrenosum.

Acute febrile neutrophilic dermatosis is considered to be in the same disease spectrum, but the clinical signs are of tumid, erythematous nodules or plaques, sometimes with bullous changes, occurring acutely in association with pyrexia, joint pains and neutrophilia. Histological examination of a skin biopsy can differentiate this reactive process from malignant skin infiltrates. The commonest malignant associations of Sweet's syndrome are with myelodysplastic disorders.[65]

KEY POINTS

Late cutaneous effects of childhood cancer include:

- cutaneous infections related to a relative state of immunosuppression;
- graft-versus-host disease;
- adoptive transfer as a result of allografting;
- adverse effects of drugs or irradiation;
- cutaneous or mucosal tumors;
- cutaneous signs of disease recurrence or progression.

REFERENCES

1. Wallace WHB, Blacklay A, Eiser C, et al. Developing strategies for long term follow-up of survivors of childhood cancer. Br Med J 2001; **323**:271–274.
2. Euvrard S, Kanitakis J, Cochat P, et al. Skin diseases in children with organ transplants. J Am Acad Dermatol 2001; **44**:932–939.
3. Benton EC. Human papillomavirus infection and molluscum contagiosum, In: Harper J, Oranje AP, Prose NS (eds). Textbook of paediatric dermatology. Oxford: Blackwell Science, 2000:307–320.
4. Hughes RG, Colquhoun M, Eccles DM, et al. Cervical intra-epithelial neoplasia in lymphoma patients: a cytological and colposcopic study. Br J Cancer 1989; **59**:594–599.
5. Leman JA, Benton EC. Verrucas: guidelines for management. Am J Clin Dermatol 2000; **1**:145–149.
6. Horn CK, Scott GR, Benton EC. Resolution of severe molluscum contagiosum on effective anti-retroviral therapy. Br J Dermatol 1998; **138**:715–717.
7. Au WY, Lie AKW, Shek TW. Fulminant molluscum contagiosum infection and concomitant leukaemia cutis after bone marrow

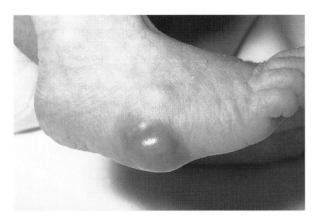

Figure 11.8 *Cutaneous metastatic deposit from a neuroblastoma. (Photograph courtesy of Dr H. Wallace.)*

transplantation for chronic myeloid leukaemia. *Br J Dermatol* 2000; **143**:1097–1098.

8. Smith K, Skelton H, Yeager J. Molluscum contagiosum – ultrastructural evidence of its presence in skin adjacent to clinical lesions in patients infected with human immunodeficiency virus type 1. *Arch Dermatol* 1992; **128**:223–227.

9. Davies EG, Thrasher A, Lacey K, Harper J. Topical cidofovir for severe molluscum contagiosum. *Lancet* 1999; **353**:2042.

10. Reusser P, Cordonnier C, Einsele H, *et al.* European survey of herpesvirus resistance to anti-viral drugs in bone marrow transplant recipients. Infectious Disease Working Party of the European Group for Blood and Marrow Transplantation (EMBT). *Bone Marrow Transplant* 1996; **17**:813–817.

11. Hughes BR. Tinea versicolor in immunosuppressed patients. *J Am Acad Dermatol* 1988; **19**:357–358.

12. Ivy SP, Mackall CL, Gore L, *et al.* Demodicidosis in childhood acute lymphoblastic leukaemia: an opportunistic infection occurring with immunosuppression. *J Pediatr* 1995; **127**:751–754.

13. Smith KJ, Welsh M, Skelton H. Trichphyton rubrum showing deep dermal invasion directly from the epidermis in immunosuppressed patients. *Br J Dermatol* 2001; **145**: 344–348.

14. Song WK, Kim YC, Park HJ, Cinn YW. Ecthyma gangrenosum without bacteraemia in a leukaemic patient. *Clin Expt Dermatol* 2001; **26**:395–397.

15. Barnes L, McCallister RE, Lucky AE, Crusted (Norwegian) scabies. Occurrence in a child undergoing a bone marrow transplant. *Arch Dermatol* 1987; **123**:95–97.

16. Duran C, Tamayo L, de la Luz Orozco Ma, Ruiz-Maldonado R. Scabies of the scalp mimicking seborrhoeic dermatitis in immunocompromised patients. *Pediatr Dermatol* 1993; **10**: 136–138.

17. Billingham RE. The biology of graft versus host reactions Harvey Lectures 1967; **62**:21–78.

18. Harper J. Graft-versus-host disease in Textbook of paediatric Dermatology Ed HarperJ, Oranje AP Prose NS Blackwell Science 2000:1700–1709.

19. Tanasescu S, Balguerie X, Thomine E, Bouillie MC, Vannier JP, Tron P, Joly P, Lauret P. Eczema-like cutaneous graft-versus-host disease treated by UVB therapy in a 2 year- old child. *Ann Dermatol Venereol* 1999; **126**:51–53.

20 Aractingi S, Janin A, Devergie A, Bourges M, Sonie G, Gluckman E. Histochemical and ultrastructural study of diffuse melanomaderma after bone marrow transplantation. *B J Dermatol* 1966; **134**:325–331.

21. Ivker RA, Woosley J, Resnick SD. Dyskeratosis congenita or chronic graft-versus-host disease? A diagnostic dilemma in a child 8 years after bone marrow transplantation for aplastic anaemia. *Pediatr Dermatol* 1985; **10**:362–365.

22. Ling NS, Fenske NA, Julius RL, Espinoza CG, Drake LA. Dyskeratosis congenita in a girl simulating chronic graft-versus-host disease. *Br Dermatol* 1985; **121**:1424–1428.

23. Jampel RM, Farmer ER, Vogelsang GB, *et al.* PUVA therapy for chronic cutaneous graft-versus-host disease. *Arch Dermatol* 1991; **127**:1673–1678.

24. Altman JS, Adler SS. Development of multiple cutaneous squamous cell cancers during PUVA therapy for chronic graft-versus-host disease. *J Am Acad Dermatol* 1994; **31**:505–507.

25. Gardembas-Pain M, Ifrah N, Foussard C, *et al.* Psoriasis after allogeneic bone marrow transplantation. *Arch Dermatol* 1990; **126**:1523.

26. Snowden JC, Heaton DC. Development of psoriasis after syngeneic bone marrow transplant from psoriatic donor: further evidence for adoptive autoimmunity. *Br J Dermatol* 1997; **137**:130–132.

27. Eedy DJ, Burrows D, Bridges JM, Jones FG. Clearance of severe psoriasis after allogeneic bone marrow transplantation. *Br Med J* 1990; **300**:908.

28. Jowitt SN, Yin JA. Psoriasis and bone marrow transplantation. *Br Med J* 1990; **300**:1398–1399.

29. Adkins DR, Abidi MH, Brown RA, *et al.* Resolution of psoriasis after allogeneic bone marrow transplantation for chronic myelogenous leukaemia. *Bone Marrow Transplant* 2000; **26**:1239–1241.

30. Tucker J, Barnetson RStC, Eden OB. Atopy after bone marrow transplantation. *Br Med J* 1984; **290**:116–117.

31. Bellou A, Kanny G, Fremont S, Moneret-Vantria DA. Transfer of atopy following bone marrow transplanation. *Ann Allergy Asthma Manual* 1997; **78**:513–516.

32. Neumeister P, Strunk D, Apfelbech U, *et al.* Adoptive transfer of vitiligo after allogeneic bone marrow transplantation for non-Hodgkin's lymphoma. *Lancet* 2000; **355**:1334–1335.

33. Latal Hajnal B, Lips U, Friednich W, *et al.* Addison's disease 10 years after bone marrow transplantation for Wiskott–Aldrich Syndrome. *Eur J Pediatr* 1995; **154**:729–731.

34. Susser WS, Whitaker-Worth DL, Grant-Kels JM. Mucocutaneous reactions to chemotherapy. *J Am Acad Dermatol* 1999; **40**:367–398.

35. Gallant C, Kenny P. Oral glucocorticoids and their complications: a review. *J Am Acad Dermatol* 1986; **14**:161–177.

36. Singal R, Tunnessen, W, Wiley JM., Hood AF. Discrete pigmentation after chemotherapy. *Pediatr Dermatol* 1991; **8**:231–235.

37. Nagore E, Insa A, Sanmartin O. Antineoplastic therapy-induced palmar–plantar erythrodysesthesia (hand–foot) syndrome: incidence, recognition and management. *Am J Dermatol* 2000; **1**:225–234.

38. Burke MC, Bernhard JD, Michelson AD. Chemotherapy-induced painful acral erythema in childhood (Burgdorf's reaction). *Am J Pediatr Hematol Oncol* 1989; **11**:44–45.

39. De Vathaire F, Schweisgath O, Rodary C, *et al.* Long-term risk of second malignant neoplasm after a cancer in childhood. *Br J Cancer* 1989; **59**:448–452.

40. Smith MB, Xue H, Strong L, *et al.* Forty-year experience with second malignancies after treatment of childhood cancer: analysis of outcome following the development of the second malignancy. *J Pediatr Surg* 1993; **28**:1342–1348.

41. Moppet J, Oakhill A, Duncan AW. Second malignancies in children: the usual suspects. *Eur J Radiol* 2001; **38**:235–248.

42. Lowsky R, Lipton J, Fyles G, *et al.* Secondary malignancies after bone marrow transplantation in adults. *J Clin Oncol* 1994; **12**:2187–2192.

43. Hughes BR, Cunliffe WJ, Bailey CC. Excess benign melanocytic naevi after chemotherapy for malignancy in childhood. *Br Med J* 1989; **299**:88–91.

44. DeWitt PE, de Vaan GA, de Boo TM, *et al.* Prevalence of naevocytic naevi after chemotherapy for childhood cancer. *Med Pediatr Oncol* 1990; **8**:336–338.

45. Baird A, McHenry PM, Mackie RM. Effect of maintenance chemotherapy in childhood on numbers of melanocytic naevi. *Br Med J* 1992; **305**:799–801.

46. Swerdlow AJ, English JA, Mackie RM, *et al.* Benign melanocytic naevi as a risk factor for malignant melanoma. *Br Med J* 1986; **292**:1555–1559.

47. Naldi L, Adamoli L, Fraschini D, *et al.* Number and distribution of melanocytic naevi in individuals with a history of childhood leukaemia. *Cancer* 1996; **77**:1402–1408.

48. Green A, Smith P, McWhirter W, *et al.* Melanocytic naevi and melanoma in survivors of childhood cancer. *Br J Cancer* 1993; **67**:1053–1057.

49. Goldes J, Holmes S, Satz M, *et al.* Melanoma masquerading as Spitz naevus following acute lymphoblastic leukaemia. *Paediatr Dermatol* 1984; **1**:295–298.

50. Bourguignon JP, Pierard GE, Ernould C, *et al.* Effects of human growth hormone on melanocytic naevi. *Lancet* 1993; **341**:1505–1506.

51. Zvulunov A, Wyatt DT, Rabinowitz LG, Esterly NB. Effect of growth hormone therapy on melanocytic naevi in survivors of childhood neoplasia. *Arch Dermatol* 1997; **136**:795–796.

52. Whitemore SE, Greer LE. Multiple neck papules in a child with acute lymphatic leukaemia. *Arch Dermatol* 1990; **126**:104–105.

53. Dinehart SM, Anthony JL, Pollack SY. Basal cell carcinoma in young patients after irradiation for childhood malignancy. *Med Pediatr Oncol* 1991; **19**:508–510.

54. Yoshihara T, Ikuta H, Hibi S, *et al.* Second cutaneous neoplasms after acute lymphoblastic leukaemia in childhood. *Int J Hematol* 1993; **59**:67–71.

55. Garcia-Silva J, Velasco-Benito JA, Pona-Ponabad C, Armijo M, Basal cell carcinoma in a girl after cobalt irradiation to the cranium for acute lymphoblastic leukaemia: case report and review of the literature. *Pediatr Dermatol* 1996; **13**:54–57.

56. Kroll SS, Woo SY, Santin A, *et al.* Long term effects of radiotherapy administered in childhood for the treatment of malignant diseases. *Ann Surg Oncol* 1994; **1**:473–479.

57. Tay YK, Weston WL, Aeling JL. Treatment of childhood cutaneous T cell lymphoma with alpha-interferon plus PUVA. *Pediatr Dermatol* 1996; **13**:496–500.

58. Stern RS, Nicholls KT. Therapy with orally administered methoxsalen and ultraviolet: a radiation during childhood increase risk of basal cell carcinoma. The PUVA follow up study. *J Pediatr* 1996; **129**:915–917.

59. Zackheim HS, McCalmont TH, Deanovic FW, Odom RB. Mycosis fungoides with onset before 20 years of age. *J Am Acad Dermatol* 1997; **36**:557–562.

60. Crowley JJ, Nikko A, Varghese RT, Kim YH. Mycosis fungoides in young patients: clinical characteristics and outcome. *J Am Acad Dermatol* 1998; **38**:696–701.

61. Van Neer FJMA, Toonstra J, Van Voorst Vader PC, *et al.* Lymphomatoid papulosis in children: a study of 10 children registered by the Dutch Cutaneous Lymphoma Working Group. *Br J Dermatol* 2001; **144**:351–354.

62. Kishimoto S, Ishii E, Murakami Y, *et al.* Cutaneous infiltration by leukaemic cells in acute promyelocytic leukaemia of a child after treatment with all-trans retinoic acid. *Pediatr Hematol Oncol* 1997; **14**:169–175.

63. Molina DN, Sanchez JL, Lugo-Somolinos A. The spectrum of cutaneous lesions in pediatric patients with leukaemia PR. *Health Sci J* 1994; **13**:247–249.

64. Graham JA, Hansen KK, Rabinowitz LG, Esterly NB. Pyoderma gangrenosum in infants and children. *Pediatr Dermatol* 1994; **11**:10–17.

65. Bajwa RP, Marwaha RK, Garewal G, Rajagopalan M. Acute febrile neutrophilic dermatosis (Sweet's syndrome) in myelodysplastic syndrome. *Pediatr Hematol Oncol* 1993; **10**:343–346.

12

Quality of life issues

12a

y of life and body image

ISER

A BRIEF HISTORY

Concerns about the quality of life (QoL) of survivors of childhood cancer have been raised since the 1970s. Opportunities for survivors to achieve good QoL may be compromised directly through physical late effects associated with the original tumor or its treatment and less directly through the practical implications of these late-effects. Thus, survivors of acute lymphoblastic leukemia (ALL) treated by chemotherapy and central nervous system (CNS) irradiation are likely to experience learning difficulties and compromised academic achievements. In the short term, these learning difficulties may reduce the child's enjoyment of and participation in school but, in the longer term, QoL may be further compromised by reducing opportunities for further education and employment. A child's learning difficulties also potentially compromise social and family life, especially where these result in the loss of age-appropriate independence and autonomy. Healthy siblings may feel upset and sometimes embarrassed by the child's behavior. As a result, the whole family may have a smaller circle of friends and relations, and enjoy fewer activities than they might have done. Thus, the ramifications of the disease are not restricted to physical symptoms but affect all aspects of the child's life. In treating a child with cancer, it is clear that the implications of the disease go beyond the impact on cell counts and spleen sizes. Children, and their families, have

dreams, goals, aspirations and feelings. Ultimately, cure is about controlling the disease, but it is also about preserving dreams and maximizing potential.

The idea that it was not enough to evaluate the implications of cancer purely in physical terms and that cure should be considered in relation to three separate components was initially formally acknowledged by van Eys.[1] These separate components included the biological (eradication of the disease), psychological (the acceptance of having had cancer as a past event without interference with normal development and schooling) and social (incorporation of the person cured of cancer into society, without consideration of past history of cancer and its therapy). This subchapter is concerned with efforts to evaluate and maximize these latter two components of cure.

One of the first papers to address the question of QoL and body image (BI) in survivors of childhood cancer was reported by Holmes and Holmes.[2] These authors identified 124 survivors, treated between 1944 and 1963, and registered with the Tumor Registry at the University of Kansas. All had survived at least 10 years from diagnosis. It is worth considering in some detail the rationale for this study, since in many ways it represents one of the first large comprehensive assessments of QoL and body image (BI) in survivors of childhood cancer:

> Little is known or has been written about the fate or rehabilitation of long-term survivors of childhood cancer. Obviously, the ultimate justification for dangerous and

drastic therapy (mutilating surgery, irradiation, and cyto-toxic drugs) is survival affording normal, near normal, or at least an acceptable life style and quality of life for some of the children treated. ... Some very basic questions remain to be answered. Is the life saved worth living? Do survivors achieve educational and economic status commensurate with their premorbid expectations? Is the development of a secondary primary malignancy likely? Do survivors marry and beget children? Do survivors' children get cancer? Do some childhood cancers recur after ten years? (Holmes and Holmes, p. 819)[2]

The results of their survey suggested that:

most survivors have made excellent adjustments and have matured to live essentially normal lives. A few with serious mental disability have not entered the mainstream of life, yet the majority have achieved their premorbid expectations, or a bit more, and a few have been true overachievers. Thus, it would appear that the drastic, dangerous and often mutilating approaches utilized in the modern treatments for cancer are justifiable. These afford permanent cure of those surviving longer than 10 years after diagnosis, and enable the overwhelming majority to enjoy a normal or nearly normal life style. (Holmes and Holmes, p. 823)[2]

While much of the sentiment expressed above remains, the language of contemporary research is considerably tempered. Changes in treatment and practice mean that the incidence of 'mutilating' surgery is much reduced. However, questions relating to achievement of premorbid potential remain pertinent. With time, attempts are being made to answer more sophisticated questions. How is it that some individuals achieve more than might be expected? How can we account for the huge variability in outcomes? What sort of help needs to be made available to facilitate optimum QoL for the greatest number of survivors? The aim of this subchapter is to describe the QoL and BI of survivors as it is currently understood. In addition, we hope to generate greater interest in this issue and suggest directions for future work.

THE SCIENTIFIC STUDY OF QUALITY OF LIFE

The scientific study of QoL is complicated by the diverse ways in which the term is used in everyday language. To many people, quality of life is about being happy. For clinicians, it is predominantly about freedom from physical symptoms. For others, QoL is about relationships with family and friends. Social historians emphasize the way in which perceptions of QoL differ over time and between cultures. Thus, perceptions of QoL are colored by the specific social, cultural and historical circumstances in which we find ourselves. The concept of *health-related*

QoL refers specifically to the impact of health and illness on the individual's QoL.

Several key ideas define the concept of QoL. First is the notion that individuals have a unique perspective on QoL, which depends on present lifestyle, past experience, hopes for the future, dreams and ambitions. Second, QoL is generally conceptualized as a multidimensional construct encompassing a number of separate domains.[3–6] These domains, as put forward by the World Health Organisation (WHO) include 'the state of complete physical, mental and social well-being and not merely the absence of disease or infirmity'.[7] The WHO goes on to describe QoL as 'the individual's perception of their position in life, in the context of culture and value systems in which they live and in relation to their goals, expectations, standards and concerns'.[7] Third, QoL can include both objective and subjective perspectives in each of these domains.[8] The objective assessment of QoL focuses on what the individual can do. The subjective assessment includes the individual's perception or appraisal of what they can do. Differences in appraisal account for the fact that individuals with the same objective health status can report very different subjective QoL. 'The patient's perceptions of and attributions about the dysfunction are as important as their existence'.[9]

A good quality of life can be said to be present when the hopes of an individual are matched and fulfilled by experience. The opposite is also true: poor QoL occurs when hopes do not meet with the experience.[10] These themes were further elaborated by Bergner[11] who suggests that QoL is enhanced when the distance between the individual's attained and desired goals is less. However, an individual's goals must be realistic in order that the gap can be narrowed. From a therapeutic point of view, it is as possible to improve QoL by helping a patient give up some dreams and accept reality (and restrictions) as well as work with another patient to achieve more realistically set goals. In both cases, the gap is narrowed. A major limitation of this approach may be in the difficulty to specify goals as realistic and achievable compared with those that are merely dreams or lack substance.[12]

There has been much criticism of the concept of QoL,[13,14] with many dismissing it as a nebulous term of little value. For others, QoL represents the single most important outcome in evaluating medical intervention. While a clinician may assess the efficacy of treatment in physiological terms (e.g. blood sugar levels within norms), this information is less useful for patients if it does not translate into feeling better. Thus, the success of growth hormone therapy (GHT) may be measured objectively in terms of increased height, but for children and their families, subjective improvements in the way they feel, their self-esteem, social acceptance or perception of future work opportunities may be equally, or even more, important. Thus, the issue may be less about how many

centimeters have been gained, but more about whether children can keep up with daily activities and enjoy life.

Measurement of QoL is further complicated because it is viewed differently by children, parents and clinicians.[15] The child who does not grow may see this to be a major impact on QoL if he wants to be in the army, while parents may feel that there are many other opportunities available.

For all of these reasons, QoL and its measurement can be dismissed as unscientific compared with traditional end-points, such as height. However, the more elusive subjective outcomes may, in the end, be as important, although raising many dilemmas in terms of measurement. In an attempt to clarify the different approaches, Gill and Feinstein[13] distinguished three ways in which QoL may be operationalized in a health context as follows.

1 In terms of *objective* measures, some researchers emphasize 'alive time' or time without symptoms or toxicity, and relapse-free time. These may include information about white cell counts, time to remission, number of episodes of neutropenia, etc.
2 QoL has also been equated with *functional* performance or activity. The assumption is that QoL is compromised where individuals are unable to participate in age-appropriate physical activity. For younger patients, this may include strenuous sports, while for older patients, the emphasis may be on the ability to perform daily self-care or live independently.
3 To account for individual differences in the meaning of physical limitations, there has been a shift to focus on *subjective* measures of QoL. Rather than emphasize what an individual can do, the focus is on feelings or *appraisal* about what can be done. Some children, the argument goes, will be distressed if they are unable to take part in sports activities, while others will be less concerned, and some may feel positively pleased!

This emphasis on subjectivity or appraisal is important but is still often restricted to physical activity. The original definition of health[7] on which many QoL measures are based emphasized that illness affects a very broad spectrum of behavior including physical, social and emotional functioning. In work with children, the need for additional domains of QoL to assess family relationships, cognitive functioning, independence, BI and opportunities for the future have been emphasized. Measurement of this very broad spectrum of behavior in the context of the developing child has proved very challenging.[16]

MEASUREMENT OF QoL

At least three approaches to measurement can be identified. These include (1) measures of social, emotional or psychological adjustment, (2) 'lifestyle' indicators, and (3) specially developed cancer-specific measures of QoL.

Social, emotional and psychological adjustment

By far the most common approach involves the use of measures developed to assess domains of physical or emotional functioning assumed to be related to QoL. In a recent review, Eiser et al.[17] identified 20 studies broadly concerned with emotional adjustment among cancer survivors. There was little consensus regarding the most appropriate way to measure emotional adjustment. QoL was inferred from assessments of self-esteem ($n = 11$), anxiety ($n = 5$), depression ($n = 3$), social skills ($n = 2$), BI ($n = 2$), loneliness ($n = 2$), mood ($n = 2$), personality ($n = 3$), coping ($n = 1$), social desirability ($n = 2$), intrusiveness ($n = 4$) and physical symptoms ($n = 2$). In recognition of the limitations of measures developed to assess concepts other than QoL, three studies used specially developed QoL interviews together with standardized questionnaires.[18–20] In four studies, post-traumatic stress disorder (PTSD) was determined (on the assumption that survivors reporting significant PTSD have poor QoL).

To a large extent, conclusions drawn were dependent on the measure of adjustment adopted and the design of the study. In many studies, no major differences were found between survivors of childhood cancer and healthy controls. However, survivors were more likely to have repeated a school grade, less likely to be drinkers and less likely to have experienced blackouts following a drinking episode than healthy controls.[18,19] Madan-Swain et al.[21] found that survivors were more likely to report BI disturbance and adjustment difficulties, and Pendley et al.[22] reported that survivors participated in fewer activities than controls. Specific symptoms of PTSD were reported in more than half their sample of survivors.[23] These included bad dreams, feeling afraid or upset when they think about cancer, feeling 'alone inside' and feeling nervous. In total, 12.5 per cent of survivors scored at a level that would indicate a clinical diagnosis of PTSD. However, Butler et al.[24] found little evidence of PTSD in a group of 42 survivors compared with children on treatment. Both Kazak et al.[25] and Barakat et al.[26] reported that the incidence of PTSD among survivors was similar to healthy controls.

It can be difficult to interpret some of these results. It might be assumed that repeating a school grade has a negative impact on QoL at least in the short term, but in the longer term it may be that repeating a school grade leads to an increase in QoL. The reduction in drinking and blackouts following drinking sessions may reflect a more positive QoL (the survivor has better things to do) or might indicate poorer QoL (few friends to go out

with). Studies that simply compare survivors with others in terms of the frequency of different activities may, therefore, offer limited insight into the impact of cancer on QoL.

QoL may well be moderated by demographic, family or clinical variables. Families with more financial resources may be able to offer opportunities to offset the limitations of disease. For example, access to a car can improve QoL for those with restricted mobility. Finally, whatever the child's demographic or family resources, QoL may be compromised by clinical variables including late effects of treatment. In general, children from families of higher social class, better family environment and whose mothers cope better appear to adjust better themselves.[27–29] The incidence of PTSD is related to family functioning and social support.[25,26]

BODY IMAGE

The emphasis which is placed in our society on conforming to norms of social attractiveness has significant implications for those who fail to reach these recognized standards.[30] Poor BI in cancer survivors may be expected, especially where patients feel that their bodies have in some way 'failed them'.

An individual's BI reflects thoughts and feelings about their body.[31] Like QoL, it is thought to be multidimensional, involving attitudes towards physical appearance, and perceptions associated with body and size. It is affected by social and cultural factors.

Cancer challenges BI in many ways. Some are temporary, such as the loss of hair following chemotherapy. Others may be longer lasting. These include changes in body shape; children treated for ALL or CNS tumors often put on weight during steroid treatment and may never regain their precancer shape. Cancer treatment can affect BI in both adults and children but, in some ways, may be more critical for children. Thus, treatment that limits growth or is associated with infertility may have negligible adverse effects for a middle-aged man who has completed his family but may be devastating for the BI of an adolescent.

A number of measures have been developed to assess BI in healthy individuals or those with special needs, such as eating disorders. Measures developed within the field of eating disorders are not ideal for children with cancer, as they often include questions about body size distortion. Perceptions of BI distortion may simply be demonstrating heightened awareness or distress related to body parts affected by the illness or treatment for those with cancer. In addition, given that eating disorders affect more females than males, measures may have less validity especially for males who are ill rather than having weight problems.

BI measures most commonly used with children include the Self-image questionnaire for young adolescents,[32] the Body Cathexis scale,[33] self-report Likert ratings of BI, the physical appearance subscale of the Self Perception Profile for Adolescents,[34] the BI Avoidant Questionnaire[35] and the Situational Inventory of BI Distress.[36] These measures, which focus on weight-related appearance, do not touch on all of the areas relevant to chronic illness. These include patient's feelings about specific body parts affected by treatment, reactions of others to visible marks of illness and feelings about how the condition affects body functioning.

In an effort to develop a more sensitive measure of BI appropriate for young people treated for cancer, Kopel et al.[37] reported a measure specifically for work with both male and female adolescents with cancer. The scale (28 items) was devised from items that were elicited from previous interviews with children in the defined age-range undergoing treatment for a number of different cancers. It assesses BI in relation to five dimensions or subscales: general appearance; body competence; others' reaction to appearance; value of appearance; and body parts. Adequate internal reliability for the subscales and the total BI score were reported.

In considering the long-term effects of treatment on QoL and BI, it is important to distinguish between those survivors who have no or little residual difficulties and those who have late effects likely to compromise BI. Early studies consistently reported more negative impact on BI compared with later studies. Fritz and Williams[38] reported BI concerns in half their sample, as well as concerns about their sexuality, attractiveness to the opposite sex and reproductive capacity. Certainly where survivors have no obvious physical problem, there is evidence that BI is not compromised. Pendley et al.[22] compared BI in 21 adolescent survivors (9 female and 12 males) and matched healthy controls, recruited from advertisements in local newspapers. In addition, objective ratings of attractiveness based on videotapes of participants were made. Although no analysis was made of the relationship between BI and QoL, the authors explored the relationship between BI and measures related to QoL including peer activities,[39] loneliness[40] social anxiety[41] and self perception.[31] No differences were found between those with cancer and controls on measures of BI, nor were there any differences in terms of objective ratings of attractiveness made by independent observers. There were no differences in terms of loneliness, social anxiety or school absenteeism. However, survivors participated in fewer activities. It should also be noted that survivors with obvious physical deformities (e.g. amputations) were excluded from this study. Given the small sample and exclusion of survivors with physical problems, it is likely that this study provides a limited view of the impact of cancer on BI.

nown to compromise QoL and
nial irradiation for example, can
l, therefore, survivors treated in
ely to have QoL and BI problems
emotherapy alone. There is some
uted in part to the smaller head
roup. In other cases, QoL and BI
promised following surgery. In the
refore, we consider in more detail
it QoL and BI following growth
(GHD), and for survivors treated

e studies

near growth is common following radi-
ation. GHD and obesity are frequently found among survivors of ALL treated with chemotherapy and cranial
irradiation.[42,43] Outcomes following treatment by chemotherapy alone are less clear, with conflicting reports regarding final height.[44,45]

Individuals differ in the importance attached to short
stature. For some it is a small price to pay for survival.
Others experience considerable distress in their attempts
to cope. Denial,[46] acting the clown[47] and acting out or
aggressive behavior[48] have all been reported.

The difficulties experienced by short children can continue or increase when they become adults. Evidence that
adults with GHD have a poorer QoL compared with others has been reported. These include increased incidences
of anxiety and depression, feelings of social isolation,
high unemployment and tendency to live longer in the
parental home.[49]

Questions about the impact of GHT on QoL among
survivors of ALL are unclear. These children will necessarily have experienced several years intensive treatment
involving frequent hospital appointments and interrupted
schooling. Recommendations about GHT will lengthen
the time the child feels a 'patient' as well as impose daily
demands and responsibilities on families. The assumption is that these short-term restrictions will lead, via
increased height, to greater QoL.

Although there have been some assessments of QoL
among children of short stature, there have been few
comparable assessments among those prescribed GHT
following malignancy. Even among normal short stature
children, the evidence for improved QoL is sparse. Pilpel
et al.[50] compared 96 children treated for a number of reasons with GHT for at least 2 years with a group of similar
children who were not treated owing to lack of resources.
QoL was measured in terms of school achievements, leisure
activities, emotional and physical self-esteem, relationship with peers and family members. No differences were
found between the groups.

As GHT is increasingly prescribed to survivors of
childhood cancer, with the goals not only to improve
height but to contribute to more general well-being, it is
increasingly important to conduct longitudinal assessments of the efficacy of the treatment. These must include
evaluation of the QoL of the survivors. Demands to
determine the benefits of GHT to QoL are also required
on economic grounds. Given the costs of GHT, some
cost–benefit analysis is critical.[51] 'Values ascribed by an
individual child to potential outcomes should be central
to the age-appropriate discussion process'. Cost–benefit
analysis requires detailed knowledge of physical (improved
height, lack of physical symptoms), psychosocial and QoL
outcomes.

Amputation versus limb salvage surgery following a bone tumor

A second example includes young people with a bone
tumor treated by amputation or limb salvage surgery
(LSS). There is considerable evidence that there are no
differences in survival between the two treatments, nor
in terms of costs to the health service.[52] However, the
social and psychological treatments for patients are quite
different. Theoretical advantages of amputation include
the fact that it is a once and for all operation, requiring
minimal additional surgery. Good mobility is possible
and, critically for some, it is possible to play contact sports,
not least because breakages can be relatively easily dealt
with. However, it is a very final procedure. The incidence
of phantom pains and the impact on an individual's BI
are primary reasons why patients may prefer LSS. For
many, then, LSS would be the treatment of choice. This
imposes much less of an obstacle to BI and is likely to be
socially more acceptable. However, risks of infection and
breakages are major obstacles to the achievement of QoL.

On the face of it, there would seem to be both QoL
and BI advantages to LSS. Efforts to determine QoL differences in physical, social or emotional functioning have
failed. Thus, although physical function was reported to
be better for the LSS group in two studies,[53] three studies
reported no differences[54–56] and one study found an
advantage for the amputee group.[57] No differences in
reported pain were noted by Rougraff et al.[53] or in emotional well-being, social well-being, love life and subjective capabilities, adjustment to illness, perceived impact
of illness and activities of daily living,[54] or for mood,
adjustment to illness or psychiatric symptoms.[53,55,56,58]
Amputees reported more work and social discrimination
compared with the limb salvage group, and were more
socially isolated.[10]

Most studies do not provide data on sexual functioning.
However, contrary to expectations, LSS patients reported
greater reduction in sexual functioning compared with

amputees.[54] Patients treated in the early days of LSS often had stiff, painful or edematous legs following radiotherapy and, for this reason, it is hoped that more recently treated patients may fare better. Most patients had sexual experience and reported few problems with sexual functioning, but amputees were less likely than limb salvage patients to have married.[57] Clearly, these data are difficult to collect and self-reports may be subject to considerable bias.

These failed attempts to establish QoL and BI differences depending on surgery raise serious questions about measurement and the assumptions underlying the concepts.

LIFESTYLE INDICATORS

Academic success and achievements

In addition to the quite extensive and detailed work involving assessments of IQ and academic functioning in survivors of ALL described in Chapter 2b,[59] a limited number of studies have described academic achievement among survivors more generally. In these cases, interest has focused on the level of achievement reached, i.e. number of examinations passed, special educational needs placement or involvement in higher education. Evans and Radford compared school achievements of 48 survivors of different childhood cancers with healthy siblings and, where possible, national statistics.[60] Slightly fewer survivors (55 per cent) compared with siblings (62 per cent) achieved recommended national standards at school leaving age. Even so, survivors were less likely to go to university. Survivors and siblings were equally likely to be involved in competitive sports and enjoyed an active social life, although more survivors than siblings had passed their driving test. Among the survivors, there were three known cases of employer prejudice. Overall, few differences were found between survivors and their siblings, and the conclusions were that survivors achieved as well (or better) than the general population at school-leaving age. Similar results were reported by Mackie et al. who found no differences between cancer survivors and controls in terms of numbers of examinations passed, or numbers entering further education.[61]

These two studies from the UK contrast sharply with findings from the USA,[62] and The Netherlands.[63] Haupt et al. compared 593 survivors of ALL with 409 sibling controls. This large sample was recruited from 23 centers specializing in care of these children in the USA.[62] Telephone interviews were conducted to determine the highest level of schooling completed, average grades obtained in high school, enrollment in special needs or gifted programs. Before diagnosis there were no differences

between the groups in special education needs. However, children with ALL were more likely to enter a special needs or learning disabled program after treatment. Relative risk was higher for females compared with males but not significantly so. Survivors diagnosed during the preschool period and those treated by larger doses of cranial irradiation were more likely to be enrolled in special needs or learning disabled programs. Despite these problems, survivors were as likely as their siblings to finish high school, go to college or gain a Bachelors degree.

Kingma et al. compared school careers of 94 children treated for ALL with 134 of their siblings. Significantly more survivors had been placed in special educational programs compared with siblings and had completed significantly fewer terms of secondary schooling.[63] However, there were no effects of gender on either of these findings. As reported previously, the group most at risk was those diagnosed at younger ages. These findings suggest that school achievements may be compromised in the ALL group, but the response rate (questionnaires by post) was not very good and the amount of detail limited.

These four studies suggest some consistent findings about educational achievement in survivors, particularly in terms of increased need for special educational placement. Some differences may reflect different organization of education services and availability of special needs programs in different cultures. Schools in the UK are often reluctant to recommend that a child should repeat a school year, and the processes involved in determining eligibility for special educational needs and referral to special schools are cumbersome.

Employment and insurance

Given that the public tends to be relatively uninformed about the cause, treatment or prognosis of childhood cancer, some workplace discrimination has to be expected. Misunderstanding and lack of knowledge may result in expectations that survivors will have unacceptably high absences, may fail to 'pull their weight' and expect to be treated differently from others. Over many years, there have been reports of discrimination in the workforce generally and the armed forces especially.[64]

Green et al. traced 227 survivors (median age 26 years) at follow-up.[65] Eleven per cent reported some work discrimination. Males were as likely to be employed as would be expected from population statistics but females were less frequently in employment. Hays et al. located 219 cancer survivors (aged between 30 and 50 years) and compared their educational, occupational and insurance status with a healthy age-matched control group.[66] Interviews were conducted by phone and covered a range of psychosocial issues. No differences were found between survivors treated between 1945 and 1975 and matched

controls on any of the variables assessed. However, those treated for CNS tumors had more limited educational achievements, lower rates of marriage and were less likely to be parents than expected. They also reported greater interpersonal problems.

In a later study that included younger survivors, Hays *et al.* conducted telephone interviews with 300 of 986 eligible survivors 20 years or older.[67] In 58 cases, where survivors were unable to participate (because of health or disability problems), a proxy was interviewed instead. Cancer survivors had completed fewer years of schooling and, therefore, had lower educational status, higher rates of unemployment, lower occupational status and lower annual incomes compared with controls. There were no differences between the two groups in terms of number of days of absence or requests for special arrangements at work. Within the group of survivors, those who had been treated by CNS irradiation had significantly lower levels of education and poorer employment compared with those not treated by CNS irradiation.

Ignorance and prejudice on the part of careers advisors can mean that opportunities that would be very possible are denied to the individual survivor. Monaco argues that careers advisors and counselors need to overcome their own prejudices, become more informed about survival in childhood cancer, and more practical and realistic in the advice they offer.[68] Eiser *et al.* reported that young people who had been treated for bone cancer had been given little realistic advice about appropriate career opportunities.[69] Information also needs to be offered to employers. Prejudices that cancer survivors will have poor attendance records need to be challenged. It is assumed that survivors of cancer are no more likely to have more days absent from work than others, but few data are available.

It is difficult to determine any underlying trend behind these figures. Since the first published studies, legislation has increasingly demanded less discrimination on the basis of disability, so that we might expect greater integration of cancer survivors in the workforce. However, employment statistics are likely to be affected by fluctuations in the economy and national employment rates. As the numbers of survivors increase, albeit sometimes with major disability, issues of vocational counseling, employment and discrimination are likely to become more pertinent.

Marriage and attitudes to parenting

The situation regarding marriage rates is unclear, since different conclusions have been reached in different studies. Lower rates of marriage and higher divorce rates compared with sibling controls or US population norms have been reported[65,70–72] and these differences may be more pronounced for males compared with females. However, no differences in marriage rates in comparison with population norms were reported by Hays *et al.*[67] or Nicholson.[73]

There are also reports that survivors worry about the health of future children.[74,75] Since many survivors should have no fertility problems, professional and sensitive counselling may be needed to allay unnecessary fears.

Comprehensive disease-specific measures of QoL

There are considerable disadvantages to the approaches to measuring QoL described above. Scales to measure social and emotional adjustment or BI tend to be very lengthy and repetitive, and may lack sensitivity to detect the specific impact of cancer on the child's QoL.[16] Lifestyle indicators, such as employment or marriage, are only useful for older survivors. In addition, lifestyle indicators are difficult to interpret, since it is not clear if the survivor is unmarried through choice or because of social prejudice. For these reasons, a number of specifically developed measures of QoL for children with cancer have been reported (see Table 12a.1).

Early measures of QoL were simple downward extensions of adult measures (e.g. Lansky *et al.*,[80] Bradlyn *et al.*[82]). More recently, the approach has been more child-centered, with researchers going to some pains to collect preliminary data from children in order to ensure that their views are represented (e.g. Eiser *et al.*,[84] Jenney *et al.*[85]).

The issue of establishing validity is problematic, since, to date, there is no widely accepted gold standard. Most new measures report validity in relation to the Play Performance Scale for Children: (PPSC).[80] Yet this scale is widely criticized, particularly in that it lacks sensitivity for work with children functioning at near normal levels, as is true for many survivors, especially of ALL. Since it is not clear that the PPSC is a comprehensive measure of QoL for children, it follows that establishing a correlation between the PPSC and any other measure does not satisfactorily establish the validity of the new instrument.

PARENT–COMPLETED MEASURES

The play performance scale for children

This is the original, most simple and most frequently cited indicator of QoL used for children with cancer.[80] It is a relatively simple 'downward extension' of the Performance Scale described by Karnofsky *et al.*[86] for work with adult cancer patients. Parents are asked to record

Table 12a.1 *Summary of the quality of life measures identified*

Measure	Respondent	Age range (years)	Number of items	Number of domains	Name of domains	Reliability	Validity	Origin
Behavioral, Affective and Somatic Experiences Scale[76]	Parent Self Nurse	5–17	38 14 38	5	Somatic distress; compliance; mood disturbance; quality of interactions; activity	Internal consistency Inter-rater	Clinical	USA
The Miami Pediatric Quality of Life Questionnaire[77]	Parent	1–18	56	3	Social competence; emotional stability; self-competence	Internal consistency Test-retest	Clinical	USA
Pediatric Quality of Life Inventory[78]	Self Parent	2–4 5–7 8–12 13–18	Core = Cancer specific =	5 + disease-specific module	Core: physical functioning; emotional functioning; social functioning; school functioning; well-being			USA
Pediatric Oncology Quality of Life Scale[79]	Parent	Pre-school–adolescence	21	3	Physical functioning; emotional distress; externalizing behavior	Internal consistency Inter-rater	Concurrent Clinical	USA
Play Performance Scale for Children[80]	Parent	6 months–16	1	1	Play	Inter-rater	Construct Clinical	USA
Health Utilities Index–Mark 3[81]	Parent		8	8	Vision; hearing; speech; ambulation; dexterity; emotion; cognition; pain/discomfort	Test–retest	Clinical	Canada
Quality of Well-Being[82]	Parent Self	0–18	3 scales and 23 symptoms	3	Mobility scale; physical activity scale; social activity scale	Internal consistency	Clinical	USA
Quality of Life[83]	Self	8–18	34	6	Autonomy; physical functioning; emotional functioning; cognition; social functioning/friends; social functioning/family; body image	Internal	Clinical	Germany

play activity in terms of ten graded statements ('fully active, normal' scored as 100 through to 'unresponsive', scored as 0). It is quick to administer and easy to score. It was originally considered suitable for a relatively wide age range (1–16 years), although it has recently been thought to lack sensitivity, particularly for older children and those functioning at near normal levels. As noted, the PPSC is frequently treated as a kind of 'gold standard' against which new measures are compared, although the wisdom of this is hard to accept, given its clear limitations.

The quality of well-being scale (QWB)[82]

This is a slightly modified version of the QWB for adults.[87] Health status is assessed in three areas; physical functioning, social/role functioning and mobility. In addition, patients are shown a list of 27 symptoms and asked to identify any that have affected them within the previous 6 days.

Evidence for the validity of the scale was provided in that lower QoL was reported for those who had experienced more surgeries and hospitalizations. Criticisms of this scale are that it involves a complex and time-consuming method of data collection (individual interview) and needs trained personnel for administration. As with the PPSC, there is no parallel form for children to make their own ratings.

Multi-attribute health status classification system[81,88]

The Multi-attribute health status classification system[88] based on the Health Utility Index (HUI)[89] has been used for work in neonatal intensive care and oncology. Feeny et al. initially asked parents of children in the general population to identify important components of health for their children.[88] Six domains were identified: sensation, emotion, cognition, mobility, self-care and pain. A seventh domain; fertility, was added, as this was felt to be important to parents of children treated for cancer, although not an issue for parents of healthy children. For each attribute, 3–5 levels of functioning were identified. The child's health status score is a computation of functioning on the different levels for each domain.

The link between these health status scores and QoL is assessed using a technique called the standard gamble. Respondents are asked to consider a specific health state. Then they must choose between remaining in this health state or take a gamble, the gamble being between sudden death and enjoying perfect health. These preferences are then varied until the respondent is unable to choose between the two. This is called the utility score; the better the state of health the higher the utility score.

There are problems with the schema itself. The attributes are not completely independent. (If you score badly on the mobility attribute, it is almost inevitable that you will also score badly in terms of self-care). In partial recognition of some of these problems, later versions dropped the self-care attribute. The system does not allow for better than average functioning, so, in terms of cognition, for example, ratings are made from severe morbidity to normality. Thus, the system does not assess well children who function better than average.

Although it has now been modified to allow completion by parents, the Multi-attribute health status classification system may not address the key component of QoL, i.e. it was not designed to tap the child's perspective but focuses on the views of the clinician. With simple modifications, however, the measure has been used successfully by Billson and Walker to elicit data directly from children.[90] The relatively simple responses required would be easy for many children and thus the measure does not need to be limited to adult views.

The main advantages of the HUI include brevity and ease of administration. It is possible for a clinician to complete the instrument within a few minutes. From this point of view, it seems ideal for work in a busy clinic. It may prove useful as a very brief screening instrument in the comparison of different therapies but is unlikely to yield a comprehensive picture of QoL unless supplemented by additional measures.

The pediatric oncology quality of life scale[79]

This is a 21-item questionnaire generated from discussions with health professionals, parents of cancer patients and patients themselves. Three components of QoL are assessed: physical functioning and restriction from normal activity, emotional distress, and response to active medical treatment.

The authors report good internal reliability for the total score and for the three separate subscales. The measure also appears to have adequate validity, at least in terms of discriminating between children, depending on time since diagnosis. In addition, scores on the subscales correlated with the validity measures as expected. For example, scores on the physical functioning subscale correlated with the PPSC[80] but not with behavior[91] or depression.[92]

This measure was designed for use by parents of children from preschool through to adolescence. Age differences on subscale scores suggest that the impact of cancer on QoL may be age dependent, at least as far as parents are concerned. There are indications that adolescents are more affected in terms of physical functioning compared with younger children, while children between the ages

of 8 and 12 years are most affected in terms of emotional functioning.

The BASES scale[76]

Phipps et al.[76] used the BASES scales to determine relationships between parent, nurse and child rating during initial hospitalization for bone marrow transplant (BMT). There are three versions of the BASES.[76] The versions for completion by parent and nurse consist of 38 items; the child version consists of 14 items. All versions examine QoL in terms of five domains: somatic distress, compliance, mood disturbance, quality of interactions, and activity. Correlations between nurse and parent ratings on day 0 were good (27 of 28 correlations were significant at the 0.05 level). On day 14, 22 out of 27 correlations were significant. Further correlations were conducted between child, nurse and parent ratings. Most correlations were in the low to moderate range, but parent–child correlations tended to be more significant than nurse–child ratings. In line with previous findings of greater concordance for observable than non-observable behaviors, agreement was higher for scales measuring somatic distress and activity compared with scales measuring mood disturbance, compliance and quality of interactions. This remains the most well-developed measure for assessing QoL during BMT.

The Miami pediatric quality of life questionnaire: parent scale[77]

This scale assesses three primary factors of QoL identified through factor analysis: self- competence, emotional stability, and social competence. The questionnaire differentiated between children treated for leukemia and those treated for solid tumors. Those treated for leukemia were rated as having a better QoL overall, and on two of the three separate factors (self-competence and social competence). There were no significant correlations between physician and parent ratings of QoL. This lack of correlation between physician and parent ratings suggests that care needs to be exercised in any study that relies exclusively on one of these sources of information. The authors state that they intend to report a child form of the measure but this is not yet available.

MEASURES FOR CHILDREN AND PARENTS

The pediatric cancer quality of life inventory (PCQOL and PCQOL-32)[78]

The PCQoL includes 84 items organized around five domains: physical functioning (8 items), disease-related and treatment-related symptoms (28 items), psychological functioning (13 items), social functioning (23 items) and cognitive functioning (12 items). Ratings are made on a series of four-point Likert scales (where 0 is never a problem and 3 always a problem) and respondents are asked to think back over a 1-month period. The PCQoL includes a child form for 8–12-year-olds, an adolescent form for 13–18-year-olds and a parallel form for parents.

Varni et al. subsequently reported a shorter form (PCQOL-32).[93] The number of items in each domain was reduced (disease and treatment related symptoms = nine items, physical functioning = five items, psychological functioning = six items, social functioning = five items, cognitive functioning = seven items). Ratings were made on four-point scales as before.

The authors report satisfactory internal consistency, clinical and construct validity, and suggest that the brief form is potentially suitable for research involving evaluation of randomized clinical trials. It should be noted that the item means were mostly under 1.0, suggesting that, at least on the domains assessed, patients did not rate the impact of cancer on their lives to be very significant. It is not clear if this is because patients included in the study were well and not severely affected, if the items used lacked sensitivity, or if children 'denied' or dismissed the importance of any difficulties. However, the standard deviations were larger, suggesting a degree of variability in response.

SYNTHESIS

The number of measures developed in recent years poses a problem for researchers and clinicians wanting to measure QoL. Decisions need to be made about the most suitable *respondent* (parents, survivor or both) and the *appropriateness* of the measure for work with survivors. Other considerations relate to the *psychometric properties* of the measure and method of development.

Respondent

Many measures are designed for parent rather than survivor report. Where measures are for use in evaluation of clinical trials following diagnosis, this may well be appropriate or, indeed, the only way to collect information, given that on diagnosis many children will be too young or too ill to respond themselves. However, differences between survivors and their parents in ratings of QoL need to be considered and, for this reason, greater attention needs to be given to development of measures for survivor completion. There is no suggestion that parent or survivor views are more accurate, but a complete picture of QoL may need to include both (see example).

EXAMPLE

Jo (16 years) was recovering from surgery to remove a bone tumor on her lower leg. The tumor had been successfully removed and the diseased bone replaced with a metal prosthesis. Six months later, according to Jo, she was making an excellent recovery. She was having difficulty running, but otherwise she was riding her bike, going out with friends and doing everything she wanted to do.

Her mother told a different story. Jo was often sick and had not returned to school full time. She could ride the stable bike in the Physiotherapy Center, but would be unable to ride a normal bike on a road. Yes, she was seeing her friends, but only when her father drove her around. The family had reorganized the house so that Jo could sleep downstairs and, therefore, not have to climb upstairs.

Psychometric properties

The critical question is how far any of these measures, whatever their psychometric properties, actually measure QoL. In simple terms, it is yet to be established that the different measures correlate significantly with one another. There is also a question of how far these measures focus on issues of concern to families. It is regrettable that new measures continue to be published even though there has been little, if any, consultation with children or their families.

THE POTENTIAL VALUE OF QoL MEASURES

Clinical trials

It is generally recognized that improvements in survival in childhood cancer have been achieved at least partly as a result of collaboration through national and international clinical trials. Given that current trials are unlikely to be associated with significant differences in survival rates, questions are raised about the most appropriate method of evaluation. QoL measures are expected to be useful in this context. Traditional end-points, such as disease free survival, need to be supplemented by outcomes reflecting the impact of treatment on the patient and their families.

Bradlyn *et al.* conducted a national survey to determine how far QoL measures were employed in Phase III clinical trials in pediatric oncology.[94] Research publications were identified in bibliographies from two major US Oncology Groups (Pediatric Oncology Group and Children's Cancer Group). They did not restrict their work to the use of comprehensive QoL measures, but

defined QoL very broadly to include any assessment of individual domains, such as mobility or relations with parents. Based on this broad definition, QoL measures were only included in 3 per cent of pediatric oncology trials. Any evaluation based strictly on the use of standardized QoL measures would suggest an even lower incidence. In adult work, despite the increasing availability of QoL measures, researchers continue to rely on *ad hoc* questions in evaluations of clinical trials.[95] The relationship between QoL during treatment with that of survivors remains a question of central interest but is, as yet, poorly understood.

Evaluating treatments

Our focus on use of QoL measures in evaluating clinical trials should not cloud the issue that the measures have other potential uses. Measurement of QoL has also been seen to be relevant in determining the efficacy of physical and psychological interventions. The development of a BMT specific measure is to be welcomed given the increasing use of BMT for children with cancer. Information about the potential impact during and after BMT on QoL may be useful for parents before beginning this treatment.

Barr *et al.* used the HUI (marks 2 and 3) to track QoL in children with ALL in remission during postinduction chemotherapy.[96] Children ($n = 18$) ranged in age from 11 months to 14 years. Ratings were made by nurses, parents and, where appropriate, by children themselves. As might be expected, the burden of morbidity is cyclical in nature, mirroring the schedule of chemotherapy. The impact on QoL was least at the onset of the treatment cycle (following a week of no treatment) and greatest at the beginning of the second week (following use of steroids). Pain was the most frequently reported indicator of morbidity, followed by emotion and mobility. This study documents the close relationship between treatment and QoL, and suggests also that HUI is sufficiently sensitive to detect these changes.

Interventions

Given the extent to which QoL is potentially affected by cancer, there is clearly ample room for interventions to improve QoL. Although there is considerable evidence that psychological interventions are helpful to reduce stress in adults with cancer, very little intervention work has been conducted with children. Some suggestion that psychological intervention may be helpful was provided by Varni *et al.*[97] These authors established a link between psychological distress and perceived stress. They argue that, unlike clinical or demographic variables, perceived

stress is potentially modifiable. Efforts to help the individual reinterpret the cancer experience and thus reduce feelings of stress should be as valuable in work with children as has been shown for work with adults.

Kazak *et al.* devised an intervention to reduce distress among children undergoing bone marrow aspirations and lumbar punctures.[98] Children were compared in two arms of a randomized, controlled prospective study. One group ($n = 45$) received a pharmacological intervention only, and the other group a combined pharmacological and psychological intervention ($n = 47$). Outcome measures included child distress, parent rated assessment of child QoL and parenting stress. Child distress was lower in the combined intervention group but there were no differences in QoL scores. (Subsidiary analyses suggested that QoL for both groups improved over the 6-month course of the study. Thus, there is evidence that this QoL measure lacks sensitivity to identify differences as a function of the intervention but may more adequately reflect changes over time).

CONCLUSIONS

Simple comparisons of survivors against healthy controls on standardized measures of anxiety, depression, self-esteem or body image point to few differences. However, different findings have emerged when other methods are used. For example, interview data can highlight problems not identified on questionnaire measures.[18,19]

Parents and teachers tend to rate survivors as having more behavior problems than controls. Certain family, demographic and clinical variables have been described as moderating outcomes, including parental distress,[27] social class and coping[28] and incidence of recurrence.[99] The incidence of PTSD is unclear. When comparisons have been made against population norms, survivors have shown more PTSD,[23] whereas when control groups are used, few differences are found.[24–26]

There is considerable clinical evidence that individual survivors experience some difficulties obtaining health and life insurance policies. However, there is minimal research in this area and data are difficult to interpret, given the time lapse between treatment and when an individual seeks insurance cover. Inevitably current information is based on survivors treated before current protocols and so the implications may be different.

Methodological limitations

All of these findings need to be considered in relation to methodological limitations inherent in current work. These particularly include difficulties in measurement of QoL and BI, and the reliance on cross-sectional rather than longitudinal designs.

Issues of measurement are not satisfactorily resolved. Many measures in common use were developed to assess symptoms generally and are not cancer specific. Some questionnaires are potentially distressing or intrusive[23] and many measures lack sensitivity because they target very wide age-ranges.

These methodological problems, including use of postal surveys and potentially distressing questionnaires, may contribute to poor completion rates. The solution has to be more focused and developmentally appropriate assessments. This can be achieved as the numbers of survivors grows and if centers are prepared to collaborate together. Pediatricians and child psychologists need to be prepared to draw on the expertise of adult clinicians in order to select measures that are appropriate for young adult survivors.

The lack of agreement about domains to be used in QoL work is highlighted by comparing the domains used in some measures with others. Thus, Armstrong *et al.*[77] identified three key domains (physical functioning and restriction from normal activity, emotional distress, and response to active medical treatment), while Bradlyn *et al.*[82] identified three others (physical functioning, social/role functioning, and mobility). Although both workers initially adopted the WHO definition of QoL, there is clear overlap only for the subscale measuring physical functioning.

Many questions remain about QoL measurement. Evaluation involves repeated assessment throughout treatment. As such, issues of sensitivity to change and practice effects of repeated administration are as vital as information about validity and reliability. Attention also needs to be given to issues of clinical rather than statistical change, i.e. what constitutes a meaningful change in QoL? Answers to these questions require a coordinated and collaborative approach. Our hope is that this review may facilitate the good will to initiate a national research agenda, which will ultimately provide us with an exemplary means of measuring child QoL. Only in this way can we achieve our aims of providing the child with quality as well as quantity of life.

Only Kupst and her colleagues have traced QoL outcomes over a significant period of time (from diagnosis for more than 10 years).[28] Longitudinal work has the important advantage over cross-sectional studies of charting changes in adjustment and functioning over time. However, using longitudinal data can also have severe shortcomings. Comparisons of group means on a variety of measures can give the impression that adjustment does not change over time, while inspection of individual scores (e.g. individuals who move from scoring at a clinically elevated level to a non-clinical level on a measure) can show a completely different pattern. Researchers should attempt more longitudinal research, while remaining alert to individual differences within the data.

Survivors with pronounced difficulties are excluded from much research with the result that perceptions of the need for services for survivors is likely to be underestimated. Survivors with obvious physical difficulties are routinely excluded and there has been very little follow-up of survivors of CNS tumors who are more likely to need educational support.

While some questions can be answered by research designs, where children with cancer are compared with healthy controls, others really cannot. Comparisons with norms (e.g. in terms of educational level) can tell us that the population has specific problems and that remedial services may be necessary. However, showing differences on a measure of self-esteem or depression tells us nothing about the processes whereby the problems arose. Indeed, taken to an extreme, this kind of approach is subject to the criticism that the differences were always there, that is, depressed children get cancer.

Perhaps the greatest problem with much research in this area is the failure of oncologists and behavioral scientists to work together to determine QoL implications of childhood cancer. The result is that many conclusions are too general and do not take into account how far QoL outcomes are moderated by differences in treatment. In the future, there must be greater collaboration between professionals so that it is possible to determine the links between physical health and QoL outcomes.

IMPLICATIONS

Current empirical work supports ideas from clinical practice that QoL outcomes in survivors of childhood cancer vary markedly. There are also considerable indications about the specific clinical, demographic and family variables that leave a survivor most at risk of compromised QoL. It is time, therefore, that the emphasis in research shifts from the focus on description of QoL outcomes to consider the potential for intervention. Based on the literature currently available, it is clear that improvements to QoL may be achieved through interventions targeted at vulnerable groups (CNS tumors) and vulnerable domains (social relationships; special education needs). As the length of survival increases, it is important to consider the needs of young adults. Some specialized vocational counseling is also needed.

Given the importance of QoL and BI for the individual survivor, it is disappointing to see that the emphasis in research remains focused on measurement. Refinements in measurement are crucial but may be facilitated by experience of how current measures work in practice.

The question of psychological outcome following the experience of a life-threatening disease and its treatment remains to be determined, but good studies are important

in order to determine the scope and range of remedial resources that are needed by some survivors. As with clinical work, these answers are most likely to be achieved through collaboration, both between professionals and internationally.

KEY POINTS

- Quality of life (QoL) is a measure of the impact of illness on the individual's physical, emotional, social and cognitive functioning.
- Measures of QoL need to be brief, comprehensive and include parallel versions for child and parent completion.
- There is wide variability in QoL and body image following treatment for childhood cancer.
- Vulnerable groups include survivors of brain tumors, those who were younger on diagnosis, and those from families who communicate less well.
- Attempts to improve QoL must begin during treatment and include efforts to offset school disadvantages.

REFERENCES

1. van Eys, J. The truly cured child? *Pediatrician* 1991; **18**:90–95.
2. Holmes HA, Holmes FF. After ten years, what are the handicaps and life styles of children treated for cancer? An examination of the present status of 124 such survivors. *Clin Pediatr* 1975; **14**:819–823.
3. Eisen M, Ware JE, Donald C, Brook RH. Measuring components of children's health status. *Med Care* 1979; **17**:902–921.
4. Aaronson NK, Meyeravitz BE, Bard M, *et al.* Quality of life research in oncology: past achievements and future priorities. *Cancer* 1991; **67**:839–843.
5. Gotay CC, Kom EL, McCabe MS, *et al.* Quality of life assessment in cancer treatment protocols: research issues in protocol development. *J Natl Cancer Inst* 1992; **84**:579.
6. Ware JE. Conceptualising disease impact and treatment outcomes. *Cancer* 1984; **53**:2316–2323.
7. World Health Organisation. *World Health Organisation Constitution.* Geneva: World Health Organisation, 1947.
8. Schipper H, Clinch JJ, Olweny CLM. Quality of life studies: definitions and conceptual frameworks. In: Spilker B (ed.) *Quality of life and pharmacoeconomics in clinical trials*, 2nd edn. Philadelphia: Lippincott-Raven Publishers, 1996.
9. Testa MA, Simonson DC. Assessment of quality-of-life outcomes. *N Engl J Med* 1996; **334**:835–840.
10. Calman KC. Definitions and dimensions of quality of life. In: Aaronson NK, Beckmann J (eds) *The quality of life of cancer patients.* New York: Raven Press, 1987.
11. Bergner M. Quality of life, health status and clinical research. *Med Care* 1989; **27**:S148–S156.
12. Hayry M. Measuring quality of life: why, how and what? In: Joyce CRB, O'Boyle CA, McGee H (eds) *Individual quality of life:*

approaches to conceptualisation and assessment. Australia: Harwood Academic Publishers, 1999.

●13. Gill TM, Feinstein AR. A critical appraisal of the quality of quality-of-life measurements. *JAMA* 1994; **272**:619–626.

●14. Leplege A, Hunt S. The problem of quality of life in medicine. *JAMA* 1997; **278**:47–50.

15. Eiser C, Morse R. Can parents rate their child's health related quality of life? Results of a systematic review. *Qual Life Res* 2001; **10**:347–357.

◆16. Eiser C, Morse R. Quality of life measures in chronic diseases of childhood. *Health Technol Assess Monographs* 2001; **5**(no. 4):1–156.

17. Eiser C, Hill JJ, Vance YH. Examining the psychological consequences of surviving childhood cancer: systematic review as a research method in pediatric psychology. *J Pediatr Psychol* 2000; **25**:449–460.

18. Gray RE, Doan BD, Shermer P, *et al.* Psychologic adaptation of survivors of childhood cancer. *Cancer* 1992; **70**: 2713–2721.

19. Gray RE, Doan BD, Shermer P, *et al.* Surviving childhood cancer: a descriptive approach to understanding the impact of life-threatening illness. *Psycho-Oncol* 1992; **1**:235–246.

20. Van Dongen-Melman JE, De Groot A, Kahlen K, Verhulst FC. Psychosocial functioning of children surviving cancer during middle childhood. In: Van Dongen-Melman JE (ed.) *On surviving childhood cancer*. Alblasserdam, The Netherlands: Haveka BY, 1995.

21. Madan-Swain A, Brown RT, Sexson SB, *et al.* Adolescent cancer survivors: psychosocial and familial adaptation. *Psychosomatics* 1994; **35**:453–459.

22. Pendley JS, Dahlquist LM, Dreyer ZA. BI and psychosocial adjustment in adolescent cancer survivors. *J Pediatr Psychol* 1997; **22**:29–43.

23. Stuber M, Christakis D, Houskamp B, Kazak A. Posttrauma symptoms in childhood leukemia survivors and their parents. *Psychosomatics* 1996; **37**:254–261.

24. Butler RW, Rizzi LP, Handwerger BA. Brief report: The assessment of posttraumatic stress disorder in pediatric cancer patients and survivors. *J Pediatr Psychol* 1996; **21**:499–504.

25. Kazak AE, Barakat LP, Meeske K, *et al.* Post traumatic stress, family functioning and social support in survivors of childhood leukemia and their mothers and fathers. *J Consul Clin Psychol* 1997; **65**:120–129.

26. Barakat LP, Kazak AE, Meadows AT, *et al.* Families surviving childhood cancer: A comparison of posttraumatic stress symptoms with families of healthy children. *J Pediatr Psychol* 1997; **22**:843–859.

27. Sloper P, Larcombe I, Charlton A. Psychosocial adjustment of five-year survivors of childhood cancer. *J Cancer Educ* 1994; **9**:581–588.

28. Kupst MJ, Natta MB, Richardson CC, *et al.* Family coping with pediatric leukemia: ten years after treatment. *J Pediatr Psychol* 1995; **20**:601–617.

29. Hill J, Komblith AB, Jones D. A comparative study of the long term psychosocial functioning of childhood acute lymphoblastic leukemia survivors treated by intrathecal methotrexate with or without cranial radiation. *Am Cancer Soc* 1998; 208–218.

30. Allport GW. *Pattern and growth in personality*. New York: Holt, Rinehart & Winston, 1961.

31. Cornwell CJ, Schmitt MH. Perceived health status, self esteem and BI in women with rheumatoid arthritis or systemic lupus erythematosus. *Res Nurs Health* 1990; **13**:99–107.

32. Petersen AC, Schulenberg JE, Abramowitz RH, *et al.* A self-image questionnaire for young adolescents (SIQY A): reliabilty and validity studies. *J Youth Adolescence* 1984; **13**:93–111.

33. Secord PF, Jourard SM. The appraisal of body-cathexis: body-cathexis and the self. *J Consulting Psychol* 1953; **17**:343–347.

34. Harter S. *Manual for self-perception profile for adolescent.* Denver: University of Denver Press, 1988.

35. Rosen JC, Srebnik D, Saltzberg E, Wendt S. Development of a body image avoidance questionnaire. *Psychol Assess* 1991; **3**:32–37.

36. Cash TF. *Body-image therapy. A program for self-directed change.* New York: Guilford, 1991.

37. Kopel SJ, Eiser C, Cool P, *et al.* Brief report: Assessment of BI in survivors of childhood cancer. *J Pediatr Psychol* 1998; **23**:141–147.

38. Fritz GK, Williams JR. Issues of adolescent development for survivors of childhood cancer. *J Am Acad Child Adolescent Psychiat* 1988; **27**:712–715.

39. Moos RH, Cronkite RC, Billings AG, Finney JW. *The health and daily living form manual,* 1984. Available from the Social Ecology Laboratory, Department of Psychiatry and Behavioral Sciences, Stanford University, Stanford, CA 94035, USA.

40. Asher SR, Hymel S, Renshaw PD. Loneliness in children. *Child Dev* 1984; **55**:1456–1464.

41. La Greca AM, Stone WL. Social anxiety scale for children-revised: factor structure and concurrent validity. *J Clin Child Psychol* 1992; **22**:17–27.

42. Davies H, Didcock E, Didi M, *et al.* Growth, puberty, and obesity after treatment for leukemia. *Acta Pediatr Suppl* 1995; **411**:45–50.

43. Schell M, Ochs J, Schriock E, Carter M. A method of predicting adult height in long term survivors of childhood lymphoblastic leukemia. *J Clin Oncol* 1992; **10**:128–133.

44. Holm K, Nysom K, Hertz H, Muller J. Normal final height after treatment for acute lymphoblastic leukemia without irradiation. *Acta Pediatr Scand* 1994; **83**:1287–1290.

45. Sklar C, Mertens A, Walter A. Final height after treatment for acute lymphoblastic leukemia: comparison of no cranial irradiation, 1800 cGy and 2400 cGy. *J Pediatr* 1993; **123**:59–64.

46. Stabler B. Growth hormone insufficiency during childhood has implications for later life. *Acta Pediatr Scand Suppl* 1991; **377**:9–13.

●47. Money J. Psychological aspects of endocrine and genetic disease in children. In: Gardner LI (ed.) *Endocrine and genetic diseases of childhood*. Philadelphia: WB Saunders, 1968.

48. Rotnem D, Genel M, Hintz RL, Cohen DJ. Personality development in children with growth hormone deficiency. *J Am Acad Child Adolescent Psychiat* 1977; **16**:412–416.

49. Bjork S, Jonsson B, Westphal O, Levin JE. Quality of life of adults with growth hormone deficiency: a controlled study. *Acta Paeditr Scand Suppl* 1989; **356**:55–59.

50. Pilpel D, Leiberman E, Zadik Z, Carel C. Effect of growth hormone treatment on quality of life of short stature children. *Hormone Res* 1995; **44**:1–5.

51. Kelnar CJH. Cost–benefit analysis is the key. *Arch Dis Child* 2000; **83**:176–177.

52. Grimer RJ. Costs and benefits of limb salvage surgery for osteosarcoma. In: Selby P, Bailey C (eds) *Cancer and the adolescent*. London: BMJ Publishing Group, 1996:120–135.

53. Rougraff BT, Simon MA, Kneisl JS, *et al.* Limb salvage compared with amputation for osteosarcoma of the distal end of the femur. *Am J Bone Joint Surg* 1994; **76**:649–656.

54. Sugarbaker PH, Barofsky I, Rosenberg SA, Gianola FJ. Quality of life assessment of patients in extremity sarcoma clinical trials. *Surgery* 1982; **91**:17–23.

55. Weddington WW, Segraves KB, Simon MA. Psychological outcome of extremity sarcoma survivors undergoing amputation or limb salvage. *J Clin Oncol* 1985; **3**:1393–1399.

56. Postma A, Kingma A, De Ruiter JH, *et al.* Quality of life in bone tumor patients comparing limb salvage and amputation of the lower extremity. *J Surg Oncol* 1992; **51**:47–51.

57. Christ GH, Lane JM, Marcove R. Psychosocial adaptation of long-term survivors of bone sarcoma. *J Psychosoc Oncol* 1995; **13**:1–21.

58. Felder-Puig R, Formann AK, Mildner A, *et al.* Quality of life and psychosocial adjustment of young patients after treatment of bone cancer. *Cancer* 1998; **83**:69–75.

59. Mulhemt R, Phipps S, White H. Neurological and special senses: neuropsycological outcomes. In: Wallace H, Green D (eds) *Late effects of childhood cancer.* London: Arnold, 2003:000-000.

60. Evans SE, Radford M. Current lifestyle of young adults treated for cancer in childhood. *Arch Dis Child* 1995; **72**:423–426.

61. Mackie ET, Hill J, Kondrynt H, McNally R. Adult psychosocial outcomes in long-term survivors of acute lymphoblastic leukaemia and Wilm's tumour: a controlled study. *Lancet* 2000; **355**:1310–1314.

62. Haupt R, Byme J, Connelly RR, *et al.* Smoking habits in survivors of childhood and adolescent cancer. *Med Pediatr Oncol* 1992; **20**:301–306.

63. Kingma A, Rammeloo LAL, van der Does-van den Berg, *et al.* Academic career after treatment for acute lymphoblastic leukaemia. *Arch Dis Child* 2000; **82**:353–357.

64. Teta MJ, Del Po MC, Kasl SV. Psychosocial consequences of childhood and adolescent cancer survival. *J Chronic Dis* 1986; **39**:751–759.

65. Green DM, Zevont MA, Hall B. Achievement of life goals by adult survivors of modem treatment for childhood cancer. *Cancer* 1990; **67**:206–213.

66. Hays DM, Dolgin M, Steele LL, *et al.* Educational achievement employment and workplace experience of adult survivors of childhood cancer. *Int J Pediatr Hemotol Oncol* 1997; **4**:327–337.

67. Hays DM, Landsverk J, Sallant SE, *et al.* Educational, occupational, and insurance status of childhood cancer survivors in their fourth and fifth decades of life. *J Clin Oncol* 1992; **10**:1397–1406.

68. Monaco GP. Socioeconomic considerations in childhood cancer survival: society's obligations. *Am J Pediatr Hemotol Oncol* 1987; **9**:92–98.

69. Eiser C, Cool P, Grimer RJ, *et al.* Quality of life following treatment for a malignant primary bone tumour around the knee. *Sarcoma* 1997; **1**:39–45.

70. Byrne J, Lewis S, Halamek L, *et al.* Childhood cancer survivors' knowledge of their diagnosis and treatment. *Ann Int J Med* 1989; **110**:400–403.

●71. Meadows A, McKee L, Kazak AE. 1989 Psychosocial status of young adult survivors of childhood cancer: a survey. *Med Pediatr Oncol* 1989; **17**:466–470.

72. Novakovic B, Fears TR, Horowitz ME, *et al.* 1997. Late effects of therapy in survivors of Ewing's sarcoma family tumors. *J Pediatr Hemotol Oncol* 1989; **19**:220–225.

73. Nicholson HS, Byrne J. Fertility and pregnancy after treatment for cancer during childhood or adolescence. *Cancer* 1993; **71**:3329–3399.

74. Weigers ME, Chesler MA, Zebrack BJ, Goldman S. 1998 Self-reported worries among long-term survivors of childhood cancer and their peers. *J Psychosoc Oncol* **16**:1–23.

75. Zevon MA, Neubauer NA, Green DM. Adjustment and vocational satisfaction of patients treated during childhood or adolescence for acute lymphoblastic leukaemia. *Am J Pediatr Hematol Oncol* 1990; **12**:454–461.

76. Phipps S, Dunavant M, Jayawardene D, Srivastiva DK. Assessment of health related quality of life in acute in-patient settings: use of the BASES Scales in children undergoing bone marrow transplantation. *Int J Cancer* 1999; **812**:18–24.

77. Armstrong FD, Toledano SR, Miloslavich K, *et al.* 1999 The Miami pediatric Quality of Life Questionnaire: Parent Scale. *Int J Cancer* 1999; S12:11–17.

●78. Varni JW, Katz ER, Seid M, *et al.* The Pediatric Cancer Quality of Life Inventory (PCQL). I. Instrument development, descriptive statistics, and cross-informant variance. *J Behav Med* 1998; **21**:179–204.

79. Goodwin DA, Boggs SR, Graham-Pole J. Development and validation of the Pediatric Oncology Quality of Life Scale. *Psychol Assess* 1994; **6**:321–328.

80. Lansky SB, List MA, Lansky LL, *et al.* The measurement of performance in childhood cancer patients. *Cancer* 1987; **60**:1656.

81. Feeny D, Furlong W, Barr RD, *et al.* A comprehensive multiattribute system for classifying the health status of survivors of childhood cancer. *J Clin Oncol* 1992; **10**:923–928.

82. Bradlyn AS, Harris CV, Warner JE, *et al.* 1993 An investigation of the validity of the quality of Well-Being Scale with pediatric oncology patients. *Health Psychol* 1992; **12**:246–250.

83. Calaminus G, Weispach S, Teske C, Gobel U. Quality of life in children and adolescents with cancer. *Klin Padiatr* 2000; **212**:211–215.

84. Eiser C, Havermans T, Craft A, Kernahan J. Development of a measure to assess the perceived illness experience after treatment for cancer. *Arch Dis Child* 1995; **72**:302–307.

♦85. Jenney ME, Kane RL, Lurie N. Developing a measure of health outcomes in survivors of childhood cancer: a review of the issues. *Med Pediatr Oncol* 1995; **24**:145–153.

86. Karnofsky DA, Abelman WH, Craver LF, *et al.* 1948. The use of nitrogen mustards in palliative treatment of carcinoma. *Cancer* 1995; **1**:634–656.

87. Kaplan RM, Anderson JP. A general health policy model: an integrated approach. *Health Serv Res* 1988; **23**:203–235.

88. Feeny D, Furlong W, Boyle M, Torrance GW. Multi-attribute health-status classification systems: health utilities index. *Pharacoeconomics* 1995; **7**:490–502.

89. Torrance GW. Utility approach to measuring health-related quality of life. *J Chronic Dis* 1987; **40**:593–600.

90. Billson AL, Walker DA. Assessment of health status in survivors of cancer. *Arch Dis Child* 1994; **70**:200–204.

91. Achenbach TM. *Manual for the child behavior checklist/4–18 and 1991 profile.* Burlington, University of Vermont, Department of Psychiatry, 1991.

92. Reynolds RV, Tobin DL, Creer TL, *et al.* A method for studying controlled substance use: a preliminary investigation. *Addict Behav,* 1987; **12**:53–62.

93. Varni JW, Katz, ER, Seid M, *et al.* The Pediatric Cancer quality of life inventory-32 (PCQL-32): instrument development, descriptive statistics, and cross-informant variance. *J Behav Med* 1998; **21**:179–204.

94. Bradlyn AS, Harris CV, Spieth LE. Quality of life assessment in pediatric oncology: a retrospective review of phase III reports. *Social Sci Med* 1995; **41**:1463–1465.

95. Sanders C, Egger M, Donovan J, *et al.* Reporting on quality of life in randomised controlled trials: bibliographic study. *Br Med J;* 1998; **317**:1191–1194.

96. Barr RD, Petrie C, Furlong W, *et al.* Health-related quality of life during post-induction chemotherapy in children with acute lymphoblastic leukemia in remission. *Int J Oncol* 1997; **11**:333–339.

97. Varni JW, Kazt ER, Colegrove JR, Dolgin M. Perceived stress and adjustment of long-term survivors of childhood cancer. *J Psychosoc Oncol* 1994; **12**:1–16.

98. Kazak AE, Penati B, Boyer BA, Himelstein B. A randomized controlled prospective outcome study of a psychological and pharmacological intervention protocol for procedural distress in pediatric leukemia. *J Pediatr Psychol* 1996; **21**:615–631.

99. Elkin TD, Phipps S, Mulhern RK, Fairclough D. Psychological functioning of adolescent and young adult survivors of pediatric malignancy. *Med Pediatr Oncol* 1997; **29**:582–588.

12b

Legal issues: US perspective

GRACE-ANN P MONACO AND GILBERT SMITH

INTRODUCTION

As childhood survivors ultimately discover, the challenges of cancer do not stop at the close of treatment. Ultimately, we are faced with a whole new set of non-treatment-related issues involving education, employment, and insurance and other benefits. Fortunately, there are federal, state and local laws that provide us with protections, and help us navigate around or through these new issues. The key, of course, is knowing that they are out there and how to best access them.

The purpose of this subchapter is to provide an overview of the laws that childhood cancer survivors can utilize as they move forward with their lives. The law is constantly changing, if not always in word, then in interpretation by the courts and regulatory agencies. That said, this subchapter is not an immutable bible. Rather it is a tool to help you recognize and address the legal issues that may confront you, and how to obtain helpful resources and a helpful network of support, should you ever need it. As a survivor, this subchapter presumes that you completed most of your treatments, with the exception of some maintenance therapy or appropriate medical follow-up guidance and participation in late effects studies. For general legal issues resources focused on patient issues, see: Childhood Cancer Ombudsman Program (CCOP);[1] The National Coalition for Cancer Survivorship (NCCS);[2] The Childhood Brain Tumor Foundation (CBTF);[3] and Candlelighters Childhood Cancer Foundation (CCCF).[4]

OVERVIEW OF LEGISLATION

Regarding education, there are three possible resources to provide a child having cancer with needed educational services:

- Federal Individuals with Disabilities Education Act (IDEA) (PL 94-142 and PL 99-457 amendments) and the respective state laws that implement this law.
- Federal Rehabilitation Act of 1973 (Rehab Act) (PL 93-112, section 504). This Act bans both public and private employers receiving public funds from discriminating on the basis of disability. Information and assistance available from the Access Unit of the Civil Rights Division, Department of Justice, Washington, DC.
- Americans with Disabilities Act of 1990 (PL 101-336).

Generally, these laws protect the rights of children with cancer who may be left with learning disabilities, attention disorders, a high risk of infection, amputations or other physical limitations that prevent use of the full range of educational programs. These laws, which apply to primary and secondary education, to infant, toddler, and preschool interventions, and to college, university and vocational education, are premised on education as a right guaranteed to every citizen regardless of physical, mental or health impairments. Although these laws have the authority of federal mandate, state governments implement them and may interpret provisions differently.

In general, as to employment, insurance and benefits, the various laws that affect the childhood cancer survivor are listed below:

- The Americans with Disabilities Act (ADA);
- Health Insurance Portability and Accountability Acts (HIPAA);
- Consolidated Omnibus Budget Reconciliation Act (COBRA);
- Employee Retirement and Income Security Act (ERISA).

Viewed *in toto* these laws represent a concerted approach on the federal level to provide a fair and equal playing field for cancer patients and survivors regarding access to employment and insurance. Listed below are some of the protections you are afforded under these laws.

- Generally, no associational discrimination is allowed. For example, denial of benefits or job to a spouse solely on his or her relationship to a person with a disability is prohibited.
- Prevention of discrimination on the basis of genetic information relating to illness, disease or other disorders.
- Ensure equal insurance to all workers and no diminution in benefits unless there is either legitimate actuarial data or reasonably anticipated experience (current statistics) that show the person is still at risk. You may have to put up with diminished benefits (a 'rated' policy) depending on when you will be a normal risk and the available actuarial data.
- If you are fired or laid-off, you have a right to continue group health coverage at your own expense and, if you are disabled, obtain coverage up to 29 months to bridge the gap to other insured employment or, depending on the nature of the disability, to bridge the gap to Medicare coverage.
- The law also provides assistance in combating discrimination in the collection of employee benefits by parents, spouse or survivor forced into retirement or fired or assigned part-time status, which would remove their insurance benefits.

EDUCATION

The Individuals with Disabilities Education Act, the ADA and the Rehab Act all apply to public schools. Specifically, Title II of the ADA, applies to state and local government, and that includes public schools. Children with cancer and other eligible disabilities are entitled to and guaranteed a free and appropriate public education. They are entitled to specially designed instruction and related services, such as occupation and physical therapy, and transportation, for example, as well as entitled to accommodation,

such as modification in policies that they may need in order to have the equal opportunity to participate in academic and athletic instruction, and extra curricular activities at school. The ADA further states the disabled cannot be forced to accept an accommodation. In other words, childhood cancer survivors cannot be forced to accept educational plans, such as separate classes, that they do not wish to take. If an appropriate public placement is unavailable, the school system must provide an appropriate private placement to substitute for or supplement the public school's package. The ADA also applies to institutions of higher education.

Children covered by IDEA are entitled to a *free and appropriate public education*. Special education means specially designed instruction based on the needs of the individual survivor, and includes related services such as transportation, counseling and physical therapy. Related services may be provided by public schools to students who are enrolled in private schools. Again the Rehabilitation Act and the ADA require schools to make accommodations so that the survivor is afforded equal opportunity to participate and benefit from his or her education.

While not all children who go off treatment will qualify under the IDEA, it is important to understand that they will all qualify under the ADA and the Rehabilitation Act because they all have a record of having survived cancer. This usually takes the form of what are known as Student-Study Teams (or Child-Study Teams) that help institute various accommodations, such as providing two sets of books, one for school and one for home. *Note that, if you are furnished with special accommodative equipment (computers, hearing aids, cochlear implants, for example) by the school system, both to obtain special assistance and to maintain or replace equipment received, it may be necessary to participate in a due process hearing, which may require limited purpose disclosure of your relevant medical records.*

It is a good idea to check with your state vocational and rehabilitation agency. Assistance may be available for state college tuition or vocational training, so the survivor could get paid to go to school and fill any educational gaps.

EMPLOYMENT AND THE AMERICANS WITH DISABILITIES ACT

Most employment rights cases will involve the ADA, which is a federal civil rights law. It prohibits discrimination by requiring that disabled people be given the same chances and the same opportunities as able-bodied people. The key word here is *same*; not special, or more, just the *same* opportunities that people who are not disabled have always received. If another federal or state law grants

greater protection to the disabled than the ADA would in certain circumstances, then that law controls. The ADA is a *floor*, not a *ceiling*. Know the provisions of your state. Your original cancer is usually considered to have substantially limited you. While, you may not presently consider yourself disabled, please note that disability is a term of art in the legal profession. In other words it does not describe your actual status but your assumed status for the purposes of the rights to which you may be entitled. ADA coverage is determined on a case-by-case basis.

The ADA is *not* an affirmative action statute; there are no quotas or goals for hiring the disabled. No one gets 'bonus points' for hiring the disabled. The disabled do not receive special job *protection* once they are hired. An employer can still decline to hire the disabled, but it has to be based on the essential functions of the job and the applicant's qualifications, not because of their disability.

The ADA applies to any *qualified* individual with a disability who can perform the essential functions of the job, regardless of whether the job applicant will need a reasonable accommodation from the employer. Reasonable accommodations are defined later in this subchapter.

Defining Disability under the ADA

Generally, a qualified individual with a disability is defined as someone who is substantially impaired in a major life activity. That means they cannot perform an activity that a normal person can. Major life activities include walking, talking, eating, breathing, seeing and hearing. For example, if disabled people use drugs or devices, such as insulin, prosthetic devices, antidepressives, to perform major life activities, and mitigate the disability, they are not automatically considered disabled. Rather, they may be considered disabled on a case-by-case basis, depending on the effect of the mitigating measure. Cancer patients and survivors are covered under other definitions of disability* discussed in more detail below. Briefly, these provisions relate to a record of a disability (substantially limited in the past) or being *regarded* in the workplace as 'having a disability' (the employer perceives the person as being substantially limited in performing a major life activity).

Most important for cancer survivors, the ADA protects someone with *a record of impairment*. Every cancer survivor has a record of substantial impairment. Consequently, the ADA will apply to them for the rest of their lives. The ADA protects cancer survivors, whether the cancer is cured, controlled or in remission. However, depending upon how successful a survivor is through the use, for example, of medicines or devices, to counter or moderate an effect of the cancer or the treatment, that survivor may not be considered to have a disability under the ADA *that requires intervention or accommodation.*

Employers can no longer discriminate against the disabled in any phase of employment: hiring, training, job assignment, classification, promotion, transfer, benefits, leave of absence, layoff or termination. While employers cannot ask about a disability, they can ask an applicant to show they would perform the essential functions of a job. An applicant might want to have a scrapbook of photographs showing him performing these or similar tasks. An applicant has a right to request a reasonable accommodation in testing, and can return to take an employment test after the accommodation has been provided.

Employers will be held to their job descriptions and advertising; survivors cannot be hired and then fired because they could not perform assumed or secondary job functions. You cannot be asked nor do you have to disclose whether you have any disability that would affect your job performance. If you can do the job – that is all that counts. This applies both to oral interviews and written applications. You do not have to explain why there are gaps in your employment history. On your job you are entitled to a non-hostile work environment free from severe and pervasive workplace harassment. However, legitimate questions concerning performance or whether health problems are adversely affecting performance are not tantamount to regarding an employee as disabled.

Additional ADA protections

ASSOCIATIONAL DISCRIMINATION

Unlike the other civil rights laws, the ADA also protects those who associate with a disabled person. The parent or spouse of a child with cancer or a cancer survivor cannot be denied employment, or fired because the employer assumes the parent or spouse will need time off to deal with treatment issues. The employer cannot refuse to hire the associated individual because of a belief that it may increase health care/insurance premium costs, and the employer cannot refuse to insure an individual because he has a disabled spouse or dependent. However, an employer does not have to provide a reasonable accommodation, such as a modified work schedule, to the associated individual.

REASONABLE ACCOMMODATION

In the workplace, the ADA requires employers to make reasonable accommodations for the disabled. This means an accommodation that would not cause undue hardship for the business. If a disabled employee requests

---

*The definition of disability under Section 501 of the Rehabilitation Act is identical to the definition under the ADA (PL 101-336).

a reasonable accommodation, the employer must analyze the possible accommodations and seek technical assistance. Failure to seek this assistance is not a defense under the law. The burden is on the employer not on the employee regarding issues relating to reasonable accommodation.

If the employee can no longer do his or her current job and there is a vacant job he or she can do with or without reasonable accommodation, reassignment may be a necessary reasonable accommodation. If the survivor is no longer able to provide his or her job function even with a reasonable accommodation and no other jobs for which the survivor is qualified are available, the employer is not required to retain the employee. For example, if the job description legitimately calls for a 55-hour week and you can only provide 40, accommodating you would destroy the nature of the position, which is not required under the ADA.

Employers are not required to provide personal aids, such as wheelchairs or hearing aids, or personal assistance. This includes assistance a disabled person might need in eating, dressing or toileting. If the employee requires some accommodation to deal with medical management of a side effect of treatment, provided the employee can still do the essential functions of the job, the ADA provides flex-time as a reasonable accommodation. Additionally, the Family and Medical Leave Act (FMLA)[5] entitles eligible employees to take up to 12 weeks of unpaid, job-protected leave and continued benefits in a 12-month period for specified family and medical reasons, including childbirth, adoption, or a family medical emergency. It also covers 'intermittent leave' time, meaning that the 12 weeks does not need to taken consecutively and can be taken a few days at a time if necessary. (An excellent source of information is the National Partnership for Women and Families.[6]) Either law, ADA or FMLA can be used to achieve family/patient needs or accommodations depending on the circumstances. If pending federal executive orders and legislative efforts prevail, they will permit unemployment benefits to be collected under the FMLA to reduce financial hardship. Check your state medical leave laws. Some may provide more coverage than the federal law. A good source of this information is the agency that enforces your state civil rights laws.

However, employment rights are always dependent upon whether the employee can do the job satisfactorily. If the employee would have been terminated but for FMLA,[7] upon return the employee would not be entitled to the same job. An employee who is unable to perform the essential functions of a job, apart from an inability to work a full-time schedule, is not entitled to an intermittent or reduced schedule leave under the FMLA. If the employee has available paid sick leave and FMLA leave, it is the employee's choice, not the employer's, which one he or she wishes to use.

HEALTH CARE, INSURANCE AND OTHER BENEFITS

In this section, we provide an overview of the various legislative acts that most significantly impact the childhood cancer survivor regarding health care, insurance and other benefits. Remember to check your state law for provisions that may expand your federal rights.

ADA protections

The ADA as it pertains to insurance is discussed under the employment section of this subchapter below. In general, on access to insurance by cancer survivors, apart from the employment protections, the ADA also requires that denials must be based on either legitimate actuarial data or the reasonably anticipated experience of the persons at risk. This means that the insurance company has to have current statistics that show that this person is still at risk.

The Health Insurance Portability and Accountability Act (Public Law. 104–191)

The Health Insurance Portability and Accountability Act (HIPAA), passed into law in 1996, allows millions of Americans with pre-existing conditions to secure comprehensive health insurance. HIPAA also helps people maintain their coverage if they need to change insurance or jobs. It makes insurance more accessible for those who work for small businesses. It expands the rights of cancer survivors. In brief, HIPAA offers the following rights, some of which overlap with the ADA.

- It prevents denial of enrollment based on health status, health factors, medical condition, claims history, medical history or genetic information.[8]
- It prevents higher premiums among workers on group plan[8] (the insurer can charge higher premiums under the individual coverage plan).
- It provides uniform benefits to all workers.
- It provides individual coverage to a person who leaves a group health plan owing to loss of employment or because the new employer does not offer insurance coverage.
- It prevents waiting periods or pre-existing condition exclusions, as long as the individual opted for and exhausted COBRA continuation coverage, has had at least 18 months of prior health insurance coverage, and there has been no gap in insurance coverage of more than 63 days, excluding employer waiting periods.
- It provides a credit for the period of time an individual was insured against the pre-existing waiting period, if an individual had prior insurance that was not in effect at the time of job switch.

- It provides for renewal of group and individual plans.
- It prevents genetic information from being used to establish a pre-existing condition unless there is a diagnosis of a related condition.

The Center for Medicare and Medicaid Services (CMS) recently released a program memorandum in which it addressed the situation where an employer with a disabled employee switches its group health insurance plan from one carrier to a new succeeding carrier. According to Program Memorandum 00-04, the new succeeding carrier cannot preclude coverage for disabled employees or dependents by using 'actively-at-work-clauses.' CMS emphasized that, under HIPAA, state-sponsored succeeding carrier laws cannot eliminate a succeeding carrier's obligation to enroll individuals who were disabled at the time that the original plan is terminated.

The Consolidated Omnibus Budget Reconciliation Act

This Act mandates that both public and private employers with 20 or more employees for half of the working days in the previous calendar year must make insurance coverage available for a limited period of time to employees and their dependents. Under COBRA employees who have been fired or laid off have a right to continue their group health coverage at their own expense and at a rate no higher than 102 per cent of the employer's group insurance premium for 18 months. Beginning in 1989, it provided the same benefits for the disabled for up to 29 months to bridge the gap to Medicare. The premium for the disabled from the 18th to the 29th month can be up to 150 per cent of the premium charged. Listed below are some important facts about COBRA.

- An employer has a duty to inform employees of their COBRA rights and to notify the group health plan of an employee death, termination or reduction in hours. Coverage may extend to a spouse, for example, after the death of an eligible employee or after divorce or legal separation, and to a dependent under the same conditions or if the child leaves dependent status during the COBRA period.
- The employee or family member has the responsibility of informing the group health plan administrator of a legal separation, divorce or of a child losing dependent status. The employee or beneficiary has 60 days from the date he or she would lose coverage to make a decision about the continuation of coverage.
- COBRA coverage is not available if the terminated employee is already covered by the spouse's plan unless the spouse's plan contains any exclusions or

limitations with respect to any pre-existing condition of the terminated beneficiary.
- COBRA coverage may be terminated if the employer stops providing employee group health insurance or if the employee becomes covered under another plan, including Medicare, or ceases payment of COBRA continuation premiums.

For further information about COBRA, contact the Pension and Welfare Benefits Administration at the US Department of Labor.

Employee Retirement and Income Security Act (ERISA)[9]

This Act prohibits an employer from discriminating against an employee for the purpose of preventing collection of health benefits under an employee-benefit plan, that is, a plan providing benefits in the event of sickness, accident, disability, death or unemployment. This protection does not apply to persons denied a 'new' job due to a history of cancer. The ADA discussion above covers this.

ERISA is an additional tool to be considered by employees facing forced retirement, firing or placement in part-time status with removal of insurance benefits. For example, a case involving an employee who enrolled in a plan with out-of-network benefits in order to continue treatment with his or her original cancer care provider. The plan refused coverage and the case went to court. The court held that, unless charges exceeded the usual and customary rates of other local comprehensive cancer centers, the insurer was required to reimburse for all charges.

Note: in all insurance cases, unless the health benefit plan waives the requirement, the employee survivor is required to exhaust administrative remedies under the plan before suit is brought. Further, arbitration cannot be compelled if it is not in your insurance contract and if you have not been notified of its inclusion in a change of benefits.

Access of benefits through employment

The ADA mandates that employers provide equal access to health care benefits for the disabled and those who associate with them. This includes disability benefits. An employer cannot consider what effect hiring a disabled person would have on their insurance premium. That also applies to considering whether to hire the parent or spouse of a cancer survivor.

The ADA permits insurers to discriminate provided that those risks that are the basis for discrimination are not inconsistent with state law and are not a means to evade the ADA's purposes. It is still unclear when and whether insurance discrimination violations will be subject to state or federal remedies.

For example, although infertility is considered a disability, an employer may offer insurance that precludes fertility coverage or some aspects thereof, for all employees providing it is done on an equal basis. However, this applies in general to fertility and, *in our opinion*, does not apply to infertility that is the result of/side effect of the treatment of a disease. Although there is no reported case law related to cancer treatment *vis à vis* infertility and its remediation, insurers and employers have permitted fertility treatment under the same scenario as they would permit breast reconstruction or hearing aids for cisplatin-related deafness.

The ADA also regulates how health care providers treat the disabled. Health care providers cannot deny medical treatment to a person with a disability if they are qualified to provide it. For example, a dermatologist can refer an HIV-positive person with a broken arm to an orthopedic surgeon, but cannot refuse to treat that person for a skin disorder.

In 2000, the Department of Health and Human Services announced[10] two new initiatives to enable people with disabilities to become and stay competitively employed. The first, the Demonstration Project to Maintain Independence and Employment will fund a cutting-edge program demonstration that enables people with chronic, disabling conditions to get medical benefits to obtain needed care without having to quit their jobs. The second, Medicaid Infrastructure Grants will help states build the systems they need to allow individuals with a disability to purchase health coverage through Medicaid. Both the grants and the demonstrations help advance the goals of the Ticket to Work and Work Incentives Improvement Act of 1999,[11] a law passed by Congress to encourage people with disabilities to work without fear of losing their Medicare, Medicaid or similar health benefits.[12] If you receive a denial, request in writing a 'Notice of Action,' which states the denial and provides appeal information and apply for a 'fair hearing' review of the denial.

There is pending federal legislation and a growing trend in state policy to require parity between medical and mental health benefits. This could benefit the childhood cancer survivor because it may enhance the ability of survivors to obtain assistance in dealing with any post-traumatic stress problems relating to cancer and its treatment.

If you are in the military or a military dependent, the Interagency Agreement between the Department of Defense and National Cancer Institute for Partnership in Clinical Trials for Cancer Prevention and Treatment 10/18/99, was expanded and made permanent under a final rule effective 3/2/01 and codified in 32 CFR 1999. Under this agreement you have the opportunity to participate in Phase II and Phase III NCI-sponsored cancer treatment clinical trials for cancer either in the direct care system or through civilian providers who are reimbursed through TRICARE/CHAMPUS. At this point, we are unaware of any effort to invoke this agreement to participate in late effects trials, but it certainly provides food for thought. In general, it may be argued that failure to cover general specialized monitoring and surveillance post cancer treatment places the survivor's life at risk much along the arguments made for coverage of mammography.

GENETIC ISSUES

An excellent source for up-to-date information on genetic issues and the status of legislation and programs relating to access and discrimination issues relating to genetics is the Council for Responsible Genetics, 5 Upland Road, Suite #3, Cambridge MA 02140. Telephone: (617) 868-0870; fax: (617)-491-5344; email: crg@essential.org.

NETWORKING

Federal Agencies involved with implementing the statutes discussed in this subchapter have experienced personnel. For example, the Equal Employment Opportunity Commission (EEOC), which handles all employment-related complaints, has lawyers and investigators in state-based offices throughout the country.[13] The same is also true of the Department of Justice (complaints against public accommodations), the Department of Heath and Human Services (police medical schools, hospitals and health care providers), and the Department of Education (oversees public schools and colleges). Remember, if gentle persuasion and education fail, the government may invoke mediation or arbitration. If all else fails, the government is ready to litigate cases. The government is also going to rely on alternative dispute resolution, such as mediation and arbitration, so it does not have to bring each complaint to court.

The governments educational effort means publications are either free or low cost, and include resource lists of companies and organizations that can help you. Material comes in Braille and audiocassette forms; the government has set up telephone lines to handle TDDs (Telecommunications Devices for the Deaf) and a computer bulletin board system.[14]

There is a national network of disabled persons who have been trained as ADA specialists. The network will provide technical assistance to businesses and government, and training on the ADA for disabled persons. Persons with complaints should contact technical assistance representatives, and centers for information and assistance.[15]

Disability organizations, both cancer and non-cancer related, may have already worked out a solution to your specific problem.

CONCLUSION

First and foremost, know your rights and what resources are available to you as you live life after cancer. Survivors of childhood cancer in the population now run into the hundreds of thousands. It is important to network with other survivors in your locality and, with the advent of the Internet, beyond. You can find other survivors through local parents groups, survivor groups and referrals from your hospital and hospital programs. You probably will find that other survivors have fought through to find solutions to the problems you may encounter, both common and unique. We need to rely on each, other than just to get through treatment, if we want to lead successful and content lives. It is our experience that survivors are more than happy to share the lessons they have learned and the information provided in this subchapter is an excellent place to start. The more networking undertaken, the richer the base of information and assistance can be available to survivors.

On a larger scale, through networking, survivors can provide the numbers of constituent voices that legislators require to sit up and take notice in crafting an agenda to further expand the rights of cancer survivors, and to make the existing laws, especially state laws, more uniform. The legal issues that affect survivors are not all that unique. They cross many different diseases, thereby providing a common bond with other childhood-focused coalitions. Collectively, we need to develop an agenda for the medical, social and political change, and the legal infrastructure to improve access to care, control of disease, cure of disease and enhancement of life expectations for our survivors.

KEY POINTS

- This subchapter, in principal part, provides an overview of the key legislation impacting the employment, insurance, education, discrimination and access issues facing survivors of childhood cancer.
- The legislation discussed does not offer special privileges for survivors, rather it intends to level the playing field for survivors, neutralize the history of cancer, and facilitate equal opportunity in obtaining insurance, employment, education and benefits for most survivors.
- In employment, survivors who can perform the essential functions of a job, with or without reasonable accommodation, are entitled to benefits equal to those offered to other workers and a fair non-hostile work environment.
- The various insurance rights conveyed by the legislation provide rights to continued insurance coverage for a time certain if a job is terminated and also provides for the portability of health insurance, which helps survivors to change jobs and helps prevent 'lockdown' or having to stay in a job just to maintain insurance benefits.
- References to associations that can help in working out special problems are provided.

ACKNOWLEDGEMENT

The authors acknowledge the research assistance of Jennifer Romero, JD, American University School of Law, class of 2002.

REFERENCES

1. Childhood Cancer Ombudsman Program (CCOP): gpmonaco@rivnet.net.
2. The National Coalition for Cancer Survivorship (NCCS). Telephone: (301) 650-8868.
3. The Childhood Brain Tumor Foundation (CBTF): cbtf@childhoodbraintumor.org.
4. Candlelighters Childhood Cancer Foundation (CCCF): info@candlelighters.org.
♦5. The Family and Medical Leave Act (29 U.S. C. Section 2612(a)(1); 5 U.S. C. Section 6282(a)(1)).
6. National Partnership for Women and Families. Telephone: (202) 986-2600.
7. 29 USCA §2614(a)(1).
8. Interim final rule, 66 Federal Register 1378, at http://www.access.gpo.gov/su_docs/fedreg/a010112c.html.
♦9. ERISA, Employee Retirement Income Security Act of 1974 as amended, 29 US Section 1001 *et seq.*
10. DHHS press release: http://www.hhs.gov/news/press/2000pres/20001025.html.
11. The Ticket to Work and Work Incentives Act of 1999 (TWWIA) (Public Law 106-170); for an overview of the Act's provisions: http://www.c-c-d.org.
12. Helpful resources: www.disability.gov; and www.business-disability.com.
13. EEOC Public Information System. Telephone: 1-800-669-4000; internet: www.eeoc.gov.
14. EEOC Publications. Telephone: 1-800-669-3362; internet: www.eeoc.gov.
15. Disability and Business Technical Assistance. Telephone: 1-800-949-4232.

12c

Legal issues: UK perspective

ALEXANDER McCALL SMITH

INTRODUCTION

Greater ability to cure many childhood cancers is overwhelmingly positive, but both parents and children have to be aware of the fact that the initial battle with disease may not be the only difficulty which they face. Alongside the implications that treatment may have for subsequent development, both physical and cognitive, the survivor of childhood cancer may have to face a number of difficulties of a psychological and social nature. Some of these may be apparent reasonably soon after the completion of treatment, while others may only become apparent many years later, when, as an adult, the patient encounters discrimination in the area of employment or insurance. This problem, of course, is one that is commonly experienced by persons with a disability of some sort and the problems faced by cancer survivors should be considered in the light of how we respond to the needs of the disabled in general. Fortunately, in many countries, attitudes towards this issue have changed out of all recognition. Issues remain, however, and the passage of enlightened legislation is no guarantee of fair treatment for those who have a physical or intellectual disability, or who are perceived to have one. The childhood cancer survivor may still find that being cured of the illness means that the consequences of the illness are still present.

HOW SERIOUS IS THE PROBLEM?

Follow-up studies of cancer patients who have been cured of their illness suggest that the child patient may expect, on statistical grounds, the life they subsequently lead to differ to some degree from that of contemporaries who have not had cancer. In a study by Ehrmann-Feldmann and others,[1] the experience of 101 cured cancer patients (adults) was compared with that of a control group of 101 who had not had cancer. A total of 18 per cent of the cured patients reported experiencing discrimination against 15 per cent of the control group making such a report. Also 10 per cent of the cured patients in this study reported experiencing discrimination by an employer after they had returned to work. This study is now quite old, and attitudes may be expected to have changed. Nor do the figures for discrimination seem unduly high. A more recent British study by Evans and Radford,[2] which focused on a group of 48 young adult survivors of childhood cancer, compared the experience of the cured patients with that of their siblings who had not had cancer. The encouraging conclusion of this study was that, in general, the cured patients in the group were coping well with their lives and, significantly, achieving what were described as the 'same lifestyle goals' as their siblings. There were, however, some differences in educational achievement and the cured patients were significantly less likely to proceed to tertiary education than their siblings.

Studies that focus on employment discrimination present a less attractive picture.[3] Discrimination is difficult to measure. Asking individuals to identify whether or not they have been discriminated against may yield an excessively high result (many people feel a vague sense that they have not been treated fairly, even if they have). Some surveys of the experience of those with a heightened risk of genetic disorder reveal a high incidence of

discrimination in employment and insurance. Equally revealing perhaps is the harsh reality of the overall levels of unemployment amongst the disabled and, in particular, the evidence obtained from the self-reported attitudes of employers, coworkers and the general public. If there is a widespread belief (as there is) amongst employers that those who have had cancer are likely to be less effective employees, discriminatory treatment of cancer survivors is likely to result unless there are strong disincentives in the shape of effective legal prohibitions of discrimination. Similarly, the attitudes of coworkers may affect employment options; in this context, one study revealed that 18 per cent of employees believed that undergoing cancer treatment precluded the ability to work and 27 per cent of employees thought that they would have to carry the work of those being treated.[4] These figures relate to adults undergoing treatment but such attitudes may be expected to affect views held in relation to the working ability of survivors.

Evidence of discrimination in the context of insurance may be obtained from applicants themselves, or from underwriting manuals or other forms of medical guidance within the insurance industry. Much of the recent evidence has come to light as a result of concern over the use in insurance of the genetic test results, some of which will, of course, concern cancers. In a study by Low *et al.* of 7000 members of British support groups for families with genetic disorders, it was found that 33.4 per cent of the sample had experienced difficulties in life insurance applications (against 5 per cent of the unaffected control group).[5] The authors suggest that this pattern of discrimination may be due more to error than to a deliberate policy of discrimination against those with genetic disorders. Even so, these findings confirm concerns that those who are perceived, correctly or incorrectly, to be at a higher risk of illness find it more difficult than do others to purchase a range of insurance policies.

It is more difficult to assess the extent to which other, possibly more subtle forms of discrimination, affect cancer survivors. Areas in which this may be exercised include the social sphere, where the day-to-day relationships of those who have had cancer might be affected by distaste for or fear of the disease. For obvious reasons, a direct legal response to such stigmatization is not feasible, as it falls within the realm of the private. Antidiscriminatory legislation, however, can have a positive effect on social attitudes; by forbidding discrimination in the public arena of formal legal relations, a strong message can be sent about the need to avoid the hurtful treatment of others. In general, though, this is a task that requires public education and social rather than legal initiatives. Social stigmatization, nonetheless, underlines the need for legal protection, where such protection is appropriate.

CONFRONTING DISCRIMINATION

The final decades of the twentieth century saw a growing awareness of the rights of disadvantaged minorities within society. This awareness was evident in a wide range of contexts, and included groups of persons affected by ill health and various forms of disability. At an international level, concrete measures aimed at preventing discrimination against disabled people included the United Nations Declaration on the Rights of Mentally Retarded Persons, adopted by the General Assembly in 1971[6] and the Declaration on the Rights of Disabled Persons of 1975.[7] This latter instrument identifies certain rights that should be the focus of national and international action. These include employment rights and, more generally, a right not to be subjected to any discriminatory action. This declaration is exhortatory in nature and does not create any convention-based rights for the individual disabled person. The claims of disabled persons, however, have been given more concrete expression in certain international conventions and in national legislation. At the international level, the European Convention of Human Rights provides protection within participating countries for a range of human rights, which may be claimed by both disabled and non-disabled alike. Of particular relevance to the disabled are the articles 2, 3, 8 and 14. Article 2, which protects the right to life, protects disabled persons against treatment decisions based on the notion that a disabled life is less valuable than one that is not disabled. Article 3 protects against inhuman or degrading treatment – a right of broad potential significance to disabled people; article 8, which creates a right to a privacy, in this context enhances rights of medical confidentiality. Finally, article 14 prohibits discrimination in the application of any of the rights recognized in the Convention. These rights apply only against public bodies, or those exercising public functions, but all legislation must comply with the terms of the Convention and this provides an important protection for persons who benefit from public services. The precise scope of Convention rights in their health setting has yet to be determined by the courts.

The more potent weapon in the fight against discrimination has been domestic legislation. There have been a number of prominent examples of such legislation. In the UK, the Disability Discrimination Act 1995 has been the principal antidiscrimination statute; in Canada, not only is there broad protection against disability-based discrimination provided by the Charter of Rights and Freedoms (a part of the Canadian constitution), but protection is also provided by the Human Rights Codes of the provinces; and in the USA, the Americans with Disabilities Act is intended to provide protection against discrimination for a wide range of conditions and disabilities, actual or perceived. The technicalities of these

statutes are beyond the scope of this discussion, but certain broad questions need to be addressed in considering how far legislation of this sort goes in addressing the particular problems of the childhood cancer survivor. In particular, the question needs to be asked as to how far difficulties faced by cancer survivors are the product of the inherent inability of legislation to deal with discrimination if employers and others are sufficiently determined to practice it, and how far continued discrimination is a result of limitations and inadequacies in the drafting of the statutes in question.

THE ADJUSTMENT ISSUE

A matter of fundamental importance in antidiscrimination legislation, at least in the context of employment, is the question of whether the legislation requires employers to make adjustments in the workplace to allow those with a disability to work safely and effectively. This is basic to an effective antidiscrimination regime; the much paler alternative is to ensure equal access to an unchanged workplace – a model that inevitably results in the exclusion of those with special needs. The latter approach would allow employers to claim that an employee with a disability simply is incapable of doing the job. The former approach requires the employer to take steps to ensure that the disabled employee has the chance to do the job.

Laws that require employers to make special arrangements for employees with a disability typically seek to reach a compromise between the employer's interest in keeping costs down and in achieving operational efficiency, while at the same time recognizing the claim of the employee to recognition of his or her special needs. Typically, legislation of this sort imposes on the employer a duty to take reasonable steps to adjust working conditions to the requirements of the disabled. This balance cannot be set out in detail in legislation itself and there has inevitably been litigation on the issue of what constitutes reasonable steps. The Canadian experience might serve as an example here. In Canada, employers are required to make adjustments in order to accommodate the needs of an employee, but they are not required to do anything that would result in undue hardship to themselves or labor unions. The unavoidable vagueness of the term 'undue hardship' has been the subject of a number of important decisions by the courts, including key decisions of the Supreme Court of Canada. In one of these cases, Central Alberta Dairy Pool v. Alberta Human Rights Commission,[8] the Supreme Court set out six factors to be taken into account when assessing whether accommodation of an employee's needs would result in undue hardship. These are cost, impact on collective agreements with the labor force, employee morale implications,

interchangeability of workers and facilities, size of the employer's enterprise, and safety. Each of these factors has its complexities and the courts have pronounced on them in a number of subsequent cases. What has emerged from the growing jurisprudence on the matter, though, is that the term 'undue hardship' means that employers may be expected to shoulder *some* degree of hardship in accommodating the disabled worker: it will only be if any accommodation makes a *significant* impact on any of these factors that an employer will be entitled to decline to adjust. Moreover, as the Supreme Court ruled in Grismer v. British Columbia Superintendent of Motor Vehicles,[9] if an appeal is being made to the cost factor, then the employer must be able to produce evidence of this fact rather than producing 'impressionistic evidence of increased expense'.

Many of the cases brought under this legislation involve an employee's difficulties in carrying out physical tasks, such as lifting or moving heavy objects. It will not be enough for an employer to argue that, if an employee lacks the strength to perform these tasks unaided, he or she cannot be employed. It will be necessary for other options to be explored, such as the provision of aids or human assistance. More than this, if it is impossible to assist in the carrying out of such work, then the employer is required to look at ways in which another position can be found for the disabled employee or to investigate whether the work can be 'rebundled' to allow for physically demanding tasks to be performed by another employee.

Canadian court and arbitration decisions in this area have created an environment in which the disabled employee can claim a considerable measure of special consideration in ensuring that he or she has a chance to work. The key to a responsive system here is insistence on flexibility on the employer's part, which means that the courts must be willing to enforce a strong vision of disabled rights in the first place.

WHAT COUNTS AS A DISABILITY

The effectiveness of disability discrimination legislation is clearly going to depend on the extent to which it embraces the wide range of conditions that may form the basis of discrimination. How a disability is defined for the purposes of this legislation is, therefore, crucial and this issue has particular implications for the cancer survivor. The history of legislation in the USA is instructive here. Until the passage of the Americans with Disabilities Act (ADA) in 1990, the employment protection given to the disabled in general in the USA was patchy and inadequate, as was acknowledged by legislators during the discussion of the ADA. The Rehabilitation Act of 1974 provided protection for those employed by organizations

receiving federal funding. This prohibited discrimination against those with a 'handicap', a category defined in the legislation as 'any person who (i) has a physical or mental impairment which substantially limits one or more of such person's major life activities, (ii) has a record of such impairment, or (iii) is regarded as having such impairment.' The difficulty with this definition is that it does not cover most cancer survivors because many of those who survive cancer treatment do not have an impairment of the sort mentioned in the legislation: their performance of any major life activity tends not to be substantially impaired. Recognition of the inadequacies of this definition when it came to cancer prompted attempts to secure specific legislation to deal with discrimination against those with a history of cancer and a Cancer Patients Employments Rights Act was, in fact, proposed but did not succeed in reaching the statute books.

The ADA, by covering private employment, represented a major extension of the protection that the law provided the disabled in the employment field. The definition of disability, however, is effectively taken from the Rehabilitation Act and, therefore, is open to the same objections that were voiced to that definition. Under the ADA, the cancer survivor who believes that he or she has been discriminated against, must first establish that he or she had a disability as defined in the Act. Although there is evidence that the legislators' intention was to include cancer survivors within the category of those who were protected by the ADA, in practice there have been numerous court decisions in which they have been excluded from the scope of the Act on the grounds that they have never had a disability in ADA terms. This has seriously restricted the efficacy of the Act for this group.

A few examples of court decisions will demonstrate the problem faced by those who have not been substantially prevented from performing life activities during the course of their cancer treatment. Such people may be able to continue with their day-to-day life (education, in the case of children, or employment in the case of adults) during the course of the treatment and may, therefore, not have a history of impairment amounting to a disability. In Nave v. Wooldridge Construction,[10] for example, the plaintiff had been treated with chemotherapy and radiation for Hodgkin's disease and had suffered from depression and fatigue following upon this treatment. He was later dismissed from his job at a time when the cancer was in complete remission. His attempt to secure protection under the ADA was unsuccessful because he was deemed not to have a disability – he was not substantially limited from working, and his time off from work was a result of a temporary condition. The legal difficulty faced by those who are able to continue working during treatment is shown in Gordon v. Hamm Associates,[11] in which the employee, who received chemotherapy for malignant lymphoma, suffered various side effects of treatment,

including weakness, swelling of ankles and hands, and vomiting. These side effects were held by the court to be physical impairments, but not impairments that substantially limited the employee's ability to care for himself or to work. There was, therefore, no disability in terms of the ADA. Disability, then, is to be distinguished from critical illness, unless the critical illness has the necessary limiting effect. This was emphasized in the case of EEOC v. RJ Gallagher Co.,[12] in which the court specifically ruled that cancer was not a disability.

Such limited interpretations of the ADA have not been universally followed, and there have been cases where the cancer survivor has succeeded in establishing that there is a disability or a history of disability in ADA terms. One such case was Mark v. Burke Rehabilitation Hospital[13] in which a doctor who was treated for lymphoma was held by the court to have been physically impaired because the condition affected his digestive system. This suggests that interference in bodily functions may be a disability, even if these functions are not connected with mobility or the performance of mental tasks. Powerful support for this view has been given by the Supreme Court in an important HIV case, Bragdon v. Abbott.[14] In this case, it was held that an asymptomatic HIV patient was held to be affected by a disability for ADA purposes on the grounds that her infected status limited her reproductive options. It is possible that this decision will make it easier in the future for cancer survivors to bring suit under the ADA in that it encourages a broader view of what amounts to a disability. The substantial limitation test is a narrow one, which recognizes some conditions as disabilities while not recognizing others that may be equally burdensome for the affected individual. Antidiscrimination legislation should ideally identify cancer and, possibly certain other conditions (such as HIV infection), as conditions that, irrespective of their impact on the daily life of the individual, should not be inappropriately taken into account in any employment or equivalent decision.

CHILDHOOD SURVIVORS AND INSURANCE

Insurance poses particular problems for the survivor of childhood cancer. It may be possible to legislate to prevent unfair discrimination in the context of employment or access to public services, but this becomes a much more difficult matter in relation to insurance. The reason for this is that insurance contracts are contracts entered into freely between an individual and companies, and while the state, through the law of contract, may be prepared to set out the broad terms of fairness that should govern such agreements, the principle of freedom of contract means that the parties should be able to create their own terms. One such term, which has traditionally been

built into insurance contracts, is that the parties deal with one another in the utmost good faith. This has been interpreted by the courts to require the full disclosure of all relevant information; a person, therefore, who conceals information that he or she knows would be a material consideration as far as the other party is concerned, may not be entitled to rely on that contract. A typical example of this would be a party to an insurance contract who, when asked to disclose tobacco use, does not mention the fact that he or she is a heavy smoker. Similarly, a person who was currently undergoing treatment for a serious condition and who fails to disclose the fact when negotiating a life insurance contract, would not be acting in the utmost good faith and risks invalidating the contract of insurance.

It is normal practice in many forms of insurance to require applicants for insurance to complete a medical questionnaire or to agree to the insurance company obtaining a medical report from their doctor. The making available to an insurance company of this information, which is normally confidential, enables the insurer to underwrite the risk in the possession of all the relevant information about the nature of that risk. If the insurer behaves correctly, the risk will be properly assessed, on the basis of medical advice and mortality figures for particular conditions. In theory, the underwriter loads the premium in accordance with the increased risk, which a particular medical history reveals or, in a case where the risk is too great, the applicant is refused cover. In practice, however, insurers may not give medical evidence its proper weight and may decline to insure those whose previous medical history includes episodes of serious illness. The task of insurance regulation then is to ensure that unjustified discrimination of this nature is not practiced – a task that is often performed by the insurance industry itself through mechanisms that require explanation of underwriting decisions. From the point of view of the survivor of childhood cancer, the issue is whether insurance decisions are made on the basis of a correct actuarial assessment of the implications of the illness. In general, state regulation of the insurance industry stops short of giving a *legal right* to fair treatment in this context and underwriting decisions may also fall outside the ambit of protection provided by the complaints procedures. In the UK, for example, the Financial Services Ombudsman does not deal with complaints about premium levels.

In the USA, the importance of health insurance is recognized under the Health Insurance Portability and Accountability Act of 1996. This Act makes it illegal to exclude a person from a group health insurance scheme on the grounds of medical history or current health problems. The legislation also prohibits the charging of any member of the group scheme a higher premium than that paid by other members. Pre-existing conditions may be excluded from coverage only for 12 months, and may

not be excluded at all if the person has been covered for that condition for 12 months or more. What this legislation achieves, then, is an equality, or near equality, which would prevent the survivor of childhood cancer from being discriminated against in such health schemes. It does not provide protection, however, to those who fall outside the ambit of a group scheme.

GENETIC INFORMATION

During the final decade of the twentieth century, the protection of personal genetic information became a major matter of public concern. With the growing ease with which DNA analysis could be carried out, and with the growing understanding of the significance of particular genes, it became apparent that information about the genetic characteristics of individuals could be sought after in a number of contexts, including those of insurance and employment. This gave rise to discussion of genetic privacy, and the right that an individual has to ensure that private genetic information is obtained and used only with his or her consent. Survivors of childhood cancers, the genetic basis of which is likely to become increasingly understood, may expect to be affected by this issue. Medical records may contain the results of genetic tests already carried out, or the survivor may have been treated for a condition for which a genetic basis has been established. In either case, the survivor may have genetic characteristics, which could form the basis for discriminatory treatment. Significantly, genetic discrimination does not base itself on symptoms but operates on the simple presence of a genetic characteristic.

Information about genetic characteristics is, in many respects, no different from any other medical information. The person to whom such information pertains, therefore, has the right to expect that it will be kept confidential and not disclosed to others except with express or implicit consent. This confidentiality is protected by the law, which provides a civil action against those who wrongfully divulge confidential information to those not authorized to receive it. Concern about the sensitivity of genetic information, however, has prompted a number of initiatives to ensure that it has a special level of protection, over and above that protection provided by the general law on confidentiality. As a result of this, personal genetic information in some countries is covered by statutory provisions governing the circumstances in which it can be obtained, passed on to others, or used for specific purposes.

A right of genetic privacy is recognized at an international level in the Universal Declaration on the Human Genome and Human Rights, which was adopted by the General Assembly of the UN in 1997, and by the European

Convention on Human Rights and Biomedicine, an international convention promoted by the Council of Europe. Both of these documents state that no person should be required to take a genetic test if they do not wish to do so, the European Convention going even further to provide that the only purpose for which a genetic test may be admitted is for the purposes of medical treatment. Domestic law provides protection against non-consensual genetic testing in that any medical procedure requires the consent of the person on whom it is performed (or, in the case of a child incapable of consenting, the consent of a parent or guardian). This protection, however, does not cover circumstances where consent is given by one who is at a position of bargaining disadvantage compared with the person asking for a test to be taken, as would be the case where the test is part of a pre-employment medical examination or where the test is required for insurance purposes. In the UK, there is no evidence of the use of genetic testing by employers, and there is no indication that this is likely to become common. In the USA, there have been instances of the use by employers of genetic testing of employees, resulting in one well-known case in successful litigation by the employees. Concern over genetic privacy, however, has resulted in legislative action in some states to ensure that no employee, or prospective employee, should be required by his or her employer to furnish personal genetic information to an employer. Such legislation may also specifically prevent an employer from firing or in any way discriminating against an employee on the basis of genetic information. The level of protection against genetic discrimination in employment differs from state to state: over 20 states have legislation aimed at protecting people from genetic discrimination in this context, and an increasing number of bills offering such protection are being actively pursued. Disability rights campaigners may find it remarkable that there should be such willingness to outlaw genetic discrimination when the courts in many states have whittled away the level of protection offered against disability discrimination in general, but there is nonetheless wide support in the disability movement for antigenetic-discrimination measures.

The use of genetic information in insurance decisions has been debated at length in a number of countries. National response to this issue has varied, which is to be expected in view of the varying roles that private insurance plays in different societies. In the UK, for example, health insurance is not of central importance, given the level of care provided by the state under the National Health Service. In the USA, where private health insurance is vital, the possibility of being excluded from cover on the grounds of genetic risk bears serious consequences. Legislation controlling genetic discrimination in such circumstances, therefore, has much more significant implications.

The impact of genetic information on underwriting decisions is at present restricted to a relatively small number of cases, given the limited number of genetic tests that are of clear predictive value. There will be comparatively few conditions in which genetic evidence will dictate the level of premium or the decision whether or not to offer cover. This, of course, is likely to change, as more tests become available that will enable conclusions to be drawn about increased risk of common conditions. From the insurance point of view, this may lead to more sophisticated mortality predictions and enable underwriting to be even more accurate. It is unlikely, though, that genetic testing will transform actuarial calculations.

The legislative response to the use of genetic information by insurance has been driven, to a large extent, by antidiscrimination feeling. It is clear that many find the notion of genetic discrimination distasteful, as has been confirmed in the UK by public opinion research supported by the Human Genetics Commission. The basis of this objection is difficult to disentangle, but it is probably connected with some notion of the random nature of the 'genetic lottery' and a belief that an individual should not be at a disadvantage because of the outcome of this lottery. That is understandable, although consistency would require such an argument to be extended to take into account many other non-genetic characteristics that are currently accepted as the basis of acceptable discrimination in many contexts, including that of insurance. We accept, for example, that insurers have the right to decline offering life insurance to those who have a non-genetic condition that will severely shorten their lives; if this is allowed, then on what basis is genetic information of the same significance, in mortality terms, not admitted? This may be difficult to defend, but the desire to take an inclusive rather than exclusive approach to genetic conditions appears to outweigh such objection. One effect of this may be to give a relative advantage to childhood cancer survivors whose cancer has an established genetic element and whose prospects of recurrence may be affected by genetic factors.

The legislative response to this issue has ranged from a complete outlawing of the use of genetic test results in insurance at one extreme, to a non-interventionist approach at the other. In between there is a central ground, in which genetic information (obtained by testing) may be used by insurers, provided that it is independently evaluated and not obtained from a test stipulated by insurers. There are also options that limit the use of DNA test result information to those policies over a high financial limit, thus restricting its use for the vast majority of life insurance policies. In the UK, following consideration of the issue by the Human Genetics Commission, the Government concluded a moratorium agreement with the insurance industry at the end of 2001, in which it was agreed that, during the moratorium period, insurers would not

make use of any DNA test results that were on the medical record of an insurance applicant, provided that the policy fell within agreed financial limits. In the USA, a relatively small number of states have legislated to control the use of genetic information in life insurance, while a much greater number – a clear majority of states – have enacted laws that provide some measure of protection against the use of genetic information in health insurance.

From the point of view of the survivor of childhood cancer, developments in the field of genetics and insurance are encouraging. The growing exclusion of genetic information from insurance decisions is moving our vision of insurance in the direction of a social good approach, under which the greater risk posed by some individuals will be absorbed in the general risk pool, even if this results, as it will, in an increased burden being placed on those who choose to take insurance cover. The objective desirability, or otherwise, of this is a matter of social policy but its effect on the 'normalization' of the position of those who have genetic characteristics that increase their chance of future ill health will undoubtedly find broad support.

ETHICAL ISSUES SURROUNDING FERTILITY PRESERVATION

In the treatment above of the employment and insurance issues, it has been assumed that the goal of the human rights and disability law should be to ensure that the survivor of childhood cancer can lead as normal a life as possible, and that social and economic institutions should be designed to facilitate this. One area of human rights law that has been increasingly under the microscope is that of reproductive rights, which have become increasingly important with the development of artificial reproductive techniques. The main focus of discussion here has been the extent to which the individual has an indefensible right to avail himself or herself of reproductive assistance, or whether social notions of what is ethically acceptable should control the availability of such techniques. These arguments have been about issues such as the artificial insemination of single women or women in lesbian relationships, the use of the stored sperm of deceased men, or the offering of *in vitro* fertilization (IVF) to women past the natural age of childbearing. The issue that affects survivors of childhood cancers is that of whether the preservation of gametes is an appropriate procedure, given the level of risk involved and given the fact that it constitutes a reproductive intervention – even if one of a special, future-oriented nature – on a person who may be incapable of giving an appropriate consent.

The techniques involved, along with the ethical issues to which these techniques give rise, have been clearly set out by Grundy *et al.*,[15] who point out that the procedures involved pose risks at different points: the risk to the child in the performance of the extraction procedure itself; the risk to the adult at the later stage, when the tissue is restored; and the risk to the offspring of the transmission of a predisposition to a particular condition. Each of these involves a quite distinct ethical problem.

Risk to the child

Many therapeutic procedures are inherently risky and need to be performed in the face of the risk. The consent of the patient legitimizes the taking of these risks and, in those cases where the patient is unable to consent, e.g. on the grounds of youth, the consent of a parent or guardian suffices both from an ethical and a legal point of view. This may apply uncontroversially to therapeutic measures but its application to research is more difficult. The use of children in medical research is subject to ethical and legal limitations. Where the research is non-therapeutic, the involvement of minors must be restricted to research procedures involving negligible risk; where the research has therapeutic possibilities for the child, then the level of permissible risk it may entail will depend on the assessment of the anticipated benefit of treatment. In conditions with a high level of mortality, for example, the acceptable levels of risk may be high.

The removal of gametes from a child with the intention of providing fertility treatment in adult life is therapy for that patient, even if the possible benefit may only be experienced many years later. Yet it is undoubtedly reasonable to anticipate that the adult whom the child stands a high chance of becoming may well wish to avail himself or herself of the possibility of stored gametes. There can be no certainty of this, of course, but evidence of the take-up of fertility treatment makes this a reasonable prediction. In these circumstances, removal of gametes is a procedure that can be described as being in the best interests of the child, recognizing that the child and the future adult have an identity of interest. There remains, however, the issue of whether the procedure is one that justifies the risk involved. Even if the risks cannot be accurately quantified, they are not thought to be great and would, therefore, be something to which a reasonable parent, acting in the best interests of the child, could consent. In addition, in the UK, there is the technical legal difficulty of the requirement of the Human Fertilisation and Embryology Authority (HFEA) that consent to the extraction of gametes be given, in writing, by the person from whom they are taken. This suggests that consent on behalf of another will not be competent. The HFEA definition of a gamete is, therefore, of paramount importance. In practical terms in the UK, the removal of ovarian cortical tissue from a young person for cryopreservation is not covered

by the HFEA Act and can be carried out if the procedure is considered to be in the best interests of the child.[16]

The risk to the adult

Adults are competent to consent to risky procedures. The reintroduction into the adult of reproductive tissue removed in childhood may involve risk of transmitting cancer cells to the recipient. At present, techniques for screening such tissue for these cells are inadequate and the nature of the risk is, therefore, unclear. This should not of itself preclude the use of such techniques, provided that the risk is not thought to be so high that the procedures would be regarded as likely to cause serious injury or death. The deciding of this issue involves the weighing of benefits against the chances of harm. If this process reveals a high chance of serious harm, the existing principles of ethical research, including the recently revised Declaration of Helsinki, would not justify the taking of such a high risk. The relevant point for assessing this risk is not the point at which the tissue is removed but the point at which fertility treatment is offered. At this point, the patient is an adult and any earlier inability to understand and consent to risk is irrelevant.

The risk to the future children

There is no evidence that the offspring of survivors of cancer are more likely to develop cancer themselves than the normal population. This is based on normal reproduction, however, and it is possible that the use of stored gametes would involve different risks. If there is no evidence that it does, then there seems to be no grounds for ethical objection to the use of cyropreserved tissue to enable reproduction. If there were to be evidence of an increased risk, then this would raise the issue of whether there are ethical objections to the making available of artificial reproductive techniques in circumstances where potentially harmful conditions may be genetically transmitted. This is a complex issue, which goes to the heart of the extent to which the individual is entitled to decide to reproduce in the face of advice that the resulting children may be affected by serious genetically transmissible conditions. The individual's right to make them currently prevails, and this would suggest that it would be ethically unacceptable to prevent the use of a technique of this nature, even if there is a heightened risk that any children so conceived would have an increased risk of a serious condition.

CONCLUSION

Survivors of childhood cancers undoubtedly face difficulties in their adult life. Medical advances are likely to progressively alleviate the physical and other limitations, which may follow from the successful treatment of cancer; legal advances are increasingly having a similar effect in limiting the effect of discrimination in the conduct of day-to-day life. The growing recognition of human rights in medicine and of the social rights of those who have been or who are affected by illness, points to a likely amelioration of the cancer survivor's later experience, even if attitudes and prejudices are slow to change.

KEY POINTS

- There is some evidence that survivors of childhood cancer find it more difficult than do others to purchase a range of insurance policies.
- Antidiscrimination legislation should ideally identify cancer as a condition, which, irrespective of its impact on the daily life of the individual, should not be inappropriately taken into account in any employment or equivalent decision.
- Survivors of childhood cancers may expect to be affected by the issue of genetic privacy. Medical records may contain the results of genetic tests already carried out or they may have been treated for a condition for which a genetic basis has been established. In either case, they have genetic characteristics that could form the basis of discriminatory treatment.
- The removal of gametes from a child with the intention of providing fertility treatment in adult life is therapy for that patient, even if the possible benefit may only be experienced many years later.
- The goal of the human rights and disability law should be to ensure that the survivor of childhood cancer can lead as normal a life as possible.

REFERENCES

1. Ehrmann-Feldmann D, Spitzer WO, del Greco I, *et al*. Perceived discrimination against cured cancer patients in the work force. *Can Med Assoc J* **136**:719–723.
2. Evans SE, Radford M. Current lifestyles of young adults treated for cancer in childhood. *Arch Dis Child* 1995; **72**:423–426.
3. Rothstein M, Kennedy K, Ritchie KS, *et al*. Are cancer patients subject to employment discrimination? *Oncology*, 1995; **9**:1303–1311.
4. Arnold K. Americans with Disabilities act: do cancer patients qualify as disabled?' *J Natl Cancer Inst* 1999; **91**:822.
5. Low L, King S, Wilkie T. Genetic discrimination in life insurance: empirical evidence from a cross sectional survey of genetic support groups in the United Kingdom. *Br Med J* 1998; **317**:1632–1635.
6. United Nations. *Declaration on the Rights of Mentally Retarded Persons.* General Assembly Resolution 2856 of 20th December 1971.

7. United Nations. *Declaration on the Rights of Disabled Persons.* General Assembly Resolution 3447 of 9th December 1975.
8. Central Alberta Dairy Pool v. Alberta Human Rights Commission, 1990, 2 SCR, 1985.
9. Grismer v. British Columbia Superintendent of Motor Vehicles, 1999, 3 SCR, 868.
10. Nave v. Wooldridge Construction, 10 National Disability L. rep. (LRP) P 183, at 607.
11. Gordon v. Hamm Associates, 100 F.3d 907 (11th Circ.1996), cert. denied, 118 S.Ct. 630, 66 USLW 3416 (1997).
12. EEOC v. RJ Gallagher Co., 959 F. Supp. 405 (1997).
13. Marke v. Burke Rehabilitation Hospital, 9 National Disability L. rep. P322, at 1155 (1997).
14. Bragdon v. Abbott, 118 S.Ct 2196 (1998).
15. Grundy R, Gosedon RG, Hewitt V, *et al.* Fertility preservation for children treated for cancer. *Arch Dis Child* 2001; **84**:355–360.
16. Wallace WHB, Walker DA. Conference consensus statement. Ethical and research dilemmas for fertility preservation for children treated for cancer. *Hum Fertil* 2001; **4**:69–76.

13

Healthy lifestyle and prevention strategies

MELISSA M HUDSON

INTRODUCTION

Childhood cancer survivors are a vulnerable and growing population. With contemporary cure rates for most pediatric cancers exceeding 70 per cent, an estimated 1 in 900 young adults between the ages of 25–45 years is a long-term survivor of a childhood malignancy, with an anticipated increase to 1 in 450 within the decade.[1,2] This population is at increased risk for late medical and neoplastic complications that adversely affect quality of life and increase the risk of early mortality.[3–9] Cancer-related sequelae are typically predisposed by specific treatment modalities and/or genetic mutations. Chronic or subclinical changes may persist following apparent recovery from cancer treatment and result in premature onset of common diseases associated with aging, including coronary artery disease, renovascular hypertension and diabetes mellitus. Maladaptive health behaviors may further exacerbate the risk of organ dysfunction and subsequent malignancy. Presently, many investigations are evaluating the efficacy of risk-adapted treatment approaches in an effort to prevent or reduce the risk of cancer treatment sequelae. In contrast, few studies have evaluated the efficacy of prevention programs targeting health education and behavioral change as a method of risk reduction. This chapter will summarize the data currently available about health behaviors of childhood cancer survivors and health promotion programs targeting this group. Health behaviors and their impact on cancer-related health risks will be discussed followed by counseling recommendations for risk reduction and health monitoring.

HEALTH BEHAVIORS AND PERCEPTIONS OF CHILDHOOD CANCER SURVIVORS

Studies of global health behavior

While substantial data are available documenting the late sequelae of childhood cancer, relatively few reports describe health behaviors of childhood cancer survivors. Early studies examined health-risking behaviors in the context of compliance to cancer treatment.[10,11] These investigators observed that non-compliance occurred more frequently in older adolescents and was attributed to underlying developmental factors common to all adolescents. Hanna speculated that participation in maladaptive health behaviors by adolescent cancer patients may be related to experimentation as part of the developmental process of identity achievement.[12] She suggested that health care professionals caring for childhood cancer patients who considered health behavior in the context of a developmental framework could facilitate adolescents' exploration of more appropriate behaviors for self-assertion and problem-solving about possible consequences of maladaptive behaviors.

More recent investigations have described health-promoting and health-risking behaviors practiced by adolescent cancer survivors. Generally, the limited studies available indicate that survivors' health practices are similar to those of adolescents who have never had cancer.[13–19] Hollen and Hobbie evaluated the quality of decision-making and prevalence of smoking, alcohol consumption and illicit drug use in a group of teen survivors and their peers.[14] Both groups exhibited comparable poor-quality

decision-making in regards to health-risking behaviors, and similar rates of cigarette smoking and alcohol consumption. Behavioral practices did not differ among survivors who did or did not receive therapy predisposing to adverse neurocognitive effects. Adherence to quality decision-making by survivors correlated with a lower likelihood of reporting health-risking behaviors.

Mulhern *et al.* compared health practices of preadolescent and adolescent survivors to those of young adult survivors and correlated results with sociodemographic variables.[15] Health practices assessed included frequency of tobacco use and alcohol consumption, as well as dietary, exercise, sleep, dental and seatbelt habits. Parents were proxy respondents for survivors aged 11–17 years. Responses to the health behavior survey indicated a similar distribution by age, race and socioeconomic level for survivors in both groups. As expected, young adult respondents were significantly older at diagnosis and time of follow-up compared with preadolescent and adolescent respondents. Preadolescent and adolescent survivors had significantly better sleep and exercise habits compared to young adult survivors. Both groups showed a greater tendency to being overweight compared with normative population standards. Health perceptions regarding the importance of health protective behaviors were positively correlated with dietary and exercise practices in the preadolescent and young adolescent survivors, but not young adult survivors. While the prevalence of alcohol and tobacco use was low in the preadolescents and adolescent survivors, the frequency of binge and heavy drinking, or drinking and driving reported by young adults was similar to median national prevalence data obtained by the Centers for Disease Control.[20] In contrast to other studies of adolescents and young adults in the general population, sociodemographic variables did not affect the practice rates of health behaviors. Interestingly, health perceptions self-reported by parents of preadolescent and young adolescent survivors and young adult survivors were inconsistent with health practices. Both groups acknowledged an increased vulnerability to health problems following cancer treatment but this perception was not correlated with their practice of health-promoting behaviors.

Hudson *et al.* observed similar findings in a more contemporary cohort of childhood cancer survivors surveyed before participation in a health-promotion trial. Self-reports of health-protective practices of this group revealed that 94 per cent abstained from tobacco use, 64 per cent practiced sun protection measures, 27 per cent performed monthly gender appropriate self-examination, 40 per cent ate nutritious diets and 52 per cent performed regular aerobic exercise.[17,19] With the exception of the lower prevalence of tobacco use, health protective behavior practice rates were similar to those reported by healthy adolescents.[21] Assessment of health perceptions in this group revealed that 58 per cent of survivors acknowledged the need to change behavior to improve their health and 57 per cent professed a desire to want to change. However, these stated health concerns by childhood cancer survivors did not motivate higher practice rates of protective behaviors compared to their peers.

Tyc *et al.* also examined the relationship of survivor health perceptions and health behaviors in a cohort of preadolescent and adolescent childhood cancer survivors with the aim of identifying potential predictors of health behavior.[18] Health perception variables including perceived vulnerability, perceived importance of health protection and health locus of control (strength of belief in ability to control health outcomes) were correlated with self-reported health habits. Survivors in this group indicated a moderately frequent practice of health protec-tive behaviors: 73.3 per cent brushed their teeth at least twice daily; 62.3 per cent ate balanced nutritious meals; 44 per cent always wore a seatbelt; 75.6 per cent slept eight or more hours nightly; and 75.6 per cent exercised three or more hours weekly. Compared to practice rates of healthy peers, the prevalence rate of risky health behaviors, such as alcohol and tobacco use, was low with only 17.2 per cent reporting tobacco use and 27.3 per cent ever using alcohol.[22] The practice of health-protective behaviors was best predicted by patient age and socioeconomic status; younger and more affluent adolescents had higher practice levels of healthy behaviors. The health perception variables examined were not significantly correlated with health-protective behaviors. Similar to earlier studies, survivors perceived themselves as more vulnerable to health problems than others not treated for cancer and recognized a need to protect their health. Importantly, they acknowledged that their behavior determined their health outcomes.

Tobacco use in childhood cancer survivors

Several studies of health behaviors have focused specifically on tobacco use prevalence in childhood cancer survivors. Smoking incidence rates of childhood cancer survivors reported in earlier studies were comparable to those of age- and gender-specific population standards and sibling controls.[23,24] In a large retrospective study, Haupt *et al.* compared the smoking habits of 1289 childhood cancer survivors diagnosed at five US cancer centers between 1945 and 1974 with those of 1930 sibling controls. Matched analyses were used to control for the influence of family factors and results indicated small to moderate differences in smoking habits between the groups.[25] The social acceptability of tobacco use during the treatment eras studied is reflected in the frequency of survivors currently smoking (28.6 per cent) and ever

smoking (57 per cent). Compared to sibling controls, survivors were 8 per cent less likely to be current smokers, 13 per cent less likely to be ever-smokers, but 12 per cent less likely to have quit smoking. Smoking practices for survivors and siblings were similar to US population rates and did not differ by gender. However, survivors diagnosed more recently (1965–1974) were significantly less likely to be current smokers compared to those diagnosed in earlier years (1945–1954), suggesting an increased awareness of the group about their vulnerability to tobacco-related health risks.

Using a more contemporary treatment cohort, Children's Cancer Group investigators described similar results after surveying the smoking habits of 592 adult survivors of acute lymphoblastic leukemia diagnosed between 1970 and 1987.[26] Compared to 409 sibling controls, survivors in this cohort were significantly less likely to have ever smoked (23.0 per cent vs. 35.7 per cent) and less likely to be current smokers (14.0 per cent vs. 20.3 per cent). Survivors were less likely than siblings to have quit smoking (26.6 per cent vs. 35.2 per cent) but this trend was not statistically significant. Smoking cessation in the survivor and control group was correlated with older age, female gender and college education. Of concern, more than 60 per cent of all study participants who were regular smokers continued to smoke at 10 years. These results indicate that young adult survivors of childhood leukemia are less likely to experiment with cigarette smoking but encounter a risk similar to their siblings of becoming habitual persistent smokers.

In the largest cohort study to date, the multi-institutional consortium Childhood Cancer Survivor Study (CCSS) examined smoking behaviors among 9709 adult study participants surviving a childhood cancer diagnosed between 1970 and 1986.[27] Predictors of smoking initiation and cessation evaluated included demographic variables (race, age, gender, education, household income, marital status) and cancer-related variables (age at cancer diagnosis, cancer histology, cancer treatment). Survivor reported rates of ever smoking (28 per cent) and currently smoking (17 per cent) were significantly lower compared to those reported for the general population over 18 years of age; this difference was significant for all survivors, as well as for male and female survivors. Further, survivors who smoked were also significantly more likely to quit smoking; this higher quit frequency was also observed for both males and females. Factors associated with a significantly higher relative risk of smoking initiation were older age at cancer diagnosis (10 years or older), lower household income (less than $20 000), less education, and cancer history not including pulmonary-related treatment or cranial radiation. Blacks were also less likely to start smoking. Factors associated with a statistically significant risk of being a current smoker were age less than 14 years at smoking initiation, not graduating from high school and

history of cranial radiation; younger age at cancer diagnosis was predictive of an increased likelihood of smoking cessation. These data provide important insights regarding the characteristics of survivors who should be targeted for smoking prevention/cessation interventions.

Health knowledge of childhood cancer survivors

Few investigations have evaluated health knowledge of childhood cancer survivors. Based on results of an early survey of 1928 adults who survived a childhood cancer diagnosed between 1945 and 1974, Byrne et al. reported that 14 per cent of survivors of malignancies other than central nervous system (CNS) tumors were not aware that they had cancer.[28] Knowledge about cancer diagnosis and treatment varied by race, the type of tumor and its treatment, the father's education level and the year of cancer diagnosis. Factors correlated with being unaware of a cancer diagnosis were not being white, having less educated parents, having a diagnosis of a 'tumor', being born in earlier years or younger at treatment or receiving less aggressive treatment. Fewer survivors of cancers designated by an eponym (Hodgkin's disease, Ewing sarcoma, Wilms' tumor) were unaware of their cancer diagnosis. The investigators speculated that racial, socioeconomic and cultural factors affected physician/family communication or treatment practices that accounted for these findings.

Hudson et al. also observed knowledge deficits about health risks following cancer in a group of 272 childhood cancer patients surveyed at baseline before participation in a multicomponent behavioral health promotion intervention.[17] A significant number of survivors underestimated their risk of several serious treatment complications, including second cancers and cardiovascular disease. In this regard, 52 per cent were unaware that their cancer treatment predisposed them to a higher risk of second malignancy. Similarly, 42 per cent indicated that they were never told about the increased risk of heart disease resulting from their cancer therapy. Notably, the development of a second cancer and cardiovascular disease were identified as the most concerning potential late effect in 48 per cent and 39 per cent of patients, respectively.

Recently, CCSS investigators evaluated the accuracy, sensitivity, specificity and predictive value of self-reported information obtained through a cross-sectional survey of 635 adult survivors of childhood cancers in their cohort.[29] Self-reported information provided by survivors was compared to medical record data. Overall, 93 per cent of participants were aware of their cancer diagnosis but only 74 per cent of respondents could provide an accurate general summary of all of the elements of their cancer history. Survivors of CNS tumors and neuroblastoma were more likely not to know their cancer

diagnosis, whereas 98 per cent of survivors of Hodgkin's disease, Wilms' tumor and bone cancers were able to name their cancer diagnosis with detail. Accuracy rates for general chemotherapy, radiation and splenectomy history were 94 per cent, 89 per cent and 93 per cent, respectively. Younger age at diagnosis, diagnosis during an earlier treatment era and history of a CNS cancer were significantly correlated with not knowing chemotherapy history. Seventy per cent of survivors treated with radiation therapy accurately reported treatment fields. Surprisingly, survivors who attended a long-term follow-up clinic or received a written clinical summary did not exhibit a greater knowledge about their cancer diagnosis and treatment. Also, survivors reporting anxiety about health problems predisposed by cancer therapy did not have a greater level of knowledge about diagnosis or therapy.

In summary, the limited studies evaluating health knowledge of childhood cancer survivors indicate knowledge deficits about cancer diagnosis, treatment and cancer-related health risks. These deficits may be related, in part, to cultural and ethnic variations in attitudes regarding medical disclosure about the diagnosis of a life-threatening illness like cancer. While some health care professionals and families still favor not 'burdening' cancer survivors with information about cancer-related health risks, more and more are recognizing the importance of health education as a prerequisite for prevention/risk reduction strategies. To make fully informed decisions about their health, childhood cancer survivors must be informed about cancer-related and behavioral factors that affect health risks. The survivor who is unaware of factors that may adversely affect health or who overlooks relevant risk information may not accurately estimate

health risks, identify appropriate health goals or practice health protective behaviors. Similarly, health care providers treating childhood cancer survivors must be knowledgeable about potential cancer-related adverse effects to prescribe appropriate monitoring and therapeutic interventions should health problems arise. With contemporary therapy, increasing numbers of childhood cancer survivors are reaching maturity and transitioning from pediatric to medical practices. To accurately evaluate the long-term effects of cancer treatment as survivors age, it is critical that survivors and health care providers be as completely informed as possible.

HEALTH PROMOTION INTERVENTIONS IN CHILDHOOD CANCER SURVIVORS

The risk of developing a cancer-related complication is determined by a complex interplay of demographic factors (age at diagnosis/treatment, race, gender, time since diagnosis), genetic factors (cancer-predisposing mutations, genetic polymorphisms), cancer treatment modalities (surgery, radiation, chemotherapy) and health behaviors (tobacco/alcohol use, sun protection, dietary/exercise habits) (Figure 13.1). Added to these factors is the relatively unknown contribution of aging to treatment-induced subclinical injury or organ dysfunction. The relationship of age at cancer treatment, gender, race and cancer treatment modality has been comprehensively evaluated for many late treatment sequelae. Conversely, relatively few studies have correlated late effects after childhood cancer with genetic mutations predisposing to carcinogenesis or

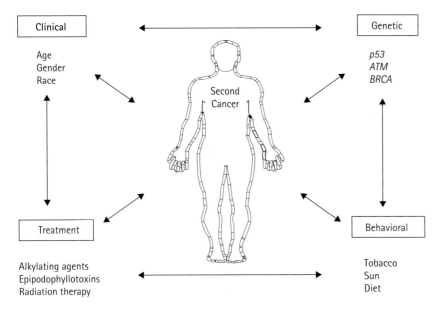

Figure 13.1 *Interaction of risk factors contributing to cancer treatment-related sequelae like the development of a second malignant neoplasm.*

genetic polymorphisms affecting drug metabolism and DNA repair.[30,31] Even fewer have explored how cancer treatment-induced changes are affected by normal physiologic processes that occur with organ senescence. For many cancer-related complications, behavioral modification is the primary means available to survivors to reduce disease risk.

Theoretically, interventions that enhance survivor knowledge about health risks following cancer and motivate them to practice health protective behaviors have the potential to reduce morbidity and mortality. Results from intervention programs targeting healthy adolescents indicate that health promotion is feasible and beneficial. Previously reported cancer prevention programs in healthy populations have used community or school-based educational interventions that focus on the long-term consequences of specific behaviors. More recent programs have evaluated psychosocial factors that influence behavior and strategies to induce behavioral change. Targeted behaviors have included tobacco use, dietary fat intake, sun exposure and compliance with medical monitoring to promote early detection of cancer. Common to these programs are components of health education, protective health behavior training and behavior modification, which have produced improvements in health knowledge and protective behavior practice.[32–36]

Using a behavioral model that focuses on the relationship between health risk perceptions and health practices is useful when developing a health-promotion intervention and interpreting its effectiveness. For example, the Health Belief Model is one of several behavioral models proposed to explain factors that influence the practice of risk-reducing health behaviors.[37,38] The model predicts that health behavior is governed by an individual's perceptions of vulnerability to an adverse health outcome, combined with perceptions of severity of the health problem, the benefits of practicing the health-protective behavior and barriers to engaging in the preventive action. If health is highly regarded, individuals will practice a health-protective behavior if they perceive that: (1) they are susceptible to the adverse health outcome; (2) the health problem is serious; and (3) the benefit of undertaking the preventive action is greater than the barriers or personal costs of taking the action. Health-promotion interventions guided by a predictive behavioral model facilitate the interpretation of the complex relationships among health behavior and personal variables, and provide insight about strategies that will motivate behavioral change.

Health-promotion approaches previously used with healthy adolescents may not be as effective with childhood cancer survivors who have unique educational needs related to their cancer experience. Tyc et al. suggest modification of the content and administration of traditional adolescent health programs to enhance their impact on childhood cancer survivors (Table 13.1).[16]

Table 13.1 *Components of health promotion interventions with adolescent cancer patients*

Inform of potential health risks
Address increased vulnerability to health risks relative to healthy peers
Provide personalized risk information relative to treatment history
Establish priority health goals
Discuss benefits of health protective behaviors
Discuss barriers to/personal costs of engaging in self-protective behaviors
Provide follow-up counseling

Reproduced with permission from Tyc et al. Health promotion interventions for adolescent cancer survivors. *Cognitive Behav Practice* 1999; **6**:128–136.

In particular, interventions that exploit survivor perceptions of increased health vulnerability may be used as a foundation to augment the impact of traditional health curricula. One must be careful with this approach as characterization of childhood cancer survivors as different from healthy peers may result in some survivors being less responsive to health-promotion efforts because of their desire to identify with peers. To avoid this, discussions about the adverse health effects of risky behaviors should be presented first as a risk for any adolescent followed by an explanation of the additional risks predisposed by the individual's cancer experience. This approach reduces anxiety and provides a more 'normalizing' experience that permits the survivor to identify with peers.[14]

The optimal timing of health risk education for childhood cancer survivors has not been previously studied. While cancer patients may be more sensitized to their health at diagnosis, the physical and emotional stresses experienced during this time may interfere with the patient's ability to focus on long-term health issues. When initiation of life-saving therapy is the priority, late health risks discussed by physicians obtaining informed consent for therapy are often understandably relegated to lower consideration. Similarly, cancer patients suffering from the acute effects of therapy may become discouraged with admonitions of potential late treatment-related health problems. Cancer patients may be more receptive to risk counseling sometime after completion of therapy when remission status appears assured. However, other clinical, developmental and psychosocial factors likely influence the optimal timing for providing health education in a given patient.

Health-promotion initiatives in healthy adolescents have been implemented in a variety of settings including community centers, schools and physician offices. Owing to the relative rarity of childhood cancer, health-promotion efforts in childhood cancer survivors have been delivered

almost exclusively in clinical settings. Education about cancer-related health risks and risk-reduction measures during routine medical examinations have several advantages. Childhood cancer patients usually have a close long-term relationship with the nurses and physicians who participated in their cancer treatment experience. Because of their credibility and medical expertise, health care providers can deliver powerful messages about survivors' increased vulnerability to health risks resulting from their cancer treatment. Further, patients may be more sensitized to their health and vulnerability when they return to the cancer center or oncologist's office, creating a 'teachable moment' during which they may be more receptive to health-promotion messages.[16] In particular, after completion of therapy evaluations for long-term survivors that focus on health surveillance rather than disease eradication provide an atmosphere more conducive to health-promotion discussions.

The increasing numbers of long-term childhood cancer survivors and awareness of cancer-related health risks have prompted the development of other health education forums, which have been most often sponsored by long-term follow-up clinics and cancer survivor advocacy groups. These include conferences and workshops, newsletters and brochures and internet-based web pages. Similar to clinician-based interventions, most feature health curricula that aim to motivate behavioral change by education about health risks following cancer. While counseling about cancer-related health risks and providing anticipatory guidance about risk-reduction methods are 'good medicine', the effectiveness of these methods to increase knowledge and change behavior in childhood cancer survivors is largely unstudied, underscoring the need for prospective controlled health education investigations.

Very few longitudinal, randomized health-promotion studies have been undertaken in childhood cancer survivors. Hudson et al. prospectively evaluated the efficacy of a multicomponent behavioral intervention to induce change in childhood cancer survivors' health knowledge, health perceptions and health-protective behavior practice.[19] Study participants were recruited from adolescent cancer survivors attending a long term follow up clinic and randomized to receive standard follow-up care or standard care plus the educational intervention. Standard care comprised: (1) self-examination teaching using a breast or testicle model; (2) targeted late effects screening; (3) a thorough clinical assessment; and (4) late effects risk counseling. Patients randomized to receive the multibehavioral intervention had standard care plus: (1) distribution and discussion of a clinical cancer treatment summary; (2) health behavior training in a health goal specified by the survivor; (3) health goal commitment to behavior practice; and (4) telephone follow-up at 3 and 6 months after the clinic visit to reinforce the behavioral training.

Baseline measures of health knowledge, perceptions and behaviors were obtained at randomization and repeated 1 year later during the survivor's annual check-up. Study results in 252 patients evaluable at both time points did not demonstrate a significant difference in change in outcome measures among patients randomized to standard care or standard care plus the behavioral intervention. However, patients who chose the health goal of breast/testicle self-examination showed improved practice of the health behavior and females in the intervention group demonstrated a greater improvement in knowledge scores than did males. Also, health perceptions about the seriousness of cancer-related risk factors were increased as a result of the intervention, although scores were not significantly different from the control group. This study demonstrated the feasibility of conducting health-promotion research in a medical setting dedicated to long-term survivor care. The limited effectiveness of the multicomponent intervention with respect to other outcome measures suggests that a brief, broad-based risk-counseling approach may not be sufficient to achieve long-term change in health knowledge, perceptions and practices in vulnerable childhood cancer survivors.

Two recent health promotion investigations aim to reduce tobacco use among childhood cancer survivors. Tyc et al. implemented a randomized study to compare a patient-centered educational/risk-counseling smoking intervention with a standard smoking advice approach in preadolescent and adolescent cancer survivors.[39] The objective of the study was to determine if the risk counseling intervention could increase knowledge and perceived vulnerability to tobacco-related health risks and decrease future intentions to use tobacco. Patients assigned to the standard advice approach were simply asked about tobacco use, advised about tobacco-related health risks and encouraged to abstain from or stop using tobacco. Patients who received the smoking education intervention received a multicomponent intervention that emphasized the cancer survivor's increased vulnerability to tobacco-related health problems compared to their healthy peers. The intervention was delivered in a single session by a psychologist followed by periodic reinforcement of tobacco abstinence goals by telephone. Childhood cancer survivors who received the tobacco intervention had significantly higher knowledge and perceived vulnerability scores, and lower tobacco use intention scores at 12 months compared to survivors receiving standard care. These results indicate that health knowledge and perceptions and tobacco use intentions can be modified by a risk-counseling intervention delivered by health care professionals in the context of a routine medical care. These investigators encouraged additional longitudinal studies to determine definitive long-term intervention effects on actual tobacco use in childhood cancer survivors.

Investigators at the Dana-Farber Cancer Institute initiated another longitudinal intervention trial to promote abstinence from tobacco among childhood cancer survivors participating in the Childhood Cancer Survivor Study.[40] The trial features a novel peer-based counseling approach implemented through telephone contacts. Eligible patients were CCSS participants who endorsed cigarette smoking ($n = 796$). The smokers were randomly assigned to receive self-help materials about tobacco cessation or a motivational intervention comprising up to six telephone calls from a childhood cancer survivor peer counselor. Telephone counseling content and supporting materials were tailored to the participant's stage of readiness to quit smoking; all participants were offered nicotine replacement therapy. Early study results at 8-month follow-up indicate a significant difference in smoking cessation among study participants who received the peer-counseling intervention (17 per cent) compared to those who received self-help materials (8.5 per cent) ($p \leqslant 0.001$). Further follow-up is under way to evaluate long-term results and cost effectiveness of the intervention.

In summary, health-promotion initiatives in childhood cancer survivors have primarily been implemented in the context of routine clinical care. Limited studies have been organized to evaluate the effectiveness of health education curricula prospectively. Longitudinal controlled trials are needed to evaluate accurately the numerous factors contributing to the success or failure of health promotion programs. The dearth of knowledge in this area underscores the need for more research to define: (1) the optimal timing of health-risk counseling relative to the time from diagnosis and completion of therapy; (2) the influence of neurocognitive function and developmental status of the patient; (3) the most feasible, cost-effective and efficacious methods and forums for health education; and (4) psychosocial and economic barriers to practice of health-protective behaviors.

HEALTH BEHAVIOR COUNSELING OF CHILDHOOD CANCER SURVIVORS

Following treatment for childhood cancer, many long-term survivors encounter an increased risk for the development of second cancers during adulthood and premature onset cardiovascular disease and other health problems associated with aging. Genetic predisposition and poor health habits can contribute to this excess risk. Clinicians should routinely counsel survivors about healthy lifestyles that reduce the risk of these complications that are discussed below.

Tobacco

Childhood cancer survivors should not smoke or use any form of tobacco. Tobacco use is the most important preventable cause of cancer in adulthood, and is also linked to an increased risk of cardiopulmonary disease including hypertension, emphysema and stroke. Tobacco has been linked to 90 per cent of cases of lung cancer, and one-third of all other cancers, including cancers of the mouth, larynx, pharynx, liver, colon, rectum, kidneys, urinary tract, prostate and cervix. Tobacco carcinogens have been associated with additive risks of lung cancer in adult cancer patients treated with thoracic radiation and specific chemotherapeutic agents.[41–43] While the additional contribution of tobacco use to the development of subsequent cancer in childhood cancer survivors has not been established, survivors should be reminded of their increased vulnerability to tobacco-related health problems if their cancer treatment included the antineoplastic therapies outlined in Table 13.2. Similarly, although the impact of environmental tobacco exposure to cancer and cardiopulmonary disease risk predisposed by cancer therapy for childhood cancer has not been established, it seems prudent to counsel avoidance of second-hand smoke as well.

Diet and physical activity

For individuals who do not smoke, diet and physical activity are the most important health behaviors that affect cancer and cardiovascular disease risk. This may be

Table 13.2 *Antineoplastic therapies with cardiopulmonary toxicities potentiated by tobacco use*

Therapy	Potential effects
Bleomycin	Pulmonary toxicity (pulmonary pneumonitis, fibrosis, restrictive lung disease)
Lomustine Carmustine Busulfan Cyclophosphamide Methotrexate Cytarabine	
Anthracyclines Doxorubicin Daunorubicin Idarubicin	Cardiac toxicity (cardiomyopathy)
High-dose cyclophosphamide	
Thoracic radiation therapy (mantle, mediastinum, lungs)	Cardiopulmonary toxicity

Reproduced with permission from Tyc *et al*. Tobacco use among pediatric cancer patients: recommendations for developing clinical smoking interventions. *J Clin Oncol* 1997; **15**:2194–2204.

Table 13.3 *American Cancer Society (ACS) individual guidelines on nutrition and physical activity for cancer prevention*

1 Eat a variety of healthful foods, with an emphasis on plant sources:
- Eat five or more servings of a variety of vegetables and fruits each day
- Choose whole grains in preference to processed (refined) grains and sugars
- Limit consumption of red meats, especially those high in fat and processed
- Choose foods that help maintain a healthful weight

2 Adopt a physically active lifestyle:
- Adults: engage in at least moderate activity for ≥30 minutes on ≥5 days of the week (≥45 minutes of moderate-to-vigorous activity ≥5 days per week may further enhance reductions in the risk of breast and colon cancer)

3 Maintain a healthful weight throughout life:
- Balance caloric intake with physical activity
- Lose weight if currently overweight or obese

4 If you drink alcoholic beverages, limit consumption

Adapted from Byers *et al. CA Cancer J Clin* 2002; **52**:92–119.

particularly important in cancer survivors treated with potentially carcinogenic and cardiotoxic cancer therapies. Certain antineoplastic therapies, e.g. cranial radiation, predispose to pituitary endocrinopathies, which adversely affect fat metabolism and insulin sensitivity. The American Cancer Society recently updated nutrition and physical activity guidelines that aim to reduce cancer risk; similar recommendations have been endorsed by the American Heart Association and the Department of Health and Human Services.[44] These guidelines, summarized in detail in Table 13.3, promote adherence to a diet with a variety of healthful foods, especially plant sources, adopting a physically active lifestyle, maintaining a healthful weight throughout life and limiting consumption of alcohol. Guidelines are presented for individual choices, as well as community action to provide environmental changes that facilitate healthy choices.

Sun protection

Recreational and lifestyle preferences have contributed to the steadily rising incidence rates of melanoma and other skin cancers.[45,46] Cumulative and excessive sun exposure has been linked to an increased risk of skin cancer and premature skin aging.[47] Childhood cancer survivors appear to have an increased risk of skin cancer. Nonmelanoma skin cancers, like basal cell carcinomas, are low-grade malignancies frequently observed in childhood cancer survivors, particularly within or near radiation treatment fields. Because basal cell carcinomas are not included in the Surveillance, Epidemiology and End Results (SEER) registries, the excess risk in childhood cancer survivors has been difficult to quantify. Nevertheless, adherence to skin cancer prevention measures recommended for healthy populations are especially important for childhood cancer survivors.[48–50] These recommendations include: (1) limiting the amount of time in the sun, especially from 10:00 am to 2:00 pm, when ultraviolet rays are most intense; (2) regularly using sunscreen with a sun protection factor of 15 or more; (3) wearing protective clothing, especially when planning extended activities in the sun; and (4) not tanning. Routine evaluations of childhood cancer survivors should include a thorough inspection of the skin, a discussion of skin cancer risk factors and symptoms, and a review of sun protection measures and their benefits.

Regular screening examinations

As many as two-thirds of childhood cancer survivors will experience adverse cancer-related effects that persist or develop beyond 5 years.[51] Numerous studies document a multitude of complications affecting virtually all organ systems. Of concern, is the fact that persistent, often initially subclinical effects, may exacerbate common diseases associated with aging. Because of the delayed onset of many cancer treatment sequelae, regular medical follow-up is crucial to provide timely interventions that reduce morbidity and mortality.

Confounding the issue of long-term follow-up is the lack of standardized screening guidelines for vulnerable cohorts of childhood cancer patients at risk for cardiovascular disease, second cancers and a variety of health problems. In some cases, for example, female patients treated with thoracic radiation during puberty, there is consensus among pediatric oncologists that breast cancer surveillance should be initiated earlier than in the general population, but the frequency and optimal screening modality has not been defined. Most pediatric cancer centers have recommended guidelines that include self-examination, more frequent clinician examinations, and earlier and/or more frequent mammographic screening. Table 13.4 summarizes the recommendations proposed by the St Jude investigators.[52] However, these and similar recommendations by other centers may not be endorsed by insurance companies and health maintenance organizations reimbursing medical care costs. Defining rational, cost-effective and universally accepted screening guidelines for at-risk childhood cancer survivors remains a significant challenge for future studies.

Nevertheless, clinicians should encourage childhood cancer survivors to pursue regular medical evaluations, and participate in cancer screening programs appropriate for their age, gender and treatment history. To provide the

Table 13.4 *Guidelines for breast cancer screening*

Age	Frequency
For all women	
BSE monthly	Beginning at puberty
Age 20–40	Breast examination by doctor every 3 years
Age 40	Baseline mammogram
Age 40–50	Breast examination by doctor every year; mammogram every 1–2 years
Over Age 50	Breast examination by doctor every year; mammogram every year
For women treated with chest radiation	
BSE Monthly	Beginning at puberty
Age 25–40	Breast examination by doctor twice a year; baseline mammogram – repeat every 3 years until 40
Age 40	Mammogram every year
Over age 50	Breast examination by doctor every year; mammogram every year

BSE, breast self-examination.

appropriate screening and health counseling, health care providers must be familiar with the survivor's cancer treatment history and its potential adverse effects. Acquisition of cancer treatment records and communication with the treating oncologist(s) will facilitate this process. In all cases, the ideal health maintenance evaluation should include a thorough physical examination, targeted screening appropriate for the patient's age, gender, treatment history, family history and health behaviors, and health education about risk reduction.

KEY POINTS

- Maladaptive health behaviors may exacerbate the risk of organ dysfunction and subsequent malignancy in aging childhood cancer survivors.
- Despite an increased vulnerability to cancer, cardiovascular diseases and other health problems after cancer therapy, childhood cancer survivors have practice rates of high-risk behaviors that are comparable to those of their healthy peers.
- A surprising number of childhood cancer survivors have knowledge deficits about their cancer diagnosis, treatment and cancer-related health risks.
- To make fully informed decisions about their health, childhood cancer survivors must be informed about cancer-related and behavioral factors that affect health risks.
- The risk of developing a cancer-related complication is determined by a complex interplay of demographic factors, genetic factors, cancer

treatment modalities and health behaviors. For many cancer-related complications, behavior modification is the primary means available to survivors to reduce disease risk.

- Health-promotion initiatives in childhood cancer survivors have been primarily implemented in the context of routine clinical care. Longitudinal trials are needed to evaluate: (1) the optimal timing of health risk counseling; (2) the influence of neurocognitive and developmental status of the patient; (3) the most feasible, cost-effective and efficacious methods and forums for health education; and (4) psychosocial and economic barriers to the practice of health-protective behaviors.

REFERENCES

1. Ries LAG, Smith MA, Gurney JG, *et al. Cancer incidence and survival among children and adolescents.* United States SEER Program 1975–1995, National Cancer Institute, SEER Program, NIH Pub. No. 99-4649, Bethesda, MD, 1999.
2. Landis SH, Murray T, Bolden S, *et al.* Cancer statistics. *CA Cancer J Clin* 1998; **48**:6–29.
♦3. Hawkins MM, Kingston JE, Wilson Kinnier LM. Late deaths after treatment for childhood cancer. *Arch Dis Child* 1990; **65**:1356–1363.
♦4. Robertson CM, Hawkins MM, Kingston JE. Late deaths and survival after childhood cancer: implications for cure. *Br Med J* 1994; **309**:162–166.
♦5. Nicholson HS, Fears TR, Byrne J. Death during adulthood in survivors of childhood and adolescent cancer. *Cancer* 1994; **7**:3094–3102.
♦6. Hudson MM, Jones D, Boyett J, *et al.* Late mortality of long-term survivors of childhood cancer. *J Clin Oncol* 1997; **15**:2205–2213.
♦7. Hudson MM, Poquette CA, Lee J, *et al.* Increased mortality after successful treatment for Hodgkin's disease. *J Clin Oncol* 1998; **16**:3592–3600.
♦8. Wolden SL, Lamborn KR, Cleary SF, *et al.* Second cancers following pediatric Hodgkin's disease. *J Clin Oncol* 1998; **16**:536–544.
♦9. Green D, Hyland A, Chung CS, *et al.* Cancer and cardiac mortality among 15-year survivors of cancer diagnosed during childhood or adolescence. *J Clin Oncol* 1999; **17**:3207–3215.
10. Baker L, Jones J, Stovall A, *et al.* Psychosocial and emotional issues and specialized support groups and compliance issues. *Cancer* 1993; **71**:2419–2422.
11. Jamison R, Lewis S, Burish T. Cooperation with treatment in adolescent cancer patients. *J Adolescent Health Care* 1986; **7**:162–167.
12. Hanna KM. Health behaviors of adolescents who have been diagnosed with cancer. *Issues Comprehens Nurs* 1993; **16**:219–228.
13. Hollen PJ, Hobbie WL. Risk taking and decision making of adolescent long-term survivors of cancer. *Oncol Nurs Forum* 1993; **20**:769–776.
♦14. Hollen PJ, Hobbie WL. Decision-making and risk behaviors of cancer-surviving adolescents and their peers. *J Pediatr Oncol Nursing* 1996; **13**:121–134.
15. Mulhern RK, Tyc VL, Phipps S, *et al.* Health-related behaviors of survivors of childhood cancer. *Med Pediatr Oncol* 1995; **25**:159–165.

◆16. Tyc VL, Hudson MM, Hinds P. Health promotion interventions for adolescent cancer survivors. *Cognitive Behav Practice* 1999; **6**:128–136.

◆17. Hudson MM, Tyc VL, Jayawardene DA, *et al.* Feasibility of implementing health promotion interventions to improve health-related quality of life. *Int J Cancer* 1999; S(12):138–142.

18. Tyc VL, Hadley W, Crockett G. Prediction of health behaviors in pediatric cancer survivors. *Med Pediatr Oncol* 2001; **37**:42–46.

◆19. Hudson MM, Tyc VL, Srivastava DK, *et al.* Multi-component behavioral intervention to promote health protective behaviors in childhood cancer survivors: the Protect Study. *Med Pediatr Oncol* 2002; **39**:2–11.

20. Anda RF, Waller MN, Wooten KG, *et al.* Behavioral risk factor surveillance, 1988. *Mort W Rep CDC Surveil Summ* 1990; **39**:1–21.

21. Kann L, Kinchen SA, Williams BI, *et al. Youth risk behavior surveillance – United States, 1997.* Atlanta, GA: Division of Adolescent and School Health, National Center for Chronic Disease Prevention and Health Promotion 1998; **47**:(SS-3):1–89.

22. Adams PF, Schoenborn CA, Moss AJ, *et al. Health risk behaviors among our nation's youth: United States, 1992.* Hyattsville, MA: US Department of Health and Human Services, Public Health Service, Centers for Disease Control and Prevention. National Center for Health Statistics, 1995; **192**:1–51.

23. Corkery JC, Li FP, McDonald JA. Kids who really shouldn't smoke. *N Engl J Med* 1979; **300**:1279.

24. Troyer H, Holmes GE. Cigarette smoking among childhood cancer survivors. *Am J Dis Child* 1988; **142**:123.

25. Haupt R, Byrne J, Connelly RR, *et al.* Smoking habits in survivors of childhood and adolescent cancer. *Med Pediatr Oncol* 1992; **20**:301–306.

◆26. Tao ML, Guo MD, Weiss R, *et al.* Smoking in adult survivors of childhood acute lymphoblastic leukemia. *J Natl Cancer Inst* 1998; **90**:219–225.

◆27. Emmons K, Li FP, Whitton J, *et al.* Predictors of smoking initiation and cessation among childhood cancer survivors: a report from the Childhood Cancer Survivor Study. *J Clin Oncol* 2002; **20**:1608–1616.

28. Byrne J, Lewis S, Halamek L, *et al.* Childhood cancer survivors' knowledge of their diagnosis and treatment. *Ann Intern Med* 1989; **110**:400–403.

◆29. Kadan-Lottick NS, Robison LL, Gurney JG, *et al.* What do childhood cancer survivors know about their past diagnosis and treatment? The Childhood Cancer Survivor Study. *JAMA* 2002; **287**:1832–1839.

30. Malkin D, Jolly KW, Barbier N, *et al.* Germline mutations of the p53 tumor-suppressor gene in children and young adults with second malignant neoplasms. *N Engl J Med* 1992; **326**:1309–1315.

31. Draper GJ, Sanders BM, Kingston JE. Second primary tumors in patients with retinoblastoma. *Br J Cancer* 1986; **53**:661–671.

32. Bruvold WH. A meta-analysis of adolescent smoking prevention programs. *Am J Public Health* 1993; **83**:872–880.

33. Fardy PS, White REC, Clark LT, *et al.* Health promotion in minority adolescents: a Healthy People 2000 pilot study. *J Cardiopulmonary Rehabil* 1995; **15**:65–72.

34. Lombard D, Neubauer TE, Canfield D, Winnett RA. Behavioral community intervention to reduce the risk of skin cancer. *J Appl Behav Analysis* 1991; **24**:677–686.

35. Williams CL, Carter BJ, Eng A. The 'know your body' program: a developmental approach to health education and disease prevention. *Prevent Med* 1980; **9**:371–383.

36. Winnett RA, Cleaveland BL, Tate DF, *et al.* The effects of the safe-sun program on patrons' and lifeguards' skin cancer reduction behaviors at swimming pools. *J Health Psychol* 1997; **2**:85–95.

37. Janz NK, Becker MH. The health belief model: a decade later. *Health Educ Q* 1984; **11**:1–47.

38. Weinstein ND. Testing four competing theories of health-protective behavior. *Health Psychol* 1993; **12**:324–333.

39. Tyc VL, Rai SN, Lensing S, *et al.* An intervention to reduce intentions to use tobacco among pediatric cancer survivors. *J Clin Oncol* 2003; **21**:1366–1372.

40. Emmons K, Park E, Puleo E, *et al.* Partnership for Health: a smoking cessation intervention trial of the Childhood Cancer Survivor Study. *Proceedings of the 23rd Annual Meeting of the Society Behavioral Medicine*, April 2002, Washington, DC.

41. Boivin J. Smoking, treatment for Hodgkin's disease, and subsequent lung cancer risk. *J Natl Cancer Inst* 1995; **87**:1502–1503.

42. Van Leeuwen FE, Klokman WJ, Stovall M, *et al.* Roles of radiotherapy and smoking in lung cancer following Hodgkin's disease. *J Natl Cancer Inst* 1995; **87**:1530–1537.

43. Kaldor JM, Day NE, Bell J, *et al.* Lung cancer following Hodgkin's disease: a case control study. *Int J Cancer* 1992; **52**:312–325.

◆44. Byers T, Nestle M, McTiernan A, *et al.* and the American Cancer Society. 2001 Nutrition and Physical Guidelines on Nutrition and Physical Activity for Cancer Prevention: reducing the risk of cancer with healthy food choices and physical activity. *CA Cancer J Clin* 2002; **52**:92–119.

45. Marks R. Prevention and control of melanoma: the public health approach. *CA Cancer J Clin* 1996; **46**:199–216.

46. Parker SL, Tong T, Bolden S, *et al.* Cancer statistics: 1996. *CA Cancer J Clin* 1996; **46**:7–29.

47. Holman CD, Armstrong BK, Heenan PJ. Relationship of cutaneous malignant to individual sunlight-exposure. *J Natl Cancer Inst* 1986; **76**:403–414.

48. Buller MB, Loescher LJ, Buller DB. Sunny days, healthy ways: a skin cancer prevention curriculum for elementary school students. *J Cancer Educ* 1994; **9**:155–162.

49. Buller DB, Callister MA, Reichert T. Skin cancer prevention by parents of young children: health information sources, skin cancer knowledge, and sun protection practices. *Oncol Nursing Forum* 1995; **22**:1559–1566.

50. Loescher LJ, Emerson J, Taylor A. Educating preschoolers about sun safety. *Am J Public Health* 1995; **85**:939–943.

51. Oeffinger KC, Eshelman DA, Tomlinson GE, *et al.* Grading of late effects in young adult survivors of childhood cancer followed in an ambulatory adult setting. *Cancer* 2000; **88**:1687–1695.

◆52. Kaste SC, Hudson MM, Jones DJ, *et al.* Breast masses in women treated for childhood cancer: incidence and screening guidelines. *Cancer* 1998; **82**:784–792.

14

Strategy for long-term follow up

14a

US perspective

KEVIN C OEFFINGER

NEED FOR FOLLOW-UP

Late effects or health problems secondary to previous treatment with chemotherapy or radiation are common. As many as two-thirds of survivors of childhood cancer will experience a late effect secondary to their previous cancer treatment.[1-4] Commonly, survivors have more than one late effect, with perhaps as many as a quarter of them experiencing one that is severe or life-threatening.[1,3,4] All organ systems are at risk, with late effects including cognitive impairment, infertility, alterations in growth and development, organ system damage and second malignant neoplasms.[5-9] The rationale for long-term follow-up of survivors of childhood cancer is based upon two assumptions: (1) screening and surveillance for late effects can lead to early diagnosis and intervention that will improve outcomes and quality of life, and (2) how and to what extent radiation and chemotherapy alter the aging process of normal tissue and how this impacts the development of other common adult health problems associated with aging is largely unknown. These two assumptions are briefly discussed in the following paragraphs.

Screening and surveillance

For screening to be effective in reducing morbidity and mortality, and improving quality of life, two criteria must be met. First, a screening test must be available that allows detection of a late effect earlier than without screening and with sufficient accuracy to avoid producing large numbers of false-positive and false-negative results. Second, screening for and treating survivors with early disease or late effects should improve the likelihood of favorable health outcomes compared to treating survivors when they present with signs or symptoms of the disease or late effect. Although there are few studies to date that have tested both of these criteria in survivors of childhood cancer, much of the work in the general population that has formed the cornerstone of preventive medicine can be applied. Four examples where studies in the general population can be applied to survivors are: (1) screening for chronic hepatitis C virus (HCV) in high-risk populations; (2) screening for skin cancer; (3) prevention of osteoporosis; and (4) early diagnosis of breast cancer.

The prevalence of circulating HCV RNA ranges from 6.6 to 49 per cent in survivors of childhood acute lymphoblastic leukemia (ALL) who were treated before current screening tests of blood products became available in the early 1990s.[10-13] An unknown, and likely sizeable, percentage of survivors have never been tested and are unaware of their risk. Chronic HCV infection develops in 75-85 per cent of persons infected with hepatitis C.[14,15] The natural history of chronic HCV in leukemia survivors has not been well characterized. In the general population, about 30-40 per cent of chronically infected persons have persistently normal alanine aminotransferase (ALT) levels and tend to have indolent disease. However, over the course of 20-30 years, 20-30 per cent of patients with untreated HCV will develop cirrhosis or extrahepatic sequelae, such as cryoglobulinemia, porphyria cutanea tarda or membranoproliferative glomerulonephritis.[16-18] Successful long-term treatment prior to liver decompensation has rapidly improved in the past decade. A sustained virologic response rate of 43 per cent has been reported in patients with chronic hepatitis secondary to HCV who were treated with 48 weeks of interferon alpha2b and ribavirin.[19] Based upon the prevalence

of chronic HCV in those given a blood transfusion prior to July 1992, the devastating consequences of liver decompensation, and the availability of treatments that significantly reduce this risk, the Centers for Disease Control and Prevention (CDC) recommend that all individuals at risk be screened, and those positive counseled regarding transmission and treatment options.[20] Thus, identification of survivors who were treated with blood products prior to 1992, determination of their HCV RNA status, assessment of the liver function of those infected, counseling regarding alcohol consumption, and appropriate treatment and follow-up is essential to reduce the risk for potentially life-threatening sequelae.

A second example is screening for second skin cancers following radiation. The epidermis, particularly the basal layer, is sensitive to radiation carcinogenesis, especially at a young age. In a study of the atomic bomb survivors of Japan, the excess relative risk for basal cell carcinoma (BCC) for children exposed prior to the age of ten was 21 [95 per cent confidence interval (95%CI), 4.1–73].[21] Moderate doses of therapeutic radiation for tinea capitis in childhood resulted in an excess relative risk of 1.7 at 1 Gy of radiation, with an absolute excess incidence of 0.31 per 1000 person-years.[22] Higher doses of radiation used in the treatment of childhood cancers, such as Hodgkin's and non-Hodgkin's lymphomas, soft tissue sarcoma, and Wilms' tumor, are associated with an increased risk for melanoma, squamous cell carcinoma (SCC) and BCC.[23,24,25] The standardized incidence ratio (SIR) of all skin cancers following treatment for childhood cancer was 4.1 in a cohort of 8602 survivors from Denmark.[24] In an analysis of 1039 patients treated for Hodgkin's disease, Swerdlow and coworkers reported an SIR of 4.0 and 3.9 for malignant melanoma and non-melanoma skin cancers (NMSC), respectively.[25] NMSC secondary to ionizing radiation occur in skin fields exposed to the radiation, which may be in an unusual or non-sun-exposed part of the body. Whether or not sun protection will confer a reduced risk in those exposed to ionizing radiation of a sun-exposed part of the body is not known.[21,22,26] Skin cancer is the most common group of cancers diagnosed in adults in the general population, accounting for nearly one-third of all cancers. Early diagnosis and treatment, particularly with melanoma, is associated with improved outcomes.[27] Public education regarding sun protection and self-examination has been associated with earlier stage of disease at diagnosis.[27] Recognizing the increased risk for skin cancer after radiation and the benefits of early diagnosis and treatment, it is important that health care providers counsel survivors regarding methods of sun protection, the ABCs of skin cancer, and the importance of periodic examination of the skin in and around the radiation field.

It appears that a large percentage of survivors of childhood cancer, including males, may be at risk for osteoporosis. Several well-designed, small to medium-sized cross-sectional studies of childhood cancer survivors, with median ages at evaluation ranging from 12 to 25 years, consistently showed reduction in bone mineral density (BMD), bone mineral content (BMC), and/or age-adjusted bone mass.[28–34] In an ongoing prospective cohort study, Atkinson et al. reported that by 6 months of therapy for ALL, 64 per cent of children had a reduction from baseline measures of BMC, and by the end of 2 years of therapy, 83 per cent were osteopenic.[35] Reduction in peak bone mass in young adults is a significant risk factor for developing osteoporosis and subsequent fracture, and measures to prevent or reverse bone loss are important. Exercise increases bone density in obese children[36] and young adults[37] and has recently been shown by meta-analysis[38] to prevent or reverse almost 1 per cent of bone loss per year in premenopausal and postmenopausal females. Long-term survivors of childhood cancer should be periodically assessed to determine their risk for osteoporosis, and counseled regarding adequate calcium intake and the benefits of exercise and avoidance of smoking.

A final illustrative example is screening for breast cancer in women who were treated with mantle or chest irradiation. The cumulative incidence of breast cancer in survivors who were treated with mantle radiation for childhood Hodgkin's disease is about 35 per cent by 20–25 years post-therapy.[39,40] In a retrospective review of 885 female Hodgkin's disease survivors, Hancock and colleagues reported a relative risk of 136 for those treated with mantle radiation prior to the age of 15 years.[41] In the Childhood Cancer Survivor Study (CCSS), Neglia and colleagues reported a SIR for breast cancer of 16.2 in a retrospective analysis of 13 581 long-term survivors.[42] Onset of breast cancer has been noted as early as 8 years post-radiation, with a median age at diagnosis of 31.5 years[39] and a median interval from radiation of 15.7 years.[42] It appears that pathologic features and prognosis for Hodgkin's disease survivors with breast cancer is similar to the general population.[43] Likewise, 5-year survival is strongly associated with stage of disease at time of diagnosis.[44] There is universal agreement that early diagnosis and treatment of breast cancer in the general population is associated with improved outcomes and reduced mortality. Screening mammography is considered a cost-effective method of early detection in women at increased risk.[45–47] Because breast cancer is common in female survivors of childhood cancer who were treated with mantle or chest/lung radiation, and early diagnosis and treatment is associated with improved outcomes in the general population, there is general consensus that periodic screening mammography be started 8–10 years after completion of therapy or around age 25.[39–41]

The intent of describing these four examples is to emphasize the potential benefits of proactive and anticipatory periodic evaluations, and counseling to reduce risk

and minimize progression of disease, rather than reacting to disease as it occurs.

Aging and the development of comorbid conditions

How radiation and chemotherapy affect the aging process and influence the development of common adult health problems is not well understood. Whether or not survivors who experience cognitive dysfunction and neuropathologic changes from cranial irradiation, such as leukoencephalopathy or mineralizing microangiopathy, will experience premature dementia-type illnesses is not known. Similarly the long-term consequences of radiation-induced skeletal delay in maturation and asymmetric growth of bone and soft tissues on the function and aging of weight bearing joints and muscle groups is not well understood. It is not known to what extent survivors will be at risk for premature joint deterioration and chronic muscle spasm/pain. Obesity and physical inactivity, prevalent in survivors of childhood ALL, are important predictors of eventual development of adult-onset diabetes mellitus, hypertension, dyslipidemia and, ultimately, cardiovascular disease. The risk for premature cardiovascular disease in leukemia survivors has not been determined. Because the population of adult survivors of childhood cancer is still relatively young, with a small percentage over the age of 40, there are no data available to answer these questions. Only through long-term follow-up of adult survivors will the impact of these types of late effects on the aging process become evident.

CURRENT STATUS OF FOLLOW-UP IN THE USA

Thus, long-term follow-up care of childhood cancer survivors provides: (1) the opportunity for prevention of and early diagnosis/intervention for late effects of the previous cancer treatment; and (2) longitudinal information to determine how these late effects modify risk for diseases associated with aging. Because there is no published literature regarding the health care access, utilization and status of long-term follow-up of childhood cancer survivors in the USA, preliminary results from two studies are provided. The first is a recently completed analysis of the Childhood Cancer Survivor Study regarding medical follow-up of 9434 adult survivors, age 18 and older.[48] The CCSS is a 25-institution, retrospective cohort study funded by the National Institutes of Health that is following over 14 000 long-term survivors of childhood cancer who were diagnosed between 1970 and 1986.[49] Baseline data were collected for participants of the study cohort using a 24-page questionnaire. The

baseline questionnaire was designed to capture a wide range of information, including demographic characteristics, education, income, employment, insurance coverage, marital status, health habits, family history, access and utilization of medical care, medication use, frequency of diagnosed medical conditions, surgical procedures, recurrent cancer, subsequent new neoplasms and off-spring/pregnancy history.

The second study, supported through the Robert Wood Johnson Foundation and directed by the author, is ongoing and aims to determine barriers to long-term follow-up from the perspective of adult survivors of childhood cancer. As part of this study, hereafter referred to as the 'Barriers study in progress', 1600 adult survivors were randomly selected from the CCSS cohort and mailed an 88-item questionnaire to determine factors associated with general and cancer-related health care utilization. The response rate of completed questionnaires is currently 70 per cent, with additional mailings in process. For the purpose of this subchapter, preliminary descriptive results from the first 441 respondents are provided.

Based upon the results of these two studies and anecdotal experience, it appears that most long-term survivors of childhood cancer do not receive cancer-related follow-up health care. In the CCSS analysis of 9434 adult survivors, only 42 per cent reported a health care visit in the previous 2 years that was related to their previous cancer treatment.[48] This percentage decreased with age, from 48.6 per cent in 18–19-years-olds to 37.8 per cent in those 35 years or older ($p < 0.01$). Factors associated with not reporting a general physical, a cancer-related visit or a cancer center visit included: no health insurance [odds ratio (OR) 2.19; 95%CI 1.89–2.53]; males (OR 1.80; 95%CI 1.60–2.02); lack of concern for future health (OR 1.56; 95%CI 1.38–1.77); and age 30 years or older in comparison with those 18–29 (OR 1.45; 95%CI 1.29–1.64). Race and ethnicity were not associated with lack of cancer-related follow-up. In the Barriers study in progress, only 26 per cent (114 out of 441) of adult survivors reported a health care visit in the previous 2 years that they thought was related to their previous cancer treatment. This lack of long-term follow-up and potential barriers are discussed in the following sections from the perspective of the cancer center, the primary care physician and the survivor (Table 14a.1).

Perspective of the cancer center

In the 1970s and 1980s, survival rates increased, the survivor population grew and the potential for late effects were recognized, leading to a gradual shift that includes not only the paradigm of cancer-free survival but also the long-term health and quality of life of survivors. As a result of this paradigm shift, many cancer centers developed

Table 14a.1 *Potential barriers and enablers of follow-up of long-term survivors of childhood cancer*

Survivor-related barriers and enablers
- Cancer experience (psychological factors, knowledge of risks)
- Core health beliefs (general motivation, perceived susceptibility to late effects, perceived seriousness of late effects)
- Internal modifying factors (sociodemographics, cultural background, spiritual beliefs, social structure)
- External modifying factors (subjective norms, cues to action)
- Health locus of control (internal, powerful others, chance)

Health care provider-related barriers and enablers
- Core preventive beliefs of health care provider
- Knowledge of risks
- Attitudes towards cancer survivors
- Organizational structure of practice

Health care system-related barriers and enablers
- Health care policies regarding survivorship
- Health care system
- Health/medical insurance

'long-term follow-up' programs to educate survivors and their families about treatment-related risks and to identify late effects. In 1997, 53 per cent of the institutions of Children's Cancer Group (CCG) and the Pediatric Oncology Group (POG) institutions had some type of long-term follow-up program for childhood cancer survivors under the age of 18.[50] However, most of these programs focused on acute problems and recurrence of disease. In 1999, each of the CCG and POG institutions was contacted to determine the type of services available for survivors (personal communication, Nancy Keene). The coordinator of each long-term follow-up program was identified and asked if the program included:

1 at least a single physician interested in late effects;
2 a nurse or nurse practitioner coordinator;
3 a dedicated time and place;
4 at least two follow-up clinics a month;
5 comprehensive care and screening for late effects based on the survivor's treatment;
6 referral to appropriate specialists; and
7 wellness education.

Only 26 programs in the USA fulfilled all of these criteria.

Few survivors entering young adulthood maintain contact with the treating cancer center. In the CCSS analysis, only 31 per cent of survivors who were 18–19 years of age at time of interview had been seen by a health care provider at a childhood cancer center in the previous 2 years.[48] This percentage steadily decreased with age of the survivor, to 17 per cent of those who were 35 years or older ($p < 0.001$). Similarly, preliminary results of the Barriers study in progress found that, although 32 per cent (143 out of 441) of adult survivors

reported a check up at a cancer center in the previous 4 years, this proportion decreased with age of survivor from 61 per cent in 18–24-year-olds to 16 per cent of survivors 35 years or older ($p < 0.001$). Only 20 per cent of respondents, regardless of age, had been seen in a children's cancer center in the previous 2 years.

In response to the growing recognition that many survivors were being 'lost to follow-up', multidisciplinary transition programs, combining the expertise of pediatric oncologists with primary care providers experienced in the needs of adult patients, were recommended as a mechanism for long-term follow-up of adolescent and young adult survivors of childhood cancer.[51–55] Three primary models have evolved and are in use in a handful of institutions in the USA:

1 continued follow-up of adult survivors at the childhood cancer center;
2 one-time evaluation of adult survivors at a childhood cancer center with a summary provided to the survivor and their primary care physician; and
3 multidisciplinary collaborative efforts between pediatric oncologists and health care providers experienced with adult health problems.

Perspective of the primary care physician

Many, if not most, adult survivors seek a primary care physician for some aspect of their health care. In the Barriers study in progress, 89 per cent of respondents (388 out of 441) reported having a regular primary care physician or site of care. However, only 30 per cent (130 out of 441) had ever seen a primary care physician for a problem they thought was related to their cancer. While 36 per cent felt that a primary care physician could usually handle a problem related to the previous cancer treatment, 28 per cent did not. Of the 110 survivors who felt they had a problem in the previous 2 years potentially related to their cancer treatment, 51 per cent saw a primary care physician as the first point of contact, while 40 per cent saw another type of health care provider and 9 per cent did not seek health care.

It should not be surprising that primary care physicians are not particularly aware of the risks of this population. Nationally recommended curricula for instruction of medical students and primary care residents do not include the topic of health care of childhood cancer survivors. Little has been written in US or Canadian primary care-based journals[56–59] or general, non-cancer-specific journals[60,61] regarding childhood cancer survivors and their long-term health care. None of the major primary care textbooks contains a section on providing health care for childhood cancer survivors. There has not been a national effort to link childhood cancer centers with primary care physicians in the transitioning process.

Also, methods to help primary care physicians navigate the complexities of the cancer center to find and communicate with the individual(s) involved in long-term care of survivors have not been developed. Compounding these issues, a typical family physician's practice only includes about 2–3 adult survivors.[58] Realizing that survivors are heterogeneous, with a variety of different cancers diagnosed at different age periods or treatment eras, and that the recommendations for screening and surveillance are constantly evolving, it is understandable that primary care provider-initiated discussions regarding appropriate cancer follow-up may be infrequent.

Perspective of the survivor

In addition to traditional barriers to health care utilization, such as sociodemographic factors and core health beliefs, other potential barriers are likely important in predicting whether or not an 'asymptomatic' survivor will seek cancer-related follow-up health care. These include psychological stresses that result from or are modified through the cancer experience, such as the perception of being well versus ill, use of avoidance as a coping mechanism, experiencing post-traumatic stress symptoms, feelings of invincibility, and developing a mistrust of doctors and the medical system.

Perhaps the most important barrier is survivors' lack of knowledge of risks associated with their cancer treatment. This is, in part, understandable. From the 1960s to the 1980s, as the survival rates were increasing, there was not the concurrent recognition of late effects. Often, parents of children who made it through their cancer were told that they had 'beat the odds' and were instructed to follow-up in 20 years; in other words, when the survivor had a problem. As the prevalence of late effects began to surface, long-term follow-up programs were developed. However, many institutions did not/do not have such programs, and care is focused on the immediate acute care needs or assessing for recurrence of the cancer. Illustrating this acute care focus, only 19 per cent (83 out of 441) of the respondents to the Barriers study in progress reported having a copy of a summary of their cancer type and previous treatment, and these were generally in medical rather than lay terms. Then, inevitably, there are the parents who listened to the discussions regarding the potential for late effects but later did not transmit this information to their child as he grew into adulthood. To date, there are no data regarding the extent to which this may or may not be a problem. Illustrating experiences common to many, one survivor stated:

> According to doctors, my heart failure was most likely caused by adding stress to a heart that was already weak from chemotherapy treatments. Although I remember being told that some of my treatments could cause heart damage, kidney failure, or bladder damage, I don't recall being told to monitor heart status after being released from treatment and especially during pregnancy. I am being compensated with medicines now. However, my doctors feel that I will probably need a heart transplant in the next two years.

Or another who said:

> I am a survivor of Hodgkin's disease diagnosed in 1971 at age 16. I was treated with high dose radiation only. I do not know my stage or level of rads. I have no documentation from [treating institution]. I asked for it a couple of years ago and they said it was in storage somewhere.

WHO SHOULD FOLLOW LONG-TERM SURVIVORS?

Ideal care of childhood cancer survivors should include the following key components:

- longitudinal care that is considered a continuum from cancer diagnosis to eventual death, regardless of age;
- continuity of care consisting of a partnership between the survivor and a single health care provider or program that can coordinate necessary services;
- comprehensive, anticipatory, proactive care that includes a systematic plan of prevention and surveillance;
- multidisciplinary team approach with communication between the primary provider/program, specialists in pediatric and adult medicine, and allied/ancillary service providers;
- health care of the whole person, not a specific disease or organ system, which includes the individual's family and his or her cultural and spiritual values;
- sensitivity to the issues of the cancer experience, including expressed and unexpressed fears of the survivor and his family/spouse.

Models for providing this type of longitudinal cancer-related health care for long-term survivors need to be further developed and compared. Two possible models, each with distinct advantages and disadvantages, are described.

First, longitudinal care can be provided through a comprehensive program in an academic health center that partners the childhood cancer center with academic primary care physicians. This route facilitates the continuum of care of the survivor within a familiar set of institutions and joins the expertise of those involved in the care of childhood cancer with those experienced in prevention and coordination of care. Further, it provides the necessary ancillary resources generally found in a medical center. Finally, this model can benefit from the

Patient's name:
SS#:

Year cancer Dx:	**Potential late effects**

Year cancer Dx:
Year off therapy:

Treatment center:

Treatment: Circle all that apply:

Cyclophosphamide   **Intrathecal medications:**
Etoposide (VP-16)   Cytarabine
Ifosfamide   Hydrocortisone
L-asparaginase   Methotrexate
6-mercaptopurine
Methotrexate
Prednisone
Vincristine

Cumulative Dose of Anthracycline (if used): _____ mg/m^2
(Daunorubicin or Doxorubicin)

Radiation?   Yes   No
     Site:
     Dose:

Blood Transfusion?   Yes   No   Unsure
     If Yes or Unsure, **Hepatitis C** status?
     Positive   Negative   Unknown

Signs or Symptoms? (circle all that apply)
   Unexplained fever   Bone pain
   Night sweats   Arthralgias
   Weight loss   Lymphadenopathy
   Weight gain   Hair changes
   Loss of appetite   Skin changes
   Weakness   Constipation
   Fatigue   Diarrhea
   Easily distracted   Menstrual abnormalities
   Difficulty with: Incoordination
     Abstract thinking   Difficulty with exercise
     Memorization   Sadness
     Handwriting   Feeling hopeless
   Visual changes   Apathy
   Bleeding gums
   Toothache
   Shortness of breath   **Smoke?**
   Dyspnea on exertion   No Yes (pk/day _____)
   Orthopnea
   Frequent coughing   **Chew/dip tobacco?**
   Chest pain   No Yes
   Hematuria
   Pain with urination   **Current exercise regimen:**
   Urinary hesitancy/frequency

Potential late effects

Alopecia	Infertility
Anxiety	Altered menarche
Cardiomyopathy	Early menopause
Cardiovascular disease	Obesity
Cataracts	Osteopenia/osteoporosis
Dental problems	Restrictive pulmonary
Depression	disease
Fine motor disturbance	Second malignancy
Gross motor disturbance	(CNS, thyroid, blood)
Growth hormone deficiency	Thyroid problems
Hepatitis C	(hypothyroid, nodules)

Late Effects Diagnosed:
1.
2.
3.
4.

Recommended tests and follow-up (risk groups)

CBC with platelets and differential	1–3 years
ALT	1–3 years
Lipoprotein analysis	1–3 years
TSH (CRT or CS-RT)	1–3 years
Urinalysis (cyclophosphamide)	1–3 years
Anti-HCV (if treated before 7/92)	Baseline
FSH, LH, estradiol (CS-RT, abdominal RT or cyclo)	Baseline and prn
Semen analysis (CS-RT, abdominal RT or cyclo)	Baseline and prn
Echocardiogram (LVF, SF) (anthracycline $\geq$ 300 mg/m^2)	Every 2–3 years
Depression and Anxiety screen	1–3 years
Referral to Dentist (CRT)	1–3 years
Counsel regarding:	Yearly

  – School/work problems
  – Exercise prescription
  – Healthy diet, calcium
  – Tabacco product use

Abbreviations:
   ALT – alanine aminotransferase
   Anti-HCV – antibody to hepatitis C
   CBC – complete blood count
   CRT – cranial irradiation
   CS-RT – cranio-spinal irradiation
   FSH – follicle stimulating hormone
   LH – luteinizing hormone
   LVF – left ventricular function
   SF – shortening fraction
   TSH – thyroid stimulating hormone

Figure 14a.1 *Putting it all together: example of a single-page medical record template. (Reproduced with permission from Oeffinger KC, Eshelman DA, Tomlinson GE, Tolle M, Schneider GW. Providing primary care for long-term survivors of childhood acute lymphoblastic leukemia.* J Family Pract *2000; 49:1133–1146.)*

integration of patient care, education and research. However, it must be recognized that most survivors do not live near an academic health center, and may prefer instead to be followed in their neighborhood near home or work.

Second, care can be provided through a primary care provider's office. To be effective, this will require development of an ongoing two-way relationship between the primary care provider and the childhood cancer center. Methods to enhance educating and updating primary care physicians about recommended guidelines and the evolving knowledge base of late effects is critical. Resources to assist with coordination of the different health care services are also important.

Regardless of model, a critical aspect in long-term follow-up is educating and empowering survivors and their families. This begins during treatment or early follow-up, and should be built upon with each visit. A medical summary in lay terms should be provided to all survivors and their families for use with subsequent medical visits. Written or electronic educational materials should be available and easily accessible.

RECOMMENDATIONS FOR FOLLOW-UP

When seeing a long-term survivor of childhood cancer for the first time or in follow-up, a systematic plan for screening and counseling is essential. The goal of such a plan is to identify modifiable risk factors for late effects or diagnose disease that is amenable to early intervention. The plan should be considered dynamic, created with the first visit and periodically updated as risks change or new information becomes available. An example of a template developed for ALL survivors is provided in Figure 14a.1. A thorough history and physical examination provides the foundation to discuss appropriate screening tests, and counsel regarding preventive and risky health behaviors. From this, an individualized plan can be developed.

History

A good history is basic to health care. That being said, it is a critical component in providing optimum cancer-related follow-up care for survivors. In addition to items in a standard history, several additional pieces of information should be elicited and documented (Table 14a.2). First, a summary of the survivor's cancer diagnosis and treatment should be created and always available. Items should include the age at and year(s) of diagnosis and completion of therapy, primary treating institution with contact information, treatment protocol (if one), and a description of the cancer therapy. Gender, age at

Table 14a.2 *Key points in the history*

Medical summary
- Age at diagnosis
- Date of diagnosis
- Date of completion of therapy
- Primary treating institution with contact information
- Treatment protocol
- Chemotherapy agents (with cumulative doses as appropriate)
- Radiation (type, site, cumulative dose)
- Surgery (e.g. nephrectomy, splenectomy, abdominal exploration)
- Blood transfusion (hepatitis C virus status)

Preventive and risky behaviors
- Physical activity level
- Calcium intake
- Testicular or breast self-examination
- Dental examinations
- Nicotine use (type, frequency)
- Alcohol use (amount, frequency)
- Illicit drug use (amount, frequency)
- Sexual history

Family history of hereditable diseases
- Cardiovascular risk factors (hypertension, diabetes mellitus, dyslipidemia, premature cardiovascular disease)
- Cancer (breast, colon, ovarian, endometrial, prostate)
- Osteoporosis
- Miscellaneous
- Extended review of systems based on cancer treatment

diagnosis, era of treatment and interval since treatment commonly modify risk for late effects. Each of the chemotherapeutic agents should be listed and include cumulative doses, when known, of agents such as anthracyclines, epipodophyllotoxins and alkylating agents. Similarly, radiation type, site and cumulative dose should be listed. Any surgeries should be noted, especially removal of an organ, such as the spleen or a kidney, or abdominal explorations, as these surgeries increase the risk for subsequent sepsis, renal problems or small bowel obstruction, respectively. Special effort should be made to ascertain if the survivor received a blood transfusion or blood product during therapy.

Documentation of preventive health behaviors and practices is an integral part of the medical record of a survivor and should include physical activity levels, calcium intake, practice of testicular or breast self-examination, and dates of routine screening tests, such as pap smears and dental examinations. Likewise, the record should include risky behaviors, such as nicotine use, excessive alcohol intake, illicit drug use and unprotected intercourse. Risk for late effects can be positively or negatively modified by these healthy or risky behaviors.

Family history of potentially hereditable diseases that may modify risk need to be part of the medical record. Preferably, a family genogram should be created and

Table 14a.3 *Treatment-specific protocol for routine screening of asymptomatic survivors seen in the After the Cancer Experience (ACE) Young Adult Program. (Reproduced with permission of John Wiley from Oeffinger KC, et al. Grading of late effects in young adult survivors of childhood cancer followed in an ambulatory adult setting.* Cancer *2000; 88:1687–1695)*

Treatment	Screening test	Frequency
Chemotherapy if patient received:		
Actinomycin or antimetabolite	ALT	Annually
	Bone densitometry	Optional
Aminoglycoside, high dose	Audiology	Annually
Anthracycline ($\geqslant$300 mg/m^2, or anthracycline	Echocardiogram	Every 3 years
administered prior to 1 year of age, or $\geqslant$ 200 mg/m^2	EKG	Optional
with radiation involving the chest)		
BCNU, CCNU, bleomycin	CXR	Baseline
	Pulmonary function tests	Baseline and as needed
Cisplatin	BUN, creatinine, magnesium	Annually
	Audiology	Optional
Corticosteroids	Bone densitometry	Optional
Cyclophosphamide	FSH, LH	Optional
	Semen analysis	Optional
	Urinalysis	Annually
	Urine cytology	Optional
Cyclosporine	Bone densitometry	Optional
Etoposide	CBC with platelets and differential	Annually
Nitrogen mustard, procarbazine	CBC with platelets and differential	Annually
	FSH, LH, estrogen	Optional
	Testosterone	Optional
Semen analysis		Optional
Vincristine	ALT	Annually
Radiation therapy if patient received:		
Cranial or craniospinal radiation	Cataract screening	Annually
	Audiology	Optional
	Dental screening	Annually
	TSH, free T4	Annually
	Lipid profile	Annually
	Bone densitometry	Optional
Mantle radiation	TSH	Annually
	Thyroid ultrasound	Optional
	Lipid profile	Annually
	Mammogram (females)	Start 8 years post-radiation, then annually
	Plain radiographs of irradiated site	Optional
Abdominal radiation	Hemoccult screening	Annually
	Urinalysis	Annually
Pelvic radiation	FSH, LH	Optional
	Semen analysis	Optional
High-dose radiation of the trunk or extremities	Plain radiographs of the irradiated sites	Optional
Surgery if patient received:		
Nephrectomy	BUN, creatinine, UA	Annually
Splenectomy	Verify immunizations	Annually
	Antibiotic prophylaxis	Optional
Miscellaneous:		
If patient received blood products before July 1992	HIV	Baseline
	Anti-HCV	Baseline

ALT, alanine aminotransferase; anti-HCV, antibody to hepatitis C; BCNU, carmustine; BUN, blood urea nitrogen; CBC, complete blood count with differential; CCNU, Lomustine; CXR, chest radiograph; ECG, electrocardiogram; FSH, follicle-stimulating hormone; HIV, human immunodeficiency antibody; LH, luteinizing hormone; TSH, thyroid stimulating hormone; UA, urinalysis.

	Treatment-related risk factors	Other risk factors	Things to do to stay healthy
Eyes	☐ Radiation to head ☐ Surgical removal of the eye ☐ Other	☐ Other	☐ Ophthalmology exams every 2–3 years to check for cataracts ☐ Other
Teeth	☐ Radiation to head/neck/mantle ☐ Chemotherapy at a young age ☐ Other	☐ Smoking ☐ Snuff/chewing tobacco ☐ Lack of dental care ☐ Other	☐ Floss every day ☐ See your dentist at least every 6 months ☐ Make a plan to eliminate nicotine ☐ Other
Thyroid	☐ Radiation to head/neck/mantle ☐ Other	☐ Family history of thyroid problems ☐ Other	☐ Have your thyroid level checked yearly ☐ Have your thyroid felt for nodules ☐ Take Synthroid as directed ☐ Other
Breasts	☐ Radiation to chest/mantle/lung ☐ Other	☐ Family history of breast cancer ☐ First child born after 30 ☐ High fat diet ☐ Late menopause ☐ Other	☐ Learn how to do a monthly breast self-exam ☐ Baseline mammogram or other imaging beginning at 25 then every 1–2 years ☐ Other
Heart	☐ Adriamycin/daunomycin/mitoxantrone/Cytoxan ☐ Radiation to the chest, thorax, mantle, TBI ☐ Other	☐ Smoking ☐ Family history of heart disease ☐ Diabetes ☐ High cholesterol ☐ Other	☐ Exercise at least 3 times per week, aerobically like brisk walking, running, bicycling, swimming ☐ Take steps to eliminate nicotine (smoking) ☐ Eat a heart healthy diet, low in saturated fat ☐ Have cholesterol panel (lipid panel) checked regularly ☐ Have blood pressure checked regularly ☐ Other
Lungs	☐ Bleomycin ☐ Radiation to chest/lungs ☐ Other	☐ Smoking ☐ Passive smoke ☐ Other	☐ Take steps to stop smoking ☐ Lung function tests as necessary ☐ Exercise 3 times per week ☐ Other
Kidneys	☐ Cisplatin ☐ Radiation to the abdomen/pelvis ☐ Surgical removal of a kidney ☐ Other	☐ Excessive alcohol ☐ Other	☐ Have urinary tract symptoms or infections treated promptly ☐ Limit salt intake ☐ Limit alcohol ☐ Check with your doctor about sports limitations ☐ Other
Bladder	☐ Radiation to the abdomen pelvis/groin ☐ Cyclophosphamide (Cytoxan), Ifosfamide, hemorrhagic cystitis ☐ Other	☐ Alcohol ☐ IV drug use ☐ Other	☐ Have a urinalysis regularly ☐ Other
Intestines	☐ Radiation to the abdomen, pelvis or groin ☐ Other	☐ High fat diet ☐ Other	☐ Stool for hidden blood every 2 years after the age of 18 ☐ Other
Liver	☐ Methotrexate, 6MP, 6-thioguanine, Vincristine, 1-asparaginase (rare) ☐ Hepatitis C ☐ Hepatitis B ☐ Radiation to the abdomen ☐ Other	☐ Alcohol ☐ IV drug use ☐ Other	☐ Minimize/eliminate alocohol because it is toxic to your liver ☐ If you have hepatitis B or C it is vital to eliminate alcohol and discuss use of common over the counter drugs with your Dr or NP ☐ Check stool for blood yearly

(continued)

	Treatment-related risk factors	Other risk factors	Things to do to stay healthy
			☐ Avoid body piercing or tattooing to decrease the risk of hepatitis ☐ Hepatitis A vaccine ☐ Other
Skin	☐ Radiation ☐ Other	☐ Sun ☐ Fair skinned ☐ Other	☐ Avoid sun exposure between 10am–2pm ☐ Wear sunscreen with a SPF of 30 or greater ☐ Try to find makeup with SPF in it ☐ Avoid tanning beds and lights ☐ Check skin for suspicious moles, marks or changes regularly ☐ Learn the 'A,B,C,D' of skin exams ☐ Pay attention to any skin changes in radiation areas
Sex Organs	☐ Radiation to abdomen pelvis, or directly to ovaries/testicles ☐ Nitrogen mustard ☐ Leukeran, procarbazine ☐ Cyclophosphamide ☐ Ifosfamide ☐ Surgical removal of ovary or testicle ☐ Other		☐ Females should see their gynecologist yearly for pap smears after the age of 18 ☐ Sperm count to check fertility as indicated ☐ Hormonal evaluations as indicated ☐ Other
Bone	☐ Cranial irradiation ☐ Chemotherapy ☐ Other	☐ Physical inactivity ☐ Smoking ☐ Family history ☐ Other	☐ Exercise ☐ Stop smoking ☐ Other
Obesity	☐ Cranial irradiation ☐ Other	☐ Physical inactivity ☐ Other	☐ Exercise ☐ Check blood pressure ☐ Check cholesterol ☐ Other
Other	☐	☐	☐

Figure 14a.2 *ACE Program health care information sheet. IV, intravenous; SPF, sun protection factor; TBI, total body irradiation. ACE Program (After the Cancer Experience: Pediatric and Young Adult Survivor Programs) January 2002.*

include cardiovascular risk factors (diabetes, hypertension, dyslipidemia, premature coronary or cerebrovascular disease), cancers (e.g. breast, colon, ovarian, endometrial, prostate, melanoma), and osteoporosis.

Finally, the history should include a few items in addition to the standard review of systems and be based upon the previous cancer treatment. For example, cognitive impairment is a common sequelae of ALL therapy, and so the survivor should be questioned about problems with abstract thinking, memorization, handwriting, mathematic skills and ability to focus on a problem. Similarly, survivors treated with head or neck irradiation are at increased risk for periodontal disease, and so should be questioned regarding dental symptoms. Screening for depression and anxiety should also be considered.

Physical examination

A few caveats regarding physical examination are important. Previous treatment with radiation increases risk for second malignant neoplasms (e.g. skin cancer, soft tissue sarcomas, adenocarcinomas), cataracts, dental problems and musculoskeletal problems. Thus, particular attention should be paid to the fields of radiation. Nevi within the field, including areas of scatter, should be inspected for dysplastic features or changes suggestive of malignant melanoma. Recognizing the increased risk for basal cell carcinomas, including in sun-protected parts of the body, unusual or atypical skin lesions should be biopsied or referred to a dermatologist. Palpable organs in the radiation field, such as the thyroid, breasts and testicles,

should be examined, along with a careful eye and oral examination.

Screening asymptomatic survivors

To date, there are few well-designed longitudinal studies with adequate power that compare different screening strategies of asymptomatic survivors. Most long-term follow-up programs have developed institution-specific protocols for screening that are largely dependent on consensus and draw from studies of other populations. As an example, the protocol used in the After the Cancer Experience (ACE) Program at Children's Medical Center of Dallas and UT Southwestern Medical Center is provided (Table 14a.3). It is important to recognize that this is an institution-specific protocol based upon available literature and resources, and should not be considered an evidence-based set of guidelines. Clinicians should be selective in ordering tests and providing preventive services, actively incorporating the patient's concerns and fears in arriving at an individualized decision on whether or not to perform a test.

Risk assessment and modification

Based on the data obtained through these steps, risk can be assessed. Survivors should be educated about late effects and counseled about ways to reduce risk. A two-page template that is used as a guide with survivors followed in the ACE Program is provided as an example in Figure 14a.2. The discussion may include counseling about methods to increase physical activity, insure adequate calcium intake, properly protect the skin from sun exposure and avoid adoption of risky behaviors. If necessary, assistance and resources should be provided to help with smoking cessation, and alcohol and drug counseling and rehabilitation. A medical summary and a systematic plan of follow-up, written in lay terms, should be provided to all survivors and updated as needed.

FUTURE DIRECTIONS

Interventions to enhance cancer-related follow-up of childhood cancer survivors need to be developed, tested and implemented. Current screening protocols are largely based on small, retrospective, single-institution studies. Federal funding is needed to support further outcome-based and cost-effective studies comparing different strategies of screening and follow-up with the goal of developing evidence-based guidelines.

KEY POINTS

- Late effects secondary to chemotherapy and radiation therapy are common.
- Optimum cancer-related health care for long-term survivors consists of proactive and anticipatory longitudinal care that includes screening and surveillance for late effects and counseling to reduce risk.
- Most long-term survivors of childhood cancer do not receive cancer-related health care.
- A minority of long-term survivors are followed at a cancer center, most primary care physicians are unfamiliar with the health care problems of this population and most survivors are not aware of their risks related to their previous cancer treatment.
- Targeted education of survivors and coordination of care with ongoing communication between cancer centers and primary health care physicians is necessary to improve longitudinal cancer-related health care of survivors.

REFERENCES

1. Garre ML, Gandus S, Cesana B, et al. Health status of long-term survivors after cancer in childhood. Results of an uniinstitutional study in Italy. Am J Pediatr Hematol Oncol 1994; **16**:143–152.
2. Vonderweid N, Beck D, Caflisch U, et al. Standardized assessment of late effects in long-term survivors of childhood cancer in Switzerland: results of a Swiss Pediatric Oncology Group (SPOG) pilot study. Int J Pediatr Hematol Oncol 1996; **3**:483–490.
3. Stevens MC, Mahler H, Parkes S. The health status of adult survivors of cancer in childhood. Eur J Cancer 1998; **34**:694–698.
4. Oeffinger KC, Eshelman DA, Tomlinson GE, et al. Grading of late effects in young adult survivors of childhood cancer followed in an ambulatory adult setting. Cancer 2000; **88**:1687–1695.
● 5. DeLaat CA, Lampkin BC. Long-term survivors of childhood cancer: evaluation and identification of sequelae of treatment. CA Cancer J Clin 1992; **42**:263–282.
6. Neglia JP, Nesbit ME Jr. Care and treatment of long-term survivors of childhood cancer. Cancer 1993; **71**(10 Suppl):3386–3391.
7. Donaldson SS. Lessons from our children. Int J Radiat Oncol Biol Phys 1993; **26**:739–749.
● 8. Meister LA, Meadows AT. Late effects of childhood cancer therapy. Curr Probl Pediatr 1993; **23**:102–131.
9. Schwartz CL. Late effects of treatment in long-term survivors of cancer. Cancer Treat Rev 1995; **21**:355–366.
10. Dibenedetto SP, Ragusa R, Sciacca A, et al. Incidence and morbidity of infection by hepatitis C virus in children with acute lymphoblastic leukaemia. Eur J Pediatr 1994; **153**:271–275.
11. Locasciulli A, Testa M, Pontisso P, et al. Prevalence and natural history of hepatitis C infection in patients cured of childhood leukemia. Blood 1997; **90**:4628–4633.
◆ 12. Paul IM, Sanders J, Ruggiero F, et al. Chronic hepatitis C virus infections in leukemia survivors: prevalence, viral load, and severity of liver disease. Blood 1999; **93**:3672–3677.

13. Strickland DK, Riely CA, Patrick CC, *et al.* Hepatitis C infection among survivors of childhood cancer. *Blood* 2000; **95**:3065–3070.

14. Alter MJ, Margolis HS, Krawczynski K, *et al.* The natural history of community-acquired hepatitis C in the United States. The Sentinel Counties Chronic non-A, non-B Hepatitis Study Team. *N Engl J Med* 1992; **327**:1899–1905.

15. Shakil AO, Conry-Cantilena C, Alter HJ, *et al.* Volunteer blood donors with antibody to hepatitis C virus: Clinical, biochemical, virologic, and histologic features. The Hepatitis C Study Group. *Ann Intern Med* 1995; **123**:330–337.

16. Tong MJ, el Farra NS, Reikes AR, Co RL. Clinical outcomes after transfusion-associated hepatitis C. *N Engl J Med* 1995; **332**:1463–1466.

17. Fattovich G, Giustina G, Degos F, *et al.* Morbidity and mortality in compensated cirrhosis type C: a retrospective follow-up study of 384 patients. *Gastroenterology* 1997; **112**:463–472.

18. Poynard T, Bedossa P, Opolon P. Natural history of liver fibrosis progression in patients with chronic hepatitis C. The OBSVIRC, METAVIR, CLINIVIR, and DOSVIRC groups. *Lancet* 1997; **349**:825–832.

19. Poynard T, Marcellin P, Lee SS, *et al.* Randomised trial of interferon alpha2b plus ribavirin for 48 weeks or for 24 weeks versus interferon alpha2b plus placebo for 48 weeks for treatment of chronic infection with hepatitis C virus. International Hepatitis Interventional Therapy Group (IHIT). *Lancet* 1998; **352**:1426–1432.

20. CDC. Recommendations for prevention and control of Hepatitis C virus (HCV) infection and HCV-related chronic disease. *MMWR* 1998; 47(No.RR-19).

21. Ron E, Modan B, Preston D, *et al.* Radiation-induced skin carcinomas of the head and neck. *Radiat Res* 1991; **125**:318–325.

22. Ron E, Preston DL, Kishikawa M, *et al.* Skin tumor risk among atomic-bomb survivors in Japan. *Cancer Causes Control* 1998; **9**:393–401.

23. Meadows AT, Baum E, Fossati-Bellani F, *et al.* Second malignant neoplasms in children: an update from the Late Effects Study Group. *J Clin Oncol* 1985; **3**:532–538.

24. Olsen JH, Garwicz S, Hertz H, *et al.* Second malignant neoplasms after cancer in childhood or adolescence. Nordic Society of Paediatric Haematology and Oncology Association of the Nordic Cancer Registries. *Br Med J* 1993; **307**:1030–1036.

25. Swerdlow AJ, Barber JA, Horwich A, *et al.* Second malignancy in patients with Hodgkin's disease treated at the Royal Marsden Hospital. *Br J Cancer* 1997; **75**:116–123.

26. Lichter MD, Karagas MR, Mott LA, *et al.* Therapeutic ionizing radiation and the incidence of basal cell carcinoma and squamous cell carcinoma. The New Hampshire Skin Cancer Study Group. *Arch Dermatol* 2000; **136**:1007–1011.

27. Rhodes AR. Public education and cancer of the skin. What do people need to know about melanoma and nonmelanoma skin cancer? *Cancer* 1995; **75**:613–636.

28. Hesseling PB, Hough SF, Nel ED, *et al.* Bone mineral density in long-term survivors of childhood cancer. *Int J Cancer Suppl* 1998; **11**:44–47.

♦29. Aisenberg J, Hsieh K, Kalaitzoglou G, *et al.* Bone mineral density in young adult survivors of childhood cancer. *J Pediatr Hematol Oncol* 1998; **20**:241–245.

30. Arikoski P, Komulainen J, Voutilainen R, *et al.* Reduced bone mineral density in long-term survivors of childhood acute lymphoblastic leukemia. *J Pediatr Hematol Oncol* 1998; **20**:234–240.

31. Nysom K, Holm K, Michaelsen KF, *et al.* Bone mass after treatment for acute lymphoblastic leukemia in childhood. *J Clin Oncol* 1998; **16**:3752–3760.

32. Hoorweg-Nijman JJ, Kardos G, Roos JC, *et al.* Bone mineral density and markers of bone turnover in young adult survivors of childhood lymphoblastic leukaemia. *Clin Endocrinol* 1999; **50**:237–244.

33. Vassilopoulou-Sellin R, Brosnan P, Delpassand A, *et al.* Osteopenia in young adult survivors of childhood cancer. *Med Pediatr Oncol* 1999; **32**:272–278.

34. Warner JT, Evans WD, Webb DK, *et al.* Relative osteopenia after treatment for acute lymphoblastic leukemia. *Pediatr Res* 1999; **45**:544–551.

35. Atkinson SA, Halton JM, Bradley C, *et al.* Bone and mineral abnormalities in childhood acute lymphoblastic leukemia: Influence of disease, drugs and nutrition. *Int J Cancer Suppl* 1998; **11**:35–39.

36. Gutin B, Owens S, Okuyama T, *et al.* Effect of physical training and its cessation on percent fat and bone density of children with obesity. *Obesity Res* 1999; **7**:208–214.

37. Valdimarsson O, Kristinsson JO, Stefansson SO, *et al.* Lean mass and physical activity as predictors of bone mineral density in 16–20-year old women. *J Intern Med* 1999; **245**:489–496.

38. Wolff I, van Croonenborg JJ, Kemper HC, *et al.* The effect of exercise training programs on bone mass: A meta-analysis of published controlled trials in pre- and postmenopausal women. *Osteoporos Int* 1999; **9**:1–12.

♦39. Bhatia S, Robison LL, Oberlin O, *et al.* Breast cancer and other second neoplasms after childhood Hodgkin's disease. *N Engl J Med* 1996; **334**:745–751.

♦40. Aisenberg AC, Finkelstein DM, Doppke KP, *et al.* High risk of breast carcinoma after irradiation of young women with Hodgkin's disease. *Cancer* 1997; **79**:1203–1210.

♦41. Hancock SL, Tucker MA, Hoppe RT. Breast cancer after treatment of Hodgkin's disease. *J Natl Cancer Inst* 1993; **85**:25–31.

♦42. Neglia JP, Friedman DL, Yasui Y, *et al.* Second malignant neoplasms in five-year survivors of childhood cancer: childhood cancer survivor study. *J Natl Cancer Inst* 2001; **93**:618–629.

43. Wolden SL, Hancock SL, Carlson RW, *et al.* Management of breast cancer after Hodgkin's disease. *J Clin Oncol* 2000; **18**:765–772.

44. Cutuli B, Borel C, Dhermain F, *et al.* Breast cancer occurred after treatment for Hodgkin's disease: analysis of 133 cases. *Radiother Oncol* 2001; **59**:247–255.

♦45. US Preventive Services Task Force. *Guide to clinical preventive services*, 2nd edn. Baltimore, MD: Williams & Wilkins, 1996.

46. Rosenquist CJ, Lindfors KK. Screening mammography beginning at age 40 years: a reappraisal of cost-effectiveness. *Cancer* 1998; **82**:2235–2240.

47. Overmoyer B. Breast cancer screening. *Med Clin North Am* 1999; **83**:1443–1466.

48. Oeffinger KC, Mertens AC, Hudson MM, *et al.* Health care of young adult survivors of childhood cancer: A report from the Childhood Cancer Survivor Study. *Ann Family Med* 2003 (in press).

49. Robison L, Mertens AC, Boice JD Jr, *et al.* Study design and cohort characteristics of the Childhood Cancer Survivor Study: a multi-institutional collaborative project. *Med Pediatr Oncol* (in press).

50. Oeffinger KC, Eshelman DA, Tomlinson GE, Buchanan GR. Programs for adult survivors of childhood cancer. *J Clin Oncol* 1998; **16**:2864–2867.

♦51. Bleyer WA, Smith RA, Green DM, *et al.* American Cancer Society Workshop on Adolescents and Young Adults with Cancer. Workgroup #1: long-term care and lifetime follow-up. *Cancer* 1993; **71**:2410–2425.

52. Rosen DS. Transition to adult health care for adolescents and young adults with cancer. *Cancer* 1993; **71**(10 Suppl.): 3411–3414.

53. Konsler GK, Jones GR. Transition issues for survivors of childhood cancer and their healthcare providers. *Cancer Pract* 1993; **1**:319–324.

54. Meadows AT, Black B, Nesbit ME Jr, *et al.* Long-term survival. Clinical care, research, and education. *Cancer* 1993; **71**(10 Suppl.):3213–3215.

55. MacLean WE Jr, Foley GV, Ruccione K, Sklar C. Transitions in the care of adolescent and young adult survivors of childhood cancer. *Cancer* 1996; **78**:1340–1344.

56. Hawkins MM. Long term survival and cure after childhood cancer. *Arch Dis Child* 1989; **64**:798–807.

57. Grossi M. Management and long-term complications of pediatric cancer. *Pediatr Clin North Am* 1998; **45**:1637–1658.

◆58. Oeffinger KC. Childhood cancer survivors and primary care physicians. *J Family Pract* 2000; **49**:689–690.

●59. Oeffinger KC, Eshelman DA, Tomlinson GE, *et al.* Providing primary care for long-term survivors of childhood acute lymphoblastic leukemia. *J Family Pract* 2000; **49**:1133–1146.

60. Meadows AT, Robison LL, Neglia JP, *et al.* Potential long-term toxic effects in children treated for acute lymphoblastic leukemia. *N Engl J Med* 1989; **321**:1830–1831.

61. Neglia JP, Meadows AT, Robison LL, *et al.* Second neoplasms after acute lymphoblastic leukemia in childhood. *N Engl J Med* 1991; **325**:1330–1336.

14b

UK perspective

CHRISTOPHER JH KELNAR AND W HAMISH B WALLACE

INTRODUCTION

The incidence of childhood cancer is 100–130 per 10^6 per annum, and 1 in 600 children under the age of 15 years will develop cancer, which is now curable in 65–70 per cent. One in 1000 young adults are now childhood cancer survivors. Leukemia (predominantly lymphoblastic) makes up approximately one-third of childhood cancers, and brain and spinal tumors about one-quarter. Childhood cancers are diverse in their site of origin and histological type, but long-term morbidity in survivors relates more to the treatment – surgery, chemotherapy, radiotherapy, bone marrow transplantation – than the cancer type or site.

With increasing understanding of the effects of these treatment modalities on tissues and organ systems, many of these treatment-related sequelae are predictable – and many are preventable or treatable with informed and careful follow-up. For the majority of those treated for cancer in childhood and adolescence, the goal is not merely long-term survival but high quality of life.

Nevertheless there is still an 11-fold increased overall risk of death in 5-year survivors of childhood cancer[1,2] with still higher risks in females (18.2-fold), those diagnosed under the age of 5 years (14-fold) and those with an initial diagnosis of leukemia (15.5-fold) or central nervous system (CNS) tumor (15.7-fold). The commonest treatment-related cause of death amongst 5-year survivors is a second malignancy (19.4-fold increased risk). Other common causes include cardiac problems (8.2-fold) and pulmonary problems (9.2-fold). While cancer recurrence is the cause of death in about two-thirds between 5 and 9 years after diagnosis, treatment-related causes of death account for about one in five deaths (second cancer, cardiac toxicity, pulmonary complications).

Treatment-related morbidity is diverse, with potential effects on the endocrine system (growth, puberty, fertility, pituitary, thyroid and other disorders), cardiovascular, pulmonary and renal complications, and cognitive, educational, psychological, social and quality of life manifestations.[3,4] Growth and endocrine function following treatment of childhood malignant disease and the effects of chemotherapy are also reviewed by Wallace[3] and Wallace and Kelnar,[5,6] respectively. Strategies for long-term follow-up have been reviewed by Wallace et al.[7]

While there is still a dearth of prospective longitudinal interventional large-scale studies of therapies designed to prevent, modify or treat morbidity in long-term survivors, there is an increasing body of evidence (descriptive, case control or cohort studies) on which scientifically sound recommendations for monitoring and follow-up can be based. The development of the Scottish Intercollegiate Guidelines Network (SIGN) guideline 'Long term follow-up of survivors of cancer in children and young people'[8] on which the present authors served, respectively, as methodologist and chairman, has provided a systematic review of the evidence in many (although not all) of these areas. Its evidence-based and graded recommendations provide a basis for the effective

informed and pragmatic follow-up of a cohort of patients who, it is estimated, will make up 1 in 250 of the adult population by the year 2010.

Areas covered by the SIGN guideline are:

1 the assessment and achievement of normal growth;
2 the achievement of normal progression through puberty and factors affecting fertility;
3 the assessment of thyroid function;
4 the early identification, assessment and treatment of cardiac abnormalities;
5 the assessment and achievement of optimal neurodevelopment and psychological health.
   Important areas not covered by the SIGN guideline include second malignancy, renal, respiratory and liver dysfunction.

Thus, long-term morbidity risks relate to treatment modality and the challenge remains to further improve survival rates while reducing the incidence and severity of such treatment-induced late effects. These can be anticipated and monitored to optimize prevention and treatment – ideally through multidisciplinary follow-up involving pediatric oncologist, pediatric endocrinologist, pediatric neurologist, radiation oncologist, pediatric neurosurgeon, clinical psychologist, specialist nurse and social worker (see below).

GROWTH IMPAIRMENT (see Chapter 8a)

Long-term effects of radiotherapy (RT) and chemotherapy (CT) on growth and endocrine function have become more obvious and important as survival following childhood cancers has improved.[9] Adverse effects on growth may result from radiation-induced hormone deficiencies, impaired spinal growth from spinal RT (and from CT), primary hypothyroidism from spinal RT, precocious or delayed puberty from abnormal gonadotrophin secretion, gonadal failure from RT or CT, and problems with nutrition or obesity.[10–12]

At diagnosis of acute lymphoblastic leukemia (ALL), there is already low bone turnover with reduced levels of collagen formation and resorption markers (PICP, PIIINP and ICTP).[13] In remission, there is further bone synthesis suppression (low levels of PICP and PIIINP) and growth suppression,[14–17] which probably relates to glucocorticoid (prednisolone) and high-dose methotrexate therapies. This suggests that there may be an increased risk of long-term osteoporosis and fractures. Comparison between countries suggests that the degree of growth impairment is proportional to the intensity of the CT regimen. CT has a disproportionate effect on spinal growth impairment, perhaps because of the large numbers of spinal epiphyses. High-dose cranial irradiation is associated with a significant potential height deficit because of the combined effects of precocious puberty and an impaired pubertal growth spurt (see below).

The hormone deficiency effects of RT will depend on the site of irradiation, total dose of irradiation, fractionation schedule and the child's age at treatment. Growth impairment will result from RT to the hypothalamo-pituitary axis (the hypothalamus is more radiosensitive than the pituitary and the growth hormone (GH) axis the most radiosensitive followed by the gonadal axis). RT to the spine (in the treatment of medulloblastomas, ependymomas, germinomas) will result in late pubertal growth failure (the spinal growth spurt occurs towards the end of secondary sexual development) and primary hypothyroidism owing to a direct effect on the thyroid gland. CT (glucocorticoids, methotrexate) will also impair growth (see above). Tumor recurrence should always be considered as a cause of growth failure in these patients.

Radiotherapy doses of >24 Gy will be associated with precocious (especially in young girls) or delayed puberty and GH deficiency within 5 years.[18] Very high RT doses (e.g. ~54 Gy used in craniopharyngioma) will cause growth hormone deficiency within 2 years. Lower doses (<24 Gy) may be associated with precocious puberty, an impaired pubertal growth spurt owing to relative GH insufficiency in that context[19] and reduced pubertal spinal growth. Total body irradiation (TBI), used as preparation for bone marrow transplantation (~7.5–15.75 Gy), may also be associated with pubertal GH insufficiency, thyroid dysfunction and a radiation-induced skeletal dysplasia.

The same total dose of RT given in several fractions minimizes GH deficiency and growth impairment and fractionated TBI produces less damage to normal tissues. Younger children (especially girls) are more likely to develop precocious puberty and a pubertal growth spurt can be mistaken for 'catch-up' growth. Obesity can normalize growth at the expense of disproportionate bone age advance and reduced height prognosis.

Clinical growth assessment should consist of the regular measurement of sitting and standing height, skinfolds, weight and calculation of body mass index (BMI), and puberty staging. It is recommended that all children who have survived childhood cancer should have their height and weight measured regularly, on and off treatment, until they reach final adult height. Sitting height should be measured in children who have received craniospinal irradiation (SIGN Grade B recommendation). Chemotherapy is also likely to have a deleterious affect on spinal growth, which may be particularly manifested by growth failure in late puberty.

Children with impaired growth velocity should have growth hormone levels measured after appropriate stimulation tests (SIGN Grade C recommendation). Other causes of poor growth, including potential deficiencies of other pituitary hormones or problems related to early or delayed puberty, should be considered and treated as

necessary (SIGN Grade B recommendation). Children with craniopharyngioma should be tested at presentation for growth and other pituitary hormone deficiencies and at regular intervals thereafter (SIGN Grade B recommendation). Young girls receiving cranial radiotherapy should be closely monitored for signs of precocious puberty (SIGN Grade B recommendation).

Children who have been treated with low-dose cranial radiotherapy are at risk of precocious puberty and growth hormone insufficiency (GHI), while those treated with higher doses are at risk of an evolving endocrinopathy with GHI developing early and in some children gonadotrophin, thyroid or cortisol deficiency developing later on.[20] Thus, laboratory assessment [baseline free thyroxine, cortisol, testosterone/estradiol, insulin-like growth factor 1 (IGF-1), etc.], physiological profiles [growth hormone (GH), gonadotrophins (GTs), cortisol, etc.] and dynamic tests [insulin hypoglycemia, gonadotrophin-releasing hormone (GnRH), human chorionic gonadotrophin (hCG), thyrotrophin-releasing hormone (TRH), synacthen, etc.] will be relevant. Nevertheless, integrating clinical and anthropometric information (plotting on appropriate growth charts, calculation of height velocity, calculation of body mass index and plotting on age-related BMI standards) as a prelude to appropriate investigation and treatment is an important role for the pediatric endocrinologist in a multidisciplinary team. Much information can be gleaned from careful anthropometry and pubertal assessment in the context of knowledge about the anti-cancer treatment received so as to minimize investigations in children who have already been through many unpleasant treatments and investigations. Interpretation of biochemical (hormonal) information must be on a background of thorough understanding of growth and puberty so that treatments can be used in timely and appropriate ways. Available treatment modalities include the use of GH for growth failure, pubertal suppression and thyroxine, glucocorticoid and sex steroids as indicated.

If a child has a good prognosis from the underlying condition 2 years from treatment, GH therapy should be given when indicated on biochemical and anthropometric grounds (SIGN Grade B recommendation). There is a high relapse rate in the first 2 years after diagnosis and it seems inappropriate to treat children with daily injections, if the prognosis is poor or while the chance of relapse is still high. There is no evidence that GH is associated with reactivation of the primary lesion[21] but GH may well be 'blamed' for any relapse. Where the cause of growth impairment is unclear, a trial of GH may be appropriate (SIGN Grade C recommendation). In cranipharyngioma, there is every reason to start GH therapy without delay once deficiency is identified – the response is excellent and on a par with that seen in other causes of GH deficiency. Management of the growth disorders secondary to treatment of childhood cancers is reviewed by Bath et al.[4]

There is accumulating evidence that childhood cancer survivors (particularly of leukemia, but also of brain tumors and craniopharyngioma), however they were treated, are at risk of obesity in adolescence and adult life.[22] The etiology is likely to be multifactorial (nutritional, psychological, lifestyle including lack of exercise, endocrine and neuroendocrine) and is difficult to prevent or treat. There are potentially severe consequences: childhood obesity may affect educational attainment and interpersonal relationships adversely, especially in boys,[23,24] may persist into adulthood, and is associated with an increased risk of hypertension, stroke, myocardial infarction or type 2 diabetes mellitus, osteoarthritis, breast and bowel cancers, skin disorders, and asthma and other respiratory problems. Hypertension, dyslipidemia and hyperinsulinemia are increasingly found in obese children, with two or more risk factors found in 58 per cent of obese children[25] with significantly increased odds ratios for raised diastolic blood pressure (BP; 2.4), raised low-density lipoprotein (LDL) cholesterol (3.0), raised high-density lipoprotein (HDL) cholesterol (3.4), raised systolic BP (4.5), raised triglycerides (7.1) and high fasting insulin (12.6). A SIGN guideline on 'Obesity in children and young people' was published in 2002 (SIGN 2002[26]) and should be consulted for further information.

Treatment for childhood cancer may result in reduced bone mineral density.[27] An increased fracture rate remains to be demonstrated but the observed decrease in bone mineral density would be expected to predict for increased fracture risk.

Children who are about to undergo head and neck cancer treatment, and their parents/carers, should be advised about the possible effects (particularly from radiotherapy) on orofacial growth and teeth, e.g. facial growth, temperomandibular joint function, enamel defects, mineralization, and development of crowns and root stunting. Specialist dentists have a role in the care of these children (SIGN Grade D recommendation). While levels of decay seem no worse than control children, treatment such as radiotherapy, which reduces saliva, may increase caries risk (see SIGN Dental Caries Guideline 2000[28]).

THYROID DISORDERS (see Chapter 8b)

Abnormalities of thyroid gland structure and function may occur following treatment for childhood cancer either due to primary damage to the thyroid gland itself, particularly from neck irradiation, or secondary to damage to the hypothalamo-pituitary–thyroid axis. Chemotherapy is an independent risk factor for thyroid dysfunction.

Groups particularly at risk of thyroid dysfunction include those treated for thyroid cancer (which is very rare in childhood) and survivors of neuroblastoma who

have received ^{131}I-MIBG. All will require thyroxine replacement therapy. Children with Hodgkin's disease treated with radiotherapy to the neck have a significantly increased risk of hypothyroidism, thyroid nodules and thyroid cancer compared to those treated with chemotherapy alone. Transiently abnormal thyroid function tests are common in the first few years after treatment but hypothyroidism may develop many years later.

Children treated with craniospinal radiotherapy (e.g. for medulloblastoma) are also at increased risk of primary hypothyroidism. Cranial radiotherapy is not associated with an increased risk of primary hypothyroidism but may cause secondary/tertiary hypothyroidism by damage to the pituitary/hypothalamus.

In the past, children were treated with low-dose radiotherapy for a variety of non-malignant disorders (e.g. skin conditions or lymphoid hyperplasia). The risk of thyroid cancer in such groups is significant (<10 per cent over 35 years[29]). That radiation is indeed an important cause of thyroid cancer in children[30] has been demonstrated by the effects of the short-lived radioactive fall-out from the1986 Chernobyl nuclear power plant accident.[31] The prevalence of thyroid dysfunction in survivors treated with total body irradiation seems variable, may be transient and can be secondary to thyroid or hypothalamo-pituitary dysfunction.[32–34]

Survivors who have received radiotherapy to the neck, brain or spine should have their thyroid function checked after completion of treatment and regularly thereafter – surveillance should be lifelong (SIGN Grade B recommendation). There are no good-quality studies that address the question of screening for thyroid nodules or second primary thyroid cancers. Although ultrasound may detect more abnormalities than simple clinical examination, their clinical significance is unclear. Survivors at risk should be advised accordingly and asked to seek urgent medical advice if they notice a palpable neck mass.

Thyroid hormone replacement is safe and effective in a dose of approximately $100\,\mu g/m^2$ per day. Although there is no high-quality evidence to support or refute the use of thyroxine in compensated primary hypothyroidism (clinical euthyroidism with normal free T4 but raised TSH levels), it is arguably sensible to treat such patients with thyroxine as persisting high TSH levels may theoretically predispose to malignant change owing to thyroid hyperstimulation in these patients.

PUBERTY AND FERTILITY PROBLEMS
(see Chapter 8c–e)

The impact of combination cytotoxic chemotherapy on gonadal function is dependent on gender and age of the child undergoing treatment, and the nature and dosage of the drugs received. Drugs known to cause gonadal damage include procarbazine, cytosine arabinoside and the alkylating agents, particularly cyclophosphamide, chlorambucil, mustine, melphalan, busulphan and the nitrosoureas. Both the testis and ovary are vulnerable to radiation damage.[35]

High dose (>24 Gy) radiotherapy to the hypothalamus/pituitary (e.g. for brain tumors) may result in delayed puberty, whereas lower doses (<24 Gy) are more commonly associated with early/precocious puberty, especially in children treated when they are very young.[36] Thus, early puberty (in boys) and frankly precocious puberty (in girls) are common sequelae in young children who have received cranial irradiation for high-risk ALL. The pubertal growth spurt can be mistaken for 'catch-up' growth.

The majority of childhood cancer survivors are fertile. There are low risks of infertility following chemotherapy for Wilms' tumor and ALL, and following cranial RT <24 Gy. Abdominal, pelvic and total body irradiation may all result in ovarian damage.[37] The human oocyte is sensitive to radiation and the risk of ovarian failure increases with increasing doses of radiotherapy.[38] Infertility or subfertility is common after CT for Hodgkin's disease RT (TBI, testicular or pelvic).[39,40] Thus, ovarian failure after TBI is common with the risk relating to age at treatment (younger children are at lower risk). Sex steroid replacement therapy is necessary if there is evidence of ovarian failure, from puberty through to at least the fifth decade, for bone mineralization and cardiovascular protection.

In young adult women, physiological sex steroid replacement therapy[41] improves uterine function (blood flow, endometrial thickness) so that these women could potentially benefit from assisted reproductive technologies.[42,43] However, they have reduced uterine distensibility with increased risk of small-for-gestational-age infants and miscarriage or preterm delivery.[37,39] They should be counseled appropriately and managed as high-risk pregnancies by an obstetrician aware of the potential problems.

In boys, the germinal epithelium is much more sensitive to radiation than Leydig cells: 1.2 Gy to the testis will result in azoospermia, whereas >20 Gy (in prepuberty) or >30 Gy (postpuberty) is necessary before Leydig cell function is damaged significantly.[44] Thus, spontaneous progression through puberty does not necessarily indicate subsequent fertility. Permanent azoospermia is likely in most patients receiving more than 4 Gy.

The current management of ALL in children in the UK includes cyclophosphamide. Although the long-term fertility for this group of patients is not known, the available evidence suggests that the total dose of cyclophosphamide $(2–3\,g/m^2)$ is unlikely to be sterilizing.[45] Treatment for Hodgkin's disease in the UK with 'ChlVPP'

(chlorambucil, vinblastine, procarbazine, prednisolone) is known to cause gonadal damage, particularly in the male, and the agents implicated are chlorambucil and procarbazine. In a recent long-term follow-up study, 89 per cent of the males treated before puberty had evidence of severe damage to the germinal epithelium and recovery of spermatogenesis is unlikely. Around 50 per cent of girls treated for Hodgkin's disease prepubertally with six or more courses of ChlVPP had raised plasma gonadotrophin levels, but longer follow-up is needed to determine whether these women have recovery of function or go on to develop a premature menopause.[46]

As part of their monitoring, childhood cancer survivors should have routine assessment of gonadal function. The majority will be fertile and the risk of infertility relates to the treatment received. In some situations, hormonal manipulation may restore fertility. Counseling is necessary for young people at high risk of infertility and sperm cryopreservation is available for postpubertal boys. Ovarian cortical strip cryopreservation is one current research technique in girls. Strategies to protect the prepubertal testis from damaging effects of CT or RT are under investigation.[47,48]

CARDIOVASCULAR MORBIDITY
(see Chapter 4a,b)

Cardiovascular disease can occur as a consequence of cancer treatment and contribute significantly to the late morbidity and mortality of disease-free survivors.[49] The majority of cardiovascular damage is the result of a direct effect by radiation and chemotherapeutic agents (particularly anthracyclines), but an indirect contribution can occur from injury to other organs.

There are no randomized controlled trials examining the cardiotoxic effects of chemotherapy and/or radiotherapy in the treatment of children and young people with cancer. However, there is strong evidence that anthracyclines, such as daunorubicin and doxorubicin, cause cardiac damage in a cumulative dose-related fashion.[50,51] The mechanism appears to be focal myocyte death with replacement fibrosis.[49] There is probably no 'safe' dose – cardiac dysfunction can occur with relatively low anthracycline doses – and adverse cardiac effects increase over time.[50,52–54] Younger age at treatment and female gender appear to be independent risk factors[53]. Higher anthracycline doses seem particularly to be associated with prolongation of the QT interval.[53]

Mediastinal irradiation increases the risk and incidence of coronary artery disease and myocardial infarction. Specific risk factors are high dose (>30 Gy), minimal protective cardiac blocking, young age at irradiation and length of follow-up.[55] Patients receiving TBI for BMT conditioning must also be considered at risk. While mediastinal radiotherapy appears to induce atheromatous lesions of the proximal coronary arteries (and similar lesions can be seen in the carotid bulb after cranial irradiation), there is no strong evidence that radiotherapy alters HDL blood lipid levels. Radiation damage has an additive effect to anthracycline cardiotoxicity.

The balance between useful and pragmatic assessment for cardiac dysfunction in those at risk is not easy to determine. The literature supports echocardiographic assessment at diagnosis and at regular intervals during treatment. Three monthly electrocardiograms (ECGs) on treatment have been suggested with yearly ECGs thereafter with more intensive and invasive tests, if abnormalities are detected.

Protective drugs (such as ICRF) are under investigation and may improve the prognosis in subclinical cardiotoxicity.[56] The data currently available do not support the routine treatment of the damaged heart with angiotensin-converting enzyme (ACE) inhibitors, such as captopril or enalapril. Although short-term improvements have been demonstrated, studies are uncontrolled and not blinded, and long-term outcomes are unknown.[56]

Lifestyle changes (smoking cessation, improved diet, appropriate exercise) should be encouraged. There is no evidence to suggest restricting employment or limiting activities is beneficial. However, the risks from competitive sporting activity and pregnancy are likely to be considerable and pre-pregnancy counseling is important so that women patients understand the risks involved.

RENAL MORBIDITY (see Chapter 6a)

Renal toxicity after successful treatment of childhood cancer is common and leads to a wide range of manifestations of variable severity and may be irreversible. There are many causes of nephrotoxicity in children treated for malignancy, including the disease itself, chemotherapy, radiotherapy, surgery, immunotherapy and supportive treatment. Assessment of renal toxicity should include both glomerular and tubular function. The two most commonly implicated agents are ifosfamide and cis-platinum. Ifosfamide nephrotoxicity usually affects predominantly the proximal tubule (causing a Fanconi syndrome) but may also impair glomerular function. Platinum nephrotoxicity (commoner after cis-platinum than carboplatin) causes glomerular impairment and hypomagnesemia due to tubular damage. Unfortunately, an incomplete understanding of the pathogenesis of ifosfamide or platinum nephrotoxicity has hindered attempts at developing protective strategies.

COGNITIVE, EDUCATION, SOCIAL, QUALITY OF LIFE AND PSYCHOLOGICAL OUTCOMES
(see Chapter 2b, 12a,b)

Although during the course of cancer treatment children can miss substantial amounts of schooling, a decline in cognitive function is neither a frequent nor inevitable consequence of treatment for childhood cancer.[57,58] There is a strong observed association between cranial irradiation and structural brain abnormalities (disruption of frontal lobe/basal ganglia connections, temporal lobe calcification and cortical atrophy).[59–62] Their functional significance is more difficult to determine, but impairment may be associated with vasculopathy, calcification and electroencephalogram (EEG) abnormalities.[59–62] Both structural abnormalities and cognitive impairment correlate positively with dose of brain irradiation and negatively with age at irradiation.

Thus, in the treatment of childhood cancer, cranial irradiation is an important risk factor for cognitive decline, particularly in high dosage and young children. Regular review for such deficits should be part of follow-up for patients at risk (SIGN Grade D recommendation). This is likely to have significant resource implications. Screening annually using the Wechsler Intelligence Scale for Children (WISC) may be practical. If a problem is suspected, the patient's cognitive function should be assessed more comprehensively.

The treatment of childhood cancer is likely to impact on educational, psychological and social functioning, and thus the impact on overall quality of life may be considerable. Studies addressing these issues are largely observational, and outcome measures range from formal psychiatric and psychological assessments through self-completed questionnaires to sociodemographic variables (e.g. marriage or employment). Adverse outcomes with regard to employment and marriage are, indeed, common findings but the risk of bias in the studies is high. Frank psychiatric disorders seem uncommon but survivors do seem to be at risk of anxiety, low mood and low self-esteem. Again, brain tumors and treatment with cranial irradiation are frequently reported risk factors for adverse psychological and social outcomes.

There are currently no prospective studies using standardized assessment measures, which address particular interventions for preventing or managing adverse quality of life outcomes in these groups of patients.

SECOND PRIMARY TUMORS AND TUMOR RECURRENCE (see Chapter 3a,b)

Current knowledge of the longer term risks of second cancers are based on treatments used many years ago,

and there will be an inevitable delay before we can assess the longer term consequences of current therapies with confidence. Nevertheless, in the UK, there is a 1 in 25 risk of childhood cancer survivors developing a second primary cancer within 25 years of the primary diagnosis – an approximately sixfold increased risk.[63] It is likely that this relates both to carcinogenic effects of anticancer therapies and genetic predisposition to cancer development. Thus, the excess risk after all childhood cancers (except retinoblastoma) is related to the carcinogenic effects of radiotherapy and alkylating agents,[64,65] and there is likely to be some element of genetic predisposition, which would include, for example, constitutional mutations of the p53 gene.[66]

The large second cancer excess after heritable retinoblastoma is attributable to the carcinogenic influence of both constitutional mutations in the RB gene, and exposure of bone to radiotherapy and alkylating agents.[64,65]

Second primary bone cancer affects about 1 in 100 survivors by 20 years from the original diagnosis.[64] Bone cancers, mostly osteosarcomas, are the most common solid second cancers observed after both heritable retinoblastoma and all types of childhood cancer except retinoblastoma.[64] About 7 per cent and 0.5 per cent (respectively) of these two groups of survivors are affected by 20 years from diagnosis of the original childhood cancer. This corresponds to about 380 and 25 times the expected number of bone cancers, respectively,[64] is attributable to the carcinogenic influence of both constitutional mutations in the RB gene, and exposure of bone to radiotherapy and alkylating agents.[64,65]

Second primary leukemia is diagnosed in about 1 in 500 of UK survivors of childhood cancer by 6 years from diagnosis of the original childhood cancer, about eight times the number expected.[67] Increased cumulative exposure to alkylating agents[68] or epipodophyllotoxins[67] increases the risk of subsequent leukemia. In addition, other topoisomerase II inhibitors, including the anthracyclines, appear leukemogenic.

There is still considerable uncertainty concerning the long-term risks of the adult carcinomas observed most commonly in the general population, including carcinomas of the lung, large intestine and breast.

FOLLOW-UP OF CHILDHOOD CANCER SURVIVORS – PRINCIPLES AND PRAGMATISM

With increasing survival rates, there is an increasingly urgent need for effective and cost-effective long-term follow-up strategies to be developed. Much of the evidence base in these areas is necessarily derived from descriptive longitudinal studies. Such studies are handicapped by the

Table 14b.1 *Possible levels of follow-up more than 5 years from completion of treatment*

Level	Treatment	Method of follow-up	Frequency	Examples of tumors
1	Surgery alone Low-risk chemotherapy	Postal or telephone	1–2 years	Wilms' Stage I or II Langerhans cell histiocytosis (single system disease) Germ cell tumors (surgery only)
2	Chemotherapy Low-dose cranial irradiation (<24 Gy)	Nurse or primary care-led	1–2 years	Majority of patients (e.g. ALL in first remission)
3	Radiotherapy, except low-dose cranial irradiation Megatherapy	Medically supervised late effects clinic	Annual	Brain tumors Post-BMT Stage 4 patients (any tumor type)

ALL, acute lymphoblastic leukemia; BMT, bone marrow transplantation.

lack of appropriate control groups and small numbers of patients in individual studies. While this introduces much greater risks of bias than from conclusions drawn from and recommendations based on well-conducted randomized controlled studies, this should not devalue the importance of the recommendations derived from such studies. Indeed, many of the studies are distinguished by meticulous attention to detail, and report patients enrolled into national and international clinical trials – high-quality information describing potential late effects of childhood cancer therapies is available. A corollary of the current dearth of high-quality interventional studies to prevent, modify or eradicate such late effects is that collaborative research will, in the future, need to be on a national or international scale.

Who should these patients be seen by? How often should they be seen? How should they be assessed and investigated? Adult cancer specialists are overwhelmed by the large numbers of patients with breast, lung and bowel cancers. In addition, the expertise for dealing with such problems is very different from that required for the appropriate follow-up of childhood cancer survivors.

It will be clear from the above discussion that the degree and nature of adverse long-term morbidity risk will depend on the site of the underlying malignancy, the type and intensity of the treatment given and the age of the child at treatment. While most childhood cancer survivors will require long-term follow-up, this has major practical (e.g. geographical) and resource (e.g. expertise and financial) implications. The British Cancer Survivor Study has been developed to obtain estimates of the risks of particular adverse health outcomes amongst survivors and their offspring, and to investigate the variation in risk in relation to the types of treatment received. Such national population-based studies will provide a basis for the further development of long-term clinical follow-up strategies. Clinically based research will require the maintenance of regular patient contact.

In the context of such developments it is likely that appropriate follow-up strategies will vary between patient/treatment groups. At one extreme, there are survivors for whom the benefit of clinical follow-up (beyond 5 years from treatment completion, which equates with 'cure') is not established and for whom annual or even 2-yearly postal or telephone contact may be all that is necessary. Such patients would include those treated with surgery alone (e.g. stage I or II Wilms' tumor survivors, some germ cell tumors) or low-risk chemotherapy (e.g. single system disease, such as Langerhans cell histiocytosis) – level 1 follow-up (Table 14b.1).

At the other extreme would be patients who have received radiotherapy [other than low-dose (<24 Gy) cranial irradiation], bone marrow transplantation, or megatherapy (e.g. brain tumors, stage IV patients of any tumor type). They should be seen in a medically supervised late effects clinic at least annually, and, until final height is achieved, 3–4 times per annum – level 3 follow-up (Table 14b.1). The majority of patients on current protocols, e.g. chemotherapy-treated or those who received low dose (<24 Gy) cranial irradiation, would fall somewhere in between. In theory, nurse- or primary care-led follow-up on an annual basis might be appropriate – level 2 follow-up (Table 14b.1). However, to give one example, it is doubtful whether such contact would detect the child who, as a consequence of low-dose cranial irradiation, develops an early puberty, becomes GH deficient at the time of the pubertal growth spurt and has a reduced late pubertal (spinal) growth spurt, in time to intervene successfully to prevent this 'triple whammy' in terms of adult height. Indeed, the 'normal' growth as a result of the early puberty might give a false sense of security to the insufficiently trained observer. Similarly, the effect of chemotherapy on spinal epiphyses resulting in greatly reduced late pubertal spinal growth can be predicted and would require 'level 3 follow-up', if the child were to be treated effectively.

What is clear is that, if late adverse effects are to be anticipated and monitored to optimize prevention and treatment outcomes, this requires a wide spread of expertise. Multidisciplinary follow-up involving pediatric oncologist, pediatric endocrinologist, pediatric neurologist, radiation oncologist, pediatric neurosurgeon, clinical psychologist, general practitioner, specialist nurse and social worker is necessary but, with so many health care professionals potentially involved, it would seem logical that there should be particularly important role for a key worker for each patient. The primary area of professional expertise will vary with the nature of the patient and their treatment, the intensity (level) of follow-up required, and local resources and practicalities. It could be a hospital specialist (e.g. pediatric oncologist), primary care doctor or specialist nurse. The latter could be a particularly appropriate coordinator for many of these patients but there is currently no formal training program or career structure for such an individual.

The further development of evidence-based therapy-based guidelines for follow-up[69] is an important prerequisite for an effective and cost-effective follow-up strategy. Further information to guide and inform the future follow-up and management of childhood cancer survivors will come from national population-based cohort studies and large multicenter clinical studies. Future randomized childhood cancer treatment trials should address systematically not only survival outcomes but also long-term treatment morbidities.

Follow-up outcomes should be audited carefully. As knowledge accumulates, it will be increasingly possible to determine and deliver appropriate levels of surveillance in relation to clinical need so as to deliver high-quality care in a targeted, and thus effective and cost-effective, manner.

CONCLUSIONS

One in 600 children under the age of 15 years will develop cancer, which is now curable in 65–70 per cent. One in 1000 young adults are now childhood cancer survivors.

KEY POINTS

- Long-term morbidity risks in childhood cancer survivors largely relate to treatment modality and the challenge remains to further improve survival rates while reducing the incidence and severity of such treatment-induced late effects.
- Treatment-related morbidity is diverse, with potential effects on the endocrine system (growth, puberty, fertility, pituitary, thyroid and other disorders), cardiovascular, pulmonary and renal complications, and cognitive, educational, psychological, social and quality of life manifestations.
- Morbidity can be anticipated and monitored to optimize prevention and treatment – ideally through multidisciplinary follow-up.
- Evidence-based and graded recommendations provide a basis for the effective, informed and pragmatic follow-up of a cohort of patients who, it is estimated, will make up 1 in 250 of the adult population by the year 2010.
- The further development of evidence-based, therapy-based guidelines for follow-up is an important prerequisite for an effective and cost-effective follow-up strategy.

REFERENCES

◆1. Mertens AC, Yasui Y, Neglia JP, et al. Late mortality experience in five year survivors of childhood and adolescent cancer. J Clin Oncol 2001; 19:3163–3172.
◆2. Moller TR, Garwicz S, Barlow L, et al. Decreasing late mortality among five year survivors of cancer in childhood and adolescence: a population based study in the Nordic countries. J Clin Oncol 2001; 19:3173–3181.
●3. Wallace WHB. Growth and endocrine function following treatment of childhood malignant disease. In: Plowman PN, Pinkerton CR (eds) Paediatric oncology: clinical practice and controversies. London: Chapman & Hall, 1997:706–728.
●4. Bath LE, Wallace WHB, Kelnar CJH. Disorders of growth and development in the child treated for cancer In: Kelnar CJH, Savage MO, Stirling HF, Saenger P (eds) Growth disorders – pathophysiology and treatment. London: Chapman and Hall, 1998:641–660.
●5. Wallace WHB, Kelnar CJH. The effect of chemotherapy in childhood on growth and endocrine function. In: Kelnar CJH (ed.) Paediatric endocrinology. Baillière's Clinical Paediatrics – International Practice and Research, Vol. 4. London: Baillière Tindall, 1996:333–348.
6. Wallace WHB, Kelnar CJH. The effect of chemotherapy in childhood on growth and endocrine function. Drug Safety 1996; 15:325–332.
◆7. Wallace WHB, Blacklay A, Eiser C, et al. Developing strategies for long-term follow up of survivors of childhood cancer. Br Med J 2001; 323:271–274.
●8. Scottish Intercollegiate Guidelines Network (SIGN). Long-term follow-up of survivors of cancer in children and young people. (SIGN 2003). Edinburgh: SIGN, 2003 (in press).
9. Sklar C, Mertens A, Walter A, Mitchell D, et al. Final height after treatment for acute lymphoblastic leukaemia: comparison of no cranial irradiation, 1800 cGy and 2400 cGy cranial irradiation. J Pediatr 1993; 123:59–64.
10. Didi M, Didcock E, Davies HA, et al. High incidence of obesity in young adults after treatment of acute lymphoblastic leukaemia in childhood. J Pediatr 1995; 127:63–67.

11. Shaw MP, Bath LE, Kelnar CJH, Wallace WHB. Obesity in leukaemia survivors – the familial contribution. *Pediatr Haematol Oncol* 2000; **17**:231–237.

12. Reilly JJ, Ventham JC, Newell J, *et al.* Risk factors for excess weight gain in children treated for acute lymphoblastic leukaemia. *Int J Obes Relat Metab Disord* 2000; **24**:1537–1541.

13. Crofton PM, Ahmed SF, Wade JC, *et al.* Effects of intensive chemotherapy on bone and collagen turnover and the growth hormone axis in children with acute lymphoblastic leukaemia. *J Clin Endocrinol Metab* 1998; **83**:3121–3129.

14. Ahmed SF, Wallace WHB, Kelnar CJH. An anthropometric study of children during intensive chemotherapy for acute lymphoblastic leukaemia. *Hormone Res* 1997; **48**:178–183.

15. Ahmed SF, Wallace WHB, Crofton PM, *et al.* Short-term changes in lower leg length in children treated for acute lymphoblastic leukaemia. *J Pediatr Endocrinol Metab* 1999; **12**:75–80.

16. Crofton PM, Ahmed SF, Wade JC, *et al.* Effects of a third intensification block of chemotherapy on bone and collagen turnover, insulin-like growth factor I, its binding proteins and short term growth in children with acute lymphoblastic leukaemia. *Eur J Cancer* 1999; **35**:960–967.

17. Crofton PM, Ahmed SF, Wade JC, *et al.* Bone turnover and growth during and after continuing chemotherapy in children with acute lymphoblastic leukaemia. *Pediatr Res* 2000; **48**:490–496.

18. Ahmed SR, Shalet SM, Beardwell CG. The effects of cranial irradiation on growth hormone secretion. *Acta Paediatr Scand* 1986; **75**:255–260.

19. Crowne EC, Moore C, Wallace WHB, *et al.* A novel variant of growth hormone insufficiency following low dose cranial irradiation. *Clin Endocrinol* 1992; **36**:59–68.

20. Shalet SM, Clayton PE, Price DA. Growth and pituitary function in children treated for brain tumours or acute lymphoblastic leukaemia. *Hormonal Res* 1988; **50**:53–61.

21. Swerdlow AJ, Reddingius RE, Higgins CD, *et al.* Growth hormone treatment of children with brain tumors and risk of tumor recurrence. *J Clin Endocrinol Metab* 2000; **85**:4444–4449.

22. Davies HA, Didcock E, Didi M, *et al.* Growth, puberty and obesity after treatment for leukaemia. *Acta Paediatr Suppl* 1995; **411**:45–50; discussion 51.

23. Wake M, Salmon L, Waters E. Health status of overweight/obese and underweight children: a population based survey. *Pediatr Res* (Suppl.) 2000; **47**(part 2):A943.

24. Gortmaker SL, Must A, Perrin JM, Sobol AM, Dietz WH. Social and economic consequences of overweight in adolescence and young adulthood. *N Engl J Med* 1993; **329**:1008–1012.

26. Scottish Intercollegiate Guidelines Network (SIGN). *Obesity in children and young people.* Guideline no. 69 (SIGN 2003) www.sign.ac.uk. Edinburgh: SIGN.

27. Nysom K, Holm K, Michaelsen KF, *et al.* Bone mass after treatment for acute lymphoblastic leukemia in childhood. *J Clin Oncol* 1998; **16**:3752–3760.

28. Scottish Intercollegiate Guidelines Network (SIGN). *Prevention of dental caries.* Guideline no. 47 (SIGN 2000). Edinburgh: SIGN.

29. Pottern LM, Kaplan MM, Larsen PR, *et al.* Thyroid nodularity after childhood irradiation for lymphoid hyperplasia: a comparison of questionnaire and clinical findings. *J Clin Epidemiol* 1990; **43**:449–460.

30. Brill AB, Becker DV. The safety of ^{131}I treatment of hyperthyroidism. In: Van Middlesworth L, Givens JR (eds) *The thyroid gland; a practical clinical treatise.* Chicago: Year Book Publications, 1986:347–362.

31. Shibata Y, Yamashita S, Masyakin VB, *et al.* 15 years after Chernobyl: new evidence of thyroid cancer. *Lancet* 2001; **358**:1965–1966.

32. Borgstrom B, Bolme P. Thyroid function in children after allogeneic bone marrow transplantation. *Bone Marrow Transplant* 1994; **13**:59–64.

33. Katsanis E, Shapiro RS, Robison LL, *et al.* Thyroid dysfunction following bone marrow transplantation: long-term follow-up of 80 pediatric patients. *Bone Marrow Transplant* 1990; **5**:335–340.

34. Thomas BC, Stanhope R, Plowman PN, Leiper AD. Endocrine function following single fraction and fractionated total body irradiation for bone marrow transplantation in childhood. *Acta Endocrinol (Copenh)* 1993; **128**:508–512.

35. Waring AB, Wallace WHB. Subfertility following treatment of childhood cancer. *Hosp Med* 2000; **61**:550–557.

36. Quigley C, Cowell C, Jimenez M, *et al.* Normal or early development of puberty despite gonadal damage in children treated for acute lymphoblastic leukaemia. *N Engl J Med* 1989; **321**:143–151.

37. Saunders JE, Hawley J, Levy W, *et al.* Pregnancies following high dose cyclophosphamide with or without high-dose busulfan or total body irradiation and bone marrow transplantation. *Blood* 1996; **87**:3045–3052.

38. Wallace WHB, Shalet SM, Hendry JH, *et al.* Ovarian failure following abdominal irradiation in childhood: the radiosensitivity of the human oocyte. *Br J Radiol* 1989; **62**:995–998.

39. Critchley HOD, Wallace WHB, Mamtora H, *et al.* Ovarian failure after whole abdominal radiotherapy – the potential for pregnancy. *Br J Obstet Gynaecol* 1992; **99**:392–394.

●40. Thomson AB, Critchley HO, Kelnar CJ, Wallace WH. Late reproductive sequelae following treatment of childhood cancer and options for fertility preservation. *Best Pract Res Clin Endocrinol Metab* 2002; **16**:311–334.

41. Critchley HOD, Buckley CH, Anderson DC. Experience with a 'physiological' steroid replacement regimen for the establishment of a receptive endometrium in women with premature ovarian failure. *Br J Obstet Gynaecol* 1990; **97**:804–810.

42. Bath LE, Critchley HOD, Chambers SE, *et al.* Ovarian and uterine characteristics after total body irradiation in childhood and adolescence: response to sex steroid replacement. *Br J Obstet Gynaecol* 1999; **106**:1265–1272.

43. Bath LE, Anderson RA, Critchley HOD, *et al.* Hypothalamic-pituitary-ovarian dysfunction after prepubertal chemotherapy and cranial irradiation for acute leukaemia. *Hum Reprod* 2001; **16**:1838–1844.

44. Shalet SM, Horner A, Ahmed SR, *et al.* Leydig cell damage after testicular irradiation for lymphoblastic leukaemia. *Hormonal Res* 1985; **30**:53–61.

45. Wallace WHB, Shalet SM, Tetlow LJ, *et al.* Ovarian function following the treatment of childhood acute lymphoblastic leukaemia. *Med Paediatr Oncol* 1993; **21**:333–339.

46. Mackie EJ, Radford M, Shalet SM. Gonadal function following chemotherapy for childhood Hodgkins disease. *Med Paediatr Oncol* 1996; **27**:74–78.

47. Meistrich ML, Wilson G, Kangasniemi M, Huhtaniemi I. Mechanism of protection of rat spermatogenesis by hormonal pretreatment: stimulation of spermatogonial differentiation after irradiation. *J Androl* 2000; **21**:464–469.

48. Kelnar CJ, McKinnell C, Walker M, *et al.* Testicular changes during infantile 'quiescence' in the marmoset and their gonadotrophin dependence: a model for investigating susceptibility of the prepubertal human testis to cancer therapy? *Hum Reprod* 2002; **17**:1367–1378.

49. Truesdell S, Schwartz CL, Clark E, Constine LS. Cardiovascular effects of cancer. In: Schwartz CL, Hobbie WL, Constine LS, Ruccione KS (eds). *Survivors of childhood cancer.* St Louis: Mosby, 1994.

50. Lipshultz SE, Lipsitz SR, Mone SM, *et al.* Female sex and drug dose as risk factors for late cardiotoxic effects of doxorubicin therapy for childhood cancer. *N Engl J Med* 1995; **332:**1738–1743.

51. Pihkala J, Saarinen UM, Lundstrom U, *et al.* Myocardial function in children and adolescents after therapy with anthracyclines and chest irradiation. *Eur J Cancer* 1996; **32A:**97–103.

52. Goorin AM, Chauvenet AR, Perez-Atayde AR, *et al.* Initial congestive heart six to ten years after doxorubicin chemotherapy for childhood cancer. *J Pediatr* 1990; **116:**144–147.

53. Mladosievicova B, Foltinova A, Petrasova H, Hulin I. Late effects of anthracycline therapy in childhood on signal-averaged ECG parameters. *Int J Mol Med* 2000; **5:**411–414.

54. Sorensen K, Levitt G, Bull C, *et al.* Anthracycline dose in childhood acute lymphoblastic leukemia: issues of early survival versus late cardiotoxicity. *Oncology* 1997; **15:**61–68.

55. Hancock SL, Tucker MA, Hoppe RT. Factors affecting late mortality from heart disease after treatment of Hodgkin's disease. *JAMA* 1993; **270:**1949–1955.

56. Wexler LH, Andrich MP, Venzon D, *et al.* Randomized trial of the cardioprotective agent ICRF-187 in pediatric sarcoma patients treated with doxorubicin. *J Clin Oncol* 1996; **14:**362–372.

57. Eiser C. Practitioner review: long term consequences of childhood cancer. *J Child Psychol Psychiat* 1998; **39:**621–633.

58. Eiser C. Children and cancer. *Pediatr Rehabil* 2002; **5:**187–189.

59. Heukrodt C, Powazek M, Brown WS, *et al.* Electrophysiological signs of neurocognitive deficits in long-term leukemia survivors. *J Pediatr Psychol* 1988; **13:**223–236.

60. Russo A, Schiliro G. Some aspects of neurotoxicity associated with central nervous system prophylaxis in childhood leukemia. *Acta Haematol* 1987; **78**(Suppl. 1):139–141.

61. Mulhern RK, Reddick WE, Palmer SL, *et al.* Neurocognitive deficits in medulloblastoma survivors and white matter loss. *Ann Neurol* 1999; **46:**834–841.

62. Moore BD 3rd, Ater JL, Copeland DR. Improved neuropsychological outcome in children with brain tumors diagnosed during infancy and treated without cranial irradiation. *J Child Neurol* 1992; **7:**281–290.

63. Hawkins MM, Draper GJ, Kingston JE. Incidence of second primary tumours among childhood cancer survivors. *Br J Cancer* 1987; **56:**339–347.

64. Hawkins MM, Kinnier Wilson LM, Burton HS, *et al.* Radiotherapy, alkylating agents and the risk of bone cancer after childhood cancer. *J Natl Cancer Inst* 1996; **88:**270–278.

65. Tucker MA, D'Angio GJ, Boice JD, *et al.* Bone sarcomas linked to radiotherapy and chemotherapy in children. *N Engl J Med* 1987; **317:**588–593.

66. Neugut AI, Meadows AT, Robinson E. *Multiple primary cancers.* Philadelphia: Lippincott, Williams & Wilkins, 1999.

67. Hawkins MM, Kinnier Wilson LM, Stovall MA, *et al.* Epipodyophyllotoxins, alkylating agents and radiation and risk of secondary leukaemia after childhood cancer. *Br Med J* 1992; **304:**951–958.

68. Tucker MA, Meadows AT, Boice JD, *et al.* Leukaemia after therapy with alkylating agents for childhood cancer. *J Natl Cancer Inst* 1987; **78:**459–464.

69. Kissen GKN, Wallace WHB. *Therapy based guidelines for long-term follow up of children treated for cancer.* Published on behalf of the late effects group of the United Kingdom Children's Cancer Study Group. Milton Keynes, UK: Pharmacia, 1995.

Index